ACSM's Resources for the Personal Trainer

SECOND EDITION

ACSM's Resources for the Personal Trainer

SECOND EDITION

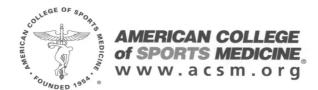

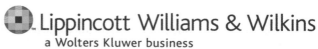

a Wolters Kluwer business

Philadelphia · Baltimore · New York · London
Buenos Aires · Hong Kong · Sydney · Tokyo

Acquisitions Editor: Emily J. Lupash
Managing Editor: Karen M. Ruppert
Marketing Manager: Christen D. Murphy
Production Editor: Paula C. Williams
Designer: Risa J. Clow
Compositor: Maryland Composition, Inc.
Printer: R.R. Donnelley

ACSM's Publications Committee Chair: Jeffrey L. Roitman, Ed.D., FACSM
ACSM Group Publisher: D. Mark Robertson

Copyright © 2007 American College of Sports Medicine

351 West Camden Street
Baltimore, MD 21201

530 Walnut Street
Philadelphia, PA 19106

Printed in China

First Edition, 2004

Library of Congress Cataloging-in-Publication Data

ACSM's resources for the personal trainer.—2nd ed.
   p. ; cm.
 Includes bibliographical references and index.
ISBN 13: 978-0-7817-9053-6
ISBN 10: 0-7817-9053-0 (alk. paper)
1. Physical education and training. 2. Sports medicine. 3. Personal trainers. 4. Exercise. 5. Physical education and training. 6. Personal trainers. 7. Sports medicine. I. American College of Sports Medicine. II. American College of Sports Medicine's resources for the personal trainer. III. Title: Resources for the personal trainer.
   [DNLM: 1. Physical Education and Training. 2. Exercise—physiology.
QT 255 A1873 2007]
RC1213.A268 2007
613.7′1—dc22   2006014956

The publishers have made every effort to trace the copyright holders for borrowed material. If they have inadvertently overlooked any, they will be pleased to make the necessary arrangements at the first opportunity.

To purchase additional copies of this book, call our customer service department at **(800) 638–3030** or fax orders to **(301) 223–2320.** International customers should call **(301) 223–2300.**

Visit Lippincott Williams & Wilkins on the Internet: http://www.LWW.com. Lippincott Williams & Wilkins customer service representatives are available from 8:30 am to 6:00 pm, EST.

For more information concerning American College of Sports Medicine certification and suggested preparatory materials, call **(800) 486–5643** or visit the American College of Sports Medicine web site **www.acsm.org**.

08 09 10
5 6 7 8 9 10 11

Foreword

In 1951, Jack La Lanne became the world's best-known Personal Trainer when he used first names to energize invisible television viewers who were huffing and puffing along to his reps and sets. For years before and after Jack, licensed physical therapists have been working, one-on-one, with each one of their patients, bringing them back to health. I speculate that at one time in the early 1980s, a gutsy Personal Trainer from California or New York broke the $100 per hour fee for a personal workout. Breaking this barrier was significant, as now you had a real profession in the making—the making of a decent living, that is.

In 1983, my first personal training client was Calvin Klein, the famous fashion entrepreneur. For three years, he helped me pay New York City rents and attend Columbia University. Yes, I was worried about what I looked like when training Calvin. My last client was Holly Brubach, a noted *New York Times Magazine* editor, author, and certifiable sports nut. At the time, she had just had a hip replaced, so thankfully I had to be more concerned about what she felt like than what I looked like when I was putting her through her paces.

Between my first high-profile client in 1983 and today, I have had the pleasure of working with hundreds of hard-working, dedicated Personal Trainers who are committed to making each and every one of their clients achieve better health one session at a time. If you too believe that *what* you do is much more important than *whom* you do and *what* you look like while doing it, then this book is for you.

The opportunities for qualified Personal Trainers are endless. Physical activity and nutrition strategies are becoming solutions of choice to combat rising healthcare costs, childhood obesity, chronic diseases such as diabetes and depression, and all-to-frequent workplace injuries to the lower back. Since 1954 the American College of Sports Medicine (ACSM) has been the leading organization in sports medicine and the exercise sciences. Now you can take advantage of their wealth of experience inside this new edition of *ACSM's Resources for the Personal Trainer*.

In the pages that follow, ACSM has orchestrated the collaboration of some of the best minds in the science of exercise and the art of personal fitness business. From initial client assessments to legal strategies that ensure business continuity, this book combines academic insight with practical examples that have been tested in real-world personal training facilities. You will learn the well-established importance of goal setting to some cutting edge concepts that involve coaching and behavioral change. Dr. Howard Zalaznik will enlighten all on what motor learning tells us about personal training, while Dr. William Kraemer will tell you all he knows about strength training (and that is a whole lot of knowing). From pre-participation waiver forms to the minute details of a periodization cycle, *ACSM's Resources for the Personal Trainer* is a how-to resource from a team of professionals who have taken great pains to provide you with their many years of experience, knowledge, successes, failures, and practical tools.

Read carefully, experiment where you can, dig deeper, formulate questions, and capitalize on the competitive advantages that you will have at your fingertips inside *ACSM's Resources for the Personal Trainer*—and hope that the competition around the corner does not.

Michael Motta
President & Founder
Plus One Health Management, New York, N.Y.
www.plusone.com

Preface

This second edition of *ACSM's Resources for the Personal Trainer* represents a wholesale revision of the successful first edition. Thanks to some very dedicated members of the ACSM Committee on Certification and Registry Boards (previously chaired by Dr. Steven Keteyian and now by Dino Costanzo) and staff of the ACSM (directed by Mike Niederpruem), the first edition was a compilation of edited select chapters of other ACSM resource books. They were effectively rewritten to make them applicable to the Personal Trainer. This second edition, while keeping constant the high standards established by the first edition, is a completely original manuscript written by the world's most respected scientists and practitioners. Many of them are pioneers in the personal training industry.

OVERVIEW

This is the first book of its kind that introduces the Personal Trainer as a recognized professional in the continuum of creating healthy lifestyles. The book is divided into six distinctly different parts, ranging from an introduction to the profession of personal training (for the professional first entering the field) to how to run your own business. In between are chapters dedicated to exercise physiology, biomechanics, anatomy, motor learning, and nutrition. Even the most experienced Personal Trainer will find the educational approach to personal training chapters to be perhaps a new way to incorporate knowledge transfer from the Personal Trainer to the client (making the personal training session more enjoyable for the client, who now knows why he or she is doing an exercise the proper way, which increases the compliance rate, making the Personal Trainer happier and perhaps even more wealthy). The middle chapters include establishing goals and objectives for clients and a "how to" manual for assessing strength, flexibility, and risk stratification. Specific chapters have been dedicated to developing resistance, cardiorespiratory, and flexibility training programs.

Specific elements in this book that will appeal to the Personal Trainer include a list of objectives preceding each chapter. There are many tables and figures that help the Personal Trainer understand the written material as well as numerous photographs. In addition, the bibliography for each chapter is contained at the conclusion of each chapter so the reader does not have to turn to the back of the book for a reference.

ORGANIZATION

The chapters are divided into six parts designed for ease of navigation through the text. We tried to keep the educational approach to personal training separated from the science, and the behavior modification separated from the business of personal training. The six parts of the book include the following.

Part I: Introduction to the Field and Profession of Personal Training. Two introductory chapters are designed to introduce the new and aspiring Personal Trainer to the profession. The first chapter provides great insight into why the health and fitness professions are some of the fastest growing industries in the world and how the Personal Trainer can capitalize on this growth. The second chapter provides a career track for the Personal Trainer. Did you ever wonder why you had an interest in personal training and if you were ever going to have a decent income? This chapter might help you answer those questions.

Part II: The Educational Approach to Personal Training. Ken Baldwin and Terry Ferebee Eckmann created the next three chapters as education-specific approaches to personal training. These approaches include some specific examples of using "teaching moments" during a personal training session. These chapters are useful if the Personal Trainer wants to "take it up a notch" (to use a very popular expression in the food preparation industry) and include educating the client and not just training him or her.

Part III: Learning the Foundations of Exercise Science and Important Related Disciplines. The six chapters in this part provide the scientific foundations for personal training. Every Personal Trainer, regardless of experience, will find these chapters helpful. For the Personal Trainer just starting out, these chapters introduce the scientific basis for exercise, psychology, motor learning, and nutrition. For the advanced Personal Trainer, these chapters serve as a foundational resource for specific lifestyle modification programs. These six chapters include exercise physiology; anatomy, kinesiology, and biomechanics; motor learning; pedagogy and the client learning program; exercise psychology, motivation, and behavior change; and nutrition.

Part IV: Initial Client Consultation, Goals/Objectives, Screening, and Assessments. This part of the book walks the Personal Trainer through a series of steps from the first client meeting through a comprehensive health-related physical fitness assessment. Capitalizing on the learning objectives of Chapter 10 (Exercise Psychology, Motivation, and Behavior Change), Chapter 13 establishes a framework for developing SMART goals, a strategic way to develop client-centered goals and objectives. While certainly not an exhaustive list of physical fitness assessments, Chapter 15 provides critical techniques to evaluate a client both in the field and in the laboratory.

Part V: Developing Your Client's Exercise Program. The first chapter of this part introduces the concept of developing a client-centered exercise program. Based on the goals established by the client and the Personal Trainer, the next three chapters (resistance training, cardiorespiratory, and flexibility programs) are specific "how to" chapters. For example, a Personal Trainer who wants to develop a resistance training program can turn to Chapter 17 and learn "how to" develop a muscle group-specific program.

Part VI: Business Principles for Personal Trainers. So, you have made the decision to start a business, which translates to "how do I make a profit in this business of personal training" (after all, we can only take altruism so far). The final two chapters, the first one written by Joan Hatfield and Neal Pire from one of the most recognized fitness management companies in the world, introduces the professional Personal Trainer to common business practices and provides information on how to avoid some of the common mistakes beginners typically make in the development of their practices.

INSTRUCTOR RESOURCES

We understand the demand on an instructor's time, so to make your job easier, you have access to Instructor's Resources upon adoption of the second edition of ACSM's Resources for the Personal Trainer. The Instructor's Resources are available online at http://thepoint.lww.com/ACSMpersonaltrainer and include the following:

➤ A Test Generator.
➤ PowerPoint slides for every chapter.

➤ An Image Bank that contains all of the figures and tables from the book.

➤ Chapter Objectives from the book.

➤ Lesson Plans to help in course preparation.

In this constantly evolving profession and increasing need for the personal delivery of health-related services, a definitive resource must be revised constantly. The ACSM welcomes your comments and suggestions on future editions.

Walt Thompson
Ken Baldwin
Mike Niederpruem
Neal Pire

Acknowledgments

The editors wish to thank the many volunteer writers and reviewers of this book. This was a major undertaking, as there were no templates to follow and no other resource books from which to gather ideas. The editors also wish to thank the many reviewers who spent countless hours ensuring that the book represented the facts, as we know them today. In all, there were more than 50 editors, contributors, and reviewers—all of them volunteers. We also thank the ACSM Publications Committee (chaired by Dr. Jeff Roitman) and ACSM Assistant Executive Vice President D. Mark Robertson for having the faith in the editorial team to complete this project in the face of some initial misfortune.

The editors wish to thank our good friends at Lippincott Williams & Wilkins, our publishing partners for this project. Specific thanks go out to our managing editor, Karen Ruppert, who not only guided us through this process but also made many editorial suggestions, making this book even better than it was before we submitted manuscript pages to her. We also thank LWW illustrator Kim Battista, acquisitions editor Emily Lupash, and Pete Darcy, executive editor, for their constant and unwavering encouragement.

Finally, this book is dedicated to the professional Personal Trainer. We remain convinced that the public health is better off today than yesterday and will be even better tomorrow because of your dedication.

Contributors

Nicki Anderson
President
Reality Fitness, Inc.
Naperville, Illinois

Shirley Archer, M.A., J.D.
Health Educator, Author, and Fitness Professional
Health Improvement Program
Stanford Prevention Research Center
Stanford University School of Medicine
Palo Alto, California

Dan Benardot, Ph.D., DHC, RD, FACSM
Laboratory for Elite Athlete Performance
Division of Nutrition
School of Health Professions
Georgia State University
Atlanta, Georgia

Christopher Berger, M.S.
Department of Kinesiology & Health Promotion
University of Kentucky
Lexington, Kentucky

Barbara Bushman, Ph.D., FACSM
Associate Dean, Graduate College
Professor, Department of Health, Physical Education, and Recreation
Missouri State University
Springfield, Missouri

Nikki Carosone, M.S.
General Manager
Personal Training Director
Plus One Health Management
New York, New York

Frank Claps, M.Ed.
Owner/Operator
Fitness For Any Body
Springfield Township, Bucks County, Pennsylvania

Shala E. Davis, Ph.D., FACSM
Associate Professor/Graduate Coordinator
Department of Exercise Science
East Stroudsburg University
East Stroudsburg, Pennsylvania

Gregory B. Dwyer, Ph.D., FACSM
Associate Professor
Department of Exercise Science
East Stroudsburg University
East Stroudsburg, Pennsylvania

Terry Ferebee Eckmann, Ph.D.
Associate Professor
Department of Teacher Education and Human Performance
Minot State University
Minot, North Dakota

Maren S. Fragala, M.S.
Human Performance Laboratory
Department of Kinesiology
University of Connecticut
Storrs, Connecticut

Lisa Todd Graddy, M.S.W., M.S.
Licensed Mental Health Therapist, LCSW
Licensed Wellness Coach
Midway, Kentucky

Disa L. Hatfield, M.A.
Human Performance Laboratory
Department of Kinesiology
University of Connecticut
Storrs, Connecticut

Joan Hatfield, M.S.
General Manager
Personal Training Director
Plus One Health Management
Seattle, Washington

Gabrielle R. Highstein, R.N., Ph.D.
Instructor in Medicine
Washington University School of Medicine
Division of Health Behavior Research
St. Louis, Missouri

Tarra Hodge
Assistant Director Fitness/Wellness
Division of Recreational Sports
Purdue University
West Lafayette, Indiana

Stanley Sai-chuen Hui, Ed.D., FACSM, FAAHPERD
Associate Professor
Department of Sports Science and Physical Education
The Chinese University of Hong Kong
Shatin, N.T.
Hong Kong, China

William J. Kraemer, Ph.D., FACSM
Professor of Kinesiology
Human Performance Laboratory
Department of Kinesiology
University of Connecticut
Storrs, Connecticut

Kate Larsen, PCC
President, Certified Coach, Lifestyle Expert
Winning LifeStyles, Inc.
Minneapolis, Minnesota

Theresa J. Lavin, B.S., M.B.A.
Licensed Wellness Coach
MGH Institute of Health Professions
Boston, Massachusetts

John Mayer, D.C., Ph.D.
Research Director
U.S. Spine & Sport Foundation
La Jolla, California

Margaret Moore, B.S., M.B.A.
Founder & CEO
Wellcoaches Corporation
Wellesley, Massachusetts

Michael Rankin, M.S.
Owner, Fitness Together
Waldwick, New Jersey

Jan Schroeder, Ph.D.
Associate Professor
Department of Kinesiology
California State University, Long Beach
Long Beach, California

Cody Sipe, M.S.
Director, A.H. Ismail Center for Health, Exercise & Nutrition
Purdue University
West Lafayette, Indiana

Barry A. Spiering, M.S.
Human Performance Laboratory
Department of Kinesiology
University of Connecticut
Storrs, Connecticut

Jakob L. Vingren, M.S.
Human Performance Laboratory
Department of Kinesiology
University of Connecticut
Storrs, Connecticut

Howard Zelaznik, Ph.D.
Professor
Department of Health and Kinesiology
College of Liberal Arts
Purdue University
West Lafayette, Indiana

Reviewers

Chris Berger, M.S.
University of Kentucky
Lexington, Kentucky

Dierdra Bycura, M.P.E.
Mesa Community College
Mesa, Arizona

Lisa Cooper Colvin, Ph.D., FACSM
University of Louisiana at Monroe
Monroe, Louisiana

Dino G. Costanzo, M.A.
New Britain General Hospital
New Britain, Connecticut
and
Bradley Memorial Hospital
Southington, Connecticut

Brian J. Coyne, M.Ed.
WellnessWorks
Ruston, Louisiana

Julie Downing, Ph.D.
Central Oregon Community College
Bend, Oregon

Shawn Drake, Ph.D.
Arkansas State University
Jonesboro, Arizona

Steven Keteyian, Ph.D., FACSM
Henry Ford Hospital
Detroit, Michigan

Marcia Mastracci-Ditmyer, Ph.D.
UNLV School of Dental Medicine
Las Vegas, Nevada

Michelle Miller, M.S.
Indiana University
Bloomington, Indiana

Madeline Paternostro-Bayles, Ph.D., FACSM
Indiana University of Pennsylvania
Indiana, Pennsylvania

William F. Simpson, Ph.D., FACSM
University of Wisconsin-Superior
Superior, Wisconsin

Paul Sorace, M.S.
Private Lifestyle Management, LLC
Florham Park, New Jersey

Jeffrey Soukup, Ph.D.
Appalachian State University
Boone, North Carolina

Michael Teague, Ed.D.
University of Iowa
Iowa City, Iowa

Michael J. Webster, Ph.D., FACSM
University of Southern Mississippi
Hattiesburg, Mississippi

Brief Contents

Expanded Contents

Introduction to the Field and Profession of Personal Training

Introduction to Personal Training

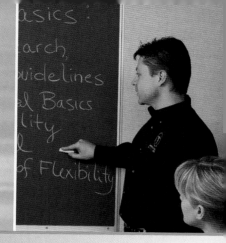

Mike Niederpruem, M.S., National Director of Certification and Registry Programs, American College of Sports Medicine, Indianapolis, Indiana.

Cody Sipe, M.S., Director, A.H. Ismail Center for Health, Exercise & Nutrition, Purdue University, West Lafayette, Indiana.

Chapter Outline

The Fitness Industry—An Overview of the Landscape

The Profession of Personal Training

- The Definition of a Personal Trainer
- Becoming a Personal Trainer
- The Backgrounds of Personal Trainers
  - Educational Background
  - Work-Related Background
  - Experiential Background

Professional Work Environments

- For-Profit
- Not-for-Profit
- Corporate

ACSM's Role and the Educational Continuum

- Identification of a Core Body of Knowledge
- Development and Continuous Revision of Knowledge, Skills, and Abilities (KSAs)

Establishing Your Knowledge Base

- The Exercise Sciences
- Developing Your Tool Kit
  - Communication Skills (Motivating and Influencing Behavioral Change)
  - Screening, Assessment, and Referrals

Ethics and Professional Conduct

- Code of Ethics for ACSM Certified and Registered Professionals
  - Purpose
  - Principles and Standards
- Principles and Standards for Candidates of ACSM Certification Examinations
- Public Disclosure of Affiliation
- Discipline

Objectives

- Describe the current state of the fitness industry as it specifically applies to personal training
- Identify professional career environments and options for Personal Trainers
- Identify future trends that will affect the fitness industry and personal training

Personal Training (practiced by one referred to in this book as the "Personal Trainer" but often described as a "fitness trainer," "personal fitness trainer," "fitness professional," or "exercise professional") is emerging as one of the fastest growing professions in the United States. According to the U.S. Department of Labor, Bureau of Labor Statistics, the job outlook for this profession is projected to "grow faster than average" between 2002 and 2012, which is further defined as an increase between 21% and 35% during this time period (1). Employment opportunities for Personal Trainers are available in more diverse settings than ever before and include (but are not limited to) the following:

➤ Commercial (for-profit) fitness centers
➤ Community (not-for-profit) fitness centers
➤ Corporate fitness/wellness centers
➤ University wellness/adult fitness centers
➤ Owner/operator (self-employed) studios, fitness centers, and in-home businesses
➤ Medical fitness centers
➤ Municipal/city recreation/public parks/family centers
➤ Governmental/military fitness centers
➤ Activity centers/retirement centers/assisted living communities for older adults
➤ Worksite health promotion programs

Each of these employment settings is reviewed in more detail later in this chapter. Indeed, these opportunities and the diversity of work settings are predicted to increase further as the population continues to both grow and age as well as transition further to a more sedentary (i.e., physically inactive) lifestyle. It appears then, that now is the best time to commit to the profession of personal training. There may be no other profession better placed to enhance the quality of life of the growing, aging, and increasingly sedentary population in the immediate future.

THE FITNESS INDUSTRY—AN OVERVIEW OF THE LANDSCAPE

Interestingly, although the population may be larger and more physically inactive than ever, the health club industry has never been in better "shape." Consider the following facts from the International Health, Racquet and Sportsclub Association (IHRSA), a trade association serving the health and fitness club industry (2, 3):

➤ 26,046   Number of health clubs in the United States (2)
➤ 39.4 million   Number of health club members in the United States (2)
➤ $4.4 billion   Total industry revenues for 2003 (2)
➤ 160,000   Number of full-time employees (3)
➤ 635,000   Number of part-time employees (3)

Although these numbers may appear impressive, the total estimated U.S. population (July 2004) is 293,655,404 (4), so only about 13% to 14% of the population are members of health or fitness clubs. Although difficult to estimate, many more individuals are physically active and do participate in various outdoor recreational or at-home physical activities on a daily or at least weekly basis. Even so, there is still a large proportion of the population that could benefit from involvement in some type of regular physical activity as part of a healthy lifestyle, whether as a member of a health club

Table 1.1	PERCENTAGE DISTRIBUTION OF OVERALL PHYSICAL ACTIVITY LEVEL FOR ADULTS 18 YEARS AND ABOVE: UNITED STATES, 2000				
Age	Never Active	Low	Medium	Medium–High	High
18–24 years	4.4	14.2	29.9	27.5	24.1
25–44 years	5.3	15.0	34.0	25.2	20.5
45–64 years	10.1	17.4	33.0	22.5	17.1
65 years and above	22.5	15.8	27.9	18.4	15.3

From Percent distribution of overall physical activity level for adults 18 years and over: United States, 2000. Source: Barnes PM, Schoenborn CA. Physical activity among adults: United States, 2000. Advance data from vital and health statistics; no. 333. Hyattsville, Maryland: National Center for Health Statistics. 2003. (public domain)

or on their own. Personal Trainers, then, are well positioned to influence public health in this regard. First, as the health club industry continues to grow, so too will the demand for highly qualified and certified fitness professionals to serve the needs of their members. Even now, competent Personal Trainers are in high demand. Second, most people are not health club members, and most likely will never become health club members. These individuals may not feel comfortable exercising in public, or perhaps a health club is not conveniently located near their home or place of work. Fortunately, these individuals can benefit just as much by in-home personal training, which is another growing segment of the Personal Trainer job market.

According to the Centers for Disease Control and Prevention (CDC), at least 50% of all U.S. adults are insufficiently active, with levels of activity decreasing with age. Over 22% of adults over the age of 65 report never being active in their daily lives (4) (Table 1.1). Even with the growth of the fitness industry and emerging opportunities for physical fitness, these numbers have not really changed in the past 20 years. As a consequence, the United States is one of the most obese nations in the world, and with record levels of childhood obesity, the trend is worsening. Schools are cutting back or eliminating physical education. Healthcare costs are rising exponentially as the medical field continues to focus more on treatment than prevention. Food portion sizes in restaurants are increasing. With these conditions, the time is right for highly qualified Personal Trainers to lead the charge toward a healthier nation.

THE PROFESSION OF PERSONAL TRAINING

As mentioned above, the profession of personal training is rapidly evolving, and employment opportunities are wide ranging and will continue to increase. But what does a Personal Trainer do? Depending on the work setting, Personal Trainers may perform any or all of the following tasks (a noninclusive list):

➤ Screen and interview potential clients to determine their readiness for exercise and physical activity
➤ Perform fitness tests or assessments (as appropriate) on clients to determine their current level of fitness
➤ Help clients set realistic goals and provide motivation for adherence to the program
➤ Develop exercise regimens and programs (often referred to as an "exercise prescription") for clients to follow and modify programs as necessary, based on progression and goals
➤ Demonstrate and instruct specific techniques to clients for the safe and effective performance of various exercise movements
➤ Supervise or "spot" (physically assisting your client with an exercise that usually involves free weights or dumbbells to minimize risk of injury) clients when they are performing exercise movements
➤ Maintain records of clients' progress or lack thereof with respect to the exercise prescription

Other responsibilities not directly involving a client may be assigned or performed as needed. These usually include administrative paperwork, maintenance of equipment, and cleaning of equipment and facilities as required.

Many Personal Trainers also obtain additional instruction or specialty certifications in areas such as yoga, aquatic exercise, wellness coaching, studio cycling, and kickboxing. These specialties should not be confused with "core" or primary certifications, such as the ACSM certified Personal Trainer^{SM}. Additional specialty certifications make you more valuable and also allow you to have a wider variety of responsibilities, such as teaching group exercise classes.

Even though more health clubs than ever before are requiring certifications for current and future employees, some health clubs still hire Personal Trainers without certifications. This does not mean that you don't need a certification! You owe it to yourself as a true professional, as well as to the clients you serve, to document your competence, and certification is the best way to accomplish this objective. Also, the health club industry is unique in that there are a large number of organizations that offer certifications in this field, and even among the health clubs that do require certifications, there isn't agreement on which ones are universally accepted. One of your first tasks in pursuing a career in personal training will be to determine which certification(s) best suit your personal and professional goals.

The kinds of fitness facilities are diverse, with the most numerous being multipurpose commercial for-profit clubs, followed by community, corporate, and medical fitness centers. Although there are many core similarities between facilities, there is also great variety in size, structure, target markets, program offerings, amenities, membership fees, contracts, staffing, and equipment. This variety is necessary to attract and serve many different populations with many different interests.

With the member retention rate varying greatly across the industry, most clubs and centers must continually recruit new members. Since many experts agree that the majority of a club's membership base will come from within a 10- to 15-minute drive time from home to the facility, clubs that are located close to one another are typically competing for the same members. This means that Personal Trainers are vying for the same clients as well. However, Personal Trainers, just like clubs, can differentiate themselves from the competition in a number of ways, such as focusing on a specific clientele (e.g., women, children, seniors, athletes), developing expertise in a given area, offering small-group training in addition to individual sessions, offering a different price point, and using multiple locations.

The Definition of a Personal Trainer

The American College of Sports Medicine (ACSM) scope of practice for the ACSM certified Personal Trainer^{SM} is

> The ACSM certified Personal Trainer^{SM} is a fitness professional involved in developing and implementing an individualized approach to exercise leadership in healthy populations and/or those individuals with medical clearance to exercise. Using a variety of teaching techniques, the Personal Trainer is proficient in leading and demonstrating safe and effective methods of exercise by applying the fundamental principles of exercise science. The ACSM certified Personal Trainer^{SM} is familiar with forms of exercise used to improve, maintain, and/or optimize health-related components of physical fitness and performance. The ACSM certified Personal Trainer^{SM} is proficient in writing appropriate exercise recommendations, leading and demonstrating safe and effective methods of exercise, and motivating individuals to begin and to continue with their healthy behaviors.

As mentioned above, the health and fitness industry is unique in that it has a wide variety of certifications available to the potential fitness professional. Organizations that offer certifications are commercial (for-profit) as well as non-profit. Some have services and benefits that facilitate your professional development, such as publications and conferences. Before committing to a specific certification, study each one for its relevance to your situation. Ask your fellow students (if applicable) or coworkers, or potential employers or talk to some professional Personal Trainers in your area for specific recommendations.

Some certification organizations recognize other certifications for the purposes of continuing education. Most legitimate certifications will require their respective certified professionals to pursue educational opportunities, commonly referred to as *continuing education units* (CEUs), or *continuing education credits* (CECs). These CEUs/CECs are required in an ongoing fashion for a certified professional to maintain his or her certification status and as one way to maintain professional competence. Some certifications are complementary to others, and again, multiple certifications could make you more valuable to a potential employer.

Becoming a Personal Trainer

Because of the large number of certification organizations, the prerequisites and eligibility requirements for becoming a Personal Trainer vary widely. Some are standalone certifications, while others, such as those offered by ACSM, are part of a progressive professional development pathway in which the scope of practice increases in both depth and scope as the prerequisites and eligibility requirements increase. For example, entry into the ACSM professional development pathway for emerging professionals does not have any formal academic requirement at this time for the ACSM certified Personal Trainer[SM], but the ACSM certified Health/Fitness Instructor® possesses at least an associate or bachelor's degree in an allied health/exercise science field, and the ACSM Registered Clinical Exercise Physiologist® requires a master's degree in exercise science, plus an additional 600 work-related hours. Therefore, it is important that you consider not only what you want to do now but in the next few years as well, as you determine your educational preparation and what certification(s) you may need to realize your career goals. Your background and interests will combine in determining how fast and by what process you can begin your career.

The Backgrounds of Personal Trainers

Because the Personal Trainer profession has evolved so rapidly, currently there is no mandatory or standardized academic preparation model, such as exists for physicians, nurses, or other allied health professionals. Because of this, certification in the fitness industry takes on greater importance. And, because of the many different types of certifications that exist, the background of today's Personal Trainer varies significantly with respect to educational preparation and work-related experience. Some individuals commit to the profession early and pursue an appropriate course of study in college. Many of these individuals actually begin working part-time at a local health club or at the university student recreation center, gaining valuable "hands-on" practical experience to complement their studies. Other Personal Trainers enter the profession later in life as a new career, or as a second career on a part-time basis while maintaining their primary career pursuit. Ideally, the Personal Trainer will have a good combination of education, work-related experience, and even first-person perspective experiences as either an athlete or former client.

EDUCATIONAL BACKGROUND

As the profession of personal training continues to evolve and grow, more and more educational opportunities become available. Many certification organizations offer workshops and online examination preparation opportunities. From a formal academic training perspective, there are certificate and associate's, bachelor's and master's degree programs available for fitness professionals. Typically, certificate programs (both in-person and online) range from 1 year to 18 months in duration. Associate degree programs range in length from 18 months to 2 years. Bachelor's degree programs are usually 4 years in duration. Master's degree programs are typically 18 months to 2 years beyond a bachelor's degree. Also, internships (typically an unpaid opportunity to work under the direct supervision of an experienced fitness professional) may or may not be part of these different types of programs. Common names for these academic programs include exercise science, exercise physiology, physical education, kinesiology, sport science, personal trainer, fitness specialist, and others.

Please note that some health clubs actually require their Personal Trainers to have degrees, and long-term employment advancement may require a degree at some health clubs. Also, most fitness directors, those individuals who have management/supervisory responsibilities over the floor staff (Personal Trainers), usually have a degree.

WORK-RELATED BACKGROUND

It is possible for Personal Trainers to obtain employment without a related degree, especially if they have one or more certifications and some prior industry-related work experience. For many individuals who want a career change, pursuing a second degree or even a first degree later in life simply is not possible. On-the-job training for many in this scenario may be an acceptable way to develop the skills necessary to be a successful Personal Trainer. Some health clubs have formal training paths and processes for their employees that may include assigning a more experienced Personal Trainer as a mentor or scheduling periodic staff training sessions, sometimes referred to as "in-services." Some health clubs may even pay for continuing education opportunities for their staff as one benefit of employment. If not, look for an experienced Personal Trainer either at your facility or elsewhere with an exemplary reputation who would consider taking on an apprentice. Many certification organizations have educational opportunities, such as workshops, which can also provide a good review of the various areas of content, especially as they relate to preparing for a certification examination. It is always advisable for all professionals working in this environment to seek a college degree whenever possible.

EXPERIENTIAL BACKGROUND

Some Personal Trainers were once college, professional, or elite athletes. Like those who are changing careers, some may not have a related academic degree, and some no college degree at all. However, their passion for a particular sport or a love of exercise in general usually motivates them sufficiently to fill in any knowledge gaps they may have as they begin their personal training career. Again, if you are one of these individuals, commit to the profession by obtaining one or more certifications from reputable organizations such as the ACSM, as well as obtaining relevant, work-related experience under the supervision of a proven, experienced (preferably degreed) Personal Trainer.

Another type of experiential background from a first-person perspective is as a former client. These individuals usually are people who had such a significant positive or transformational experience that their lives were changed for the better. Think of an obese patient who loses hundreds of pounds and now thinks of himself or herself as healthy, or the previously sedentary individual who now competes in marathons regularly. Much like the professional athlete, these individuals feel strongly about reproducing their positive experience for others but may not have a college degree. Similarly, by being proactive from a self-study perspective, obtaining one or more certifications and combining these with work-related experience, these individuals can become competent professional Personal Trainers over time.

Regardless of your background, starting down the career path as a Personal Trainer doesn't have to be complicated. To get started, determine from where you are starting, and then where you want to be professionally in one, two, or five years' time. Ask yourself the following questions:

➤ Do I have a college degree related to the field?
➤ If not, is it feasible for me to go back to obtain a certificate or degree on either a part-time or full-time basis?
➤ Was I ever a client of a Personal Trainer, and did I have a positive experience in achieving my goals?
➤ Do I have experience as a college, professional, or elite athlete that provides me with some first-person experiences?

> ➤ Which certifications are appropriate for me to pursue now and in the future?
> ➤ Which certifications have study materials and/or workshops to help me accumulate a core body of knowledge?
> ➤ Where can I begin obtaining the necessary skills, either by observing a more experienced Personal Trainer or by volunteering at a local health club?
> ➤ Which certifying organizations and, specifically, which level of certification do potential employers in my city expect to see when hiring Personal Trainers for their clubs?

PROFESSIONAL WORK ENVIRONMENTS

For-Profit

Commercial clubs dominate the fitness landscape and include independents, chains, licensed gyms, and franchises. Many opportunities for gainful employment exist within the commercial club industry. Most clubs advertise employment opportunities locally or regionally, while some also post them on their corporate websites. It is wise to thoroughly investigate a company's policies concerning compensation, benefits, policies, and opportunities for advancement before accepting a position.

Licensed gyms and franchises have been a popular choice for a new club. The benefits of choosing a franchise include brand recognition, access to proven operational systems, logo usage, marketing templates, in-depth training, and ongoing support. Franchisers then retain the right to dictate most aspects of the facility, including colors, layout, décor, equipment, programs, and product sales. Initial fees for fitness franchises can range from $10,000 to over $100,000, and equipment may or may not be included in the cost. There is also a monthly franchising fee, which is either a set amount or a percentage of gross revenue (typically about 5%). Licensed gyms operate on a much simpler model. A fee is paid to use (license) the name and logo. Licensees typically have much more flexibility in how they operate the facility than do franchisees, but they also do not receive as much operational support.

Not-for-Profit

Not-for-profit (or non-profit) organizations with fitness centers make up a large proportion of the total market. According to the International Health, Racquet and Sportsclub Association (IHRSA) Fair Competition Annual Report (5), approximately 38% of the total membership in health clubs is from the non-profit sector. Some examples of the larger non-profit organizations in which fitness professionals can find relevant employment include the YMCA (Young Men's Christian Association), JCCs (Jewish Community Centers, medical fitness centers, and college/university recreation centers.

Personal Trainers may find that some non-profits may not have rates of pay comparable to those of their for-profit counterparts but at the same time may provide better benefits. Non-profit work (regardless of the industry) creates a strong sense of mission throughout the organization and carries a significant commitment to service with respect to their specific members or constituents. Non-profit fitness centers fill a significant role in the fitness professional job market, and it is ultimately up to the individual to determine the most appropriate place of employment for his or her personal and professional goals.

The growing relationship between the fitness industry and the healthcare field is evidenced by the steady growth of medical fitness centers (MFCs) and the establishment of the Medical Fitness Association. The numbers of MFCs and the number of members they serve have seen a compounded annual growth rate of 15% since 1985. Conservative projections (assuming a growth rate of 7.5%) estimate over 3 million members and 1150 MFCs by the year 2010. While it is true that there are a number of extremely large MFCs, approximately 30% to 50% of the current 715 centers are less than 10,000 to 20,000 square feet, with a heavy concentration of all centers in the Southeast and upper Midwest sections of the United States. Although they offer a number of clinical and wellness services not typically found in traditional clubs, personal training tops the list of reported non-membership fee services, with 78% of centers offering such a program. In addition, 80% report being owned by a hospital or health system, and 67% report holding not-for-profit status (5).

A central mission of many MFCs is integration of services for both the "sick" and the "healthy." It is not uncommon for patients in cardiovascular rehabilitation or physical therapy programs to exercise next to healthy community members. Using the same space and equipment saves on overhead, space, and staffing needs. While there currently are not any specific guidelines for hiring Personal Trainers with specific degrees or certifications in these facilities, the focus on transitional programs may require a Personal Trainer to have higher qualifications than usual.

Corporate

More than 50% of business profits are spent annually on employees' and dependents' healthcare (6). Worksite health promotion (WHP) can be defined as "a combination of educational, organizational, and environmental activities and programs designed to motivate and support healthy lifestyles among a company's employees and their families" (7). The three chief goals of WHP programs are to:

➤ Assess health risks
➤ Reduce those health risk factors that can be reduced
➤ Promote socially and environmentally healthy lifestyles

However, only about 55% of companies have a comprehensive WHP program. The National Employee Service and Recreation Association estimates that there are more than 50,000 organizations with on-site physical fitness programs in the United States and nearly 1,000 employing full-time program directors.

The kinds of fitness-specific offerings vary greatly in WHP programs, ranging from pedometer-based walking programs to group exercise classes to fully equipped health clubs. One of the primary determinants of facility and program size is the number of employees. Companies with more than 1000 employees working in a central location (building or campus) are much more likely to offer traditional fitness facilities, because they have the financial means to do so and it makes economic sense. Smaller companies with a smaller employee base are much less likely to offer a WHP, especially one that includes fitness facilities.

Many corporate fitness programs are outsourced to companies that specialize in facility and program management. This makes it somewhat easier for the corporation because it can rely on someone else's expertise instead of having to develop it from within. Some choose to avoid development and management altogether by setting up a corporate account with an existing local fitness facility. A reduced membership fee is negotiated, and the company reimburses employees a portion or all of the fees. It is common, though, for the company to dictate that an employee must visit the facility a certain number of times per month to qualify for reimbursement.

Corporate fitness opportunities exist for Personal Trainers within both large and smaller companies. For larger companies, the typical route is to work as a traditional employee or independent contractor in the fitness center. For smaller companies, a more entrepreneurial approach is usually taken. Personal Trainers will typically need to approach the management about offering on-site services to the employees with the employer absorbing some of the cost. Since employers are often very cost-conscious and are typically unsure about investing in preventive programs, Personal Trainers will need to educate them about the benefits of their services to the health and well-being of their employees. Reporting client results, such as weight loss, reductions in blood pressure, and other health factors, also has a positive impact on their thinking and decision-making. Because individual sessions are the most expensive option, small-group training sessions are potentially more appealing to the employer.

ACSM'S ROLE AND THE EDUCATIONAL CONTINUUM

The ACSM is a 501(c)(3) professional member association composed of a multi-disciplinary mix of more than 20,000 exercise science researchers, educators, and practitioners. More specifically, member categories include physicians, nurses, athletic trainers, exercise physiologists, dietitians, and physical therapists, as well as many other allied health professionals with an interest in sports medicine and the exercise sciences. The mission statement for ACSM is:

> ACSM promotes and integrates scientific research, education and practical applications of sports medicine and exercise science. To maintain and enhance physical performance, fitness, health, and quality of life.

ACSM was founded in 1954, was the first professional organization to begin offering health and fitness certifications (in 1975), and continues to deliver the most respected certifications within the health and fitness industry. Because of the multi-disciplinary nature and diversity of its members, ACSM has evolved into the unique position of an industry leader for creating evidence-based best practices through the original research of its members, as well as disseminating this information through its periodicals, meetings and conferences, position stands and consensus statements, and certification workshops.

Identification of a Core Body of Knowledge

Shortly after ACSM began offering certifications, the first edition of *ACSM's Guidelines for Exercise Testing and Prescription* (8) was published along with its companion publication *ACSM's Resource Manual for Guidelines for Exercise Testing and Prescription* (9). These publications included, for the first time anywhere, the consensus of subject matter experts and so defined the core body of knowledge with respect to standards and guidelines for assessing fitness and prescribing exercise. Generally, all professions, regardless of the industry, have a core body of knowledge that provides guidance and clarity and also helps establish a specific profession's scope of practice. This initial publication proved so effective for practitioners that periodic review and revision of this book now takes place every 3 to 5 years. The year 2005 marks the publication of the 7th edition of *ACSM's Guidelines for Exercise Testing and Prescription,* celebrating its 30th anniversary.

Development and Continuous Revision of KSAs

Included in the appendices of every edition of *ACSM's Guidelines for Exercise Testing and Prescription* is a comprehensive list of knowledge, skills, and abilities (KSAs) relative to each ACSM certification. These KSAs represent the specific attributes necessary for success as a practitioner and usually are categorized across different areas of content. The general process for the ongoing revision and/or addition to the KSAs follows industry-accepted best-practice models for ongoing quality assurance. First, a group of appropriate subject matter experts (SMEs) is convened to review the current set of KSAs. These SMEs represent practitioners, academicians, researchers, and even potential employers. After their first round of review and revision, the first draft of updated KSAs are evaluated through a "job task analysis," in which a large number of randomly selected practitioners and employers further comment on the importance, frequency, and relevance of each specific KSA compared with the typical job demands and requirements in the real world setting. Additionally, the participants in the job task analysis phase can comment and suggest other appropriate attributes as new KSAs, not appearing within the current KSA list.

Once the job task analysis results are compiled, the original group of SMEs further revises the KSAs as needed, based on the results and comments from the job task analysis. Finally, the KSAs are assigned to their appropriate content areas, and a certification examination blueprint is developed that represents the combined work of the SMEs and the results of the job task analysis. This examination blueprint is the basis of the certification examination. The

Table 1.2 ACSM CERTIFIED PERSONAL TRAINER^SM EXAMINATION BLUEPRINT

The approximate percentage of questions from each content area is as follows:

Percentage	Content Areas
28%	Exercise Prescription (Training) and Programming
24%	Exercise Physiology and Related Exercise Science
13%	Health Appraisal and Fitness Exercise Testing
10%	Clinical and Medical Considerations (risk factor identification)
9%	Nutrition and Weight Management
8%	Safety, Injury Prevention, and Emergency Procedures
4%	Program Administration, Quality Assurance, and Outcome Assessment
4%	Human Behavior
Total 100%	

current examination test blueprint for the ACSM certified Personal Trainer^SM is found in Table 1.2.

ESTABLISHING YOUR KNOWLEDGE BASE

Everyone has strengths and weaknesses with respect to how much he or she knows or doesn't know about any given topic, including Personal Trainers. Even fitness professionals with college degrees have content areas that they are more knowledgeable in than others. Part of your commitment to the profession is to continuously evaluate your educational foundation, or knowledge base. One way to focus on an action plan for your specific continuing education needs is to use the KSAs as your knowledge map.

Begin by performing a thorough review of the KSAs, rating your familiarity and competence against each specific KSA. Next, use this checklist to prioritize the KSA content areas from weakest to strongest. Over the course of a year, seek out and participate in continuing educational opportunities that focus on your weakest content areas. You should do this on a yearly basis, at a minimum, as content areas that were once weak may become stronger for you over time, especially as you devote additional study to these areas and, more importantly, develop a client base in which some content areas are relied upon more than others. If you can do this consistently one year to the next, recertifying becomes a pleasure as opposed to a chore. Some Personal Trainers procrastinate, waiting until the last minute to accumulate the required number of CEUs/CECs. Not only does this create a great deal of stress for you, but also it is not a very effective way to expand your knowledge base as a Personal Trainer.

The Exercise Sciences

The competent Personal Trainer should have a strong knowledge foundation in the exercise sciences. Exercise science is a broad term that includes multiple disciplines. These disciplines often include anatomy and physiology, exercise physiology, motor learning/motor control, nutrition (dietetics), biomechanics/applied kinesiology, and exercise (sports) psychology. Good quality educational programs (workshops or online opportunities offered by certification organizations or curriculums offered by academic institutions) may offer a course of study that includes content or courses dedicated to helping the Personal Trainer develop an understanding of these more specific disciplines.

Developing Your Tool Kit

In addition to a strong knowledge foundation in the exercise sciences, effective Personal Trainers are constantly adding skills to their "tool kit." Additional tools include:

➤ Effective communication skills
➤ Ability to motivate appropriately
➤ Ability to influence behavior change
➤ Effective interviewing and screening
➤ Effective use of goals and objectives
➤ Effective exercise program design
➤ Ability to instruct appropriate exercise movements
➤ Using a business model

These are the minimum tools you should not only include in your tool kit but also master using effectively, either individually or in combination with others. As you progress through your professional career, you should be continuously adding tools to make you more effective as a Personal Trainer.

COMMUNICATION SKILLS (MOTIVATING AND INFLUENCING BEHAVIORAL CHANGE)

Perhaps the most overlooked yet important skill for the Personal Trainer tool kit is that of communication. Communication is more than just verbal, as it includes non-verbal elements such as visual (what is observed) and kinesthetic (what is felt). Additionally, effective communication involves much more than information exchange. Communication also relies on the emotional state of both individuals. For example, is the client "ready" to accept information or is there temporary resistance to the new information being provided? Likewise, are you an effective motivator who can create an optimal emotional state for clients so they are not only ready to take in the information that you are providing but also to put it to good use? As a complex and important skill, communication is discussed throughout this book.

SCREENING, ASSESSMENT, AND REFERRALS

Another set of tools required for the Personal Trainer includes interviewing, screening, risk stratification, and the ability to recognize when to refer a client to a medical healthcare provider such as a physician or registered dietitian. When health screening forms are used appropriately, these tools help establish a foundation of trust that facilitates the development of the trainer/client relationship. Combined with effective communication skills, these tools further improve the possibility of achieving the client's goals.

Typically, a Personal Trainer conducts an initial interview with a potential client in which basic demographic information is obtained, along with the client's heath history. Two types of forms are used at a minimum: the health history form and the PAR-Q$^{©}$ form. (Examples of these and other forms are available in Chapter 16, "Screening and the ACSM Risk Stratification Process.") In addition, it is appropriate during this initial interview to ask clients about their specific expectations for working with a Personal Trainer, what initial goals they may have, as well as any other lifestyle information they can share. Examples include:

➤ Recent and past history of physical activity (if any)
➤ History of previous injuries (if any)
➤ Level of social support from family and friends
➤ Potential stressors that may impose challenges on their exercise regimen, such as excessive work hours, physically demanding work, multiple recurring commitments within the community or with family

Finally, this initial consultation should be used to synchronize the Personal Trainer/client expectations, obtain or request any medical clearance forms (if required), as well as obtain signatures on required waivers, informed consent forms, and/or other contractual forms and agreements as required by your employer.

Risk stratification (ranking the client into a category of "low," "medium," or "high" risk, based on the presence or absence of various risk factors for cardiovascular disease) of your new client is the next step and should be based on the ACSM's risk stratification system (8), which is described in detail in Chapter 16. It is important to note that Personal Trainers do not diagnose or treat disease, disorders, injuries, or other medical conditions under any circumstance. The presence of specific and/or multiple risk factors requires that the Personal Trainer refer the client to the appropriate medical/healthcare provider for additional guidance and/or a medical release before designing and implementing an exercise program. Also, even if the client fails to initially disclose information that becomes known at a later time, the Personal Trainer still has a legal obligation to refer the client to his or her healthcare provider before additional training guidance can be provided. Personal Trainers who provide services outside their scope of practice place both themselves and their clients at risk.

Assessments are tests and measurements that Personal Trainers use with their clients to evaluate their current physical and functional status. Assessments may include:

➤ Resting heart rate
➤ Resting blood pressure
➤ Body weight and height
➤ Body composition estimates using skinfold calipers, etc.
➤ Circumference measurements of limbs, hips, and waist
➤ Calculation of body mass index (BMI)
➤ Calculation of waist-to-hip ratio
➤ Measurements of flexibility
➤ Tests for muscular strength/muscular endurance
➤ Tests for cardiorespiratory fitness

Assessments provide a current snapshot of the functional ability of your client. When combined with the data from the PAR-Q© and other health-related questionnaires, the Personal Trainer can begin developing a draft of a customized exercise regimen for the client.

ETHICS AND PROFESSIONAL CONDUCT

Ethics can be described as standards of conduct that guide decisions and actions, based on duties derived from core values. Specifically, core values are principles that we use to define what is right, good, and/or just. When a professional demonstrates behavior that is consistent, or aligned, with widely accepted standards in their respective industry, that professional is said to behave "ethically." On the other hand, "unethical" behavior is behavior that is not consistent with industry-accepted standards. As a fitness professional, you have an obligation to stay within the bounds of the defined scope of practice for a Personal Trainer, as well as to abide by all industry-accepted standards of behavior at all times. Furthermore, as a certified or registered professional through ACSM, it is your responsibility to be familiar with all aspects of the ACSM's Code of Ethics for certified and registered professionals.

Code of Ethics for ACSM Certified and Registered Professionals

PURPOSE

This Code of Ethics is intended to aid all certified and registered American College of Sports Medicine Credentialed Professionals (ACSMCPs) to establish and maintain a high level of ethical conduct, as defined by standards by which ACSMCPs may determine the appropriateness of their conduct. Any existing professional, licensure, or certification affiliations that ACSMCPs have with governmental, local, state, or national agencies or organizations will take precedence relative to any disciplinary matters that pertain to practice or professional conduct.

This Code applies to all ACSMCPs, regardless of ACSM membership status (to include members and non-members). Any cases in violation of this Code will be referred to the ACSM Committee on Certification and Registry Boards (CCRB).

PRINCIPLES AND STANDARDS

Responsibility to the Public

➤ ACSMCPs shall be dedicated to providing competent and legally permissible services within the scope of the knowledge, skills, and abilities (KSAs) of their respective credential. These services shall be provided with integrity, competence, diligence, and compassion.

➤ ACSMCPs provide exercise information in a manner that is consistent with evidence-based science and medicine.

➤ ACSMCPs respect the rights of clients, colleagues, and health professionals, and shall safeguard client confidences within the boundaries of the law.

➤ Information relating to the ACSMCP/client relationship is confidential and may not be communicated to a third party not involved in that client's care without the prior written consent of the client or as required by law.

➤ ACSMCPs are truthful about their qualifications and the limitations of their expertise and provide services consistent with their competencies.

Responsibility to the Profession

➤ ACSMCPs maintain high professional standards. As such, an ACSMCP should never represent him/herself, either directly or indirectly, as anything other than an ACSMCP unless he/she holds other license/certification that allows him/her to do so.

➤ ACSMCPs practice within the scope of their knowledge, skills, and abilities. ACSMCPs will not provide services that are limited by state law to provision by another healthcare professional only.

➤ An ACSMCP must remain in good standing relative to governmental requirements as a condition of continued credentialing.

➤ ACSMCPs take credit, including authorship, only for work they have actually performed and give credit to the contributions of others as warranted.

➤ Consistent with the requirements of their certification or registration, ACSMCPs must complete approved, additional educational course work aimed at maintaining and advancing their knowledge, skills, and abilities.

Principles and Standards for Candidates of ACSM Certification Examinations

Candidates applying for a credentialing examination must comply with candidacy requirements and, to the best of their abilities, accurately complete the application process. In addition, the candidate must refrain from any and all behavior that would be interpreted as "irregular."

Public Disclosure of Affiliation

➤ Any ACSMCP may disclose his or her affiliation with ACSM credentialing in any context, oral or documented, provided it is currently accurate. In doing so, no ACSMCP may imply college endorsement of whatever is associated in context with the disclosure, unless expressly authorized by the college. Disclosure of affiliation in connection with a commercial venture may be made provided the disclosure is made in a professionally dignified manner; is not false, misleading, or deceptive; and does not imply licensure or the attainment of specialty or diploma status.

➤ ACSMCPs may disclose their credential status.

➤ ACSMCPs may list their affiliation with ACSM credentialing on their business cards without prior authorization.

➤ ACSMCPs and the institutions employing an ACSMCP may inform the public of an affiliation as a matter of public discourse or presentation.

Discipline

Any ACSMCP may be disciplined or lose his or her certification or registry for conduct that, in the opinion of the Executive Council of the ACSM Committee on Certification and Registry Boards (CCRB), goes against the principles set forth in this Code. Such cases will be reviewed by the ACSM CCRB Ethics Subcommittee, which will include a liaison from the ACSM CCRB executive council, as appointed by the CCRB chair. The ACSM CCRB Ethics Subcommittee will make an action recommendation to the executive council of the ACSM CCRB for final review and approval.

SUMMARY

The rapidly expanding fitness industry offers Personal Trainers many potential work environments in which to gain experience and to develop a career, including commercial clubs, not-for-profit clubs, university recreation centers, corporate fitness centers, medical fitness centers, and more. Although compensation varies greatly for trainers, they are overall very satisfied with their career choice and see opportunities for advancement and growth. With a nation on the verge of a healthcare crisis due primarily to the prevalence of lifestyle-related conditions, highly qualified and motivated Personal Trainers are needed now more than ever to lead individuals down the road to good health and well-being. As the fitness industry grows and the demographics/characteristics of the population continue to change, it is likely that the role of Personal Trainers will change too. This changing role will likely be an expansion of Personal Trainers' scope of practice, so that Personal Trainers may soon be seen as allied health professionals. In the future, Personal Trainers may be commonplace in areas where they are seldom seen now, such as medical clinics specializing in preventive and rehabilitative medicine, as one example. As an emerging professional in this rapidly growing field, you can contribute to this expanding sphere of influence by being the utmost professional at all times, for your clients and for the best interests of the profession.

REFERENCES

1. Bureau of Labor Statistics, U.S. Department of Labor. Occupational Outlook Handbook. 2004-05 ed. Recreation and fitness workers. Online at http://www.bls.gov/oco/ocos058.htm. Accessed February 26, 2005.
2. International Health, Racquet and Sportsclub Association. Online at http://cms.ihrsa.org/IHRSA/viewPage.cfm?pageId=149. Accessed February 27, 2005.
3. International Health, Racquet and Sportsclub Association: The US Health Club Industry (Industry estimates for 2001–2002). Online at http://cms.ihrsa.org/IHRSA/viewPage.cfm?pageId=654. Accessed February 27, 2005.
4. United States Census Bureau: American FactFinder. Online at http://factfinder.census.gov/servlet/SAFFPopulation?_sse=on. Accessed May 19, 2005.
5. International Health, Racquet and Sportsclub Association Fair Competition Annual Report (2003). Online at http://download.ihrsa.org/gr/faircomp.pdf. Accessed February 27, 2005.
6. The Ethics Resource Center. Online at http://www.ethics.org/faq.html#eth. Accessed February 27, 2005.
7. Chenowith D. Worksite Health Promotion. Champaign, IL: Human Kinetics, 1998.
8. American College of Sports Medicine. ACSM's Guidelines for Exercise Testing and Prescription. 7th ed. Baltimore: Lippincott Williams & Wilkins, 2005.
9. American College of Sports Medicine. ACSM's Resource Manual for Exercise Testing and Prescription. 5th ed. Baltimore: Lippincott Williams & Wilkins, 2005.

2 Career Track for Professional Personal Trainers

Nicki Andersen, President, Reality Fitness, Inc., Naperville, Illinois

Kenneth E. Baldwin, M.Ed., A.H. Ismail Center for Health, Exercise & Nutrition, Department of Health and Kinesiology, College of Liberal Arts, Purdue University, West Lafayette, Indiana

Chapter Outline

Becoming a Personal Trainer
Organizing Your Career Pathway
Education
Continuing Education
Developing Business Relationships
Establishing a Client Base

Community Involvement
Medical Affiliations
Building a Solid Professional Foundation
Personal Trainer's Role As Teacher and Educator
Being Well-Rounded – It's More Than Counting Reps
Practices, Standards, and Ethics

Objectives

- **Choosing a career as a professional Personal Trainer**
- **Determining your area of specialization**
- **Setting a timeline**
- **Deciding on your educational options**
- **Developing a successful professional foundation**
- **Dedicating yourself to excellence**

Although fitness professionals have been providing exercise advice for decades, the reality is that the term "Personal Trainer" did not become popular until the late 1970s. In the early days, the only prerequisite for a Personal Trainer was a decent personality and the physical appearance of being "fit." Today, however, a career in personal training is positioned to evolve into a highly respectable profession.

As the personal training industry grew, so did the number of untrained, uneducated, but well-intended people wanting to teach others how to get fit regardless of their academic training or experience. Even though the early Personal Trainers had a knowledge base that was minimal at best, the training business continues to expand.

The personal training field is expected to grow 44% by 2012 (1). Between large corporations seeking health professionals to keep employees well and more people becoming aware of the need for becoming physically fit, a career in personal training is positioned for an exciting growth trend.

This chapter covers many of the areas that you should consider if you choose to pursue a career in personal training. The following questions may help you to determine your career interest.

1. **Why do I want to become a Personal Trainer and what are my specialty options?** As with any profession, it is important that you be clear about your reasons for wanting to dedicate your life to a particular career. Did you decide to become a Personal Trainer because you have had your own experience that drew you into the health and fitness business? Do you know someone who is involved in the industry? Are you at a place in your life where a career in personal training seems like a great fit? Do you want to help people? Whatever your objectives, make sure that they resonate with your personal values. The exciting part about becoming a Professional Personal Trainer is that your specialty options are endless (2), as discussed in this chapter.

2. **Do I possess the compassion and empathy that are required in a profession that deals with peoples' physical and mental strengths and weaknesses?** Being a Personal Trainer requires that you have a well-developed capacity to connect with people. This skill will enhance your success as well as that of your clients. You must also be able to understand where and when clients need support at various points in your relationship. You may have clients who are focused and clear about their goals, while others will struggle with the whole idea of making lifestyle changes. Whatever the situation, you must be prepared to deal with client frustrations and disappointments to help them move forward with optimism rather than feeling defeated, frustrated, and isolated.

3. **What specific area of personal training holds the greatest interest for me?** Begin by asking yourself what part of personal training most interests you. If you enjoy working with seniors, then concentrate your efforts there. You may like the idea of a large commercial health club, which provides numerous training opportunities, or you may prefer working with children in an after-school program. Whatever your choice of specialization, you should take the time to explore the options and where and when you want to work with your client.

4. **Do I have superior time management skills?** When you begin creating your own personal training business or managing your own schedule, time management is crucial. There is a direct correlation between time management and high performance. Time management skills are critical when it comes to scheduling clients. Clients generally seek times that are convenient

for them, and they count on you to keep their appointments consistent (3). If you fail to keep consistent client schedules or don't keep appointments because you are unable to manage your time efficiently, you will soon find yourself with no clients. Being well prepared at each training session (which takes time and organizational skills) is something your clients appreciate (and deserve), and this is one of the secrets to growing a successful personal training business.

5. **Do I pay close attention to details?** Many people believe that being a Personal Trainer means creating an exercise program and counting the reps—nothing could be further from the truth. In the personal training field, for safety purposes as well as for legal purposes, you must pay attention to your client's every move during each session and make sure that he or she is committed to following your directions (4). Details must be carefully noted after each session so that you can track client results. In addition to the training sessions and depending upon your field of specialization, there will be daily responsibilities such as maintaining records, phone calls, and billing. If you own your own facility, the list will include equipment upkeep, marketing, advertising, and payroll. No matter what your role, each area of responsibility must be attended to in precise detail to meet the needs of your clients and grow a successful business.

6. **What traits do I possess that will contribute to my success as a Personal Trainer?** As a Personal Trainer, you are required to teach. You are there to provide your client with all the necessary information that will enhance his or her overall health. If you are able to communicate efficiently the information your client needs to know, your success rate as well as that of your clients will be impressive. Motivation is a key part of your communication skills set. You must ask yourself if you can adequately motivate your clients to do the work necessary to achieve their goals. Whether it is a client wishing to lose weight or a runner intent on improving his or her speed, you will need to provide the necessary motivation to help them succeed. Another key trait is self-discipline. Being a Personal Trainer requires that you not only maintain a dedication to your own health but also to the health of your clients. Leading a healthy lifestyle is not possible without self-discipline.

7. **What strengths do I have that can contribute to the fitness industry?** Regardless of your career path, it's helpful to know what strengths you bring to your chosen profession, so that you can build on them and facilitate your growth personally as well as professionally. The more you know about your industry, the more you will be able to grow your business given the insight you gain from your involvement. Very often people are so consumed by their day-to-day activities (a result of poor time management) that they find they have little time or energy to participate in extracurricular events that can have a positive impact on their professional success. There are many different ways that you can become involved in the fitness industry. For example, if you believe you have strong writing skills, why not share your expertise and experience with magazines and journals? Publications in the health and fitness field are always looking for writers who can provide timely and insightful articles. If writing is a strength of yours, explore the possibilities. Perhaps you have strong public speaking skills. Find an opportunity to speak or be a panel member at industry conferences. Becoming a speaker is a great way to enhance your credibility, as it shows your clients that you have the knowledge necessary to teach others. In addition, your public speaking skills may lead you to local organizations, which will raise your profile and again allow the opportunity for business growth.

8. **Are you passionate about your chosen career?** Publisher and philanthropist Malcolm Forbes once said, "Success follows doing what you want to do. There is no other way to be successful" (5). Nothing lays the foundation for success better than being passionate about your chosen profession. Because the personal training industry is relatively new and has grown so rapidly, there are many Personal Trainers who jumped aboard strictly because of the money-making potential. It doesn't matter how much money you make; if you are not passionate about your career choice, it will come across in your business interactions. Your clients will pick up on the fact that your focus is not on their success but on your own personal gain. This is one of the fastest ways to lose clients and your credibility.

9. **Am I willing to take responsibility as a role model and mentor?** This is a question that needs serious consideration. As a Personal Trainer, you are setting an example in the fitness industry. People will be looking to you as a model of what constitutes health and fitness.

10. **Am I committed to excellence?** Once you have decided whether a career as a Personal Trainer is for you, the next step is determining if you are willing to give 100% to your chosen profession. Whether it is a training session, your business cards, your customer service, or your interaction with other Personal Trainers, you must always avoid cutting corners and always overdeliver.

BECOMING A PERSONAL TRAINER

As you consider a career as a Personal Trainer, it is always recommended that you learn as much as you can about the fitness industry. You can set this process in motion by setting up interviews with health and fitness professionals. Sitting down one-on-one with a qualified expert in the field is a great starting point, as it will provide insight that you typically cannot get through formal academic training or in a classroom setting. Attending industry conferences and taking advantage of continuing education opportunities and interactions with others will also help to enhance your knowledge.

According to the U.S. Department of Labor, Bureau of Labor Statistics (6), more and more employers are requiring fitness employees to have a bachelor's degree in a health- or fitness-related field such as exercise science or physical education. Some employers accept certification in lieu of a college degree, while others may require both certification and a college degree.

The Personal Trainer gains increased credibility by seeking out high-quality certification and formal education. In addition, don't lose sight of the value of meeting and networking with other health professionals. It is always recommended that you do so and that you look beyond health clubs and include hospitals and educational environments in your networking activities. The more insight you gain into the various areas of the business, the greater the chance you will discover the direction that is most appropriate for you. Remember that continuing education is required with or without a degree. Commit yourself to learning as much as you can about physiology, kinesiology, biomechanics, and the inner workings of the body, to add to industry know-how, good interpersonal skills, and a desire to be your best.

ORGANIZING YOUR CAREER PATHWAY

As you begin to develop your career pathway, it is important to understand what your objectives are and decide on your specific area of interest. You may want to complete your studies at a four-year university with an emphasis on exercise science. Or, you may already hold a degree in another field and simply want to complete a credible certification in the industry. Either way, you should explore your options and begin with a certification. Refer to the career path flowchart to determine your educational options (Box 2.1).

Consider looking to colleges and universities that provide specialized curriculum and education in personal training and the exercise sciences that meet your career needs (7). Note that some universities may have ACSM's university endorsement or accreditation, which can add significant value to your educational pursuit.

Focus on the aspect of the industry that interests you most and in which you can see yourself being involved. Your area of specialization should engage your passion and dedication to becoming the best in your chosen field. As mentioned above, don't dismiss the value of connecting with experts in the area you would like to pursue. The more you learn from them, the better prepared you will be to lay out a realistic career path and timeline.

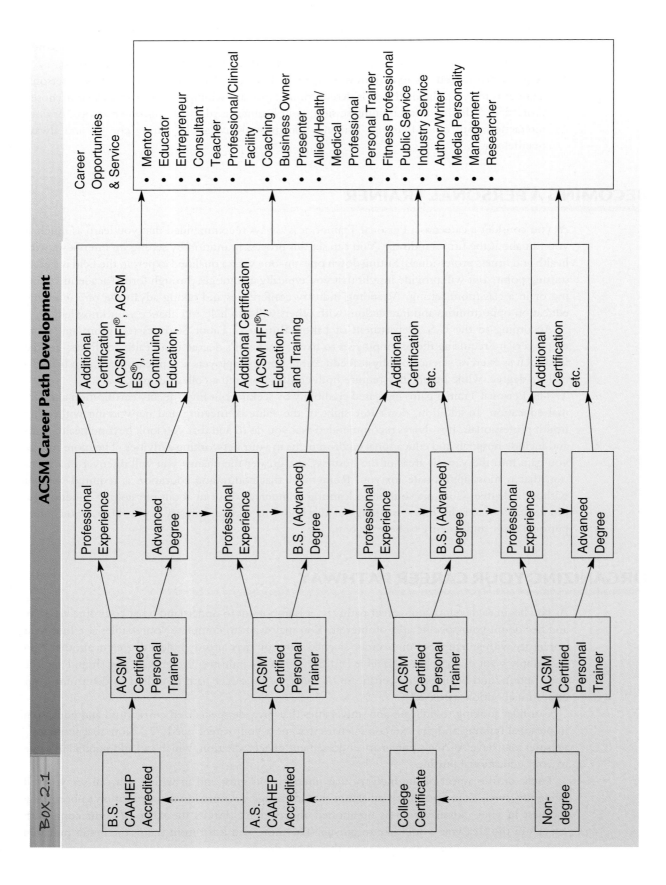

BOX 2.1

ACSM Career Path Development

It is best to start by setting up a timeline outlining the steps you need to take to reach your desired goals. Keep in mind that your educational/career path should match your goals. For example, if your goal is to work in a hospital environment, you should begin by speaking with individuals in that environment and discover what credentials will best support your goals. Once you gain a clear idea about what is involved by speaking to others, you can begin to develop a specific timeline.

By referring to the career pathways of Personal Trainer A and Personal Trainer B in Box 2.2, you will see two vastly different approaches for two people involved in the same industry. This contrast may help to illustrate the different options available to you as you organize your own career path.

Box 2.2	Career Path Contrast

Personal Trainer A

B.A. degree – Finance

Master's degree in Education, specialization in Biomechanics

Pursuing a Ph.D.

ACSM Health/Fitness Instructor® certification

Started personal training and fitness consulting business

Medically based affiliations

Community/professional affiliations

Local/international presenter and writer

Volunteer for IDEA Committee

Former Chair of the Senior Fitness Subcommittee Governor's Council on Physical Fitness and Sports

Recognitions: Personal Trainer of the Year award, nationally and internationally

Program Coordinator for College of Extended Studies Certificate program for Personal Fitness Training

Program Coordinator for four-year college—undergraduate degree in Personal Fitness Training

Committee member for numerous health and fitness organizations

American Alliance for Health, Physical Education, Recreation & Dance (AAHPERD) Exercise Science Committee

Author of books and instructional videos/DVDs

Personal Trainer B

Health Club Manager/Personal Trainer (2 years)

Associate's degree in Fitness Management (2 years)

Fitness Practitioner certification (1 year)

AFAA Certification, ACE certification

Research and study of physiology, kinesiology, biomechanics, and anatomy (ongoing)

Started in-home personal training business

NASM certification

Opened personal training studio

Contributing writer for major industry magazines

Health and fitness columnist for suburban newspaper

Family fitness columnist for major e-zine

Author of health and fitness book published by large publishing firm

Presenter at numerous health and fitness conferences

Numerous Awards for Excellence in business, management, and customer service

Active member of numerous health and fitness organizations

Note that although their paths are different, they both became certified, which is a vital part of the Personal Training profession.

EDUCATION

Among the many certification options available to you, you may choose to consider one from the ACSM. You can research which certification program is best for you by visiting the ACSM website. If you are reading this book, you are probably studying for ACSM's Certified Personal Trainer[SM] examination (considered by many in the fitness industry to be the most rigorous) or studying for some other ACSM certification. The ACSM programs are often viewed as one of the best measures of competence and require a high level of knowledge, skills, and abilities.

ACSM provides an internal recognition system of academic programs through its University Connection Endorsement program. As of this printing, there are more than 50 undergraduate and graduate programs nationwide with "ACSM-Endorsed" status. In addition to its own endorsement program, ACSM is also a sponsoring organization of the Committee on Accreditation for the Exercise Sciences (CoAES) of the Commission on Accreditation of Allied Health Education Programs (CAAHEP) (8). The primary role of the CoAES is to establish standards and guidelines for academic programs that facilitate the preparation of students seeking employment in the health, fitness, and exercise industry. The CoAES also works to establish and implement a process of self-study, review, and recommendation for all programs seeking CAAHEP accreditation (8). Academic program accreditation through CAAHEP is specifically intended for exercise science or related departments (e.g., physical education, kinesiology) with a professional preparation track designed for students seeking employment opportunities in the health, fitness, and exercise industry. CAAHEP reviews and accredits more than 2000 educational programs in 21 health science occupations across the United States and Canada. Accreditation in the health-related disciplines serves an important public interest. Along with certification and licensure, accreditation is a tool intended to help ensure a well-prepared and qualified workforce providing healthcare services. Research your local academic institutions that offer the appropriate programs to help you achieve your career goals. If you are looking for colleges and universities in which to pursue your career, the following courses are examples of some that help prepare you for a personal training career:

➤ Applied anatomy and kinesiology
➤ Exercise physiology
➤ Biomechanics
➤ Motor skills and learning
➤ Exercise psychology
➤ Health & fitness in clinical/worksite settings
➤ Health behavior and health promotion
➤ Health screening and fitness evaluation & prescription
➤ Health & fitness program management
➤ Exercise program development
➤ Professional development and internship in health & fitness
➤ Clinical practices in personal training

Whether you are seeking certification through ACSM, are currently ACSM certified, or hold an undergraduate degree in the exercise sciences, it does not mean that you are finished with your education. You should make a commitment to education and continued learning. One degree or one certification is not all that is required to succeed. You should keep up with the industry through continuing education classes, business relationships, your client base, community involvement, and medical affiliations.

CONTINUING EDUCATION

The reality is that you need to make continuing education a part of your commitment right from the start. You should read good-quality professional periodicals that offer CEUs or CECs that are designed to inform you of not just the physical changes in the industry but also the business changes. Get involved in conferences that put you in touch with different aspects of the industry and provide you with opportunities for meeting and networking with people in your field.

DEVELOPING BUSINESS RELATIONSHIPS

There is no better way to understand the nuances of a business than through the voice of experience. Talking with seasoned professionals can help you avoid the mistakes they made and teach you the secrets to building a successful career. It is important to meet new business contacts throughout your career, not just in the beginning. For example, if you are interested in writing for health and fitness journals and you read an article that focuses on sports-specific training and it piques your interest, why not contact the author? By contacting the author, you will have a chance to ask specific questions and have the author elaborate not only on the article but also on how he or she got into writing for health and fitness journals.

ESTABLISHING A CLIENT BASE

To develop a client base, you need to determine the type of client you are seeking. This can only be done if you have contact with people of varying ages and personalities who have different needs, goals, and other physical challenges. Once you have established the clientele with whom you are interested in working, you need to find a venue that hosts that type of clientele. For example, if you like working with seniors, you will most likely find them at a community center, senior center, or health club. Once you have found a location with the clientele you are seeking, see if you can gain employment there on a full- or part-time basis. Create business cards, as mentioned above, offer to do public speaking as a way to introduce yourself to your community, and establish yourself as a health and fitness expert. Consider writing articles or a column for a local newspaper as another way to raise your profile and credibility within the community.

If you start working the floor at a health club, it is a great opportunity to meet members and to introduce yourself. When members see your enthusiasm for assisting them, they will remember when they are seeking a qualified Personal Trainer. Teaching large groups is also a great way to develop relationships and to establish yourself in a new facility. The more you are able to engage with your potential clients, the greater the likelihood of attracting and retaining a healthy clientele.

COMMUNITY INVOLVEMENT

It is unfortunate that many believe that community involvement is only for those who have a lot of time. It is not uncommon for people to get so caught up in their business, that they lose sight of the industry and the community that supports their vocation. Overlooking the value of working within your community or industry might be the difference between a successful business and a marginal business. Look into donating your time at a senior center teaching group classes or after-school programs for kids. You will find literally hundreds of opportunities within your community that will enable you to get involved. A community that knows who you are and sees that you are involved will become one of your best business referral sources.

MEDICAL AFFILIATIONS

Another great way to help develop a client base is forming partnerships with professionals in the health field such as a Registered Dietician, a physician, a mental health specialist and others, all of whom can have a profound effect on the development of your business. You can offer to train these professionals so that they are able to see your capabilities or you can offer to present a program on developing a sound fitness program for their patients and/or clients. Establishing relationships with allied professionals serves to elevate your credibility within the community and the fitness industry. Set aside time to sit and discuss your philosophies and find out how you can develop a reciprocal relationship.

BUILDING A SOLID PROFESSIONAL FOUNDATION

One of the best ways to establish yourself as a professional is to develop a reputation that is credible and respected. Your reputation will be based upon the perception of how well you work with your clients and how you have positioned yourself within the community and within the fitness industry.

PERSONAL TRAINER'S ROLE AS TEACHER AND EDUCATOR

Excellent communication skills are an absolute necessity to enhance your role as a Personal Trainer. Personal Trainers must be able to teach with a clear and succinct message. This book will show how you, as Personal Trainers, can create and develop personal training sessions that have a sound educational, scientific, and practical approach. Unfortunately, there is a glut of bogus health and fitness information in the media. It is the responsibility of Personal Trainers to be able to disseminate correct and scientifically valid information and avoid the fads and gimmicks that detract from professional and client success.

BEING WELL-ROUNDED—IT'S MORE THAN COUNTING REPS

A Personal Trainer who is simply counting repetitions has no business in an industry that requires focus, listening, and leadership skills. From the time a personal training session starts to the time it is completed, the job of a Personal Trainer is to guide a client through a series of exercises that are designed to help that client achieve his or her stated goals. To do this effectively, it is important to have interpersonal skills that will allow your client to feel comfortable and safe in the knowledge that you are committed to their success. One of the most valuable skills that a Personal Trainer can have is the ability to know when to talk and know when to listen. Whether it is reviewing client goals and training them accordingly or laying out specific guidelines, being able to provide your client with a personalized effort will make you a successful Personal Trainer.

PRACTICES, STANDARDS, AND ETHICS

Part of what creates a successful and rewarding career is a clear understanding of ethical practice and standards. To run a business with integrity, you must follow clear guidelines of standards and ethics.

SUMMARY

It is an exciting time to be a part of the personal training industry. Make sure that you do your homework and assess all of the different options available to you before selecting an area of specialization.

The field is vast, so take the time to explore it. Regardless of the career path you choose, it is important to take the necessary steps to position yourself for a long and successful career. The Personal Trainer makes a commitment to excellence in the areas of education, community/industry involvement, customer service, and time management and embraces the highest ethical standards. If you pay close attention to each of these aspects of your career, you will find yourself in a business that is rewarding and satisfying and ultimately successful.

REFERENCES

1. IDEA Fitness Journal 2004;Nov/Dec:13.
2. Kravitz L, Rochey C. Career growth tips for the 21st century: a resource guide to career opportunities. Online at http://www.unm.edu/;lkravitz/article%20folder/career.html. Accessed March 27, 2005.
3. Cooper J, Fazio R. A new look at dissonance. Adv Exp Psychol 1984;17:229–266.
4. Herbert DL, Herbert WG. Legal considerations. In Roitman JL,Kelsey M, eds. ACSM's Resource Manual for Guidelines for Exercise Testing and Prescription. 3rd ed. Baltimore: Lippincott Williams & Wilkins, 1998:614.
5. Klein A. The Change-Your-Life Book. New York: Gramercy Books, 2000:116.
6. Bureau of Labor Statistics, U.S. Department of Labor. Occupational Outlook Handbook, 2004–05 ed, Recreation and Fitness Workers. Online at http://www.bls.gov/oco/ocos058.htm. Accessed February 26, 2005.
7. Prime Media Business Magazines and Media Inc. Club Industry's Fitness Business Pro. Purdue to Offer 4-year Degree in Personal Training. September 28, 2004. Online at http://fitnessbusiness-pro.com/news/dyndicate/purdue_personaltraining_092804/. Accessed March 27, 2005.
8. Commission on Accreditation of Allied Health Education Programs (CAAHEP). Online at www.caahep.org. Accessed March 27, 2005.

The Educational Approach to Personal Training

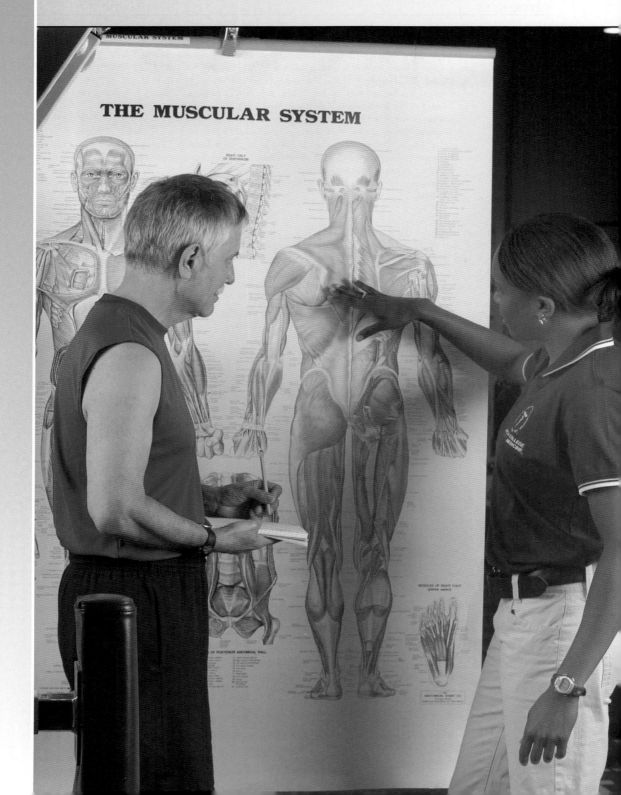

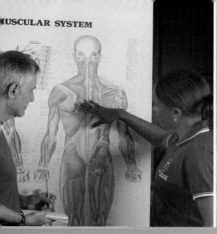

Education-Based Personal Training Programs

Kenneth E. Baldwin, M.Ed. A.H. Ismail Center for Health, Exercise & Nutrition, Department of Health and Kinesiology, College of Liberal Arts, Purdue University, West Lafayette, Indiana

Chapter Outline

- **Understand the value of the education-based approach to personal training**
- **Know the basic elements of successful education**
- **Understand the educational components of Sequential Exercise Training**
- **Understand the application of Sequential Exercise Training to the session plan and flowchart**
- **Design and implement education-based personal training sessions**

The purpose of this book is to provide Personal Trainers with knowledge on the foundations of the exercise sciences, program design, and learning principles so that they can become skilled personal training educators. Personal training involves a learning, or educational, process on the part of the trainer and the client. Traditional personal training, however, generally has not incorporated basic education methodologies commonly used in other fields of learning to the process of exercise and fitness. This stems from the difference in the concepts of training and education. Training implies the repetition of a certain behavior to instill a new habit or skill in the person being trained. Education, however, typically involves a different level of learning, one that involves intelligence not only of the body but also of the mind. Since clients of Personal Trainers are, in effect, students of exercise and fitness, the trainer's approach to the client will be more successful if it is based on both education and training principles. The quality of the training session improves greatly when the trainer approaches exercise and fitness as an educational process and not simply as a "training session."

Consequently, Personal Trainers need to be good educators, and good education depends on a knowledge and understanding of effective teaching methods. Much research over the last 40 years has greatly increased educators' understanding of how people learn. One of the primary goals of this book is to apply some of the basic results of this research to personal training and exercise program development. The term "clients" will often be supplemented with the term "students," an expansion of the usual way in which Personal Trainers may have related to their clients in the past. This broadening of the Personal Trainer's perspective in relating to the people you serve is the first step in refocusing your approach to those who have come for assistance with health, exercise, or fitness questions. When you shift your perspective from "training" to "education" you will take the first step toward the creation of a strong teacher/student relationship with your personal training clients.

To get a better grasp of this approach, a refresher on the definitions of the terms "education" and "training" is helpful. "Training" means "to teach one to be qualified, proficient, and prepared (as by exercise) for a test of skill or with an emphasis on performance" in relationship to a set standard (1). "Education" means "an activity undertaken by an individual or group designed to obtain knowledge" and understanding of a given subject or ability (1). The educator presents the knowledge or skill for the student to learn and master according to his or her own abilities. "Education-based training" is the combination of these two terms.

WHY FOCUS ON A PROCESS OF EDUCATION FOR YOUR CLIENTS?

Your clients have a wide diversity of personal needs, goals, and objectives, as well as differences in kinesthetic awareness, learning skills, performance abilities, and learning style preferences. The education-based approach to personal training considers the client's educational needs and presents information to clients that honors their learning style and performance ability as well as individual goals and health and medical history. The Personal Trainer can develop an inclusive training session model tailored to a client's specific learning styles and abilities. By taking a proactive approach to gaining more knowledge and expertise as an education-based Personal Trainer, only then can you truly begin to expand the repertoire of skills and knowledge that you can bring to your client.

THE PERSONAL TRAINER AS EDUCATOR

Personal Trainers are most effective when they view themselves as teachers and educators, and they need to remember that their clients are also learners and students. Coaching, motivating, and encouraging clients are all important components of personal training, but they will always be most effective when used for the higher goal of imparting information to, and educating clients in, ways that best allow them to learn the skills, techniques, and knowledge required to exercise in a smart and productive way throughout their lives.

THE EDUCATIONAL MODEL

The field of educational psychology has extensively researched the use and benefits of educational models in the process of learning and course instruction. As a field of study, it has much to offer personal training as a resource for better understanding of how clients learn and how to improve health and fitness education.

Educators commonly group related concepts together in easy-to-understand frameworks known as models. These models are different from a common list in that they work together as an integrated system in which all the parts necessary to complete the whole process are represented. They can also have a sequential relationship to each other; steps in an educational model are one of the most effective ways for human beings to learn new information. In their book *Educational Psychology,* Gage and Berliner explain that the use of models as learning aids has two primary benefits (2). These models provide accurate and useful representations of knowledge that is needed when solving problems in some particular area or domain. Here, in this book that seeks to teach an education-based approach to personal training, the benefit is two-fold:

➤ As a Personal Trainer, this book will help you to learn and to organize the information you teach. This mental organization will provide for you a strong background and support to your successful work as an education-based Personal Trainer.
➤ For your personal training clients, you can provide them with an organized way of learning the knowledge and skills of personal training through visual representation, stimulating their motivation and success in their training programs.

Thus, when you as a trainer have an organized mental picture of what you are teaching your clients, your clients will also obtain an organized perspective of their training process. This will ensure a sustained positive motivation for you as Personal Trainer and for your clients.

Gage and Berliner further explain that a model makes the process of understanding a domain of knowledge easier because it is a visual expression of the topic. The authors found that students who study visual models before a lecture may recall as much as 57% more on questions concerning conceptual information than students who receive instruction without the advantage of seeing and discussing models. Alesandrini came to similar conclusions when he studied different pictorial–verbal strategies for learning (3). Therefore, the use of models in this book seeks to facilitate your learning as a Personal Trainer and teach you how to educate your clients in a similar, mentally organized manner. Lastly, research on the effectiveness of pictorial learning strategies indicates that learning is improved when pictures supplement verbal materials, when learners draw their own pictures while studying, and when learners are asked to generate mental pictures while reading or studying (3).

The educational model allows the student to visualize the steps of a process before actually doing them. This mental internalization of information establishes the content as well as the ordering of that content in an organized way within the student's mind. The process of learning with models, however, requires planning and time to implement. When this time is allotted, the results are positive, and the success rate of students is greatly increased.

In Chapter 2 of his book *Designing and Assessing Courses and Curricula,* Diamond (4) suggested that there are four advantages to developing a specific curriculum and the two educational models below exemplify these characteristics. Specifically, it:

➤ Identifies the key factors that you should consider in a sequential order
➤ Serves as a procedural guide
➤ Allows you to understand where you are in the process, and if others are involved, their role in it
➤ Improves your efficiency by reducing duplication of effort and ensuring that critical questions are asked and alternative solutions explored

Bloom's Mastery Learning Model

The pioneer of educational research, Benjamin Bloom, developed one of the early educational models, the elements of which are still primary to high-quality educational presentations (5). High-quality instruction had the following characteristics, according to Bloom's model:

➤ Organize subject matter into manageable learning units
➤ Develop specific learning objectives for each unit
➤ Develop appropriate formative and summative assessment measures
➤ Plan and implement teaching strategies, with sufficient time allocations, practice opportunities, and corrective reinstruction for all students to reach the desired level of mastery

Gage and Berliner's Model

Educational researchers Gage and Berliner (2) developed a model for successful learning that demonstrates the above characteristics. They based their model on the question "What does a teacher do?" and found that an ordered sequence of five tasks are central to the instructional/learning process. This process consists of the following five sequential steps:

1. Objectives: The instructor needs knowledge of the student's goals and objectives.
2. Instruction: The presentation must be organized and in harmony with the student's goals.
3. Students' characteristics: The presentation must reflect the student's abilities and preferences.
4. Evaluation: The process must be reviewed to see if it met the student's goals and objectives.
5. Re-teaching: If unclear areas of understanding remain, the instruction needs to be adjusted and/or repeated.

Gage and Berliner point out that the objectives and the evaluation phases are linked by the instruction phase, and instruction is based on the instructor's knowledge of the student's characteristics. The re-teaching phase involves the repetition of the process "[If] the evaluations do not demonstrate that the desired results have been achieved." This shows how important the *sequence* of the various steps is to the success of the model. It also demonstrates a point that Diamond makes in his book: "Although the overall flow of the model is generally followed, the steps in the model may overlap. This allows for flexibility. The steps in the flow of the model, although generally followed, may overlap in time". For example, the process of learning the student's objectives may also provide information about the student's characteristics. The model acts as a type of checklist so that if the first step did not provide the information needed, the second step will cover that point. In this way the basic order has a certain flexibility that contributes to the model's success.

THE PRIMARY ELEMENTS OF SUCCESSFUL EDUCATIONAL MODELS

Through his work with his Mastery Learning Model, Bloom (5) found that "Mastery Learning's basic principle is that almost all students can earn A's if:

1. Students are given enough time to learn normal information taught in school, and
2. Students are provided quality instruction."

An immense number of educational models have been developed since Bloom began his research in the 1950s. Educational researchers have studied these models and have found that certain basic elements continue to recur. The following discussion of the results of some of this research is included so that you can understand how it can be implemented in designing successful personal training programs for your clients. As Gage and Berliner (2) advise, "the teacher should use research and principles from educational psychology to develop proper teaching procedures to obtain optimal results." Students wishing to enter the personal training profession can benefit greatly from the knowledge of this research in designing education-based training sessions for clients.

The Nine Principles of Learning

Noted training educator and consultant Gary Kroehnert has identified nine principles fundamental to learners common to most "methods instruction" courses containing many of Bloom's original observations (6). This means that high-quality educational presentations are characterized by these nine elements:

➤ Recency: Reinforces information so that clients remember what they have learned
➤ Appropriateness: Teaches information that is appropriate for the need and the level of the student
➤ Motivation: Instructs students that want to learn information that is relevant and meets their needs
➤ Primacy: Teaches that information taught first in a session is more likely to be remembered by a student
➤ Two-Way Communication: Identifies a teaching session that has built-in two-way communication and interaction between the teacher and students (*Fig. 3.1*)
➤ Feedback: States that both the teacher and the student need information from each other to verify that needs and objectives are being met by both parties

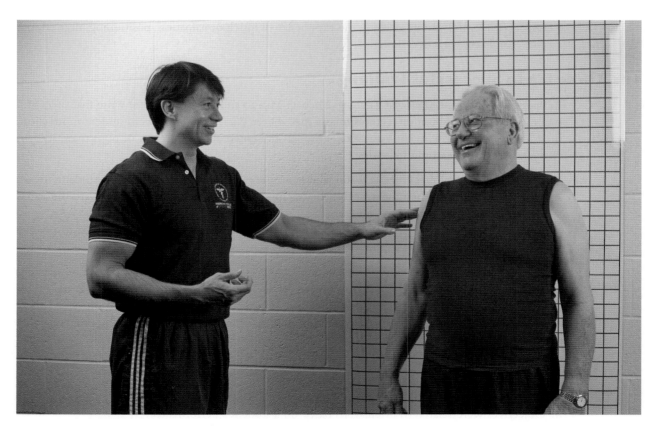

FIGURE 3.1. Two-way communication between a Personal Trainer and his client discussing proper posture and body alignment.

➤ Active Learning: Establishes that students learn more when actively involved in the process

➤ Multiple-Sense Learning: Identifies that learning is more effective if students use more than one of their five senses

➤ Exercise: Students who repeat, perform, and practice information will retain it more effectively

These nine principles, when applied to the personal training session design, may enhance the client's learning and mastery of exercise and fitness because they affirm Bloom's as well as Gage and Berliner's educational models.

The VAK Learning Preferences: Visual, Auditory, and Kinesthetic Learners

In their book *Accelerated Learning for the 21st Century*, Rose and Nicholl (7) found that people of all ages have preferences for how they best learn. These learning propensities, or styles, occur in three basic ways: visual, auditory, and kinesthetic (VAK).

Attention to the client's learning preferences addresses several points that Bloom cites as essential to the education process, those being attention to objectives, learning strategies, and time allocations. The VAK learning preferences are critical to Gage and Berliner's point that requires teachers to be familiar with "Student's Characteristics." The VAK learning preferences are discussed in more detail in Chapter 5 but are presented here as they provide an important structural component to your client's education:

➤ **V**isual—learning through seeing. Visual learners prefer to learn through reading and/or viewing pictures, flowcharts, demonstrations, diagrams, and/or drawings. They also learn well from note taking, alignment cueing, and watching television/video.

➤ **A**uditory—learning through hearing. Auditory learners prefer to learn by hearing audiotapes, lectures, spoken explanations, note taking, and verbal instruction.

➤ **K**inesthetic—learning through physical activities and through direct involvement. Kinesthetic learners prefer movement, feeling, the experience of touch or palpation, positioning, note taking, and "hands-on" practice/doing.

The Three E's to Successful Training

In their book, *Designing Powerful Training*, Michael Milano and Diane Ullius (8) write that successful training seminars and business lectures follow the "Three E's." Directed toward student motivation, these clearly dovetail with the educational models presented above in terms of objectives, student characteristics, and learning strategies:

➤ **E**ffective: Accomplishes objectives and whether those objectives are relevant to the students' needs

➤ **E**fficient: Maximizes the time available for teaching and educating the student toward the stated learning objectives and desired outcomes

➤ **E**ngaging: Creates an interactive and engaging teacher–student relationship designed to involve the student directly in the learning process

These three qualities of well-received educational presentations clearly overlap and complement the elements discussed above. Client motivation is critical to the completion of exercise and fitness programs, and these three elements have been found to be essential to that motivation.

Hannun and Briggs in 1980 (9) analyzed instructional systems designs (or teaching programs) that summarized the information presented above. They found that the instructional models they studied shared "seven common elements":

1. Teachers understood models and how they work.
2. Teachers taught material specific to the needs of the student.
3. Objectives were related to evaluations based on a student's performance.
4. Learning strategies were related to goals and objectives.

5. Preparation was not overlooked and was thorough.
6. Student's quality of performance was measured, and the outcome was related to the review of the training/instruction.
7. Attention was given to individual learning preferences, abilities, and objectives.

The nine learning styles, the VAK learning preferences, the Three E's, and the Hannun and Briggs analysis are just four of many summaries of educational models. Each offers elements that can improve the quality of personal training sessions, provided the Personal Trainer understands the basics of education-based training session design, which is outlined below. This design provides the framework needed to accurately incorporate the rich and varied amount of educational psychology's resources for educational presentations.

THE EDUCATION-BASED PERSONAL TRAINER

When Personal Trainers incorporate the principles of learning into their training repertoire, more effective and rewarding personal training is possible. Box 3.1 provides a profile of the education-based Personal Trainer that incorporates the VAK learning preferences and the nine learning styles into the Personal Trainer's exercise and fitness skills.

EDUCATION-BASED TRAINING PREPARATION

Learning models include goals and objectives. This implies that the learning process involves a preparation phase to fulfill the goals and objectives requirement. The need for adequate preparation cannot be underestimated. It allows the Personal Trainer to determine content and organize it in such a way that it efficiently and effectively complies with the learner's desired outcomes.

Personal Training Is a Sequential Process

The models and plans developed for learning share a common theme: they are "sequential." Trainers need to develop exercise sessions with proper progression or sequence based on different client factors, including their learning preferences, current physical status, goals, and abilities. This means that the order, or sequence, in which each part of the training is presented matters very much to the success of each session as well as to the whole exercise training program.

BOX 3.1	The Education-Based Personal Trainer

- The education-based Personal Trainer is an instructor, educator, and teacher who designs comprehensive exercise programs based on the assessed health needs, capabilities, and goals of an individual client that incorporate the principles of learning.
- To design these programs, the Personal Trainer incorporates knowledge from areas of study such as anatomy, kinesiology, exercise physiology, motor learning, neurology, biomechanics, training theories and techniques, nutrition, lifestyle and stress management, and the psychology of behavioral change.
- Through a balanced blend of these disciplines, the Personal Trainer evaluates, creates, and implements a unique plan for guiding, motivating, and educating individuals to improve their health and fitness levels with the goal of enhancing the quality of their lives.
- The Personal Trainer communicates this knowledge to others in an empathetic and dynamic style that is taught in educational format based on the student's learning preferences and through the implementation of the principles of learning (10).

Every training session has three basic components that occur in the following sequence:

➤ Initial client consultation
➤ Exercise implementation and practice
➤ Assessment of achieved objectives

The goal of education-based personal training preparation is to make the trainer and the client aware of these three phases and to thoroughly prepare them in conjunction with the client's goals and objectives. With this in mind, the trainer can prepare sessions that incorporate learning principles that fully serve the learning needs of the client. The trainer can develop and enhance the three personal training components through the creative application of learning models so that the client achieves the maximum benefit from the personal training experience.

THE NEED FOR ADEQUATE TRAINING SESSION PREPARATION

For clients to succeed, the design of the personal training program must be based on planning organized, sequential training sessions. Many Personal Trainers are never able to develop successful personal training careers because they offer their clients unorganized and poorly structured training sessions that leave clients feeling lost, frustrated, and confused. Even if the client is attentive and has a good rapport with the trainer, all can be lost if the personal training session lacks proper structure and planning.

Advanced preparation and design of the content of the personal training session plan or program is based on creating a "big picture"—a visual schematic of how the program will help the client achieve his or her desired results. From there, a detailed session-by-session breakdown is created that clarifies the program's content and increases the effectiveness of skill development as well as the client's ease in the learning process. Proper exercise program design solves many of the problems that a client might confront before the problems occur. Preparation and design of detailed exercise plans allows you to evaluate clients' success in achieving objectives for all levels of abilities and learning preferences. Box 3.2 describes the four components of training session preparation. The consequences of poorly structured personal training sessions, regardless of the Personal Trainer's educational level, become evident when clients are confused, frustrated, and performing exercise movements below expectations. Exercise program preparation carefully considers these questions:

➤ Does the sequence of exercise seem reasonable, with most movements leading clearly to the ones that follow in a building block fashion?
➤ Do the exercises support the training goals and objectives of the client?
➤ Does the order of exercise provide options where appropriate?

| BOX 3.2 | **The Four Components of Training Session Preparation** |

THE FOUR COMPONENTS OF TRAINING SESSION PREPARATION
1. Achievable Goals: sensitive to abilities of the Personal Trainer, their clients, and to their time and schedule constraints
2. An Intelligent Plan: allows the Personal Trainer and the client/student to visualize and understand the entire exercise program process
3. Client Learning Style: gives considerable attention to the planning of the instructional strategy used to communicate how the content of sessions are prepared and organized
4. Effective Assessment: provides the Personal Trainer with guidelines to analyze and grade their clients' performance of exercise movements

➤ Do you allow enough time between practicing exercise movements taught previously and teaching new exercises?

➤ Do you take the teaching style and learning preference of the client into consideration in developing the exercise program?

➤ Does the client practice movements on his or her own between sessions and return to the next training session performing the movement poorly?

SOME EXAMPLES OF PREPARATION-RELATED TRAINING PROBLEMS

Imagine watching a movie in which the reels are projected out of sequence. You don't have the information you need to understand the characters' actions, motives, or emotions. You lose interest in the story because you cannot find the logical progression of events. Your mind wanders. You become bored and restless.

In contrast, the solidly designed training program presents the "reels of the story" of each session in logical sequence so the student/client can follow the "plot" step by step and gets caught up in the logic and inevitability of each progressive stage. Consequently, the client's learning is a vicarious product of the trainer's well-organized presentation. If it was prepared in advance and makes sense, the student will learn it and also enjoy the process.

POOR PREPARATION: THE PROBLEMS THAT COULD HAVE BEEN AVOIDED

Unfortunately, many trainers have a tendency to make three fundamental mistakes that largely are the result of a lack of adequate education and training:

1. Personal Trainers don't give clients enough time to learn. Trainers try to teach too much content in any given session without giving the client adequate time to learn, practice, or perfect a movement.
2. Personal Trainers ignore teaching basic skills. As a result, Personal Trainers cannot safely progress a client into advanced exercise skills. The client never learns basic core, posture alignment-enhancing exercises that allow him or her to perform complex and difficult exercises requiring more enhanced motor skills.
3. Personal Trainers lose focus and direction during the course of the session. Trainers can undermine the client's goals and objectives.

For example, imagine that a Personal Trainer has trained a client for two sessions and in the third session decides to teach the client how to perform a dumbbell chest press. At this point in the client's training program, the client has only performed the seated chest press machine on two occasions, both in the first session. The Personal Trainer describes how to perform the exercise correctly and even demonstrates the movement perfectly. The client now tries the movement. The client first moves into position by moving from sitting on the edge of the bench to a supine position on the bench. He moves downward in an awkward and unbalanced way and, before his back is fully on the bench, starts doing repetitions. The Personal Trainer can see that the repetitions look erratic, off the line of resistance, in bottom phase, and the dumbbells are lowered beyond a safe range of motion. The client performs 10 repetitions and the Personal Trainer asks him to stop and sit up again. The Personal Trainer reviews the exercise with the client and suggests some points to make the movement more controlled and coordinated. The Personal Trainer thinks that with more practice the client will eventually get the movement down. The main problem the Personal Trainer fails to address, however, is whether or not the client has performed the proper exercises to develop the strength and agility to be strong and coordinated enough to manage the dumbbell chest press in the first place. In this scenario, the client is having trouble because the movement was introduced too early in the training process for the client to have a chance at performing the exercise correctly the first time.

Foremost on the Personal Trainer's mind must be the following questions, "Has this client been strengthened enough to be able to manage the next level of difficulty? Does the client have an adequate level of neurological and motor ability to perform the exercise movement with a reasonably high success rate? Have I set my client up to fail?" Clearly, if the Personal Trainer does not have a defined plan of development for the client, these questions may be difficult if not impossible to answer. Answering each question clearly is the only way to keep the client motivated enough to return for the next session.

Here is another scenario of poorly prepared instruction. In this case, an exercise is presented when the client is not prepared to advance to its more challenging movement. It occurs often because many Personal Trainers put their own teaching desires ahead of their clients' needs and abilities. Or, Personal Trainers choose exercises for the client simply because they are in vogue (i.e., trainers feel they have to teach the new fad training program or work with the newest exercise machine). This is usually a recipe for disappointment and possibly serious injury. Let's say a trainer goes to a personal training conference and discovers new exercise movements that incorporate the use of a stability or physioball. She decides it's perfect for doing crunches and can't wait to use it with clients when she gets home. One of the clients she is currently training has only trained four times and still has not perfected performing the basic trunk flexion exercises (crunches) on the floor comfortably. The trainer senses the client may not be ready for the physioball but is so eager to introduce it, she goes ahead with her instruction anyway. Predictably, the client becomes frustrated and confused. He gets discouraged because he can't master the routine and forgets what progress he has made in performing the exercise on the floor. He comes to avoid the crunch, now a dreaded exercise. The trainer may become frustrated with the client and/or lose confidence in her abilities to teach. She may give up on the physioball for *all* her clients, even though it may be perfectly appropriate for some of them. The whole situation could have been avoided if she had put her student's needs and learning abilities ahead of her own enthusiasm and teaching desires.

By trying to put so much content into a session, clients are consistently not being trained correctly, and trainers are wasting precious time as a result. Going more slowly and taking your time through a well-thought-out and adequately prepared sequence of exercise will let the client safely and effectively achieve his or her fitness goal. As an example of using education methods, consider the SET program: Sequential Exercise Training. This program incorporates the educational methodology reviewed above in this chapter into a Personal Trainer model. A SET training session starts with a planned sequence of organizational steps and exercises.

With the SET as a model, you are developing a sequence of exercises that complements your student's ability to control, perfect, and memorize movement patterns. Its logical sequence, or "map," leads a client from initial structure-enhancing exercises to movements that require more sophisticated kinesthetic awareness and cognitive training abilities. The information is taught in a fashion that allows the client to absorb, comprehend, and retain the content. And, of course, the content and learning activities support the exerciser's goals and objectives. This type of detailed preparation, tailored to the needs of the client, ensures that the client will maintain motivation throughout the program you have designed and will be happy with the successful results.

Session mapping provides two advantages:

1. Increased confidence: The client's confidence in you is established, for you show the qualities of an organized, detailed-oriented, and competent Personal Trainer.
2. Increased motivation: The client is personally engaged in his or her own training process because the trainer has prepared in advance the general content and structure of the upcoming 5 to 10 individual personal training sessions.

SET is a sequentially organized teaching model used to provide an education-based learning process to teach and train clients. SET incorporates elements based on the research of learning principles and models reviewed above. The model is continuous, ever-changing, and dynamic. As

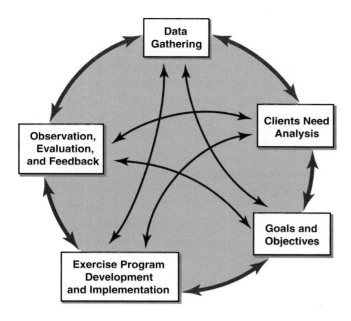

FIGURE 3.2. The Sequential Exercise Training Model.

the client's goals, health, and fitness level change, the overall exercise program design and plan will be able to adapt to the client's needs. SET takes the Personal Trainer through the components involved in the preparation and design of cohesive and coherent education-based personal training. Its five-stage process facilitates the successful design of coherent personal training sessions with achievable outcomes. Figure 3.2 and Box 3.3 describe the five components of SET.

BOX 3.3	**The Five Components of Sequential Exercise Training (SET)**

1. Data Gathering: The first component of SET involves information gathering during the client's initial consultation and includes a health and medical history questionnaire, client goals, ACSM Risk Stratification, health and fitness assessments, learning preference assessment, and client's skill level (observational).
2. Client Needs Analysis: The second component collates information on the client's health and fitness evaluation, risk stratification, learning preferences, goals, and skill level for the Personal Trainer to develop an initial exercise program. This evaluation will determine the starting level of the training. Advancement and progression will be measured from this point forward.
3. Goals and Objectives: The third component accomplishes specific goals requested by the client and establishes objectives developed by the Personal Trainer that are relevant to a client's success in a timely and systematic manner.
4. Exercise Program Development and Implementation: The fourth component ensures that the exercise program has a logical sequence and progression of information that includes teaching clients the foundations of exercise science and exercise movements based on the client's current level of knowledge, skills, and abilities. Personal Trainers prepare the SET Session Plan and SET flowchart to allow the personal training client the opportunity to visualize the entire exercise program process. Each training session must present content in a logical order that will advance the client toward his or her goals.
5. Observation, Evaluation, and Feedback: The fifth component of SET focuses on teaching trainers to develop observation, evaluation, and feedback strategies to be used before, during, and immediately after the training session. The Personal Trainer Observation Plan, Points of Evaluation, and the Exercise Grading System are an integral part of the observation, evaluation, and feedback process that measures the changes and the success in a client's performance of exercise movements.

1. Data Gathering

A primary responsibility for a Personal Trainer is design coherence and structure within the framework of the client's exercise session and program. The content of the exercise program should flow logically from one session to the next and from one exercise movement to the next, with each new body of knowledge or skill built upon the preceding information or skill taught. To design personalized exercise programs, information and data must be collected during the initial client consultation (11). Data are gathered in six areas from the client's life experience and exercise familiarity. The six areas of data gathering include:

➤ History: Current and past medical, health, and fitness history
➤ Disposition: Attitudes and behaviors about exercising
➤ Outcomes: Goals, desires, and expectations
➤ Observations: Trainer's observations of client assessment performance and results
➤ Approach: Client learning preferences through assessment and trainer observations
➤ Skills: Skill level and knowledge of exercise movements

By gathering this information, the Personal Trainer is able to begin formulating and visualizing an initial strategy and plan in determining the client's needs (12). This information is also essential when developing the Personal Trainer's objectives and predicting client outcomes based on your program design. Box 3.4 provides a complete review of what the initial screening and assessment process could cover. Part IV of this book reviews the initial client consultation and assessment process in more detail. After the data have been gathered and processed, the Personal Trainer then begins to analyze the information to create an exercise plan based on the client's needs. The next component of SET outlines the "Client Needs Analysis" process.

2. The Client Needs Analysis

For training to be effective, efficient, and engaging, the focus of exercise programs is based on the *needs* of the client. The Personal Trainer determines those needs from the initial client consultation

BOX 3.4	History: Screening and Health and Fitness Assessments

- Review Health and Physical Activity Questionnaire:
  Prior health history
  Injuries or other orthopedic limitations
  ACSM Risk Stratification
  Lifestyle and nutrition
  Review past exercise behavior patterns
  Learning preferences assessment
  Objectives, goals (short- and long-term), and interests
- Perform Health and Fitness Assessments:
  Resting heart rate
  Blood pressure
  Body fat composition, waist-to-hip ratio, and BMI analysis
  Circumference measurements
  Joint range-of-motion measurements
  Postural analysis and body alignment assessment
  Cardiovascular assessments

and health and fitness assessment. In other words, to improve alignment, balance the muscular system, and decrease body fat, Personal Trainers first must gather accurate information and figure out each client's individual personal training "starting line." A detailed needs assessment compares "what is the current state of the client" with "what is the desired state" (i.e., goal setting as further described in Chapter 13). The line connecting the starting level with the objective—the route to be followed, in other words—is guided by the client's needs. After assessing the client, when the trainer is certain of these needs, he or she can design the appropriate program to lead to the desired results. Mack points out that the screening and needs analysis creates an "observation platform" identifying weaknesses and strengths prior to engaging the exercise strategy (13). With the specific information identified in the Client Needs Analysis, the Personal Trainer designs exercise programs that are suitable and appropriate for the client to achieve the knowledge, skills, and mastery of exercise movements based on his or her abilities and history.

The Client Needs Analysis is developed by the Personal Trainer to identify the subject matter needed to be taught during a given training session and throughout the entire program. For example, during a client's initial consultation, screening, and health and fitness assessment the Personal Trainer may have determined the following:

➤ Posture and body alignment shows an exaggerated kyphotic curve in the thoracic area
➤ Right glenohumeral joint is 2 inches (5.1 cm) lower than the left and has excessive internal rotation
➤ Range of motion is below average on both the right and left side of the body in glenohumeral abduction, glenohumeral external rotation, and hip flexion
➤ Body fat composition is 10% above normal
➤ The client has made numerous attempts to make exercise a regular habit but has failed to do so
➤ The client has time to train only 1 day per week with the Personal Trainer and 2 days independently, for a total time of 4 hours per week
➤ The Personal Trainer previously observed the client improperly performing basic exercise movements
➤ The client's learning preference style leans more toward the visual and kinesthetic
➤ The client's primary goal is to get in better shape for a 25th high school reunion

Based on the information gathered, a complete client's needs analysis is created for both the client and the Personal Trainer to achieve their agreed upon goals and objectives. Once the information is gathered, the Personal Trainer must process it. The Personal Trainer then begins to draft the foundations of the exercise program and session plans that are appropriate and that address the client's needs. By carrying out a client's needs analysis, the Personal Trainer is able to target those areas that need to be addressed initially in the exercise program to build a foundation that will yield success. The specific exercises, including sequence and order of instruction, need to be accurately recorded. This information will define the SET Session Plan content and the sequence of the SET Flowchart.

3. Goals and Objectives

The third component of SET is setting goals and objectives based on the client's screening and needs analysis. Remember, the client's goals and objectives are important for both the student and the trainer. As the Personal Trainer, synthesize your own vision, goals, and strategies with the exercise programs you teach your clients. The trainer's objectives for the client should be well defined and clearly stated for the client in terms that the client can understand. There are five factors that Personal Trainers should consider in achieving a client's objectives. They include:

1. Skill level of trainers: Does the trainer have the necessary knowledge, education, skills, and expertise?

2. Equipment and facilities: Does the trainer have the necessary equipment and/or the use of a facility to support the training needs?
3. Trainer–client agreement: Are the client and trainer clear and in agreement about the client's performance goals and objectives?
4. Trainer's understanding of the client: Has the trainer learned the student/client's capabilities, health levels, skills, and learning preferences?
5. Time: Is there adequate time to teach the knowledge and skills required?

It is logical that the first task to be undertaken in any training design would be defining objectives. Designing a program without defining objectives would be like mapping out a vacation trip by car without knowing the final destination. Personal Trainers and health professionals commonly think in terms of objectives, but if these objectives are vague and not precisely articulated, evaluating progress and achievement of goals becomes a matter of guessing instead of accurate progress evaluation.

Defined training objectives answer two basic questions:

1. What will the student know and be able to perform as a result of his or her training?
2. How will the trainer know if the student has achieved this knowledge and the required performance level?

Clients themselves are negatively affected by a lack of specificity in the details of what they can expect to receive from personal training. How will you and your client know that what was intended to be taught has in fact been learned? Has the client achieved his or her personal goals? Only with a clear statement of objectives can these questions be answered. Factors that limit training objectives include:

➤ Inadequate time or training sessions to achieve the client's objectives
➤ Weak client motivation to learn the new knowledge and skills you are teaching
➤ Inadequate time to design a well-defined training program based on the client's skills and learning preferences

Goal-oriented Personal Trainers will tell you that achieving client objectives does not happen without a well-designed plan in place. Trainers need to state clearly in their exercise plans, and for their clients, what changes their bodies should be making, the precision with which they should perform each exercise, and what skills and knowledge they can expect to have acquired at the end of each session. Precisely defined objectives will assist the trainer and student by doing three things:

➤ Set up clear and realistic expectations: The statement of objectives tells the client clearly what to expect from the training program
➤ Provide a client–trainer agreement, or "contract": They serve as a kind of informal contract between client and trainer
➤ Tell client the skills that will be mastered: Well-defined objectives prepare students for what they will be able to do at the end of each session and the program

The information covered in learning preferences and educational models may be implemented when establishing objectives for those delivering personal training programs. This process has identified several points that can help deliver clear and achievable outcomes in training sessions.

The importance of having well-defined and measurable objectives at the start of the training process should now be evident. Personal Trainers are hired to deliver a service, and part of that service is providing a format for client's exercise so that they can achieve their goals. By delivering a clear statement of objectives, with specific skills and knowledge that the client can learn, the Personal Trainer can then focus on the task of teaching exercise. Box 3.5 provides some examples of personal training objectives.

BOX 3.5	**Statement of Personal Training Objectives**

Clients will:

1. Sequentially gain more knowledge in the "Foundations of Exercise Science": anatomy, kinesiology, biomechanics, exercise physiology, motor learning, neurology, pedagogy, and nutrition.
2. Learn to develop goal-specific exercise programs that incorporate resistance, flexibility, cardiovascular, and other modes of training.
3. Learn to perform exercise movements accurately and correctly with the visible results of improved posture, body alignment, and physique.
4. Feel empowered and confident because of their new ability to train safely and effectively on their own. Experience benefits to their health and wellness that will lead to improved performance of activities of daily living and a sensitivity for ergonomically correct work environments.

4. Exercise Program Development and Implementation

Many advantages result from using effective educational models in personal training session and exercise plan design, especially a straightforward, visual "road map" that allows clients to understand the process their Personal Trainers are using to develop an organized, detailed, thoughtful, and goal-oriented exercise plan. The advantages to such a format include first, the identification of the key factors that the client should consider and their sequential order. As such, this type of plan serves as a procedural guide. Second, it allows the Personal Trainer and the client to track the client's stage of development in the personal training process. And finally, this organization of the client's exercise program improves your ability to measure, evaluate, and grade client performance.

Remember, SET establishes guidelines intended to facilitate an evolving exercise development and implementation process. If your client performs a movement correctly the first time he or she does it, you cannot assume that the client has mastered the exercise, but he or she has a pretty good start. Designing an exercise program involves going back and re-enforcing information on both an educational and a performance level. Do not anticipate that clients will be bored with going over an exercise if you explain to them that you want to make sure it is in place and has been well established before you move on to the next step or exercise. This type of repetition and review is a little like applying a second or third coat of paint to make sure that the wall is properly covered.

Initially, it does not benefit you to have your clients practice complicated movements on their own. The chances are good that they will perform the exercise incorrectly and with difficulty, leading to frustration, lowered self-esteem, improper movement patterns, and possible physical injury. During the next session, you may end up spending the bulk of your time having the client "unlearn" the incorrect information he or she re-enforced during the practice sessions. Wait until an evaluation has been conducted to determine if the client is doing the movement correctly before advising to practice it without the Personal Trainer present.

Learning is best when it is logical and progressive, but it almost never happens in a straight line. Accept this fact and turn it into an advantage. SET is designed so you can move back and forth between sessions to be constantly practicing and perfecting movements at each session. Details of designing and implementing exercise programs are discussed and elaborated on in Chapter 16.

5. Observation, Evaluation, and Feedback

The observation, evaluation, and feedback process requires detail, precision, and implementation on the part of the Personal Trainer. Imagine a golf professional working with two students. The first student hits the ball easily, and it lands on the green. The second student cannot hit the ball straight down the fairway in the first 10 attempts. The motor control and precision required to hit a golf ball straight down a fairway may be easy for some, but more difficult for others. With golf there is roughly one swing motion that needs to be "grooved" or perfected, but it has multiple variations depending on the desired distance. In contrast, personal training and exercise requires the Personal Trainer to have and perfect a multitude of movements for different body parts. Evaluating the many details of personal training requires specific strategies.

Why is precision important? Stresses placed on the body while exercising must be correctly managed or they can cause serious injury or damage. The trainer's goal is to exercise the musculoskeletal system in the safest and most effective manner. Education-based personal training sessions require, and therefore ensure, that the Personal Trainer is actively discerning the difference between a client's "actual performance" and "required performance" (14). Often, a large gap exists between the way a client performs a movement the first time and the Personal Trainer's expectations. Without proper observation, evaluation, and feedback from the trainer, the client may never attain an adequate performance, and in the process, the client may be exposed to potential and multiple injuries.

Personal Trainers can protect their clients and themselves from costly errors by being able to accurately observe the difference between an ability and a skill. Clients will differ in their initial abilities and skills. The word "ability" is defined as "natural aptitude or being genetically determined and largely unmodified by practice or experience" (15). On the other hand, "skill" is defined as "dexterity or coordination especially in the execution of learned physical tasks" that "are chiefly developed as a result of practice" (16). A skill can be a complex sequence of phases or stages of a movement. The Personal Trainer can move a client successfully from ability to skill only with accurate observation and evaluation of the client. It is up to the Personal Trainer to teach exercise movement skills, and the best way to do this is through an education-based approach to client evaluation.

SESSION OBSERVATION

Quantitative and qualitative methods can be implemented to observe and analyze movements. Quantitative analysis often uses machines, computers, and numerical information to analyze human movement. Qualitative analysis is used most often through visual observation and evaluation of movement. For personal training professionals, qualitative analysis is often the choice to ensure that clients perform each exercise correctly, and it does not require the use of machines or equipment.

As personal training professionals observe a client's movements, Wuest and Bucher (16) suggest that the Personal Trainer needs prerequisite knowledge and understanding of the exercise being performed from which to create a mental image of the ideal performance of the given movement. The trainer can then perform an analysis that notes the differences between the required or ideal performance and the actual performance. This will then allow the trainer to know what is necessary to close the gap between the actual and the desired movement.

Adrian and Cooper (17), Brown (18), and Wuest and Bucher (16) recommend several observational and visualization techniques for Personal Trainers to use in performance assessment. These suggestions can be incorporated into a framework specifically for Personal Trainers, called the Personal Trainer Observation Plan (Box 3.6).

Observational skills that use qualitative analysis allow Personal Trainers to develop exercise programs that enable clients to move safely, efficiently, and effectively. Personal Trainers who develop observational and analytical skills and the ability to accurately evaluate and prescribe corrective ways to improve the client's specific exercise, sports skill, or activities of daily living are well-equipped to serve the public.

After completing the observational and analytical processes, Personal Trainers should summarize what has been evaluated and identify areas in need of correction and improvement, with constructive feedback and positive reinforcement. The Personal Trainer's enthusiasm in the evaluation phase

BOX 3.6	**Personal Trainer Observation Plan**

1. Observe and gather information about the movement from an effective position, angle, and vantage point to make accurate readings. Proper location allows the trainer to view the complete movement, the client's anterior, posterior, and lateral positions. Trainers should view the movement from several different perspectives.
2. Observe the sequence and timing of the complete musculoskeletal system moving in relation to other body structures. Observe the range of motion and coordination of movement; check that the postural alignment is in a safe and correct movement position.
3. Focus on the implement or equipment being used to aid or perform the movement. Be sure that the parts of the equipment are in proper sequence and position to allow the client to perform movements properly.
4. Implement the Points of Evaluation (as described in Box 3.7) as a checklist to guide your observation and to ensure that no items are overlooked or forgotten.
5. Recall previous observational experiences that accurately perceived, predicted, and anticipated critical features and errors that frequently occurred during a given movement to be prepared with the proper advice to correct the errors.
6. Observe several repetitions of the movement before providing advice to correct form or alignment. Advice given too frequently hinders the learning process. Do not wait to advise if the client is doing something that could hurt a muscle or joint structure.
7. Give evaluation and feedback during or after phases of movements have been completed.

can make or break a client's will to continue in the personal training process. Give the client a sense that the next step is doable and that he or she is successfully on the way to completing the "road map" that is leading toward the established goals.

EVALUATION

Personal Trainers are responsible for evaluation of outcomes, results, and feedback. In the best of circumstances, evaluation is a complex process. Whenever you design and implement personal training programs, you have an opportunity to evaluate. Each objective, every exercise chosen, the sequence of the knowledge and skills taught, can be evaluated.

The points of evaluation described in Box 3.7 focus on two key elements. First, attention must be given to the outcomes that the personal training is achieving and whether or not these are meeting the overall program objectives. Second, the evaluation process needs to include a student and trainer self-evaluation of the training process.

Training results are normally the most important factor to be evaluated, based on the following questions:

1. Have students gained knowledge about exercise and made improvements both physically and mentally?
2. Are they able to apply what they learned to their own workouts and daily lives?
3. How effective have the trainer's teaching methods been?
4. Is the client performing the exercise movements correctly, consistently, and efficiently?
5. Is the client satisfied with the knowledge gained and the level of improvement in the quality of the workouts?

Instruction is first planned to improve the client's knowledge and skills. Evaluation determines whether the instruction was successful. In determining whether the program design was effective

---

BOX 3.7	**Points of Evaluation**

Five Points to Monitor & Evaluate Body Alignment and Muscular Coordination during Movement Activities

1. Joint position, range of motion, and integrity maintained (19–21)
2. Muscle position, balance, and fiber direction (22, 23)
3. Muscular balance observed and monitored through palpation (tension created to specific primary mover and force production and relaxation of secondary movers and joints) (24)
4. Observe the control of coordinated exercise movement patterns (25–30)
   - Regulation of speed, rhythm, and fluidity
   - Path/line of motion consistent and precise
   - Transitions coordinated, consistent, and precise between preparatory, central, and terminal phases
5. Posture and body alignment stabilized and in the required position during motion (31–34)

---

and is achieving its objectives, evaluation works hand in hand with instruction. Evaluation allows the trainer to plan the next step in the client's exercise process.

Effective evaluation lets the trainer and the client measure performance during the session. They include activities such as the Points of Evaluation and the Exercise Grading System (see Chapter 17) that allow clients to test their progress toward stated objectives and to provide feedback for both Personal Trainer and client. As a result, both parties can better determine where to focus further practice, training, and retraining.

FEEDBACK

After the Personal Trainer conducts the observation and evaluation, the client needs to receive feedback on his or her performance results. Schmidt and Wrisberg (35) and O'Sullivan and Schmitz (36) suggest several factors helpful in providing client feedback. Personal Trainers should consider these questions before providing feedback:

➤ What information does the feedback need to include?
➤ How much of the information can the client absorb?
➤ How specific should the feedback information be?
➤ How often should feedback be offered?

The feedback information that the trainer gives to the client is beneficial when it considers the following content guidelines:

➤ Feedback about the sequencing during the performance of a movement will affect the coordination or motor program.
➤ Specific corrective feedback about posture, alignment, and body and hand positions is sometimes difficult for the client to absorb but is extremely important to achieve the desired corrections and improvements.
➤ Feedback about the speed of the movement, whether it is slow, medium, or fast, often can be easily applied by the client.
➤ Feedback that is prescriptive and specific in the trainer's directions for movement changes achieves better results than descriptive feedback that tells clients only about the errors they are making. For example: "You can improve your posture by relaxing your shoulders" instead of "Your shoulders are tense."

Feedback needs to correlate with the instruction, guidance, and direction provided by the trainer. Here are some important points concerning the selection and progression of exercise movements in relation to the feedback necessary to exercise instruction:

➤ Feedback can be presented more frequently when teaching a client new movements but could be provided less frequently as the client becomes more skilled in the performance of the movement. As your client becomes more precise in a movement pattern, your observations to correct errors will naturally be reduced.

➤ The amount of feedback information is reduced as the complexity of the exercise movement increases. This is only possible if the client has received sequential and progressive instruction that honors his or her step-by-step learning process. If the trainer is consistently correcting a client, chances are that the movement the client is attempting is too difficult. In this case, the Personal Trainer needs to discontinue the difficult movement, reassess the client's skill level, and suggest an alternative exercise that will build the skills needed to achieve the more difficult level of performance.

THE SESSION PLAN

The Session Plan is an organized personal training session or client meeting with established objectives that will be covered in the course of the meeting. Similar to a class curriculum plan, the Session Plan is designed to present the client with a detailed exercise format incorporating the best practices of exercise science and learning principles and models. By implementing the plan, the trainer is establishing a visual presentation or format allowing the client to see and understand the education-based personal training process.

Each personal training session is usually 1 hour in length. This does not give the Personal Trainer much time to go over all the exercises he or she may want a client to perform, along with educating the client in the science of exercise. Remember to factor in practice time to perform movements taught in the previous session, teaching clients new exercise movements, yet allowing the client to feel that he or she has gotten a good workout.

Individual plans are created for each session of the program because they all have their own objectives and each requires separate planning, as described below in Box 3.8. As you become fa-

BOX 3.8	Session Plan Contents (6)

- Session content
- Session focus or identity
- Defined session objectives
- Session's total time allocation
- Trainer's knowledge of the client's health and fitness history, goals, skills, and abilities
- Knowledge of the prior session's content and presentation
- Time for a verbal or visual overview of the session plan
- Structure of the session
- Planned use of fitness equipment
- Planned use of designated fitness areas or locations
- Planned transition timing between exercises performed or information taught
- Recap of the session performance and new information learned
- Preview of the next session

BOX 3.9　　**Sample Session Plan (Session 1 of Multiple Sessions)**

SESSION TITLE: INTRODUCTION TO HEALTH, FITNESS, AND EXERCISE
Time: 1 Hour

A. Objectives:
1. Review with the client his or her health history and goals and recap assessment results (if applicable)
2. Review the day's Session Plan
3. Provide an overview of the foundations of exercise science and teach exercise movements
4. Review posture and body alignment

B. Exercise Content
1. Perform cardiovascular warm-up: 10 to 15 minutes
   a. Teach the use of one piece of cardiovascular equipment
   b. While client is warming up, the trainer can discuss the following:
      1) The order and sequence of what will happen during the session
      2) Basic exercise science information including the benefits of exercise adaptation to the muscular, cardiovascular, and skeletal systems
      3) The trainer's plan to implement the clients Visual, Auditory, and Kinesthetic (VAK) learning preferences within the session
      4) The four points of posture and proper body alignment
2. Flexibility and Stretching Exercises: 10 minutes
   a. Provide an overview of flexibility and stretching
   b. Provide the order and format in which flexibility will be performed, including pre-stretches, inter-stretches, and post-stretches
   c. Teach the client the following flexibility movements:
      1) Windmills
      2) Chest stretch
      3) Standing back stretch
      4) Rotator cuff stretch
      5) Hamstrings and quadriceps stretch
      6) More back stretches (if applicable)
3. Resistance Training Exercises: 30 minutes
   a. Provide an overview of resistance training exercises, VAK learning preferences, and posture and body alignment
   b. Teach the following four resistance training movements:
      1) Seated back row; followed by an inter-stretch
      2) Standing trapezius (shoulder) dumbbell shrug; inter-stretch
      3) Seated chest press; inter-stretch
      4) Dumbbell lateral raises; inter-stretch
      5) Leg extensions (time permitting)
      6) Leg curl (time permitting)
      7) Basic abdominal (trunk flexion) crunch (time permitting)

C. Session Conclusion: 5 to 10 minutes
1. Trainer provides insight to observations and evaluations of the client's performance of movements
2. Trainer recaps what was learned, taught, and practiced and reminds the client not to practice movements between sessions at this point in the program
3. Trainer reminds the client about being aware of posture and body alignment between sessions
4. Trainer provides an overview of what will taught and practiced at the next session
5. Trainer prepares the client to perform additional cardiovascular training (if applicable) on the same piece of equipment the client was on earlier
6. Trainer shows the client where workout card is filed

BOX 3.10	**Advantages of the Session Plan**

For the education-based Personal Trainer:
- Ensures that the Personal Trainer's objectives for the session are established before the beginning of the client's session
- Verifies that the exercises chosen are relevant to the client's needs
- Enables the trainer to check that the sequence of exercises planned properly builds on the previous sessions
- Ensures that all necessary fitness equipment will be available to conduct the session

For the client:
- Provides the client with an understanding of the session and helps the client establish an internal plan and focus in preparation for the session
- Requires the client to adequately achieve objectives before moving on to more challenging movements and confirms that the client understands information previously learned
- Protects the client from injury due to exercises that are too difficult
- Builds client self-confidence and strengthens motivation

Other significant advantages:
- Gives the trainer a list of specified exercise movements and client information set down in a logical order, sequenced appropriately for the client's needs, and provides a detailed allocation of time to accomplish each item on the list
- Allows Personal Trainers the flexibility to make changes prior to each meeting and allows other trainers on staff to conduct the session effectively if you are absent
- In view of the litigious nature of the health and fitness industry, the Session Plan provides professional documentation of the client's exercise program that may be used as a point of reference for legal purposes should they arise (17)

miliar with the development of personal training session plans, you can begin to create flowcharts, forms of multiple session plans created 5 to 15 sessions in advance (see Chapters 20–22 for a more detailed discussion). The Session Plan allows trainers to design the content of one individual session taking into consideration various factors as outlined in Box 3.9.

With a clearly delineated Session Plan, Personal Trainers can relax into a professional teaching pattern that will be successful and rewarding for themselves as well as for their clients. The Session Plan also provides the client with a general understanding of the session and helps the client establish an internal plan and focus in preparation for the exercise session.

The Session Plan has many advantages for the Personal Trainer and for the client (Box 3.10) and is an essential tool for the Personal Trainer. It provides a template or guide to sequence and establish a format with objectives for the overall exercise session. The best way to know if a Session Plan works is to create one and practice using it. See if what you had planned to cover in the session was actually achievable for the client and for yourself. As you become proficient in designing individual session plans, progress to creating the Flowchart as outlined in the next section, which consists of 5 to 15 sessions planned in advance. This will be the next step to providing education–based personal training sessions for clients.

THE FLOWCHART

A flowchart is a schematic map of a sequence of events that tells us two things. First, it tells us in detail all the content that must be covered to train the student from his or her starting point through to the accomplishment of the training objective. Second, it shows the logical sequence in which content needs to be delivered from one point to the next in the exercise program.

Everything in the session must connect and make sense. It is this process that transforms what trainers know into a viable learning tool for the student. The way you organize what you know is extremely important to the students' ability to understand what you are teaching them. Flowcharts can help trainers be better teachers because flowcharts organize the content of the training session into a clear picture of session formats and sequencing for the client. A flowchart consists of six steps, as shown in Box 3.11.

Building a flowchart is an evolutionary process. It is built in layers, and as you move through each layer, what is discovered there influences the layer before it. You may find that you are coming up with new and important knowledge and skills. This can be added into the flowchart any time. Figure 3.3 provides an example of a flowchart outlining sessions 2, 3, and 4.

The flowchart is an integral part of an education-based personal training approach. Clients can see their entire training program, from start to finish, much the way travelers can see the route of their journey by looking at a map. Clients learn the relationship between movements, the overall design of their training experience, the logic of their exercise regimens, and the way their progress is being observed and measured.

A flowchart has two basic phases: (1) program design and (2) program production, implementation, and evaluation. The process is sequential, and yet it allows great flexibility. Although the overall flowchart is pre-planned, certain stages may be repeated or moved through more rapidly than originally anticipated. Again, think of it as a map. You can set the stages of your trip, but you might decide to spend an extra night in one city along the way or spend only a few hours in a place where you had planned to stop for several days.

The exercise program design process begins with the stated goals and needs of the student and ends with observations, evaluations, and feedback by the Personal Trainer. The design of each session, the selection of instructional methods, and student assessments will be based on the stated objectives and goals. Design and implementation of the session plans and flowcharts are presented in more detail in Chapters 20–22.

BOX 3.11   A Flowchart in Six Steps

Step 1: Identify the goals and objectives sought by the client and the trainer: Incorporate the Personal Trainer Objectives Statement

Step 2: Determine the session content and break it down into parts: knowledge and skills required, core and foundation-building exercises, and simple to complex exercises

Step 3: Sequence the practice time: Provide time during and following the session to practice and reinforce previous knowledge and skills learned before progressing to more challenging movements

Step 4: Sequence new exercises: Provide time during the session to teach, practice, and reinforce new exercises

Step 5: Observation of progress: Implement the Personal Trainer Observation Plan to observe and monitor the client's performance

Step 6: Evaluate progress: Evaluate the client with the Points of Evaluation and adjust the session plans and flowchart accordingly for cohesiveness and sequence; analyze the content of each session from point to point, adding any additional skills or knowledge necessary to achieve the objective

Session Two: Fundamentals to Exercise — 1 hour

— Objectives
Practice session one exercises
Teach new exercise movements

— Exercise content
Perform cardiovascular warm-up: 10 minutes
Perform cardiovascular warm-up on same piece from session one

Flexibility and stretching exercises: 10 minutes
Practice session one exercises
Teach new flexibility exercises including:

- Triceps stretch
- Biceps stretch
- Cat stretch
- Knees to chest
- More back stretches (if possible)

Resistance training exercises: 35 minutes
Practice session one exercises
Teach new resistance movements that include:

- Leg extensions
- Leg curl
- Leg press
- Dumbbell biceps curl
- Triceps extension with straight-bar

— Session conclusion: 5 minutes
Overview of what was taught and practiced
Remind client to practice proper posture
Tell client what to expect at the next session
Request that the client perform two 20-minute cardiovascular sessions before session three

Session Three: Fundamentals to Exercise — 1 hour

— Objectives
Practice session two exercises
Teach new exercise movements

— Exercise content
Perform cardiovascular warm-up: 10 minutes
Teach client a new cardiovascular warm-up exercise

Flexibility and stretching exercises: 10 minutes
Practice session two exercises
Teach new flexibility exercises including:

- Hamstrings
- Calves

Resistance training exercises: 35 minutes
Practice session two exercises
Teach new resistance movements that include:

- Chest press
- Standing body weight calf raises

— Session conclusion: 5 minutes
Overview of what was taught and practiced
Remind client to practice proper posture
Tell client what to expect at the next session
Request that the client perform two 20-minute cardiovascular sessions before session four

A

FIGURE 3.3. Example of a flowchart outlining sessions 2, 3, and 4.

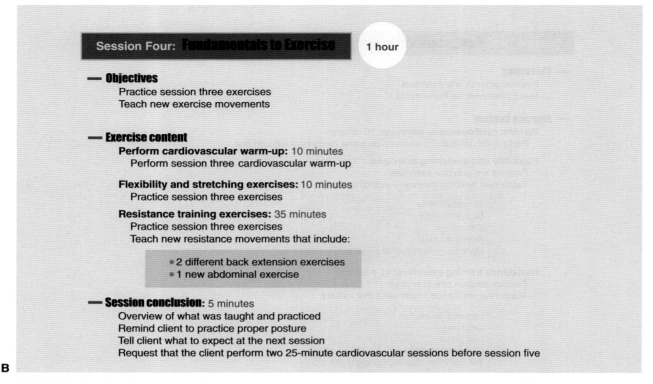

B

FIGURE 3.3. Continued.

SUMMARY

The preparation and design of education-based personal training programs are a tremendous responsibility but also an incredible opportunity to help change your clients lives for the better. With so much exercise science-related research being performed on healthy and diseased populations, from children to older adults, the opportunity to train someone from every walk of life is available if you have the training preparation to do so. As Personal Trainers using the suggestions outlined in this chapter, you will be able to formulate creative, well-designed personal training programs that are tailored specifically for your clients. Your personal training programs will not only help you get your clients healthy and fit but also make you knowledgeable and educated in exercise planning and technique.

The five components presented in this chapter will help you progress from performing a detailed screening and needs assessment to providing ongoing evaluations before, during, and after the training program. Using these models over time, you will appreciate the help of "visual" memory in originating and constructing personal training programs. The evaluation methods quantify time and interrelate knowledge and practice within each session. At its best, personal training is a transformational and educational process for the client when the Personal Trainer is committed to helping and motivating people. Successful personal training can make a positive difference in the lives of the people when practiced with integrity and responsibility.

REFERENCES

1. Merriam-Webster. Merriam-Webster Online Dictionary. Online at http://www.m-w.com/dictionary.htm. Accessed December 24, 2004.
2. Gage N, Berliner D. Educational Psychology. 6th ed., New Jersey: Houghton Mifflin, 1998.
3. Alesandrini K. Pictorial-verbal and analytic-holistic learning strategies in science learning. J Educ Psychol 1981;73(3):358–368.
4. Diamond R. Systematic Design: Model and Benefits. Designing and Assessing Courses and Curricula. 2nd ed. San Francisco: Jossey-Bass, 1998.

5. Bloom B. Taxonomy of Educational Objectives, Handbook 1: The Cognitive Domain. New York: Addison-Wesley, 1956.

6. Kroehnert G. The principles of adult learning. In: Bourma C, ed. Basic Training for Trainers. Dubuque: McGraw-Hill, 1994.

7. Rose C, Nicholl M. Accelerated Learning for the 21st Century. New York: Dell, 1997.

8. Milano M, Ullius D. Powerful training. In: Alexander L, ed. Designing Powerful Training. San Francisco: Jossey-Bass, 1998.

9. Hannun W, Briggs L. How does instructional systems design differ from traditional instruction? Chapel Hill: School of Education, University of North Carolina, 1980.

10. IDEA The Health and Fitness Source, News Release, 1998.

11. Diamond R. Gathering and analyzing essential data. Designing and Assessing Courses and Curricula. 2nd ed. San Francisco: Jossey-Bass, 1998.

12. Griffin JC. Setting priorities and measurable objectives. In: Wilgren S, Mustain E, Graham M, eds. Client-Centered Exercise Prescription. Champaign, IL: Human Kinetics, 1998.

13. Mack G. Assessing the Post-Rehab Client. IDEA Personal Trainer, 1999.

14. Kroehnert G. Session plans. In: Bourma C, ed. Basic Training for Trainers. Dubuque, IA: McGraw-Hill, 1994.

15. Schmidt R, Wrisberg C. Individual differences and motor abilities. In: Wright J, Park J, Alexander L, eds. Motor Learning and Performance. 3rd ed. Illinois: Human Kinetics, 2004.

16. Wuest D, Bucher C. Biomechanical foundations. In: Malinee V, Seely C, eds. Foundations of Physical Education, Exercise Science, and Sport. 14th ed. New York: McGraw-Hill, 2003.

17. Adrian M, Cooper J. Biomechanics of Human Movement, 2nd ed. In: Spoolman S, Klein J, eds. Biomechanics. Dubuque, IA: McGraw-Hill, 1997.

18. Brown EW. Visual evaluation techniques for skill analysis. J Phys Educ Recreation Dance 1982;53(1):21–26.

19. Norkin C, Levangie P. Joint structure and function. In: Joint Structure and Function. Philadelphia: F.A. Davis, 1992.

20. Hall SJ. The biomechanics of human articulations. In: Malinee V, Huenefeld L, eds. Basic Biomechanics. New York: McGraw-Hill, 2003.

21. Norkin C, White D. Measurement of Joint Motion 3rd ed. In: Biblis M, Seitz A, eds. Philadelphia: F.A. Davis, 2003.

22. Norkin C, Levangie P. Muscle structure and function. In: Joint Structure and Function. Philadelphia: F.A. Davis, 1992.

23. Luttgens K, Hamilton N. Moving objects: throwing, striking, & kicking. In: Dorwick T, Malinee V, Turenne M, eds. Kinesiology. 10th ed. New York: McGraw-Hill, 2002.

24. Rothenberg B, Why does stt work? In Frey R, Curry A, Giles E, eds. Touch Training for Strength. Champaign, IL: Human Kinetics, 1995.

25. Adrian M, Cooper J. Biomechanics of exercise. In: Spoolman S, Klein J, eds. Biomechanics of Human Movement. 2nd ed. Dubuque, IA: McGraw-Hill, 1997.

26. Enoka, RM. Movement Analysis. Neuromechanical Basis of Kinesiology. Champaign, IL: Human Kinetics, 1994.

27. O'Sullivan S, Schmitz T. Application of therapeutic exercise techniques to stages of motor control. In: Fithian M, ed. Physical Rehabilitation Assessment and Treatment. Philadelphia: F.A. Davis, 1994.

28. Luttgens K, Hamilton N. Introduction to the study of kinesiology. In: Dorwick T, Malinee V, Turenne M, eds. Kinesiology. 10th ed. New York: McGraw-Hill, 2002.

29. Floyd RT, Thompson C. Muscular analysis of the upper extremity. In: Malinee V, Martin M, eds. Manual of Structural Kinesiology. 14th ed. New York: McGraw-Hill, 2001.

30. Aaberg E. Exercise form and technique. In: Barnard M, Enderle K, Flaig A, eds. Resistance Training Instruction. Champaign, IL: Human Kinetics, 1999.

31. Luttgens K, Hamilton N. The standing posture. In: Dorwick T, Malinee V, Turenne M, eds. Kinesiology. 10th ed. New York: McGraw-Hill, 2002.

32. Lehmkuhl LD, Smith LK, Weiss EL. Standing and walking. In: McNichol CS, ed. Brunnstrom's Clinical Kinesiology. 5th ed. Philadelphia: F.A. Davis, 1996.

33. Enoka, RM. The Motor System. Neuromechanical Basis of Kinesiology. Champaign, IL: Human Kinetics, 1994.

34. Rothstein J, Roy S, Wolf S. Musculoskeletal anatomy and orthopedics. In: Spraggins C, Gabbay R, eds. The Rehabilitation Specialist's Handbook. Philadelphia: F.A. Davis, 1998.

35. Schmidt R, Wrisberg C. Providing feedback during the learning experience. In: Wright J, Park J, Alexander L, eds. Motor Learning and Performance. 3rd ed. Champaign, IL: Human Kinetics, 2004.

36. O'Sullivan S, Schmitz T. Motor learning approach. In: Fithian M, ed. Physical Rehabilitation Assessment and Treatment. Philadelphia: F.A. Davis, 1994.

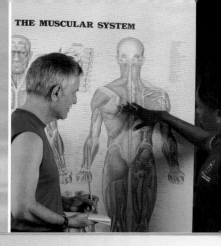

THE MUSCULAR SYSTEM

CHAPTER

4

The Education-Based Personal Trainer–Client Relationship

Kenneth E. Baldwin, M.Ed., A.H. Ismail Center for Health, Exercise & Nutrition, Department of Health and Kinesiology, College of Liberal Arts, Purdue University, West Lafayette, Indiana

Terry Ferebee Eckmann, Ph.D., Associate Professor, Department of Teacher Education and Human Performance, Minot State University, Minot, North Dakota

Chapter Outline

- **Value the importance of an open, communicative attitude toward clients**
- **Understand and apply the VAK Learning Preferences**
- **Successfully motivate clients to take charge of their fitness and exercise programs**
- **Understand the application of learning models to personal training**
- **Design personal training sessions that empower clients as learners**

In the previous chapter, learning principles and educational models are presented relating to training and education. These principles established the guidelines and provide the foundation for Personal Trainers as they develop education-based personal training sessions. This chapter outlines additional perspectives on learning models, client motivation, and learning style preferences. As a Personal Trainer, a familiarity with learning preferences and styles can provide guidance in the creation of successful programs for your clients. Basing your sessions on the principles of learning will ensure variety in your training sessions so that your clients will feel that their individual needs and learning preferences are being satisfactorily met. Additional conceptual tools are presented in this chapter as well, to support Personal Trainers as communicative and responsive educators within the context of personal training. A strong emphasis is placed on the importance of client motivation to the success of personal training.

THE CLIENT AS A STUDENT

Given the perspective that the Personal Trainer is an educator, the client in turn is seen as a student. Clients are simultaneously students who are in a learning role and who are reliant on the Personal Trainer for their education in fitness and exercise. Therefore, the terms "client" and "student" are used interchangeably throughout this text.

ESTABLISH TEACHING AND LEARNING STRATEGIES

Teaching makes learning more probable or more predictably successful. Simple change, such as increased muscle strength, is not learning. Learning is described as any change in behavior that is not maturational or due to a temporary condition. Learning involves a conscious process of education, or a strategy. The strategic approach to learning allows students to feel empowered, motivated, and in charge of their learning. Many experts have concluded that the more a student feels actively involved in the educational process, the better he or she learns. Teaching and learning strategies shared by teacher and student support student learning. Learners' value problem-solving and cooperative learning, and they benefit most from active participation in the learning process.

ESTABLISH THE LEARNING CLIMATE

It has been well established that people learn best under the following conditions:

1. Flexibility in the learning environment, because of their many time constraints
2. Individualized learning and responding better to it
3. Face-to-face learning (in most cases)
4. Activities that include experiences and interactions

Another basic area of learning is the learning environment in which the teacher expects the student to work and to learn. The character of the teacher–student relationship largely shapes this environment. Incumbent on 21st century educators is the care and concern for the learning relationship and the environment it creates. Stroot has made the following observations of successful learning environments (1):

1. People learn better when the atmosphere is one of support and encouragement.
2. A climate that fosters trust and respect will better facilitate learning.
3. People learn best if they are encouraged to express their views.
4. People prefer a learning environment in which expectations are clear.

The Personal Trainer must build a trusting relationship with the personal training client. If the relationship is based on trust, the learning environment will be conducive to communication that enhances the training process. A Personal Trainer who is open to input from the client will have greater success. The Client Learning Profile discussion below addresses the elements necessary to building the healthy training education environment.

ESTABLISH THE FOCUS OF INTELLIGENT LEARNING

The more an educational process allows for the internalization of knowledge learned, the more effective it will be. Learning involves human intelligence, and the more intelligent personal training makes the client feel, the better the client will take in the health and fitness approach not only to exercise, but to daily living as well. However, even though we assume that clients are intelligent, they also must have the neurological ability and kinesthetic awareness to improve movement patterns. The Personal Trainer should sequence the appropriate exercise movements based on the client's ability to "memorize" a movement and subsequently improve his or her muscular balance and structural alignment. When called upon to reflect on their own performance and progress, clients feel involved in their training and empowered to self-observe and self-correct their movements according to their Personal Trainer's instruction. Therefore, the following can be summarized about learning and the learning environment:

1. Learners benefit most from instructional methods that assist them in processing their experiences through reflection, analysis, and critical examination.
2. People value teaching methods that respect their autonomy as learners.
3. Practical "how-to" learning motivates most learners.

The Student As Learner: Learning Principles Applied to Personal Training

Knowles identified six assumptions regarding learners (2):

1. The need to know
2. The learners' self-concept
3. The role of experience
4. Readiness to learn
5. Orientation to learning
6. Motivation

As a result of this type of research, the education-based Personal Trainer has a large amount of information available to integrate into his or her training approach and methods. Below is an example of a way in which the above elements of learning can be incorporated into personal training.

The six assumptions of learning, when applied as follows to fitness training, can improve and enhance the education-based personal training process:

1. *The need to know.* People need to know why they need to learn something before they will invest a great deal of time and effort into the learning process. A Personal Trainer can effectively address this principle by educating clients about why they are doing what they are doing in the training

program. For example, if the client experiences low back pain, the Personal Trainer may focus on core training and describe the muscles of the core and explain how stretching and strengthening specific muscles can help to alleviate back problems. Educating clients with pertinent information enables them to understand exactly why they need to do a given exercise and how they will benefit.

2. *The learners' self-concept.* People conceive of themselves as individuals responsible for their own decisions and lives. They will resent and resist situations in which they feel they have no choice in what they are doing and/or if they feel they are expected to follow instruction blindly. In such situations, people are less likely to learn. The goal-setting process applies to the assumption that individuals need to be in charge of their own learning. Training goals are best accomplished when they are client-centered and written by the client, with guidance from the Personal Trainer.

3. *The role of experience.* People bring a great variety and a large amount of educational experiences to their personal training education. The fitness training experiences each client has will vary greatly. If clients have had a negative experience with physical education or sports activities in their formative years, the Personal Trainer must deal with the client's fears and misconceptions that have resulted from these experiences. The Personal Trainer must help to facilitate new thinking and a positive attitude about the present situation. If a client learned to do exercises incorrectly, the client must unlearn old motor patterns and replace them with new ones. A client with limited experience with exercise equipment might be overwhelmed with too much technical information as the training process begins. The Personal Trainer must make an effort to understand a client's previous experiences and adjust the presentation of information accordingly.

4. *Readiness to learn.* People will generally be ready to learn what they need to know to make their lives better. A client who has hired a Personal Trainer is very likely to be in the preparation or action stage of change. According to Prochaska, there are stages of change beginning with Precontemplation, the stage at which an individual is not thinking about change, but other people in that person's personal and professional life are encouraging them to make behavior changes (3). At the second stage, Contemplation, the individual is considering a behavior change. The next stage of change is Preparation, which takes you from the decision to change behavior to beginning to take the steps you need to solve the problem during the fourth stage of change, which is Action. A client who has hired a Personal Trainer on the advice of family and/or friends and not because that person is ready to make a change may not be as ready to learn or change and, therefore, may be less successful. The Personal Trainer needs to be aware of the things that have motivated the client to seek out personal training, for the way the Personal Trainer incorporates this into the sessions will greatly affect the chances of the client's success. Personal Trainers need to guide their clients into their own, individual desire to succeed and out of their family and friends' desire for them to succeed. See Chapter 11 of this book for greater detail about the stages of change.

5. *Orientation to learning.* Learning experiences are often life-centered or problem-centered. A life-centered learning experience is focused on making life improvement, and a problem-centered decision to learn is focused on learning to solve a problem. Problem-centered exercise often has a negative focus that is trying to get rid of the problem of an out-of-shape body. The client feels bad about this condition, and a client who keeps this orientation will have difficulty following through with the program. A life-centered orientation has a positive focus that seeks to add something new to one's life, in this case, a strong, healthy body. If the client can approach the training process as an opportunity to reach for something new and beneficial, the likelihood of success is far greater.

6. *Motivation.* People are responsive to external motivators like job promotions and higher salaries, but the most effective motivators are internal benefits such as a sense of self-improvement, increased self-esteem, a more enjoyable quality of life, and increased job satisfaction. In the case of personal training, internal motivators for clients are also related to self-esteem; people want to feel good about the way they are taking care of their health and fitness, and above all, they want

to feel good about their physical appearance. Physical fitness can also improve your clients' ability to successfully participate in the lives of those around them, such as playing active games with co-workers, significant others, children, and grandchildren, or practice sporting and recreational activities that improve one's overall quality of life. The physical ability to participate fully with others greatly improves one's sense of self-esteem and social belonging.

BUILDING THE CLIENT'S LEARNING PROFILE

Whether you are just entering the fitness industry, are a current Personal Trainer gaining advanced knowledge, or are any other allied health/medical/fitness professional, Personal Trainers have the most success when they view their clients as individual students of health, fitness, and exercise (4) and not as random people that enough repetitive motion will somehow "train."

Before the specific details of a client's exercise program are addressed, consider who your clients are as people by making a client learning profile. The learning profile includes the "big picture" of a client's life insofar as it affects the client's personal training. The type of work a person does, hobbies and recreational activities, and professional goals, all can have an impact on the client's success in training and exercise. Personal Trainers need to develop a broad perspective of their clients and their varied backgrounds, not only in terms of their age and health histories, but also in terms of their cultural and professional experiences.

At the center of the learning profile is the Personal Trainer's need to understand the client's reasons and motivations for employing a Personal Trainer, which is one of the keys to the success of the training process. The client may have a variety of goals in hiring a Personal Trainer ranging from health and fitness, to weight management and improved self-esteem at home and work. As a Personal Trainer, when you get to have a basic profile of the client's lifestyle, you are better equipped to frame the information you are teaching to that particular client's perspectives.

Also, a client's readiness for change is an important part of the client learning profile and is essential to the personal training process. A Personal Trainer who is aware of the client's true reasons for engaging in the personal training experience will achieve more success. Once a Personal Trainer understands what the client wishes to achieve, realistic goals can be set, and accurate strategies for achieving goals can be documented. As you take an educated interest in the client's goals and objectives, the client also can take more personal responsibility toward achieving the goals chosen in collaboration with the Personal Trainer.

Personal Trainers who are just starting to build a practice can benefit greatly when they become aware of the need for an adequate client learning profile as they begin to establish themselves in their personal fitness communities. Personal Trainers just starting out need to be prepared to teach within a wide continuum of clients, such as children, homemakers, corporate executives, and older adults, as well as athletes. When Personal Trainers have gotten to know the learning profiles of many different clients, they can begin to narrow the range of their clientele and focus on the needs of a specific population(s) that most interests and motivates them.

Remember, as a Personal Trainer, you must also be motivated to work with the clients you train. If you come from a family of avid golfers, you will likely be motivated to work with golfers in personal training. If you formerly worked at a desk job, you might have a great deal to offer office workers seeking personal training. This type of focus, however, is best achieved after the Personal Trainer has worked with a wide variety of clients. This allows for the development of solid knowledge of the information and skills needed to function professionally as a Personal Trainer.

It is up to you as a Personal Trainer to consider ways in which you can inspire and motivate your clients. As you read through this chapter and book, think about the vast array of clients you might come across over the course of your career and consider how as a Personal Trainer you can be better prepared to educate and motivate people to learn the knowledge, skills, and abilities needed to succeed in fitness and exercise training.

HOW CLIENTS LEARN: THE VAK LEARNING PREFERENCES

This section reviews the initial presentation of the VAK learning preferences outlined in Chapter 3. As part of your client learning profile, the manner in which your clients and students take in new information needs special attention. Every person, including you, has a specific learning style that enables information to be received and processed. Researchers in education have determined that the intake of learning occurs in three primary ways: visual (seeing), auditory (hearing), and kinesthetic (through action or movement or participation) (5). One caveat to these three preferences is the Personal Trainer's need to expect interesting combinations of learning styles in clients. No person's sensory system operates distinctly in one learning style. They occur together, with one having an emphasis. Observation is not enough for the Personal Trainer to learn the client's preference. The Personal Trainer needs to ask the client if a given approach is effective and follow the client's direction even if it seems inconsistent with what the Personal Trainer observed (6).

When you identify and understand the client's learning preference, your client's sessions will improve and so will the client's motivation and commitment to complete the exercise program. Personal Trainers can inadvertently offend or discourage clients by consistently presenting information in a learning style that does not match the client's. Teachers typically will choose presentations based on their own learning preferences, and this greatly limits the potential of the Personal Trainer's success as a teacher. A Personal Trainer can learn to adjust to the client because the Personal Trainer has developed flexibility in his or her teaching styles. The chances increase greatly that clients will "get" what the Personal Trainer is saying and experience more success in their exercise programs:

➤ **V**isual—Learning through seeing. Visually oriented clients appreciate reading about the training process and can benefit from articles or books about the subject. Images and diagrams of exercise movements and exercise equipment also are welcomed. Watching a video of an exercise sequence, Personal Trainer demonstrations, and taking notes of these activities are advised for visual learners. Anatomical diagrams of proper alignment followed by cuing also support visual learners (*Fig. 4.1*). Environments that are too stimulating visually, however, can distract visual learners. The training center television can be a welcomed, or problematic, distraction to visually oriented people—a point that Personal Trainers need to keep in mind.

➤ **A**uditory—Learning through hearing. Auditory learners will be more sensitive to the Personal Trainer's tone of voice and pace of speech than other clients. Verbal cuing can motivate auditory learners when done with a clearly positive tone. It may not be as effective if done with a bland tone, and it can noticeably damage client motivation if done with a negative tone. Clear verbal presentations combined with note taking can be very helpful. If a lecture or presentation is being

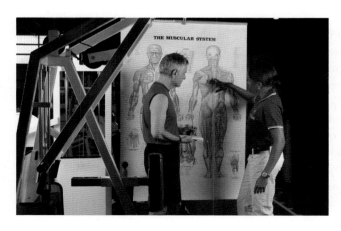

FIGURE 4.1. A Personal Trainer educating her client on musculoskeletal locations.

held, auditory learners can benefit. Loud music or the sound of a television can be a welcome, or an irritating, distraction. Personal Trainers need to pay attention to the noise levels in the training center, for some clients are too shy to ask to have music turned down and will listen politely and then lose the information the Personal Trainer has prepared.

➤ **K**inesthetic—Learning through physical activities and through direct involvement. Kinesthetic learners will learn exercises best when the verbal explanations are short and concise followed by immediate "hands-on" practice of the movement. They will benefit from lively verbal cuing of their movements as they are exercising. After asking the client's permission, kinesthetic learners often benefit when the Personal Trainer palpates the muscle being exercised with the fingers or the palm of the hand so that the client can actually sense the muscle as it contracts and relaxes. This sets up a neurological feedback link that tells the client that the muscle is being activated. The Personal Trainer can position kinesthetic learners with good results, and they also benefit from writing down the things they learned after they have done them to reinforce their new exercise experience.

Benefits of an awareness of the VAK learning preferences include:

➤ Client/Personal Trainer communication is more interactive, effective, and efficient
➤ Clients "get," or absorb, knowledge, skills, and abilities more quickly and easily
➤ Clients appreciate and value the personalized training they receive and complete their fitness programs

Careful observation of the ways the three learning preferences appear in the way clients learn provides powerful support. This knowledge will guide the Personal Trainer to provide a more personally tailored training environment and help him or her improve client performance during the training session.

Learning Style Preference Assessment

Figure 4.2 contains an example of a Learning Style Preference Assessment that Personal Trainers can give to their clients during an initial client consultation. This Learning Style Preference Assessment provides a rating system that calculates the learning style of your client. Students or current Personal Trainers reading this book can take the assessment as well to determine their preferred personal style of learning. This will help to adjust or change your learning style so that it does not conflict with or hinder the client's learning style. In greater or lesser degrees, everyone has all three, but one learning style is generally most used. Many individuals will use a combination of the three styles, depending on the learning situation. The Learning Style Preference Assessment determines where the client's strongest preference lies and which two are less favored. The client also may have two lesser, but equally strong styles, and some clients may have equal visual, auditory, and kinesthetic intake preferences. In the United States, about 60% of learners are visual learners, 15% are auditory, and 25% are kinesthetic (7).

Upon completing the Learning Style Preference Assessment, the Personal Trainer who identifies and understands a client's personal learning style will be a more effective teacher when communicating instructions and information to current or future clients. It is important to recognize, regardless of the preferred learning preference of the client, that it is best to incorporate all possible types of learning methods (7). No matter what the client's specific learning style, the Personal Trainer needs to realize that although clients are initially trained in their primary preference, the Personal Trainer is advised to use the other two preferences as well as a means of broadening the client's learning perspective. If a client does not have very good kinesthetic awareness initially, for example, it can be developed over time by incorporating education-based personal training sessions and optimal learning strategies discussed in more detail in Chapter 5.

Each individual has a different learning preference. The following assessment will help you understand your learning style and will assist your Personal Trainer in how he/she will teach, educate, and design your exercise sessions. Please complete the following assessment to allow your Personal Trainer to develop an education-based personal training session specifically for your preferred learning style.

Score each of the statements below by the following grading system:

(1) Never   (2) Occasionally   (3) Frequently   (4) All the time

1 I draw pictures/diagrams to illustrate concepts.

2 I like to write things down to plan events.

3 I can memorize information best if I write it down several times.

4 I can put something together after viewing directions or diagrams.

5 I usually look around while I'm driving.

6 I like doodling while someone is talking to me over the phone.

7 I enjoy watching movies more than listening to the radio.

8 I like to read and write when waiting for an appointment.

9 I like to read the newspaper or other materials in my spare time.

10 I prefer to look at a map rather than read written directions.

11 I prefer someone talk to me at a medium pace so I can understand them.

12 I prefer someone talk to me without a lot of hand gestures.

13 I like when someone reads to me rather than having to read it myself.

14 I like to give verbal directions.

15 I like getting my news from the radio.

16 I would rather hear a story on audio tapes than having to read a book.

17 I like to talk to myself when alone.

18 I can memorize information best if I say it out loud several times.

19 I like to talk on the phone a lot.

20 I express my thoughts through language and am well spoken.

21 I enjoy doing physical activities in my spare time.

22 I like working or doing things with my hands.

23 I move around a lot when in meetings or just sitting still.

24 I could learn better by flashcards than by listening to audio tapes.

25 I have good body awareness and can sense when someone is close to me.

26 I prefer to not sit in meetings and hear someone speaking.

27 I like touching things and feeling different textures.

28 I prefer to learn by practicing or trying something using my body.

29 I have good balance and am well coordinated.

30 I like to pace when I am talking, thinking, working, or studying.

From: **Human Behavior in Organization**, Fourth edition. Author: Sinclair, Cuttell, Vandeveer, Menefee, Pearson Custom, 2002 and **Accelerated Learning for the 21st Century,** by Nicholl and Rose, Dell Publishing 1997.

A

FIGURE 4.2. Learning Style Preference Assessment. (Adapted from Human Behavior in Organizations Fourth Edition by Sinclair, Cuttell, Vandeveer, Menefee, Pearson Custom, 2002 and Accelerated Learning for the 21st Century by Nicholl and Rose, Dell Publishing, 1997.)

Scoring

Visual-Spatial (total for questions 1-10)

Auditory-Verbal (total for questions 11-20)

Kinesthetic-Bodily (total for questions 21-30)

The highest score achieved on the Learning Style Preference Assessment test is your preferred learning style. Your personal trainer will direct his/her teaching style toward your preferred learning preference implementing different strategies for you to learn information and perform movements more successfully.

• Visual-Spatial

Show you the SET Sessions Plan and SET Flowchart.
Demonstrate exercise movements for you slowly and properly.
Visualize performing exercise movements correctly and precisely.
Recopy your notes after the training session.
Draw Free Body Diagrams to assist with remembering exercises.

• Auditory-Verbal

Read your written notes over to memorize and learn the information.
Discuss with your trainer what you have just learned.
Discuss the material you are learning with your Personal Trainer.
Tape your training sessions and listen to them again.

• Kinesthetic-Bodily

Watch your trainer demonstrate movements of what you need to learn and practice under the trainer's observation.
The trainer will outline muscle structures on you that are being trained.
Palpate muscle structures of primary and secondary muscle groups.
Think of practical uses of learning exercise movements.
Become aware of your posture and body alignment through the Four Points of Posture.

From: **Human Behavior in Organization**, Fourth edition. Author: Sinclair, Cuttell, Vandeveer, Menefee, Pearson Custom, 2002 and **Accelerated Learning for the 21st Century,** by Nicholl and Rose, Dell Publishing 1997.

B

FIGURE 4.2. *Continued.*

THE LEARNING-MOTIVATED CLIENT

Motivation Part 1: The Academic Motivation Model (ARCS)

Motivation is a state of need or desire that activates a person to do something that will satisfy a need or desire (7). Many Personal Trainers find that the client's motivational level is the single most important factor to a client's success. This model speaks directly to client motivation in personal training (8). How well clients are motivated to become healthy and fit depends on the Personal Trainer's skills in motivating clients to succeed. When aware of their motivational role, and when they take responsibility for it, education-based Personal Trainers can effectively set the stage for motivated, continual, and successful client learning. Through the study and application of motivational techniques as outlined below, most Personal Trainers can achieve improved motivation in their clients. Keller's model (8) outlines four different types of motivation necessary for successful learning and how to incorporate these elements into one's instruction:

➤ Attention
➤ Relevance
➤ Confidence
➤ Satisfaction

The ARCS Model and Personal Training

1. Gain the *attention* of the client.
   Maintain a high level of attention and enthusiasm throughout the training. Attention is the basic element of enthusiasm, and good client attention sustains the exercise effort throughout the training. The Personal Trainer can successfully sustain a high level of attention from the client because each training session can challenge the client with new knowledge, skills, and movements.
2. Keep the instruction *relevant* to the client.
   Keller (8) states that students will not consider instruction relevant and, therefore, do not absorb it when they do not sense that it pertains to them. Therefore, Personal Trainers who focus on designing the training session so that it is relevant to achieving their client's goals will retain their client's motivation. If you know the client's learning profile well, you will know how to keep each training session clearly focused on the client's achievement of his or her goals.
3. Create and maintain client *confidence*.

For clients and students to be highly motivated, they need to feel that the goal of personal exercise and fitness is attainable. They must feel confident that the training they are learning is leading them toward the mastery of exercise movements and knowledge.

CLIENT CONFIDENCE

Two situations can arise when a client either (a) lacks confidence or (b) is overconfident:

➤ Clients who lack confidence, especially if they have dropped an exercise program in the past or know that they do not have the skills to do movements well at first, need to shift their perspective to see that they do have the resources to succeed. Personal Trainers need to realize that most of the clients that come to them will not be confident in their current fitness level and/or how they have trained in the past. Therefore, the Personal Trainer's role is to teach the client during the initial client consultation about the education-based personal training process. By bridging the gap between their past experience and how the Personal Trainer teaches a step-by-step process, clients often gain the confidence they need to succeed. They appreciate the detailed process the Personal Trainer uses to guide and instruct them toward their goals.

➤ The other extreme occurs when clients are overconfident or feel that they already have a high level of knowledge and expertise in exercise and fitness. These clients are easily disappointed and lose confidence when they discover that they are not as capable as they thought. Overly confident clients must be politely reminded from the beginning that more information and skills still exist for them to master. If, however, a client has in fact obtained a certain level of precision in exercise, then it is the Personal Trainer's responsibility to challenge the client with more advanced instruction and training to keep the client's motivation high. When overly confident clients can be humbled by rigorous training demands that they have helped to create, their desire to accomplish these goals will likely increase, along with their appreciation for their Personal Trainer's guidance.

ASK QUESTIONS

Keller recommends that you ask your clients questions before you design their personal training program. This corroborates the discussion above regarding the client's learning profile. Here are the questions Keller (8) recommends to help with the client–Personal Trainer relationship. During the initial client consultation, Personal Trainers can ask these questions to assist in developing goal-oriented training sessions tailored to the client's interests:

➤ How important is it for you to learn to perform exercise movements precisely and accurately? What do you hope to gain from your personal training experience?
➤ Are you confident that you can successfully learn to perform the required movement correctly? If not, what would help you feel more confident?
➤ Are you interested in learning a process that can help you achieve your goals?
➤ How satisfied would you be if you could achieve your goals? How will you know that you have achieved your goals?

The answers to the Personal Trainer's questions will provide a picture of what your client's hopes and expectations are for the training experience and assist you in developing an education-based exercise program.

Motivation Part 2: Six Variables of Motivation (7)

Because motivation involves the learner's mental attitude, Personal Trainers must concern themselves with creating an environment and the circumstances that will affect the client's desire to learn and work to achieve goals. Hunter (7) has developed six variables of motivation theory to increase the probability of client learning and success. These variables are level of concern, feeling tone, interest, success, knowledge of results, and reward:

1. Level of Concern
   Clients are more likely to be motivated to learn or do something about which they are concerned. By focusing the training process on client goals, each exercise and behavior change can be supported as it aligns with client goals. For example, if a client goal is to increase lower body strength and to lose weight, a Personal Trainer can identify the top five exercises for the lower body. The Personal Trainer can teach the client those exercises while implementing them in the training program.

2. Feeling Tone
   Feeling tone is the atmosphere or climate in the training environment that results from the Personal Trainer's attitude and training style. It can be pleasant, unpleasant, or neutral. Motivation to learn is most likely to take place when the feeling tone is pleasant. Emotion is tagged with learning, so pleasant feeling tones produce more zest for learning. The Personal Trainer's voice, mannerisms, body language, listening skills, choice of words, and interest in the client will all contribute to creating feeling tone.

3. Interest

   Interest can be cultivated by promoting the client's self-interest and by making the training experiences novel and vivid. The client's self-interest can be promoted by focusing on the client's interest and goals. The training sessions can be novel and vivid by implementing variety, adding humor when appropriate, including fitness facts that support the training, and keeping the training interesting with simple changes (for example, a change in sequence of activity). Sharing success stories of previous clients may also cultivate interest and remembering and relating instances in which the client did something well in a previous session also serve to stimulate the client's interest.

4. Success

   A client who feels successful will be more likely to learn. The Personal Trainer can increase the possibility of success by choosing the correct level of difficulty and intensity of an exercise. The client's ability and effort level will play a major role in feelings of success.

5. Knowledge of Results

   Knowledge of results is the process of giving the client the feedback necessary to know how well he or she is doing. The most valuable feedback is immediate, specific, and precise.

6. Rewards

   Hunter (7) describes rewards as the relationship between the learning activity and the return the learner receives from the learning experience. He maintains the same points as Keller (8) on intrinsic or extrinsic rewards and also emphasizes their importance to motivation.

THE ANTICIPATORY SET

Hunter has done extensive research on lesson design (7). His model has eight steps for designing effective teaching. These eight steps begin with the anticipatory set. Personal Trainers can effectively apply the anticipatory set to prepare the client with an overview of the focus of the training session. The anticipatory set begins with the greeting that welcomes the client to the training session, setting a positive feeling tone. The anticipatory set can also include an overview of the previous training session, reflection of client goals, and a brief introduction of what the immediate session plan will include. This type of conscious conversation at the beginning of the session brings the client's focus from his or her busy day to the exercise session. It also boosts the client's motivation and ensures a greater chance of client success.

Motivation Part 3: Galbraith's Motivational Strategies

According to Galbraith certain motivational strategies are known for their success in enhancing instruction (9). These strategies are well documented in the educational psychology literature and are often used by therapists and counselors as well as human resources departments in business and industry. These motivational strategies are adapted below to fit the personal training experience:

Prepare to meet the client
- Commit yourself to success in the learning and training process.

Meet the client
- Get to know the client's visual, auditory, and kinesthetic learning modalities.
- Learn the client's needs and limitations. Help the client identify strategies based on those needs and limitations to help him or her achieve goals.

Session preparation
- Provide the client with proper sequencing and progression of movements.
- Make the training goals specific, measurable, action-based, realistic, and associated with a timeline.
- Personalize the training experience for each client.
- Plan variety into the training process.

The exercise experience
- Make the first training experience safe, successful, and interesting.
- Give the client ownership of learning, changing behavior, and performance.
- Consider the multiple intelligences occurring in the training process: bodily-kinesthetic, verbal, logical-mathematical, interpersonal, intrapersonal, naturalistic, musical, spatial. Use these observations to shape the content of the client's training program as it progresses.

Evaluation and feedback
- Provide the client with specific and immediate feedback regarding performance.
- Encourage the client with a discussion of positive attitude and effort in the process of success.

Motivation needs to be considered in the preparation of each personal training session. As research in learning has shown, incorporating any one or a combination of motivational strategies into your training sessions can inspire your clients to meet their training objectives. It will help make the training experience a rewarding one.

SUMMARY

Successful Personal Trainers have a sincere interest in their client's individual needs and preferences as well as their training goals and objectives. A Personal Trainer who understands the client on the client's terms can successfully design a training program that will engage and motivate the client to achieve his or her fitness goals and objectives. Good communication skills on the part of the Personal Trainer are essential in the process of building a thorough client profile. This, in conjunction with the VAK learning preferences and the 3 E's for sustained motivation, are tools that can greatly facilitate the training process. With a clear understanding of the client's individual characteristics and learning styles, the Personal Trainer can successfully develop an education-based personal training program that fully involves clients and empowers them to take charge of their own training development.

REFERENCES

1. Stroot S, et al. Peer Assistance and Review Guidebook. Columbus, OH: Ohio Department of Education, 1998.
2. Knowles M. The Learner: A Neglected Species. Houston, TX: Gulf Publishing, 1990.
3. Prochaska J. Changing for good. New York: William Morrow, 1994.
4. Farquharson A. Viewing Clients and Patients as Learners. Teaching in Practice: How Professionals Can Work Effectively with Clients, Patients, and Colleagues. San Francisco: Jossey-Bass, 1995.
5. Nicholl MJ, Rose C. Acquiring the Information. Accelerated Learning for the 21st Century. New York: Dell, 1997.
6. Russell L. Learning to take more in. In: Holt M, Ullius D, eds. The Accelerated Learning Field Book. San Francisco: Jossey-Bass, 1999.
7. Hunter M. Mastery Teaching: Increasing Instructional Effectiveness in Elementary and Secondary Schools, Colleges, and Universities. Thousand Oaks, CA: Corwin Press, 1982.
8. Keller JM. Strategies for stimulating the motivation to learn. Perform Instruct 1987;26(8):1–7.
9. Galbraith M. Learning Methods: A Guide for Effective Instruction. Malabar, FL: Robert Krieger Publishing, 1990.

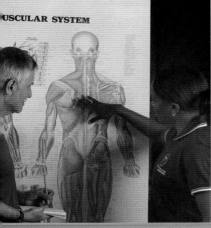

USCULAR SYSTEM

CHAPTER

Education-Based Personal Trainer Development

5

Kenneth E. Baldwin, M.Ed., A.H. Ismail Center for Health, Exercise & Nutrition, Department of Health and Kinesiology, College of Liberal Arts, Purdue University, West Lafayette, Indiana

Terry Ferebee Eckmann, Ph.D., Associate Professor, Department of Teacher Education and Human Performance, Minot State University, Minot, North Dakota

Chapter Outline

Objectives

- **Practice improved listening and communication skills**
- **Apply basic communication skills to client sessions**
- **Understand how the VAK learning preferences and optimal learning strategies apply to personal training sessions**
- **Combine and apply the VAK learning preferences with optimal learning strategies**
- **Understand how to implement exercise demonstrations and conduct exercise practice sessions**

The education-based Personal Trainer has the skills of a good educator. This chapter focuses on developing your educational skills so that you can effectively teach the knowledge you have of anatomy, kinesiology, and exercise science. First in the toolbox of the good educator are well-practiced communication skills. This chapter will provide you with the basic elements of good communication skills so that you can successfully communicate your knowledge and confidently educate your clients (*Fig. 5.1*). It also provides a more detailed study of the VAK learning preferences and optimum learning strategies, which are tools that expand your understanding of how your clients learn and how you can best teach them the rubrics of personal training. Finally, the education-based movement demonstration is explained in detail. This integrative tool synthesizes all of your knowledge of exercise science, your communication skills, and your client learning analysis. It provides you as a personal training educator with an informative and effective means of teaching your clients exercise movements and ensuring your clients' success in their personal training.

MORE SKILLS FOR THE EDUCATION-BASED PERSONAL TRAINER

Communication Skills and Education-Based Personal Training

Personal Trainers rely and depend on good communication skills when dealing with colleagues, in the workplace environment, and with clients one-on-one or in small groups. Good communication skills are essential to establishing and maintaining the teamwork required during the personal training program. The effective Personal Trainer has a good understanding of communication skills and techniques.

Communication is the giving and receiving of information. When the sender of information (the Personal Trainer) sends a message to the client, the message is then sent in the most appropriate form (1). To be understood by both parties, both the communicator and receiver need to be clear in the messages being sent. Feedback through a confirmation by all participants is recommended.

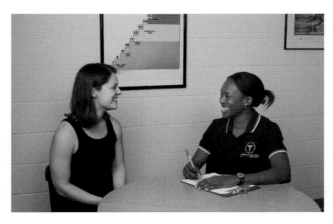

FIGURE 5.1. A Personal Trainer and her client communicating effectively.

Personal Trainers will not only have to communicate with clients in person. In addition to spoken communication, Personal Trainers may also communicate with clients through gestures, writing, e-mail, text messaging, or voicemail. Whatever the mode of communication, miscommunications can occur. Miscommunication is one of the main problems Personal Trainers can face when dealing with scheduling clients or booking appointments. Personal Trainers can be misunderstood or they can misinterpret client information. By remembering the importance of clear communication, Personal Trainers will have the motivation to communicate clearly with clients and colleagues in the workplace.

Developing Your Communication Skills

Communication is one of the most important skills in life. The four basic modes of communication are reading, writing, speaking, and listening. People spend up to 75% of their waking hours doing these four things. Almost 50% of our communication time is spent listening, yet most people have very limited formal training in how to listen. Covey (2) identifies five levels in the continuum of listening:

➤ Level One: Ignoring, not making an attempt to listen
➤ Level Two: Pretend listening, which is the form of listening that patronizes the speaker by appearing to listen when our thoughts are elsewhere
➤ Level Three: Selective listening, which occurs when we listen to what we want to hear, often engaging the speaker with eye contact and even nods of the head
➤ Level Four: Attentive listening, which is characterized by eye contact, head nods, and listening to the words of the speaker while waiting for our turn to talk as we organize our thoughts for a response
➤ Level Five: Empathetic listening, in which the listener strives first to understand and then to be understood; his or her mind is not full of thoughts that do not pertain to the client; attention is relaxed and receptive to what the client has to say and the listener can hear the client's message from the client's point of view

Empathetic listening is the most effective level of listening. It is an essential skill for a Personal Trainer. The Personal Trainer who listens with empathy will pay close attention and learn the underlying reasons why a client has hired a Personal Trainer, find out how a client feels about his or her body, understand issues the client has that may create barriers to exercise or healthy lifestyle habits, and as a result, design a training program within the client's frame of reference. When the Personal Trainer can be an empathetic listener, the client's needs become clear easily and directly. The Personal Trainer then has the information to estimate what the client can accomplish and develop ways to effectively guide the client from his or her own perspective toward his or her own goals.

DEVELOP EMPATHETIC LISTENING SKILLS

When developing empathetic listening skills, there are a number of key points to remember:

1. Be sincerely open and listen to the client so that you can reach an understanding of what clients think and why they think the way they think.
2. Interpret the meaning of the client's information and experiences through your own prior personal experiences. Stand in the client's shoes as best you can. A Personal Trainer who strives to understand the perceptions of the client will be more effective (remember that many clients may have had unpleasant experiences that create distrust, discomfort, and fear with Personal Trainers, exercise, and/or physical education in school).
3. There is more than one way to interpret information and experiences. Personal Trainers must first understand the client's perspective and do their best to make sure that the clients understand what the Personal Trainer is teaching them throughout the training process.

4. Most communication breakdowns are based on semantics and how people define words. The Personal Trainer who focuses on understanding meaning will have fewer problems with semantics. However, the Personal Trainer must make sure that the vocabulary used in the training session is understood. Not everyone knows the definition of highly technical terms.

Speakers and listeners attach their own meaning to everything they hear. Everyone has different values, attitudes, beliefs, interests, and experiences that influence the way things are heard. One person hears things differently from the next person. To bridge this gap, good communicators assume that no individual reality is right or wrong. A person has only his or her individual perception of things and, for this reason, listening for understanding the other person's point of view is essential.

Empathetic listening often involves a paradigm shift. Speakers typically seek first to be understood, and listeners usually listen with the desire to reply. Empathetic listening, on the other hand, is a type of selfless listening that is not driven by one's own personal need to be heard. Personal Trainers can continually improve listening by practicing the following skills:

➤ Be aware of listening behaviors; continually identify when you take over the conversation from the client, and when you listen well.
➤ Check for understanding by re-stating, make sure that what you heard was what was meant.
➤ Watch your nonverbal communicators; tune in to your body language while you listen (e.g., are your arms crossed, are you looking out the window).
➤ Do not assume, jump to conclusions, or overreact. People often attach old meanings to new situations, and this can cause confusion.
➤ Want to listen: Think of the benefits to you, the listener, and your organization.
➤ Ask questions to clarify your understanding of the message.
➤ Make sure you stay focused on the speaker.
➤ Be aware of when you are not really listening and waiting for your turn to talk.
➤ Refocus and place your attention again on what the speaker is telling you.

ESSENTIAL ELEMENTS OF PERSONAL TRAINER COMMUNICATION SKILLS

Personal Trainers want information and knowledge to be communicated effectively to clients and others. Communication is the effective process of giving and receiving information, but to be effective, the message must be understood by both parties. As a Personal Trainer, ask the question "Is this the best possible way for me to get my message across clearly so that both of us understand my message?" Even communication that a Personal Trainer may feel is clear enough, stated simply, or not necessary may be extremely important from the client's perspective. Most of the time, asking the client is the only way to know if one's message has been correctly received. The following essential communication points can help Personal Trainers improve their communication skills (1):

➤ *Using new or scientific terms and information.* Personal Trainers should talk in layman's terms in the beginning and progressively build the vocabulary of terms and information for the client to easily understand. If the information becomes too complicated in the beginning, clients stop listening effectively because they are overwhelmed and confused. If the information is complex, teach it progressively over the course of the sessions in small increments. This will guide the client along through the process sequentially and avoid unnecessary backtracking to re-explain things. By breaking the information into small, compartmentalized sequences, the client will absorb and retain the information with greater accuracy and success. Before continuing to the next exercise or session, the Personal Trainer can confirm with the client that the new information or movement has been understood and find out whether the client has any questions.
➤ *Using jargon terms.* Jargon such as "lats, bi's, tri's, quads, hams," should be avoided unless specifically relevant to the training. Jargon is often difficult to notice because it can be used automatically. Clients might not ask the Personal Trainer to clarify a given term or word for fear

of appearing and/or feeling unintelligent. Clearly communicate information to the client in full and simple terms, and give the client a chance to ask questions.

➤ *Verbal cues.* Verbal cues or verbal instructions can provide too little or too much information. To provide a balance, Personal Trainers using verbal cues should keep them concise and short to prompt key movement skills. Research studies have shown that cues facilitate the teaching of new skills or reviewing previously learned ones (3).

➤ *Listen to hear the client.* Personal Trainers need to hear what clients tell them. Effective communication for the personal training relationship is not complete unless the Personal Trainer understands the client's message regarding his or her exercise goals and objectives.

➤ *Nonverbal messages.* Personal Trainers can create confusion if the nonverbal message does not match the verbal communication. If you are standing too close or too far away, not making eye contact, or looking through a file while you are talking with your client, you may send an undesired nonverbal message to which the client does not know how to respond.

➤ *Training aids.* The Personal Trainer's use of training aids such as anatomy charts, exercise diagrams, and other informational tools for the intended purpose of educating the client can be very helpful to client learning.

➤ *Interesting creates motivated.* For effective communication, a Personal Trainer must offer positive reinforcement to students during the session. Personal Trainers must be enthusiastic and energized during the session. A client who senses that the Personal Trainer is bored or uninspired will lack motivation and not be interested in the training session. Learning and exercise performance may be too challenging, if not impossible, for the client.

➤ *Personal trainer assumptions.* Personal Trainers need to know, not assume, the client's current level of knowledge and ability before the first training session. Very often, clients consider their level of expertise higher than it really is. The Personal Trainer, then, is responsible for giving the client accurate feedback to correct this inaccurate self-assessment.

➤ *Tone of voice.* Personal Trainers can affect the meaning of information through the projection and inflection of voice and tone. Establish an even, positive communication tone for clients that is not loud or demanding. Avoid yelling orders to the client instead of providing instruction.

➤ *Client preconceptions.* The client and Personal Trainer need to be on the same page concerning the design and goals of the exercise program. The client must have a thorough understanding of any preconceived ideas before the personal training begins. Confirm with the client that the designed exercise program is accurate and clear before training begins. Disagreements or confusion regarding the client's potential accomplishments should be decreased or eliminated from the onset of the training relationship.

Basic Preparation of the Personal Training Session

Personal Trainers as educators are faced with the challenge of providing clients with engaging and productive training sessions that consistently improve performance. This will ensure that their practice sessions on their own are also contributing to the overall improvement the client is seeking. A Personal Trainer needs to rely on a process of providing instruction through a number of available methods. A well-structured training session provides several techniques and methods to educate a client on such knowledge and abilities. A format developed to provide Personal Trainers with instructional methods that teach knowledge, information, and a process to increase client skill level is presented below (4):

➤ Prepare information on the design of the exercise program, SET Session Plan/Flowchart, and the methods of instruction to be presented at the initial client consultation and throughout the training program.

➤ Implement the optimal learning strategies to enhance a client's learning experience.

➤ Provide new exercise demonstrations and practice times.

➤ Develop additional movements based on the client's progression and skill level and performance achievement.

Personal Trainers can evaluate the client's current movement performance in relation to the desired or required level of performance. Points to observe include muscular balance, posture, and body alignment. This observation and evaluation needs to occur on a continuous basis. When observing and evaluating performance, consider and/or use the following:

➤ The goal of the movement or skill acquisition
➤ The current or actual level of the movement performed and the required performance level of the movement determined by the Personal Trainer
➤ Provide proper instructional feedback that meets the needs of the client and the situation

THE VAK LEARNING PREFERENCES COMBINED WITH OPTIMUM LEARNING STRATEGIES

After reading Chapter 4 of this book, the Personal Trainer will have a better understanding of the client's individual learning preferences. When these learning styles are applied to specific learning activities, various strategies may be used by Personal Trainers to instruct and educate their clients. These strategies are a set of optional teaching tools or techniques that Personal Trainers can use to present information or exercise techniques that allow clients to take in information on the basis of their learning preference. Each strategy is designed to match the preferred learning preferences of the client. Personal Trainers can use one or all of the strategic options and through observations and evaluations determine which tend to work best for each of their clients. Each strategy for the visual, auditory, and kinesthetic learner is listed below and then followed by a more specific explanation of how each of them can be applied (5).

Strategies for the Visual Learner

Visual learners benefit from presentations that use the following techniques to teach exercise movements:

➤ Have clients watch you carefully and have them take brief notes of each exercise being taught before practicing the exercise. Encourage them to make simple diagrams of the movement and/or exercise machine. After the session, have the client type the notes in detail and bring them to the next session for review and correction.
➤ Bring or place an anatomical chart on your clipboard. Before teaching a movement pattern, point out all the primary muscular and joint structures being trained to perform that specific exercise. After you have explained the primary structures to the clients, you can later teach them about secondary and stabilizing structures (at an appropriate time).
➤ Trace, on the client or you, the muscle(s) or joint structures involved in the movement (ask permission from the client first before tracing the muscle on a specific muscle area or region).
➤ Demonstrate the movement correctly.
➤ Demonstrate the way the movement looks when it is performed incorrectly. This will allow the client to notice the differences between the correct movement and the incorrect way that the client may have seen it done by others.
➤ Draw a diagram of proper joint and body alignment in the client's notebook during the preparation, central, and terminal phases of an exercise movement as shown in Figure 5.2.
➤ Use imagery to describe how to perform an exercise.
➤ Provide visual cues such as pointing to proper body alignment and positioning, while demonstrating a movement.

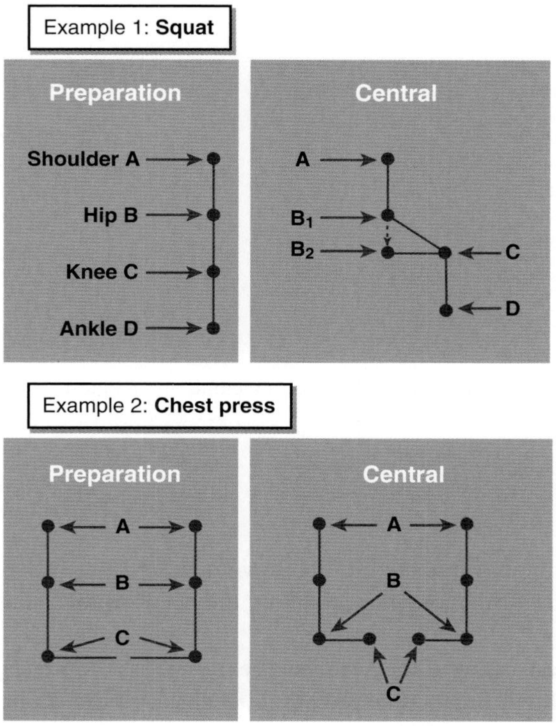

Example 1: Squat

Preparation

Shoulder A ⟶ ●
Hip B ⟶ ●
Knee C ⟶ ●
Ankle D ⟶ ●

Central

A ⟶ ●
B_1 ⟶ ●
B_2 ⟶ ● ⟵ C
● ⟵ D

Example 2: Chest press

Preparation

● ⟵ A ⟶ ●
● ⟵ B ⟶ ●
● ⟵ C ⟶ ●

Central

● ⟵ A ⟶ ●
● B ●
● ●
C

FIGURE 5.2. Examples of Free Body Diagrams of two exercises: a squat and chest press. Example 1 demonstrates a squat movement's preparation and central phase. A Personal Trainer may recommend that the beginning client not go any lower than point B_1 (the hip joint). Example 2 shows a chest press preparation and central phase. A Personal Trainer may point out to the client that points A and B will move and that point C (the shoulder joint) should remain stable during the movement.

➤ Have clients perform exercise movements in front of a mirror whenever possible, allowing for immediate visual feedback.

➤ Provide handouts of pictures or diagrams demonstrating how to perform the exercise correctly.

➤ Recommend videos, CDs, or DVDs of performing exercise movements correctly that can be viewed in the client's spare time.

➤ After being shown how to perform the movement correctly, have the client mentally visualize the movement being performed correctly.

➤ After the Personal Trainer has shown the client how to perform the movement correctly, have the client practice the movement without the use of resistance or equipment to establish the proper movement patterns.

➤ Have clients bring a friend or family member to take photos or make a video of them as they exercise that the clients can view later and keep as a record of their improvement.

Strategies for the Auditory Learner

➤ Always attempt to use a consistent tone of voice for all clients, and speak slowly, clearly, and pause frequently between thoughts or sentences.

➤ Have clients listen carefully to your instructions and take brief notes on each exercise as you explain it before they do the exercise. After the session, have clients type the notes in detail and bring them to the next session for review and correction.

➤ Have your clients audiotape your sessions with them so that they can play the sessions back on their own. This reinforces that information and helps improve retention. Additional notes can be taken from the tapes.

➤ Locate your training session in a quiet place where loud music is not a distraction and the client can always hear what you are saying. Ask clients if they can hear you adequately.

➤ Keep your body language to a minimum (keep arms and hands at your side) so the client can focus on your voice.

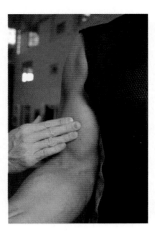

FIGURE 5.3. A client being palpated in the biceps muscle. Palpation technique is a kinesthetic teaching strategy.

Strategies for the Kinesthetic Learner

➤ Outline on the client the muscle(s) or joint structures involved in the movement.

➤ Palpate the primary muscle structures involved in the movement to allow the client to focus on specific locations and areas (*Fig. 5.3*) (6).

➤ When you are palpating the muscle structure, ask clients if they can feel the muscle as it contracts through the different phases—preparation, central, final—thus providing feedback to the client and to you.

➤ Have the client take detailed notes of each exercise *after* doing it. Encourage the client to use directional arrows to indicate the spatial directions of the exercise movement. After the session, have the client type the notes and bring them to the next session for review and correction.

➤ Guide clients physically through the proper movement so they can memorize the correct positioning of the body during an exercise. Do this several times so they can "lock in" the correct movement pattern.

➤ After you have shown the clients how to perform a movement correctly, have them practice the movement standing, sitting, or lying down without the use of resistance or equipment to review the proper movement patterns.

As discussed in Chapter 4, it is recommended that you incorporate instruction that uses a combination of all three learning styles of the VAK learning preferences. No matter what the client's specific learning style, the Personal Trainer needs to realize that although clients are initially trained in their primary preference, the Personal Trainer is advised to use all three learning strategies as an optimal means of broadening the client's learning perspective.

THE EDUCATION-BASED MOVEMENT DEMONSTRATION

Personal Trainers, as part of the education-based personal training process, can practice and implement a process of demonstrations to help their clients learn to perfect exercise movements. The word "modeling" is defined as the use of demonstration as a means of conveying information about how to perform a skill (4). The word "demonstration," therefore, refers to the modeling of a given action or behavior. Since the word "demonstration" is more applicable to the context of performing exercise movements, this term is used in the chapter. As movement practitioners, a number of strategies and techniques provide clients with the foundational skills and aptitude to achieve the desired results.

The demonstration process includes four phases (7). The first two involve the Personal Trainer's demonstration of the movement, and the second two involve the client's practice of the movement. These phases include preparation; demonstration; client practice; and observation, evaluation, and feedback.

Preparation

In the preparation phase, the Personal Trainer provides a foundation of initial information about the exercise movement before demonstrating it. This is not intended to be a comprehensive list of information to be discussed by the Personal Trainer in preparation for an exercise. However, it does show that the Personal Trainer is prepared and professional. Depending on the client's learning preferences, you can introduce additional preparation information before demonstrating the movement. The preparatory information introduced to the client includes the following:

➤ The Personal Trainer prepares an introduction to the exercise movement to gain the attention of the client. The introduction provides the core body of information, knowledge, and instructions necessary to perform the movement.

➤ The client needs to bring a pen and notepad to each meeting with the Personal Trainer so that he or she can take notes on how to perform the movement. The client also needs to be reminded to type them up before the next session and to bring them and the notebook along to the next session (*Fig. 5.4*).

➤ Provide all support materials, such as a handout, to visually show the proper movement sequence or an anatomical chart on which the Personal Trainer identifies the primary, secondary, and stabilizing muscle(s) being trained during the movement.

➤ Let the client know the muscle structure that will be palpated while the client is performing the movement. Ask permission to palpate before moving forward. *Note:* An overview of the palpation process should be addressed in initial client consultation as part of the Personal Trainer's teaching approach.

➤ Outline on the client or yourself the muscle(s) or joint structures involved in the movement. Ask permission to outline the muscle structure before moving forward.

➤ Explain to the client in advance that every exercise has three phases—preparation, central, and final—and that he or she will learn these phases for each exercise movement.

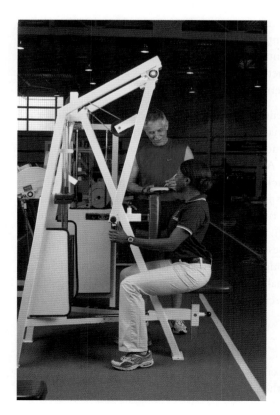

FIGURE 5.4. A client taking detailed notes on how to perform a seated row based on her Personal Trainer's recommendation.

Demonstration

In the demonstration phase, the teacher/Personal Trainer should to be able to perform the movement accurately, precisely, and correctly. A client cannot be expected to perform a movement correctly if the Personal Trainer cannot do it or explain it well. The demonstration allows the client to observe what the exercise movement or performance involves. The sequence for demonstrating a movement is as follows (4):

➤ Demonstrate at normal speed: Demonstrate the movement correctly at normal speed so the client can see its required performance and the Personal Trainer's expectations. The Personal Trainer here is using observational learning, the process by which students acquire the capability for movement skills by observing the performance of others (8).

➤ Demonstrate the movement again slowly and in phases. Demonstrate for the client at a slower speed and perform the movement in the three phases: preparatory, central, and final. Present the movement for 5 to 15 repetitions and explain the important details about the movement in the different phases. Allow clients to observe the phases and give them enough time to ask questions. The Personal Trainer can have a script of information to present the key points, details, and safety considerations of the movement.

➤ Have the client repeat verbal instructions. Have the client describe the correct sequence and proper performance of the movement in all three phases. The Personal Trainer or client now performs the movement (without resistance or equipment) as the client verbally describes the details of the exercise. This final "walk through" confirms whether clients understand the fundamentals of the exercise before performing it themselves with resistance. The Personal Trainer needs to encourage clients to ask any final questions about the exercise before practicing it.

Client Practice

In the practice phase, the client practices the movement for the first time. The objective of the practice with the Personal Trainer is to ensure that the client has learned and will perform the exercise correctly. A client cannot be expected to perform a movement precisely at 100% accuracy the first time, and Personal Trainers often allow clients to practice an exercise when the client is not fully capable of doing it well. Regardless of the client's skill performance, however, encourage him or her with positive, motivational feedback to practice and try the exercise again while you are watching (9). The process to practice a movement correctly is as follows:

➤ Use a slow and controlled performance. The client performs the movement at a controlled pace and with a low level of resistance during the initial stage of learning to acquire a general idea of the movement. The client needs to perform the movement as perfectly as possible, with attention set to memorize the proper movement patterns. As the client is performing the movement, the Personal Trainer provides some initial feedback to the client to make any corrections or adjustments. The challenge for Personal Trainers is to provide enough instruction and adequate feedback to allow the student to achieve the recommended standards required to perform movements safely, effectively, and efficiently (10).

➤ The client's solo exercise session is next. The session plan typically includes exercises that are perfected by the client, new exercises that are being introduced, and previous exercises that need to be practiced under the attention of the Personal Trainer. Approximately 50% of the session is allocated to practice while the client is building a repertoire of exercises that can be correctly solo-practiced for the next and future sessions (9).

Observation, Evaluation, and Feedback

➤ *Observation*. The Personal Trainer carefully observes the client's performance of the exercise movement. The Personal Trainer takes note of the client's posture and alignment as well as the actual exercise movement. The Personal Trainer continually observes and evaluates the client performing every exercise and each repetition of it (11). Only with effective observation of the client's movement can the Personal Trainer accurately evaluate the client's performance.

➤ *Evaluation.* The evaluation system introduced in Chapter 18 can be used to determine a grade for the client's performance. Based on this system, only when a client is able to perform an entire set correctly, consisting of 15 repetitions, at a grade of 90% or above, may the Personal Trainer progress a client to a new exercise movement using that same muscle group.

➤ *Feedback.* Using clear and uncomplicated terms, the Personal Trainer can then tell the client, or provide feedback, about how well the client performed the movement. The Personal Trainer should mention one to three positive things that the client did correctly, followed by one to three points that need improving. Pointing out too many negative points all at once can destroy the client's motivation. The Personal Trainer should focus on the point that the client is capable of improving first and needs to work on first to bring the exercise one step closer to being mastered. One small step at a time builds client confidence and, in the end, ability.

Anticipating Your First Client

The education-based Personal Trainer makes an effort to anticipate and answer certain key questions before starting a training session, especially when the Personal Trainer is new to personal training. Asking and answering the following questions helps to prepare the Personal Trainer with the basic information needed to begin a training program successfully. The questions that Personal Trainers should to be able to answer before training (or educating) a client include:

➤ What kind of teaching approach will I take?

➤ What established methods of instructions will I prepare and implement?

➤ What will I do to make each client's training session efficient, effective, and engaging?

➤ How will I establish achievable goals for my clients?

➤ How will I demonstrate and teach an exercise movement to my client?

➤ How will I organize and structure my client's practice session?

➤ What observation, evaluation, and feedback tools will I use to assess and teach a client's required skill level?

➤ How will I measure outcomes and the quality of my client's learning experience?

When these questions can be answered effectively, the Personal Trainer is ready to meet the client. Such preparation will increase the Personal Trainer's self-confidence and give the client the confidence that the Personal Trainer is informed, reliable, and responsible. This will increase the Personal Trainer's and the client's ability to work as an effective exercise and fitness team.

SIX STEPS TO BECOMING AN EDUCATION-BASED PERSONAL TRAINER (12)

Personal Trainers, like teachers, are in the business of helping people change behavior through learning and training experiences. Personal Trainers need to know the principles of exercise science to design effective exercise programs. Personal Trainers also need to have a solid understanding of the science of teaching so they know how to design the training program and deliver it in a way that is effective for the client (the learner). The following six steps presented below will prepare individuals to be effective Personal Trainers and educators over the course of their careers.

Step One: Personal Trainers need to view themselves as teachers who provide strategies and support for the improvement of exercise design, the incorporation of adult learning principles into the client's program, and the management and planning of sequential training sessions based on the client's learning abilities, knowledge, and goals.

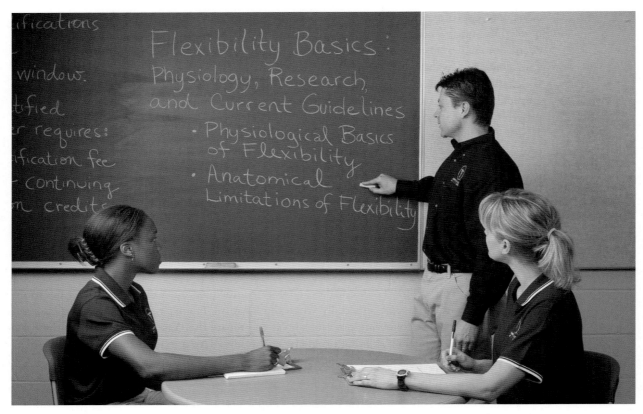

FIGURE 5.5. ACSM Certified Personal Trainer^{SM} learning skills to become better education-based Personal Trainers.

Step Two: Personal Trainers need to seek improvement of their own teaching and delivery style. A Personal Trainer who makes a conscious effort to study, learn, and practice tried and tested as well as new adult learning models can continue to develop teaching and communication skills to deliver successful instruction to the client.

Step Three: Personal Trainers develop observation, evaluation, and feedback strategies necessary for the improved teaching and learning outcomes of clients. Incorporate educational opportunities to assist Personal Trainers in evaluating the exercise program and effectively measuring objectives and providing proper feedback to help clients achieve their objective and improve their performance.

Step Four: Personal Trainers inspire, encourage, and motivate their students to learn new information and develop healthy behavior patterns (13). Think creatively and be aware of your client's individual goals so that you can think of ways to inspire the client to succeed.

Step Five: Personal Trainers should focus on finding new ways to integrate teaching, mentoring, and leadership skills into the profession by being role models for others seeking careers as Personal Trainers.

Step Six: Personal Trainers should continue learning the exercise sciences and keep up to date with trends in the industry and new exercise techniques (*Fig. 5.5*).

SUMMARY

The better the Personal Trainer teaches information, the more the client's skill level will improve. Personal Trainers, as well as their clients, benefit greatly when the Personal Trainers work on improving teaching and communication skills. The application of the VAK learning preferences in conjunction with learning strategies and techniques allows the Personal Trainer to develop an informed perspective on the client's approach to learning. By designing the client's exercise program in conjunction with a practical understanding of the client's learning characteristics, the Personal Trainer can significantly enhance the client's ability to succeed in his or her training program. The well-prepared exercise demonstration is a highly recommended tool in fitness training that Personal Trainers need to learn and incorporate into their sessions. With practiced communication skills, methods to understand a client's individual learning styles, and well-prepared demonstrations of exercise movements, the Personal Trainer becomes a skilled educator who can effectively teach the science of fitness and exercise.

REFERENCES

1. Kroehnert G. Barriers to effective communication. In: Bourma C, ed. Basic Training for Trainers. Dubuque, IA: McGraw-Hill, 1994.
2. Covey S. The 8th Habit. New York: Free Press, 2004.
3. Magill RA. Demonstrations and verbal instructions. In: Malinee V, Seely C, eds. Motor Learning and Control. New York: McGraw-Hill, 2001.
4. Schmidt R, Wrisberg C. Facilitating learning and performance. In: Wright J, Park J, Alexander L, eds. Motor Learning and Performance. 3rd ed. Champaign, IL: Human Kinetics, 2004.
5. Russell L. Learning to take more in. In: Holt M, Ullius D, eds. The Accelerated Learning Field Book. San Francisco: Jossey-Bass, 1999
6. Rothenberg B, Why does it work? In: Frey R, Curry A, Giles E, eds. Touch Training for Strength. Champaign. IL: Human Kinetics, 1995.
7. Kroehnert G. Demonstrating a skill. In Bourma C, eds. Basic Training for Trainers. Dubuque, IA: McGraw-Hill, 1994.
8. Schmidt R, Wrisberg C. Supplementing the learning experience. In: Wright J, Park J, Alexander L, eds. Motor Learning and Performance. 3rd ed. Champaign, IL: Human Kinetics, 2004.
9. Schmidt R.,Wrisberg C. Providing feedback during the learning experience. In Wright J, Park J, Alexander L, eds. Motor Learning and Performance. 3rd ed. Champaign: Human Kinetics, 2004.
10. Schmidt R, Wrisberg C. Structuring the learning experience. In Wright J, Park J, Alexander L, eds. Motor Learning and Performance. 3rd ed. Champaign, IL: Human Kinetics, 2004.
11. Wuest D, Bucher C. Biomechanical foundations. In: Malinee V, Seely C, eds. Foundations of Physical Education, Exercise Science, and Sport. 14th ed. New York: McGraw-Hill, 2003.
12. Farquharson A. Helping through Teaching: Enhancing Professional Practice. Teaching in Practice: How Professionals Can Work Effectively with Clients, Patients, and Colleagues. San Francisco: Jossey-Bass, 1995.
13. Knowles MS, Holton EF, Swanson RA. Theories of Teaching. The Adult Learner. Houston, TX: Gulf Publishing, 1998.

Learning the Foundations of Exercise Science and Important Related Disciplines

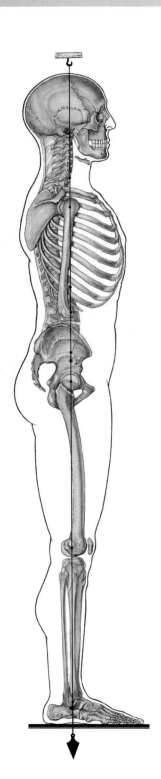

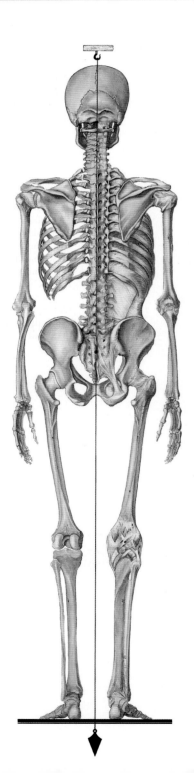

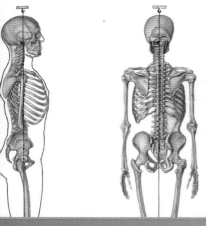

Exercise Physiology

Stanley Sai-chuen Hui, Ed.D., FACSM, FAAHPERD, Associate Professor, Department of Sports Science and Physical Education, The Chinese University of Hong Kong, Shatin, N.T., Hong Kong, China

Chapter Outline

Objectives

- Provide fundamental background about the biological structure of the human body
- Introduce the physiological mechanism of various systems of the body and how they relate to exercise training
- Identify key elements that the body reacts and adapts to exercise stimulus so that effective exercise training can be prescribed

A thorough understanding of exercise physiology is essential to the success of a Personal Trainer. A solid foundation in exercise physiology principles is important for the Personal Trainer to prescribe appropriate exercise training programs to clients and to explain the rationale, process, and effects of the program for improving fitness. The Personal Trainer needs to provide brief and precise explanations about the physiological mechanisms involved in the activities and do so in a professional manner. During physical training, the exercise stimulation acts on a human body, creating significant physiological changes. Understanding these physiological changes and mechanisms allows a Personal Trainer to better understand the exercise and movement that has been prescribed to a client so that effective training that is safe and appropriate can be achieved. In this chapter, we attempt to introduce some basic but essential concepts of exercise physiology. Specifically, various biological systems such as the cardiovascular system, respiratory system, energy system, muscular and skeletal systems, and neurological system and their roles during exercise performance are presented.

OVERVIEW OF EXERCISE PHYSIOLOGY

Among the various disciplines in exercise science, exercise physiology perhaps is one of the most important for fitness professionals. Since exercise physiology is the study of the mechanism and effects of exercise on the body, it is important to enable a Personal Trainer to prescribe safe and effective exercise for improving physical function and fitness. Exercise physiology takes into account the effects of exercise on various systems of the body, such as the cardiovascular or circulatory systems, respiration, muscles and bones, and the nervous system. These systems work together interactively to respond to an exercise stimulus, so that an efficient and effective exercise outcome is produced. The Personal Trainer needs to understand all aspects of the body and the interaction of these systems as well as the nature of the exercise stimulus given to the body. For example, when a Personal Trainer needs to prescribe an exercise to improve the quadriceps muscles, knowledge of muscular structure would allow the Personal Trainer to identify the correct location and action associated with that muscle group. Then, the understanding of muscular contraction would allow the Personal Trainer to determine the appropriate types of exercise for the quadriceps. Knowledge of energy metabolism and adaptation of the muscle would allow the Personal Trainer to determine the suitable frequency, duration, and intensity of the exercise training.

Another example is the exercise prescription for a weight loss program. The important concept of energy metabolism allows a Personal Trainer to determine the appropriate type of exercise that is oxidative in nature and uses fat as the major energy source. The efficiency of such fat-burning mechanisms relies on the effectiveness of the cardiovascular system in maintaining blood circulation and the respiratory system in maximizing blood oxygenation. Understanding factors that limit or enhance these systems would allow a Personal Trainer to adjust the exercise training program as needed. Today, because of the rapid advances in technology and research, the depth and breadth of knowledge in exercise physiology is growing rapidly. Many of the more traditional beliefs of physiological concepts are being challenged, and new ideas and concepts are being generated every year. A Personal Trainer not only needs to master the foundations in all aspects of exercise physiology, but also needs to pay attention to the development of current concepts of exercise physiology, to be a capable fitness professional of the 21st century.

DEFINITION OF EXERCISE PHYSIOLOGY

Exercise physiology is the study of the body's responses and its adaptation to the stress of exercise. Exercise physiology involves the scientific study of how exercise alters human systemic and cellular physiology both during and immediately after exercise, as well as in response to exercise training (1). Both the immediate (acute) and long-term (chronic) effects of exercise on all aspects of body function are fundamental concerns in exercise physiology. Many systems (muscular, skeletal, energy, cardiovascular) do not work independently but interactively to create the most efficient and effective responses to exercise demands.

CARDIOVASCULAR SYSTEM

The study of cardiovascular exercise physiology is one of the more prominent subdisciplines of exercise physiology. It examines how oxygen and other important nutrients are transported by the cardiovascular system and used by the muscles during exercise. The cardiovascular system consists of the heart and the blood vessels. There are more than 60,000 miles (96,000 km) of blood vessels in the body, which originate from and terminate at the heart and are structured in a continuous closed circuit (2). The primary purpose of the cardiovascular system is to deliver nutrients to and remove metabolic waste products from the tissues. The cardiovascular system assists with maintenance of normal function at rest and during exercise. The cardiovascular system performs the following specific functions (3):

1. Transports deoxygenated blood from the heart to the lungs and oxygenated blood from the lungs to the heart
2. Transports oxygenated blood from the heart to tissues and deoxygenated blood from the tissues to the heart
3. Distributes nutrients (e.g., glucose, free fatty acids, amino acids) to cells
4. Removes metabolic wastes (e.g., carbon dioxide, urea, lactate) from the periphery for elimination or reuse
5. Regulates pH to control acidosis and alkalosis
6. Transports hormones and enzymes to regulate physiological function
7. Maintains fluid balance to prevent dehydration
8. Maintains body temperature by absorbing and redistributing heat

The Heart

Figure 6.1 shows the anatomy of the heart. The heart is positioned at an angle within the chest cavity with the larger left ventricle (LV) pointed toward the left foot. It is anterior to (in front of) the thoracic vertebral column and posterior to (behind) the sternum. The lungs flank the heart on both sides and slightly overlap it. The heart has four chambers. The two upper chambers are the atria and the two lower chambers are the ventricles. The external deep grooves of the heart (called sulci) define the boundaries of the four chambers of the heart (4). The coronary sulcus separates the atria from the ventricles; the interventricular sulcus separates the LV and the right ventricle (RV). The sulci also contain the major arteries and veins that provide circulation to the heart.

The heart has a base and an apex. The base consists mainly of the left atrium (LA), the right atrium (RA), and parts of the proximal portion of the large veins that enter the heart from behind. It is located above and close to the right sternal border at the level of the second and third ribs. The apex of the heart is located below the base at the level of the fifth intercostal space.

Tissue Coverings and Layers of the Heart

The heart is covered by a double-walled, loose-fitting membranous sac called the pericardium. The outer wall of the pericardium has both a fibrous (tough) layer and a serous (smooth) layer.

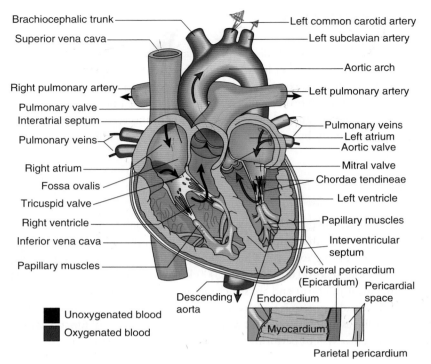

FIGURE 6.1. Anatomy of the heart and direction of blood flow. (From Smeltzer SCO, Bare BG. Brunner and Suddarth's Textbook of Medical-Surgical Nursing. 9th ed. Philadelphia: Lippincott Williams & Wilkins, 2002.)

The interior lining of the heart is the epicardium. The thickest layer of tissue in the heart is the myocardium. The myocardium is the cardiac muscle. Within the myocardium is a network of criss-crossing connective tissue fibers, called the fibrous skeleton, separating the atria from the ventricles. This skeleton provides support for the myocardium and the valves of the heart.

Chambers, Valves, and Blood Flow of the Heart

The heart is two pumps in a single unit with four chambers, or cavities. The right heart (RA and RV) and the left heart (LA and LV) make up the two pumps. The right side of the heart collects deoxygenated blood from the periphery and pumps it through the lungs (pulmonary circuit). The left side of the heart collects blood from the lungs and pumps it throughout the body (systemic circuit) (5).

The heart has four valves whose function is to maintain blood flow in one direction. The atrioventricular (AV) valves separate the atria from the ventricles. The semilunar valves separate the ventricles from the aorta and pulmonary artery. The right AV valve has three cusps and is called the tricuspid valve, while the left AV valve has only two cusps and is called the mitral (or bicuspid) valve. The tricuspid valve controls the flow of blood from the RA to the RV, while the mitral valve controls blood between the LA and LV. The chordae tendineae and papillary muscles help the AV valves stay closed, preventing them from swinging back into the atria, which would result in reversed blood flow (6).

There are two semilunar valves in the heart. The pulmonic valve lies between the RV and the pulmonary artery. The aortic valve is between the LV and the aorta. The cusps of the semilunar valves prevent the backflow of blood to the ventricles. Blood flow through the heart is accomplished by the following sequence of events, beginning with the return of systemic blood from the body to the RA:

1. Deoxygenated blood flows into the RA through the superior and inferior vena cavae, the coronary sinus, and anterior cardiac veins.
2. The RA contracts, and blood moves through the tricuspid valve into the RV.

3. The RV contracts, the tricuspid valve closes, and blood flows through the pulmonic valve into the pulmonary arteries and the branches of the respiratory system.
4. Blood enters the alveolar capillaries from the pulmonary arteries, where gas exchange occurs. Oxygen is absorbed and carbon dioxide is removed.
5. Blood flows back to the LA through the pulmonary veins.
6. The LA contracts, and blood flows through the mitral valve and into the LV.
7. The LV contracts, the mitral valve closes, and blood flows through the aortic valve into the aorta and its branches, where it is distributed to the coronary circulation and the systemic circulation (6).

Cardiac muscle has unique properties that allow it to contract without an external nervous system impulse. The components of the heart's conduction system include the sinoatrial (SA) node, atrioventricular (AV) node, AV bundle (bundle of His), right and left bundle branches, and the Purkinje fibers. The electrical impulse, which initiates cardiac contraction, begins at the SA node (the intrinsic pacemaker) of the heart. The electrical impulse is delayed at the AV node for approximately 0.13 seconds to allow the atria to contract and fill the ventricles with blood. The impulse then moves rapidly through the bundle of His, through the right and left bundle branches, and through the network of Purkinje fibers in the myocardium of both ventricles. This rapid conduction allows the two ventricles to contract at approximately the same time.

The Blood Vessels

After blood flows from the heart, it enters the vascular system, which is composed of numerous blood vessels. The blood vessels form a closed system to deliver blood to the tissues; help promote the exchange of nutrients, metabolic wastes, hormones, and other substances with cells; and return blood to the heart. Arteries carry blood away from the heart. Large arteries branch into smaller arteries and eventually to smaller arterioles. Arterioles branch into capillaries, which allow the exchange of blood and other nutrients with various tissues (e.g., digestive system, liver, kidneys). On the venous side of the circulation, capillaries converge into small venules, which converge to form larger vessels called veins. The largest veins return blood to the heart.

Arterioles play a major role in regulating blood flow to the capillaries because of their ability to vasoconstrict (narrow the opening of the blood vessel) or vasodilate (widen the opening of the blood vessel). Capillaries form dense networks that branch throughout all tissues. The average capillary is 1 mm in length and 0.01 mm in diameter. This is just large enough for a single red blood cell to pass through (7). Capillaries have extremely thin walls and are the site of exchange of nutrients between blood and the interstitial fluid. Veins receive blood from the venules. In general, the veins are thinner and more compliant than arteries and act as blood reservoirs. The walls of some veins, such as those in the legs, contain one-way valves that help maintain venous return to the heart by preventing backward blood flow even under relatively low pressures.

Cardiac Function

HEART RATE

Heart rate (HR) is the number of heart beats per minute. The average normal resting HR is approximately 60–80 beats per minute (bpm). The resting HR in women is typically 10 bpm higher than that in men. Children have higher HRs than adults, while elderly people have lower HRs. In the same age group and gender, fit individuals have a lower resting HR than do unfit individuals because of a larger stroke volume of the heart as a result of exercise training, so that the heart does not have to pump as many times as before to maintain the same cardiac output (8). HR can be measured by counting the number of pulses over a given time period.

BLOOD PRESSURE

The heart is an autonomic organ that contracts and relaxes alternatively throughout life. When the left ventricle of the heart muscle contracts, a surge of blood is propelled into the aorta and arteries. The pressure being exerted on the arterial wall during contraction is the systolic pressure (SBP), whereas the pressure during the relaxation phase of the ventricles is termed diastolic pressure (DBP). An average resting blood pressure is 120 mm Hg for SBP and 80 mm Hg for DBP. When the SBP persistently exceeds 140 mm Hg or the DBP exceeds 90 mm Hg at rest, a medical condition known as hypertension may present.

STROKE VOLUME

The amount of blood ejected from the LV in a single contraction is called the stroke volume (SV). SV is equal to the difference between the end-diastolic volume (EDV) and end-systolic volume (ESV). EDV and ESV are the total volume of blood in the ventricles at the end of diastole and systole, respectively. In an upright posture, SV is lower in untrained than in trained individuals. The SV of men is usually greater than that of women because of their larger heart size. SV is also sensitive to body position. In the supine or prone postures, SV increases.

CARDIAC OUTPUT

Cardiac output ($\dot{Q}$) is the volume of blood pumped by the heart per minute and is calculated by multiplying the HR by the SV. The resting $\dot{Q}$ for adults, both trained and untrained, is approximately 4 to 5 liters per minute. However, the maximal $\dot{Q}$ is higher in trained than in untrained individuals.

Measuring Pulses

Exercise professionals often measure peripheral pulses to obtain an index of resting HR or exercise HR. Large, superficial (close to the surface) arteries are preferred for pulse determination because they are easily palpable (easy to locate and feel). The most common palpation sites are the radial, brachial, and carotid arteries.

RADIAL PULSE

The radial artery is located on the lateral (thumb side) aspect of the forearm and becomes superficial near the distal head of the radius (9) near the wrist. Gently pressing the first two fingers over this region palpates the radial pulse. Figure 6.2 illustrates this location. Radial pulses may be difficult to obtain in individuals with large amounts of subcutaneous fat over the palpation site.

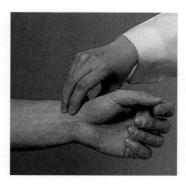

FIGURE 6.2. Radial pulse used to assess heart rate. (From Bickley LS, Szilagyi P. Bates' Guide to Physical Examination and History Taking. 8th ed. Philadelphia: Lippincott Williams & Wilkins, 2003.)

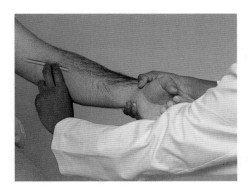

FIGURE 6.3. Palpation of the brachial pulse. (From Bickley LS, Szilagyi P. Bates' Guide to Physical Examination and History Taking. 8th ed. Philadelphia: Lippincott Williams & Wilkins, 2003.)

BRACHIAL PULSE

The brachial artery is located through a groove formed between the triceps and biceps brachii muscles on the medial aspect (inside) of the arm anterior to the elbow. It should be palpated with the first two fingers in the medial part of this groove. See Figure 6.3 for an indication of location.

CAROTID PULSE

The right and left common carotid arteries are located on the anterior portion of the neck in the groove formed by the larynx and the sternocleidomastoid muscles (large muscles on the lateral sides of the neck) just below the lower jaw (9). Figure 6.4 illustrates the location. The carotid pulse is taken by placing the first two fingers in the groove and pressing gently inward. Take care when using this site, since baroreceptors in the carotid sinus may be sensitive to pressure and result in a dramatic reduction in HR in some individuals (10). Baroreceptors are sensory nerve endings that are stimulated by changes in pressure and are found in the walls of the atria of the heart, vena cavae, aortic arch, and carotid sinus. In extreme cases, blood flow may be occluded to the point that lightheadedness or fainting may occur. This is probably a concern mainly when taking the pulse immediately after exercise, less so at rest or during physical activity (11).

TAKING PULSES

To obtain a pulse rate, the following can be done:

1. Locate a pulse with the index and third finger of one hand.
2. Count the number of pulsations in a given time period.
3. For the highest precision, if timing is initiated simultaneously with a pulsation, this first pulsation is counted as 0. If a second person is keeping time or if there is lag between the initiation of timing and the first pulsation that is felt, the first pulse is counted as 1.

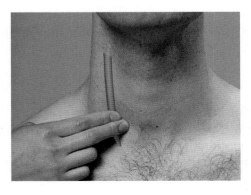

FIGURE 6.4. The carotid pulse. (From Bickley LS, Szilagyi P. Bates' Guide to Physical Examination and History Taking. 8th ed. Philadelphia: Lippincott Williams & Wilkins, 2003.)

4. To determine the pulse rate in beats per minute, multiply the number of pulse beats by the number of counting intervals in 1 minute.

    10 seconds = 6 intervals (multiply pulse beats by 6)

    15 seconds = 4 intervals

    20 seconds = 3 intervals

    30 seconds = 2 intervals

The number of seconds a pulse is counted depends on the purpose of the pulse count and the degree of accuracy needed. For instance, during a 6-second pulse count, an error of one beat translates to an error of 10 beats per minute (bpm); during a 10-second count, a one-beat error equals a 6-bpm error; and during a 15-second count, a one-beat error means a 4-bpm error. At rest and during exercise, 15-second pulse counts are advisable, although it is difficult to obtain a pulse count during many forms of exercise. Therefore, the exerciser may have to stop and take a pulse immediately post-exercise. Because heart rates decrease quickly after exercise, a 6-second or 10-second pulse count is suggested. Heart rate monitors are commonly used and can be helpful in training, particularly for those desiring frequent, immediate feedback regarding exercise heart rate.

Acute Response to Cardiovascular Exercise

Many mechanisms function collectively to support the increased aerobic requirements of physical activity. The overall effect of changes in HR, SV, $\dot{Q}$, blood flow, blood pressure, arteriovenous oxygen difference, and pulmonary ventilation is to supply oxygenated blood that is delivered to the active tissues. As exercise intensity increases, oxygen consumption and carbon dioxide production by working muscles increase. The cardiorespiratory system is required to deliver oxygen to, and transport carbon dioxide from, these tissues in an attempt to maintain cellular homeostasis. The central nervous system responds by increasing neural ventilatory and cardiac drive, resulting in increased activity of cardiac and respiratory muscles.

The lungs are largely passive, and the increased ventilatory and cardiac drives result in increasing blood and air flow and increased rate of transfer of oxygen and carbon dioxide across the gas-exchanging surfaces of the alveoli. However, limits to the degree to which increased air flow and blood flow can be supported can lead to pulmonary limitations to exercise either from mechanical ventilatory constraints or from compromised gas exchange. These limitations are generally not manifested in healthy individuals except in elite or older athletes.

HEART RATE

HR increases in a linear fashion with the work rate and oxygen uptake during dynamic exercise. The magnitude of the HR response is related to age, body position, fitness, type of activity, presence of heart disease, medications, blood volume, and environmental factors such as temperature and humidity. In contrast to SBP, which usually increases with age, maximum attainable HR decreases with age. The equation max HR = 220 − age provides an approximation of the maximum HR in healthy men and women, but the variance for any fixed age is considerable (standard deviation ∼ ±10 bpm) (12).

STROKE VOLUME

During exercise, SV increases curvilinearly with the work rate until it reaches a near-maximal level equivalent to approximately 40–50% of aerobic capacity, increasing only slightly thereafter (13). When SV reaches maximum, the increase in oxygen demand is met by increasing the HR. At a higher HR, SV may actually decrease because of the disproportionate shortening of diastolic filling time (12) in the heart.

CARDIAC OUTPUT

$\dot{Q}$ in healthy adults increases linearly with increased work rate. However, maximum values of $\dot{Q}$ depend on many factors, including age, posture, body size, presence of cardiovascular disease, and the level of physical conditioning. At exercise intensities up to 50% of maximum, the increase in $\dot{Q}$ is facilitated by increases in HR and SV (13). Thereafter, the increase results almost solely from the continued rise in HR.

ARTERIOVENOUS OXYGEN DIFFERENCE (a-$\bar{v}$ O$_2$ DIFFERENCE)

Oxygen extraction by tissues reflects the difference between oxygen content of arterial blood and the oxygen content of venous blood, yielding a typical a-$\bar{v}$ O$_2$ difference at rest of 5 mL O$_2$ · dL^{-1} of blood. This approximates a use coefficient of approximately 25%. During exercise to exhaustion, the mixed venous oxygen content typically decreases to 5 mL O$_2$ · dL^{-1} of blood or less, thus widening the a-$\bar{v}$ O$_2$ difference from 5 to 15 mL O$_2$ · dL^{-1} of blood, corresponding to a use coefficient of 75% (13).

BLOOD FLOW

At rest, 15–20% of the $\dot{Q}$ is distributed to the skeletal muscles; the remainder goes to visceral organs, the heart, and the brain (14). However, during exercise, as much as 85–90% of the $\dot{Q}$ is selectively delivered to working muscles and shunted away from the skin and the splanchnic, hepatic, and renal vascular beds. Myocardial blood flow may increase four to five times with exercise, whereas blood supply to the brain is maintained at resting levels (15).

BLOOD PRESSURE

There is a linear increase in SBP with increasing levels of exercise. Maximal values typically reach 190–220 mm Hg (16). Nevertheless, maximal SBP should not exceed 250 mm Hg (17). DBP may decrease slightly or remain unchanged. This is due to the decrease in peripheral resistance caused by the vasodilation of arterioles in the active muscles during exercise (18). An SBP that fails to rise or falls with increasing work loads may signal a plateau or decrease in $\dot{Q}$ (19). Exercise testing should be terminated in persons demonstrating exertional hypotension (a decreasing SBP).

MAXIMAL OXYGEN CONSUMPTION

The most widely recognized measure of cardiopulmonary fitness is the aerobic capacity, or $\dot{V}O_{2max}$. This variable is defined physiologically as the highest rate of oxygen transport and use that can be achieved at maximal physical exertion. Oxygen consumption ($\dot{V}O_2$) may be expressed mathematically by a rearrangement of the Fick equation (5):

$$\dot{V}O_2 \text{ (mL} \cdot \text{kg}^{-1} \cdot \text{min}^{-1}) = \text{HR (bpm)} \times \text{SV (mL} \cdot \text{beat}^{-1}) \times (\text{a-}\bar{v} \text{ O}_2 \text{ diff)}$$

Thus, it is apparent that both central (i.e., $\dot{Q}$) and peripheral (i.e., a-$\bar{v}$ O$_2$ diff) regulatory mechanisms affect the magnitude of $\dot{V}O_2$. $\dot{V}O_{2max}$ may be expressed on an absolute or relative basis. Absolute $\dot{V}O_{2max}$ usually uses the units of "liters per minute," reflecting total body energy output and caloric expenditure (i.e., 1 L $\approx$ 5 kcal), and does not account for differences in body weight. Relative $\dot{V}O_{2max}$ divides the absolute $\dot{V}O_{2max}$ value by body weight in kilograms (and is typically reported in mL · kg^{-1} · min^{-1}, or METs). Because large persons usually have larger absolute $\dot{V}O_2$ by virtue of a larger muscle mass, the latter expression allows a more equitable comparison between individuals of different body masses. This measure is widely considered the single best index of physical work capacity or cardiorespiratory fitness (20). In terms of cardiovascular fitness, the larger the $\dot{V}O_{2max}$, the better.

RESPIRATORY SYSTEM

The respiratory system consists of the nose, nasal cavity, pharynx, larynx, trachea, bronchial tree, and the lungs. The primary function of the respiratory system is to filter air that enters the body and allow for gas exchange within microscopic air sacs in the lungs called alveoli. The structure of the respiratory system is illustrated in Figure 6.5. The lungs are situated inside the chest cavity above the diaphragm and are protected by the ribs and pectoral muscles. The lungs are enclosed by a set of membranes called pleura. The breathing mechanism of the lungs is passively controlled by the involuntary movements of the respiratory muscles and diaphragm. The pressure inside the pleura cavity (intrapleural pressure) is less than atmospheric pressure and becomes even lower during inspiration, causing air to inflate the lungs, and prevents the collapse of the fragile air sacs within the lung. These pressure differences reverse during exhalation.

Control of Breathing

Respiratory muscles lack the ability to regulate their own contractions; therefore, the control of breathing in an awake person results from the interplay of brainstem and other respiratory pathways (21). Autonomic control structures are located in the brainstem, and voluntary control structures are located in the cerebral cortex of the brain.

Distribution of Ventilation

Ventilation of the pulmonary system is accomplished in two major divisions, the upper and lower respiratory tracts, illustrated in Figure 6.5.

UPPER RESPIRATORY TRACT

The upper respiratory tract, which includes the nose, sinuses, pharynx, and larynx, acts as a conduction pathway for the movement of air into the lower respiratory tract. The function of these

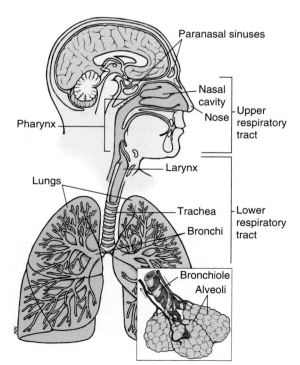

FIGURE 6.5. The structures of the respiratory system (anterior view). (From Stedman's Medical Dictionary. 27th ed. Baltimore: Lippincott Williams & Wilkins, 2000.)

structures is to purify, warm, and humidify air before it reaches the gas exchange units. During normal quiet breathing, inspired air is heated to body temperature, and the relative humidity is increased to more than 90% during passage through the nose.

The pharynx is divided by the soft palate into the nasopharynx and the oropharynx. The epiglottis, located at the base of the tongue, protects the laryngeal opening during swallowing. The larynx contains the vocal cords, which contribute to speech and participate in coughing. Receptors throughout the upper respiratory tract may initiate a cough response. Coughing is produced by closure of the vocal cords along with contraction of the expiratory muscles to create increased intrathoracic (within the chest cavity) pressures. With sudden opening of the vocal cords, the positive airway pressure forces into the atmosphere air carrying any mucus or particles from the tracheobronchial tree. A cough can move gas from the lung at rates up to $10 \ L \cdot s^{-1}$ during the expulsion phase.

LOWER RESPIRATORY TRACT

The lower respiratory tract begins in the trachea just below the larynx and includes the bronchi, bronchioles, and alveoli (*Fig. 6.6*). There are approximately 23 generations (divisions) of airways; the first 16 are conducting airways, and the last 7 are respiratory airways ending blindly in approximately 300 million alveoli, which form the gas exchange surface. The structural components of the airways coincide with their functional properties. For example, the volume of the conducting zone is approximately 1 mL of air per pound of body weight and does not contribute to gas exchange, whereas gas exchange areas occupy a proportionately greater volume in the lungs. The trachea begins at the base of the neck and extends approximately 4–4.5 inches (10–12 cm) before it divides into the right and left main bronchi. It is anterior to the esophagus. The trachea consists of a series of anterior horseshoe-shaped cartilaginous rings and a posterior longitudinal muscle bundle.

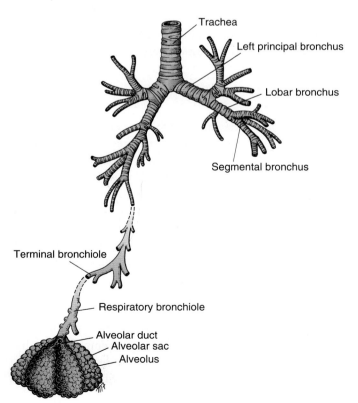

Trachea

Left principal bronchus

Lobar bronchus

Segmental bronchus

Terminal bronchiole

Respiratory bronchiole

Alveolar duct
Alveolar sac
Alveolus

FIGURE 6.6. Trachea, bronchi, bronchioles, alveolar ducts, alveolar sacs, and alveoli. Note the path taken by inspired air from the trachea to the alveoli. (From Snell RS. Clinical Anatomy. 7th ed. Baltimore: Lippincott Williams & Wilkins, 2003.)

The major bronchi contain cartilage that keeps the airway open as well as large numbers of mucous glands that produce secretions in response to irritation, infection, and/or inflammation. In the large airway, irritant receptors initiate the cough reflex when stimulated. The right main bronchus divides into three lobar bronchi: upper, middle, and lower. The left main bronchus divides into two lobar bronchi, upper and lower. Fissures separate the two lobes with two layers of visceral pleura. The lobar bronchi divide into segmental bronchi and segments, 10 on the right and 10 on the left.

Columnar cells lining the epithelium (inner lining) of the bronchi consist predominantly of ciliated cells that contain motile cilia, which move or beat in a coordinated manner to move the mucous layer toward the mouth ("mucociliary escalator"). The columnar epithelium is an important barrier for lung defense. Goblet cells interspersed among the ciliated cells secrete mucus. Segmental bronchi divide further into the terminal bronchioles, which have a diameter of about 1 mm. Beyond the terminal bronchioles are respiratory bronchioles, alveolar ducts, and the alveoli. Air flows through the conducting airways and at the level of the alveolar ducts and alveoli. Movement of air or gas is by diffusion.

Ventilatory Pump

The ventilatory pump consists of the chest wall, the respiratory muscles, and the pleural space.

CHEST WALL

The chest wall includes muscles of respiration (primarily intercostal muscles) and bones (spine, ribs, sternum). The ribs are hinged on the spine by ligaments and cartilage so that the ribs move upward and outward during inspiration and downward and inward during expiration. The hinging movement results in a change in thoracic volume and pressures. At rest and at the end of a normal expiration the elastic properties of the chest wall exert an outward (expansion) force, whereas the elastic properties of the lung structures exert an inward (recoil) force. Inspiration (airflow into the lungs) occurs by activation of the respiratory muscles, particularly the diaphragm, which creates a more negative pressure in the pleural space and the lungs than that in the atmosphere. Air enters the lungs until the intrapulmonary gas pressure equals atmospheric pressure. During expiration, when the respiratory muscles relax, air flows from the lung into the atmosphere because of the positive pressure generated by the elastic recoil of the lungs.

RESPIRATORY MUSCLES

The muscles of respiration are the only skeletal muscles essential to life. The diaphragm, the major muscle of inspiration, is innervated by the phrenic nerve, which originates from the third to fifth cervical spinal segments. Spinal cord transection as a result of injury at or above this level compromises respiratory muscle function and consequently ventilation. An illustration of the role of the diaphragm in breathing is displayed in Figure 6.7. The diaphragm consists of a flattened centralized portion and vertical muscles called the costal portion. The diaphragm functions as a piston, with contraction and relaxation of the vertical muscle fibers. With contraction, the crural portion, or dome, moves downward and displaces the abdominal contents so that the abdomen moves outward, as does the chest wall. Expiration is normally passive under quiet breathing because of elastic recoil of the lung; it requires no work and is therefore passive. However, during active breathing, when ventilatory requirements are increased (e.g., during exercise), the muscles of expiration are recruited. The major muscles of expiration are the internal intercostals and the abdominal muscles (rectus abdominis, external and internal oblique, and transverse abdominis). In clients with airflow obstruction (e.g., acute bronchoconstriction in asthma or emphysema), hyperinflation of the lungs stretches the lung tissue and leads to additional elastic recoil, forcing the crural portion of the diaphragm downward and shortening the vertical muscle fibers. This impairs the diaphragm's ability to contract.

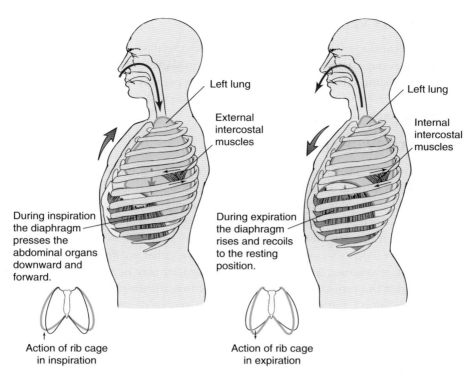

FIGURE 6.7. Mechanics of normal—not deep, not shallow—inspiration *(left)* and expiration *(right)*. (From Weber J, Kelley J. Health Assessment in Nursing. 2nd ed. Philadelphia: Lippincott Williams & Wilkins, 2003.)

PLEURA

The visceral (inner layer) and parietal (outer layer) pleura are thin membranes between the lung and the chest wall (22). The pleural space, which lies between the visceral and parietal pleura, contains a small amount of fluid. Because the pleural space is airtight and the chest wall and lung tissue pull against each other across the pleural space, negative pressure is produced at rest. During inspiration, both the visceral and parietal pleura expand outward and more negative pressure develops in the pleural space. Air can enter the pleural space (i.e., pneumothorax) by trauma to the chest wall (e.g., a fractured rib with penetration of the parietal pleura). With a pneumothorax, the lungs collapse while the chest wall expands because of its intrinsic elastic properties. The parietal pleura contains abundant pain fibers, and irritation of this membrane by a pneumothorax or inflammation produces local chest pain exacerbated by motion of the pleura (e.g., deep inspiration).

DISTRIBUTION OF BLOOD FLOW

The lungs receive blood from the pulmonary arteries, which contain systemic venous blood from the RV and bronchial arteries. The pulmonary artery emerges from the RV and divides into the right and left main pulmonary arteries. The pulmonary arteries divide into branches corresponding to the divisions of the bronchial tree and supply the pulmonary arterioles. The pulmonary circulation is a low-pressure system with a normal mean pressure of approximately 15 mm Hg at rest. Most blood flow to the alveoli is derived from the pulmonary circulation, whereas the bronchial arteries supply the walls of the bronchi and bronchioles to the level of the alveoli. Pulmonary arterioles divide into pulmonary capillaries that form networks in the walls of the alveoli, where gas exchange occurs. The pulmonary veins carry oxygenated blood from the pulmonary capillaries. These veins converge to form the main pulmonary veins, which empty into the LA.

PULMONARY VENTILATION

Pulmonary ventilation (VE), the volume of air exchanged per minute, is approximately $6 \text{ L} \cdot \text{min}^{-1}$ at rest in the average sedentary adult male. At maximal exercise, however, VE often increases 15- to 25-fold over resting values. Pulmonary ventilation is perhaps regulated more by the requirement for carbon dioxide removal than by oxygen consumption and that ventilation is not normally a limiting factor to aerobic capacity (23).

RESPIRATORY CHANGES

Several respiratory adaptations result from physical conditioning regimens. Although ventilation generally does not limit exercise in apparently healthy individuals, the limits of ventilation may be reached at $\dot{V}O_{2max}$ in elite athletes (24). Ventilation increases linearly with $\dot{V}O_{2max}$ up to about 50% $\dot{V}O_{2max}$, after which the increase is proportionately greater than the increase in work rate (24). Physically trained persons demonstrate larger lung volumes and diffusion capacity at rest and during exercise than their sedentary counterparts. Ventilation is either unaffected or only modestly affected by cardiorespiratory training. Maximal ventilatory capacity may be increased by exercise training, but it is unclear that this provides any advantage other than increased buffering capacity for lactate. Submaximal ventilation is probably not affected, but it may be decreased in some circumstances because a decrease in the production of lactate coincides with a decrease in the need to buffer lactate, which results in decreased ventilation.

ENERGY SYSTEMS

Energy is essential to produce mechanical work, maintain body temperature, and fulfill all biological and chemical activities inside the body. To release energy, foodstuff that is consumed, particularly protein, carbohydrate, and fat, must be metabolized to yield a high-energy compound called adenosine triphosphate (ATP). In the human body, all mechanical work that involves physical activity relies on the continuous supply of ATP. The manufactured ATP is stored inside muscles so that this immediate source of energy can be used for producing movement when a stimulus is given to the muscles. The storage of ATP in the muscles, however, is limited. If ATP were the only form of energy available, mechanical movement would last for only a few seconds because of this limited storage capacity. Therefore, for movement that lasts longer than a few seconds, ATP must be furthered manufactured through the immediate breakdown of carbohydrate (in forms of glycogen and glucose inside muscle tissues).

This process of immediately breaking down muscle carbohydrate does not require the presence of oxygen and would provide an additional few minutes of ATP supply. This process is termed "anaerobic metabolism," or "anaerobic glycolysis." However, the metabolic end-product of lactate and resulting localized intramuscular acidosis limits muscular performance. Hence, anaerobic glycolysis is also called the "lactic acid system." With continuous movement lasting longer than a few minutes, the increased demand for ATP must be fulfilled by a greater capacity for energy production. Carbohydrate and fat can be broken down in the presence of oxygen, resulting in an abundant supply of ATP. This process is known as aerobic metabolism, or oxidative phosphorylation. Only two molecules of ATP can be generated from breaking down a glucose molecule in anaerobic metabolism, whereas the aerobic metabolism of a glucose molecule yields 36 ATP molecules (38 ATPs when starting with glycogen). The process of generating ATP aerobically, however, is a much slower process. The relationship between exercise duration and energy sources is illustrated in Figure 6.8.

Aerobic and Anaerobic Metabolism

The energy requirements of exercising human muscle increase substantially in the transition from rest to maximal physical exertion. Because the available stores of ATP are limited and capable of providing energy to maintain vigorous activity for only several seconds, ATP must be constantly

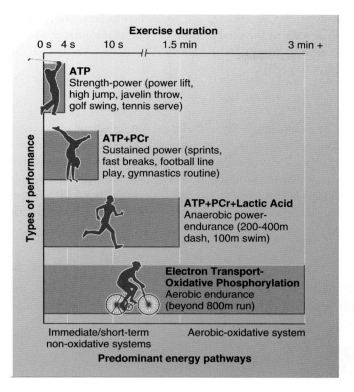

FIGURE 6.8. Comparison of activity with the energy pathways used. *ATP,* adenosine triphosphate; *PCr,* creatine phosphate; *ATP+PCr+Lactic Acid,* anaerobic glycolysis; *Electron Transport-Oxidative Phosphorylation,* aerobic oxidation. (From Premkumar K. The Massage Connection, Anatomy and Physiology. 2nd ed. Baltimore: Lippincott Williams & Wilkins, 2004.)

resynthesized to provide continuous energy production. Therefore, exercising muscle must possess a large capacity of energy to produce sufficient ATP so that increased activity can continue. Energy production relies heavily on the respiratory and cardiovascular systems for the delivery of oxygen and nutrients and for the removal of waste products to maintain the internal equilibrium of cells.

Adenosine Triphosphate (ATP)

ATP serves as the ideal energy-transfer agent that powers all of the cell's energy needs (25). The energy released through hydrolysis of the high–energy compound ATP to form adenosine diphosphate (ADP) and inorganic phosphate (Pi) powers skeletal muscle contractions. This reaction is catalyzed by the enzyme ATPase:

$$\text{ATP} \xrightarrow{\text{(ATPase)}} \text{ADP} + \text{Pi} + \text{energy}$$

The amount of ATP directly available in muscle at any time is small, so it must be resynthesized continuously if exercise lasts for more than a few seconds. Muscle fibers contain the metabolic machinery to produce ATP by three pathways: creatine phosphate (CP), anaerobic glycolysis, and aerobic oxidation of nutrients to carbon dioxide and water.

Creatine Phosphate (CP)

The CP system transfers high-energy phosphate from CP to rephosphorylate ATP from ADP (using the enzyme creatine kinase) as follows:

$$\text{ADP} + \text{CP} \xrightarrow{\text{(Creatine kinase)}} \text{ATP} + \text{C}$$

This system is rapid because it involves only one enzymatic step (i.e., one chemical reaction). How–ever, CP exists in finite quantities in cells as well, so the total amount of ATP that can be produced is limited. Oxygen is not involved in the rephosphorylation of ADP to ATP in this reaction, so the CP system is considered anaerobic (without oxygen).

Anaerobic Glycolysis

When glycolysis is rapid, it is capable of producing ATP without the involvement of oxygen. Glycolysis, the degradation of carbohydrate (glycogen or glucose) to pyruvate or lactate, involves a series of enzymatically catalyzed steps. Although glycolysis does not use oxygen and is considered anaerobic, pyruvate can readily participate in aerobic production of ATP when oxygen is available in the cell. Therefore, in addition to being an anaerobic pathway capable of producing ATP without oxygen, glycolysis can also be considered the first step in the aerobic degradation of carbohydrate (26) (*Fig. 6.9*).

Aerobic Oxidation

The final metabolic pathway for ATP production combines two complex metabolic processes, the Krebs cycle and electron transport chain residing inside the mitochondria as illustrated in Figure 6.9.

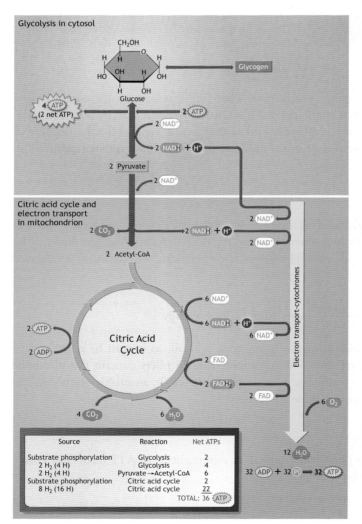

FIGURE 6.9. A net yield of 36 ATPs from energy transfer during the complete oxidation of one glucose molecule in glycolysis, the citric acid cycle, and electronic transport. (From McArdle WD, Katch FI, Katch VL. Exercise Physiology: Energy Nutrition, and Human Performance. 5th ed. Baltimore: Lippincott Williams & Wilkins, 2001.)

Oxidative phosphorylation uses oxygen as the final hydrogen acceptor to form water and ATP. Unlike glycolysis, aerobic metabolism can use fat, protein, and carbohydrate as substrates to produce ATP. Conceptually, the Krebs cycle can be considered a primer for oxidative phosphorylation. The primary function of the Krebs cycle is to remove hydrogens from four of the reactants involved in the cycle. The electrons from these hydrogens follow a chain of cytochromes (electron transport chain) in the mitochondria, and the energy released from this process is used to rephosphorylate ADP to form ATP. Oxygen is the final acceptor of hydrogen to form water, and this reaction is catalyzed by cytochrome oxidase (27). Although not all ATP is formed aerobically, the amount of ATP yielded by anaerobic glycolysis is extremely small (25). Nevertheless, anaerobic mechanisms provide a rapid source of ATP, which is particularly important at the beginning of any exercise bout and during high-intensity activity that can only be sustained for a brief period. As the duration of exercise increases, the relative contribution of anaerobic energy sources decreases (26).

The aerobic system requires adequate delivery and use of oxygen and uses glycogen, fats, and proteins as energy substrates, sustaining high rates of ATP production for muscular energy over long periods of time. The relative contributions of anaerobic and aerobic metabolism depend on oxygen exchange (respiration), delivery (cardiovascular), and use (muscular extraction) at rates commensurate with the energy demands of activity. The energy to perform most types of exercise does not come from a single source but from a combination of anaerobic and aerobic sources. The contribution of anaerobic sources (CP system and anaerobic glycolysis) to exercise energy metabolism is inversely related to the duration and intensity of the activity. The shorter and more intense the activity, the greater the contribution of anaerobic energy production. The longer the activity, however, and the lower the intensity, the greater the contribution of aerobic energy production. Although proteins can be used as a fuel for aerobic exercise, carbohydrates and fats are the primary energy substrates during exercise in a healthy, well-fed individual. In general, carbohydrates are used as the primary fuel at the onset of exercise and during high-intensity work (28). However, during prolonged exercise of low-to-moderate intensity (longer than 30 minutes), a gradual shift occurs from carbohydrate toward an increasing reliance on fat as a substrate.

Recovery from Exercise

Oxygen uptake remains elevated above resting levels for several minutes during recovery from exercise. This elevated post-exercise oxygen consumption is referred to as excess post-exercise oxygen consumption (EPOC) (29). In general, post-exercise metabolism is higher following high-intensity exercise than after light or moderate work. Furthermore, EPOC remains elevated longer after prolonged exercise than after shorter term exertion.

MUSCULAR SYSTEM

All human movements require muscular action. Muscular action is illustrated through continuous alternations of muscular contraction and relaxation. There are three major types of muscles in the body: skeletal, smooth, and cardiac. Skeletal muscle is the muscle that attaches to the skeleton so as to produce physical movements. It is also called "striated muscle" because its fibers are composed of alternating light and dark stripes. Smooth muscle is the muscle that forms the internal organs. Cardiac muscle is the muscle of the heart. Skeletal muscle is voluntary muscle because it can be controlled, for the most part, by the individual. Smooth muscle and cardiac muscle are involuntary muscle because they are controlled by the autonomic nervous system, the involuntary division of the nervous system. All three kinds of muscles possess characteristics of extendibility, elasticity, excitability, and contractility. In this chapter, the focus is placed on skeletal muscle because it is strongly related to human movement during exercise.

Skeletal Muscles

Figure 6.10 shows the structure of skeletal muscle. Individual skeletal muscles are composed of a varying number of muscle bundles referred to as "fasciculi" (an individual bundle is a fasciculus). Fasciculi are likewise covered and thus separated by the perimysium. Individual muscle fibers are enveloped by the endomysium. Immediately beneath the endomysium is the thin, membranous sarcolemma, the cell membrane that encloses the cellular contents of the muscle fiber, nuclei, local stores of fat, glucose (in the form of glycogen), enzymes, contractile proteins, and other specialized structures such as the mitochondria.

Muscle Contraction

The smallest contractile unit of a muscle cell is the sarcomere. A sarcomere is composed of two types of muscle protein called "actin" (the thin filament) and "myosin" (the thick filament). Actin contains two other components called "troponin" and "tropomyosin." Myosin contains many cross bridges. Figure 6.11 illustrates the relationship between muscle contraction and microscopic action within the sarcomere. Two major principles describe the mechanism of muscle contraction: the "sliding filament theory" and the "all-or-none principle."

The sliding filament theory describes the events that occur between the actin and myosin filaments during muscle contraction and relaxation. When a nerve impulse is received, the cross bridges of the myosin will pull the actin filaments toward the center of the sarcomere and tension is created. The sliding motion between the actin and myosin causes the shortening of a sarcomere and subsequently the entire muscle fiber. Moreover, the nerve impulse that applies to the muscle

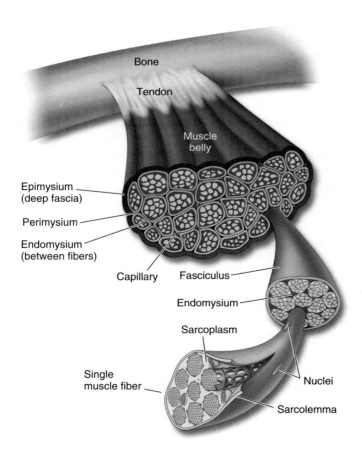

FIGURE 6.10. Macroscopic structure of skeletal muscle. (From McArdle WD, Katch FI, Katch VL. Essentials of Exercise Physiology. 2nd ed. Baltimore: Lippincott Williams & Wilkins, 2000.)

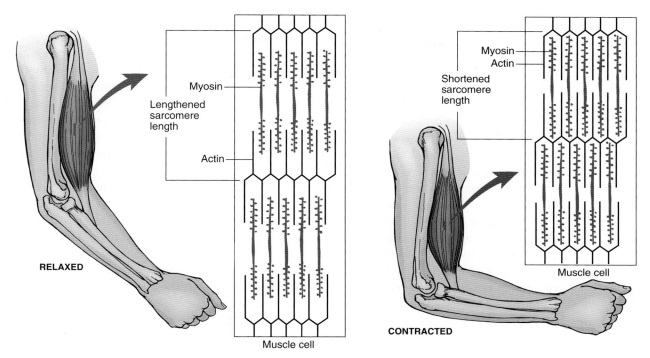

FIGURE 6.11. The sliding filament model (contraction of skeletal muscle results from the sliding of the actin chains on the myosin chains). (From Oatis CA. Kinesiology—The Mechanics and Pathomechanics of Human Movement. Baltimore: Lippincott Williams & Wilkins, 2004.)

cell, regardless of its "strength," causes the sarcomere to contract maximally or not all. This is called the all-or-none principle. The length of a muscle fiber during a contraction is determined by the number of sarcomeres being recruited for the contraction. The more sarcomeres recruited for contraction, the shorter the muscle length. The amount of force that is produced from a muscle contraction is determined by the number of motor units (one motor nerve together with all the muscle fibers that it innervated) that are recruited and the number of fibers contained in each motor unit (30).

Muscle Contraction and Training

During static (isometric) contractions, the muscle or muscle group maintains a constant length as resistance is applied, and no change in joint position occurs. Research has demonstrated that static training produces significant improvements in muscular strength. The strength gains, however, are limited to the specific joint angles at which the static contractions are performed (31–33). As a result, static training may have limited value in enhancing functional strength. Functional strength is defined as performing work against a resistance specifically in such a way that the strength gained directly benefits the execution of activities of daily life (ADLs) and movements associated with sports. Static training has also been associated with short-term elevations in blood pressure, perhaps because of increased intrathoracic pressure during static contractions. Despite the limitations, static training appears to play a positive role in physical rehabilitation. For example, it is effective in maintaining muscular strength and preventing atrophy associated with the immobilization of a limb (e.g., application of a cast, splint, or brace) (31–34).

Dynamic (isotonic) resistance training is another common method. If movement of the joint occurs during contraction, it is dynamic. If force is sufficient to overcome resistance and the muscle shortens (e.g., the lifting phase of a biceps curl), the contraction is concentric. When resistance is greater than force and the muscle lengthens during contraction, it is eccentric (e.g., the lowering phase of the biceps curl). Most dynamic resistance training includes both concentric and eccentric actions. Significantly heavier loads can be moved eccentrically; in fact, in unfatigued muscle, the ratio of eccentric to concentric strength can be as high as 1.4:1 (31, 34). For example, maximal eccentric weight is 1.4 times the maximal concentric weight in the same muscle group/movement. Furthermore, at the onset of fatigue, the relative level of eccentric strength and eccentric–concentric ratio increases even more. Greater force production during eccentric contraction than with the concentric contraction probably results from more motor units being recruited and a slow movement velocity. Individuals who are eccentrically trained are often subjected to delayed-onset muscular soreness (DOMS) (35). Eccentric training can, however, play an important role in preventing or rehabilitating certain musculoskeletal injuries. For example, eccentric training has been demonstrated to be effective for treating hamstring strains, tennis elbow, and patellofemoral pain syndrome (36).

The other major type of resistance training, isokinetic exercise, entails constant-speed muscular contraction against accommodating resistance. The speed of movement is controlled, and the amount of resistance is proportional to the amount of force produced throughout the full range of motion. The theoretical advantage of isokinetic exercise is the development of maximal muscle tension throughout the range of motion. Research documents the effectiveness of isokinetic training (31, 32). Strength gains achieved during high-speed training (i.e., contraction velocities of $180° \cdot s^{-1}$ or faster) appear to carry over to all speeds below that specific speed (37). Improvement in strength at slow speeds of movement, however, has not been shown to carry over to faster speeds.

Muscle Fiber Types

The human body has the ability to perform a wide range of physical tasks, combining varying composites of speed, power, and endurance. No single type of muscle fiber possesses the characteristics that would allow optimal performance across this continuum of physical challenges. Rather, muscle fibers possess certain characteristics that result in relative specialization. For example, certain muscle fibers are selectively recruited by the body for speed and power tasks of short duration, while others are recruited for endurance tasks of long duration and relatively low intensity. When the challenge requires elements of speed or power but also has an endurance component, yet another type of muscle fiber is recruited. These different fiber types should not be thought of as mutually exclusive. In fact, intricate recruitment and switching occurs in muscle over the performance of many tasks, and fibers designed to be optimal for one type of task can contribute to the performance of another. The net result is a functioning muscle that can respond to a wide variety of tasks, and while the composition of the muscle may lend itself to performing best in endurance activities, it still can accomplish speed and power tasks to a lesser degree (38).

Over the years, there has been a fair amount of controversy about the classification of muscle fiber types (7). In addition, there are questions about whether these types can change in response to an intervention such as endurance training (39). In either case, there is general agreement that relative to exercise performance, two distinct fiber types (type I or slow twitch and type II or fast twitch, with their proposed subdivisions) have been identified and classified by contractile and metabolic characteristics such as the chemical breakdown of carbohydrate, fat, and protein for energy within the muscle cell (40).

TYPE I MUSCLE FIBERS

The characteristics of type I muscle fibers are consistent with muscle fibers that resist fatigue. Thus, type I fibers are selected for activities of low intensity and long duration. Within whole muscle, type I motor units contract, but the units do not all contract at the same time. In addition to their inherent fatigue resistance, endurance is prolonged by the constant switching that occurs to ensure freshly charged muscle as the exercise stimulus continues. Sedentary persons have approximately 50% type I fibers, and this distribution is generally equal throughout the major muscle groups of the body (41). In endurance athletes, the percentage of type I fibers is greater, but this is thought to be largely a genetic predisposition, despite some evidence suggesting that prolonged exercise training can alter fiber type (42). Essentially, those most successful at endurance activities generally have a high proportion of type I fibers, and this is most likely due to genetic factors supplemented through appropriate exercise training. From a metabolic perspective, type I fibers are those frequently called "aerobic," since the generation of energy for continued muscle contraction is met through the ongoing oxidation (chemical breakdown using oxygen) of available energy substrates. Thus, with minimal accumulation of anaerobically (chemical breakdown without oxygen) produced metabolites, continued submaximal muscle contraction is favored in type I fibers.

TYPE II MUSCLE FIBERS

At the opposite end of the continuum, those who achieve the greatest success in power and high-intensity speed tasks usually have a greater proportion of type II muscle fibers distributed through the major muscle groups. Since force generation is so important, type II fibers shorten and develop tension considerably faster than type I fibers (43). These fibers are typically thought of as type IIB fibers, the "classic" fast-twitch fiber. Metabolically, these fibers are the classic anaerobic fibers, because they rely on energy sources from within the muscle, not the fuels used by type I fibers. When an endurance component is introduced, such as in events lasting upward of several minutes (800- to 1500-m races, for example), a second type of fast-twitch fiber, type IIA, is recruited. The type IIA fibers represent a transition of sorts between the needs met by the type I and type IIB fibers. Metabolically, while type IIA fibers have the ability to generate a moderately large amount of force, they also have some aerobic capacity, although not as much as type I fibers. This is a logical and necessary bridge between the types of muscle fibers and the ability to meet the variety of physical tasks imposed. Reference to the existence of the type IIC fiber is necessary in a complete description of human muscle fiber types. The IIC fiber has been described as a rare and undifferentiated muscle fiber type that is probably involved in reinnervation of damaged skeletal muscle (44).

Neuromuscular Activation

Physical activity involves purposeful, voluntary movement. The stimulus for voluntary muscle activation comes from the brain. The signal is relayed through the brainstem and spinal cord and transformed into a specific motor unit activation pattern. To perform a specific task, the required motor units meet specific demands for force production by activating associated muscle fibers (45).

MOTOR UNIT ACTIVATION

The functional unit of the neuromuscular system is the motor unit (30). It consists of the motor neuron and the muscle fibers it innervates. Motor units range in size from a few to several hundred muscle fibers. Muscle fibers from different motor units can be anatomically adjacent to each other, and therefore a muscle fiber may be actively generating force while the adjacent fiber moves passively with no direct neural stimulation. Several nomenclatures have been used to classify skeletal muscle fibers, including color (red or white), action speed (fast or slow twitch), oxidative or glycolytic enzyme content (fast glycolytic, fast oxidative glycolytic, or oxidative), combination schemes (fast glycolytic), and myosin adenosine triphosphatase (ATPase) content. When maximal force is required, all available motor units are activated. Another adaptive mechanism affected by heavy resistance training is the muscle force effected by different motor unit firing rates and/or frequencies.

SKELETAL SYSTEM

Beyond supporting soft tissue, protecting internal organs, and acting as an important source of nutrients and blood constituents, the bones are the rigid levers for locomotion. The skull, vertebral column, sternum, and ribs are considered the axial skeleton; the bones of the upper and lower limbs make up the appendicular skeleton. An outer fibrous layer of connective tissue attaches the bone to muscles, deep fascia, and joint capsules. Just beneath the outer layer is a highly vascular inner layer that contains cells for the creation of new bone. The outer and inner layers that cover the bones constitute the periosteum. The periosteum, continuous with tendons and adjacent articulated structures, anchors muscle to bone. Tendons are likewise continuous with the epimysium, the outer layer of connective tissue covering muscle.

Structure and Function of Joints in Movement

The effective interaction of bone and muscle to produce movement depends somewhat on joint function. Joints are the articulations between bones, and along with bones and ligaments, they constitute the articular system. Ligaments are tough, fibrous connective tissues that connect bone to bone, whereas tendons connect muscle to bone. Joints are typically classified as fibrous, in which bones are united by fibrous tissue, cartilaginous (with cartilage or a fibrocartilaginous anchor), or synovial, in which a fibrous articular capsule and an inner synovial membrane lining enclose the joint cavity. The cavity is filled with synovial fluid, which provides constant lubrication during human movement to minimize the wearing effects of friction on the cartilaginous covering of the articulating bones. Joints are typically well perfused by numerous arterial branches and are innervated by branches of the nerves supplying the adjacent muscle and overlying skin.

Proprioception is defined as the receipt of information from muscles and tendons that enables the brain to determine movements and position of the body and its parts. Proprioceptive feedback is an important joint sensation, as is pain, owing to the high density of sensory fibers in the joint capsule. This feedback has obvious importance in regulating human movement and in preventing injury. The degree of movement within a joint is typically called the range of motion (ROM). ROM can be active (AROM), the range that can be reached by voluntary movement, or passive (PROM), the range that can be achieved by external means (e.g., an examiner or device). Joints are typically limited in range by the articulations of bones (as in the limitation of elbow extension by the olecranon process of the ulna), ligamentous arrangement, and soft tissue limitations, as occurs in elbow or knee flexion. Movement at one joint may influence the extent of movement at adjacent joints, as a number of muscles and other soft tissue structures cross multiple joints. For example, finger flexion decreases in the presence of wrist flexion, because muscles that flex both the wrist and fingers cross multiple joints.

NEUROLOGICAL SYSTEM

In the earlier discussion of a muscle contraction, we described the contraction as triggered by a nervous impulse of a motor unit. The nervous impulse is released from a motor neuron, which originates from the anterior horn of the spinal cord. The spinal cord is a part of the central nervous system, which controls all of the peripheral and internal organs. All muscular movements are controlled by the nervous system. To understand the complex control of human movement, understanding neural control is essential.

The nervous system consists of the brain, spinal cord, and peripheral nerves and is divided into the central nervous system (CNS) and the peripheral nervous system (PNS). The CNS consists of the brain and spinal cord, whereas the PNS consists of all other peripheral nerves of the voluntary system (*Fig. 6.12*) (3).

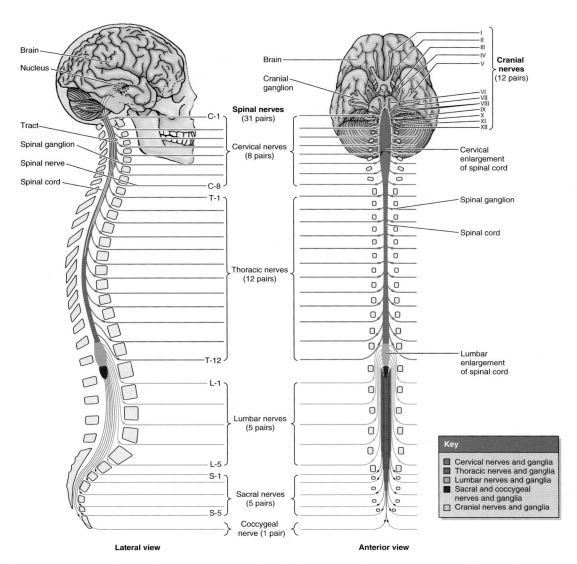

Lateral view

Anterior view

FIGURE 6.12. Basic organization of the nervous system. The brain and spinal cord constitute the CNS. A collection of nerve cell bodies in the CNS is a nucleus, and a bundle of nerve fibers connecting neighboring or distant nuclei in the CNS is a tract. The PNS consists of nerve fibers and cell bodies outside the CNS. Peripheral nerves are either cranial or spinal nerves. A collection of nerve cell bodies outside the CNS is a ganglion (e.g., a cranial or spinal ganglion). (From Moore KL, Dalley AF II. Clinical Oriented Anatomy. 4th ed. Baltimore: Lippincott Williams & Wilkins, 1999.)

Central Nervous System

The brain is the most important part of the CNS system and is surrounded and protected by the bony skull. The spinal cord is the extension of the brain, which runs along and is surrounded and protected by the vertebral column. The CNS is the body's central control center where sensory stimuli are received, integrated, analyzed, and interpreted, and finally relayed as nerve impulses to muscles and glands for taking action.

Peripheral Nervous System

The PNS is composed of the cranial nerves associated with the brain and the spinal nerves associated with the spinal cord, as well as groups of nerve cell bodies called "ganglia." In other words, the

PNS is made up of the nerve cells and their fibers that lie outside the brain and spinal cord (46). The PNS allows the brain and spinal cord to communicate with the rest of the body. There are two types of nerve fibers in the PNS, the afferent, or sensory, fiber and the efferent, or motor, fiber. The sensory nerve fiber is responsible for carrying nerve impulses from sensory receptors in the body to the CNS. Once the received signal is processed and analyzed in the CNS and an action is determined, then the motor nerve fiber is called to convey the nerve signal from the CNS to the effectors, either the muscles or other organs. The PNS can be subdivided into two functional branches, the somatic nervous system and the visceral nervous system. Both systems are composed of an afferent division and an efferent division. The somatic nervous system primarily regulates the voluntary contraction of the skeletal muscles, whereas the visceral system involves the motor activities that control internal organs such as the smooth (involuntary) muscles, cardiac muscle, and glands of the skin and viscera. The latter is also termed the "autonomic nervous system" (ANS).

Autonomic Nervous System

The ANS regulates visceral activities such as heart rate, digestion, breathing, and the secretion of hormones. These activities normally are operated subconsciously and continue to function throughout life. However, they can also be altered to a certain limit consciously. These activities can be carried out even if the organs are deprived of innervation by the ANS. The ANS includes two pathways, the sympathetic pathway and the parasympathetic pathway, which complement each other. The sympathetic pathway stimulates visceral activities under stressful (or alarm) conditions, which results in acceleration of metabolism, heart rate, and breathing and adrenal hormone release. Exercise can be treated as a stressful stimulus to the body that triggers the sympathetic pathway for generating more energy and muscular force. When the stressful stimulus subsides, the parasympathetic pathway brings the visceral activities back to normal, for example decreasing heart rate and breathing, relaxing the muscles, and increasing gastrointestinal activities. The parasympathetic pathway helps to conserve and restore body resources.

Neuromuscular Control

The information transmitted and relayed by the sensory and motor nerves is in a form of electrical energy referred to as the "nerve impulse." The sensory stimulation received through vision or touching is transmitted to the CNS. A motor command is then released after the integration and decision making of the motor cortex of the brain. A nerve pulse is then transmitted to the targeted muscles through an efferent neuron for activating muscle contraction. The functional unit of the neuromuscular system is the motor unit (47). It consists of the motor neuron and the muscle fibers it innervates. When maximal force is required, all available motor units are activated. Another adaptive mechanism affected by heavy resistance training is the muscle force affected by different motor unit firing rates and frequencies (48).

Motor unit activation is also influenced by the size principle. This principle is based on the observed relationship between motor unit twitch force and recruitment threshold. Specifically, motor units are recruited in order according to recruitment thresholds and firing rates, resulting in a continuum of voluntary force. Whereas type I motor units are the smallest and possess the lowest recruitment thresholds, type IIa and IIb motor units are larger in size and have higher activation thresholds. Therefore, as force requirements of an activity increase, the recruitment order progresses from type I to IIa to IIb motor units. Thus, most muscles contain a range of motor units (type I and II fibers), and force production can span wide levels. Maximal force production requires not only the recruitment of all motor units, including high-threshold motor units, but also recruitment at a sufficiently high firing rate. It has been hypothesized that untrained individuals cannot voluntarily recruit the highest-threshold motor units or maximally activate muscles. Furthermore, electrical stimulation has been shown to be more effective in eliciting gains in untrained muscle or injury rehabilitation scenarios, suggesting further inability to activate all available motor units. Thus, training adaptation develops the ability to recruit a greater percentage of motor units when required.

Other than the motor unit, muscular contraction is also affected by specialized sensory receptors in the muscles and tendons that are sensitive to stretch, tension, and pressure. These receptors are termed "proprioceptors." A sensory receptor called a "muscle spindle" is sensitive to the stretch of a muscle and is embedded within the muscle fiber. The muscle spindles provide sensory information regarding the changes and rate of change in the length and tension of muscles fibers. Their main function is to respond to stretch of a muscle and, through reflex action, to initiate a stronger muscle action to reduce this stretch (5). This is known as the "stretch reflex." In contrast to the muscle spindles, the Golgi tendon organs are another type of specialized proprioceptor that attaches to the tendons near the junction of the muscle. These receptors detect differences in the tension generated by active muscle rather than muscle length. When excessive tension is detected by the Golgi tendon organs, a continuous reflex inhibition signal is fired to prevent the muscle from contracting. Hence, the Golgi tendon organs serve as a protective sensory system to prevent muscle injury resulting from over-contraction.

EXERCISE SYSTEM ADAPTATIONS— STRENGTH, CARDIOVASCULAR, FLEXIBILITY

Long-term exercise training is important to overall health and physical fitness. A sound exercise training program leads to long-term physiological changes (adaptation), particularly improvement in muscular strength and endurance, cardiovascular function, and musculoskeletal flexibility. These improvements allow one to enhance athletic performance, engage in physically active leisure-time pursuits more efficiently, perform daily activities more easily, and maintain functional independence later in life.

Resistance Training

Resistance training is an effective exercise mode to improve muscular strength and endurance. Strength improves when sufficient tension is applied to the muscle fiber and its contractile proteins. The tension required for strength gain is about 60–80% of the muscle's maximum force (31). Fleck and Kraemer (31) recommended a range of 75–90% of one repetition maximum contraction (1RM) for optimizing strength gain. For improvement to take place, the resistance work against a muscle must be large enough to impose a demand on the body system. This is the so-called overload principle. Overload is accomplished when a greater than normal physical demand is placed on the muscles. The amount of overload required depends on the current level of muscular fitness. To enhance muscular fitness, the muscular system must be progressively overloaded (e.g., increased resistance, repetitions, sets). The adaptation to strength training includes increase in muscular size, a condition called "hypertrophy." Hypertrophy is one of the most prominent adaptations among all other physiological changes. Increased muscle size is generally attributed to hypertrophy of existing muscle fibers. It is thought to occur through remodeling of protein within the cell and an increase in the number of myofibrils.

Strength training also improves aerobic enzyme systems. Increases in aerobic enzyme activity are reported with isokinetic and isometric training in humans and with isometric training in rats (49). Moreover, increases in oxidative enzymes have been demonstrated to be higher in type IIA fibers than in type IIB fibers. The increase in oxidative metabolism of muscles after long-term strength training is also associated with increases in capillary supply and the concentration of cellular mitochondria. Capillaries per unit area and per fiber are significantly increased in response to varying types of heavy resistance training (such as a combination of concentric and eccentric resistance exercise). Increased capillary density may facilitate performance of low-intensity weight training by increasing blood supply to active muscle. It also increases the ability to remove lactate and thereby improves the ability to tolerate training under highly acidic condition. All of these changes promote oxygen delivery and use within the muscle fiber, thereby improving muscular endurance (50).

Part of the strength gain resulting from strength training is attributed to changes in the nervous system. This is especially true during the early stages of strength training. Training tends to reduce the neuromuscular inhibition in both the CNS and proprioceptors (Golgi tendon organs). Other neural factors include the increased neural drive to muscle, increased synchronization of motor units, and increased activation of the contractile apparatus.

Chronic Adaptations to Cardiovascular Exercise

Physical inactivity is now classified as a major contributing risk factor for heart disease, with an overall weight for preventive value similar to that of elevated blood cholesterol, cigarette smoking, and hypertension (51). Moreover, longitudinal studies have shown that higher levels of aerobic fitness are associated with lower mortality from heart disease even after statistical adjustments for age, coronary risk factors, and family history of heart disease (52). These findings and other recent reports in persons with and without heart disease have confirmed an inverse association between aerobic capacity and cardiovascular mortality (53).

Endurance exercise training increases functional capacity and provides relief of symptoms in most clients with coronary artery disease (CAD). This is particularly important because most clients with clinically manifest CAD have a subnormal functional capacity (50–70% age, gender-predicted), and some may be limited by symptoms at relatively low levels of exertion. Improvement in function appears to be mediated by increased central and/or peripheral oxygen transport and supply, while relief of angina pectoris may result from increased myocardial oxygen supply, decreased oxygen demand, or both.

Most exercise studies on healthy subjects demonstrate 20% ($\pm$10%) increases in aerobic capacity ($\dot{V}O_{2max}$), with the greatest relative improvements among the most unfit (54). Because a fixed submaximal work rate has a relatively constant aerobic requirement, the physically trained individual works at a lower percentage of $\dot{V}O_{2max}$, with greater reserve after exercise training. Enhanced oxygen transport, particularly increased maximal stroke volume and cardiac output, have traditionally been regarded as the primary mechanism underlying the increase in $\dot{V}O_{2max}$ with training.

The effects of long-term exercise training on the autonomic nervous system act to reduce myocardial demands at rest and during exercise. Exercise bradycardia may be attributed to an intracardiac mechanism (an effect directly on the myocardium, for example, increased stroke volume during submaximal work) or an extracardiac mechanism (for example, alterations in trained skeletal muscle) or both. The result is a reduced heart rate and systolic blood pressure at rest and at any fixed oxygen uptake or submaximal work rate.

The increased oxidative capacity of trained skeletal muscle appears to offer a distinct hemodynamic advantage. Lactic acid production and muscle blood flow are decreased at a fixed external work load, whereas submaximal $\dot{Q}$ and oxygen uptake are unchanged or slightly reduced. As a result, there are compensatory increases in a-$\bar{v}$ O_2 difference at submaximal and maximal exercise.

Cardiovascular Adaptations

OVERALL CHANGES

The heart rate response plays a critical role in the delivery of oxygen to working skeletal muscle. The resting heart rate decreases by approximately 10–15 bpm as a result of cardiovascular training (55). Stroke volume will increase both at rest and during exercise up to a point, as a result of long-term cardiovascular training. $\dot{Q}$ will increase during exercise but will not change significantly at rest in cardiovascularly trained individuals. The a-$\bar{v}$ O_2 difference increases with long-term cardiovascular training, particularly near maximal exertion. Both resting SBP and DBP may decrease (if elevated

Table 6.1	PHYSIOLOGICAL RESPONSES TO AEROBIC CONDITIONING IN UNTRAINED INDIVIDUALS	
Variable[a]	**Unit of Measure**	**Response**
$\dot{V}O_{2max}$	mL/kg/min	↑
Resting heart rate	beats/min	↓
Exercise heart rate (submax)	beats/min	↓
Maximum heart rate	beats/min	↔ (or slight ↓)
a-v̄ O_2 diff	ml O_2/100 mL blood	↑
Maximum minute ventilation	L/min	↑
Stroke volume	mL/beat	↑
Cardiac output	L/min	↑
Blood volume (resting)	L	↑
Systolic blood pressure	mm Hg	↔ (or slight ↑)
Blood lactate	mL/100 mL blood	↑
Oxidative capacity of skeletal muscle	Multiple variables[b]	↑

[a] At maximum exercise unless otherwise specified.
[b] Represents increase in skeletal muscle mitochondrial number and size, capillary density, and/or oxidative enzymes.
↑, increase; ↓, decrease; ↔, no change.

consistently prior to starting regular cardiovascular training) with long-term cardiovascular training. Resting lactate levels remain relatively unchanged with long-term cardiovascular training (56). As a result of proper cardiovascular training, less lactic acid will be produced at submaximal workloads during exercise (57). For responses to aerobic conditioning in untrained individuals, see Table 6.1.

GENDER-SPECIFIC IMPROVEMENT

The salutary effects of chronic endurance training in men are well documented (Table 6.2). Numerous studies now provide ample data on $\dot{V}O_{2max}$, cardiovascular hemodynamics, body composition, and blood lipids as well as changes with physical conditioning of middle-aged and older women. The results demonstrate that women with and without CAD respond to aerobic training in much the same way as men when subjected to comparable programs in terms of frequency, intensity, and duration of exercise (58). Improvement is negatively correlated with age, habitual physical activity, and initial $\dot{V}O_{2max}$ (which is generally lower in women than in men) and positively correlated with conditioning frequency, intensity, and duration (59). There are, however, large differences between individuals in the effects of physical conditioning independent of age, initial capacity, or conditioning program. These individual variations in response to aerobic exercise training may result from childhood patterns of activity, state of conditioning at the initiation of the program, or degree of physiological aging. Body compositional differences in trainability may also play an important role with respect to the results of physical conditioning. Obese women demonstrate lower aerobic capacity (per kilogram body weight), altered cardiovascular hemodynamics, and elevated serum lipids than leaner women (60). This initial varied profile may serve to modify the outcome of an aerobic conditioning program with respect to the magnitude of quantitative change.

Flexibility

Flexibility is another important, yet often neglected, component of health-related physical fitness. The level of flexibility is greatly reduced with age and physical inactivity. Lower back problems have been associated with poor flexibility of the lower back and hamstring muscles and weak abdominal

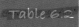

Table 6.2	**BENEFITS OF INCREASING CARDIORESPIRATORY ACTIVITIES AND/OR IMPROVING CARDIORESPIRATORY FITNESS**

Decreased fatigue in daily activities

Improved work, recreational, and sports performance

Improved cardiorespiratory function
  Increased maximal oxygen uptake
  Increased maximal cardiac output and stroke volume
  Increased capillary density in skeletal muscle
  Increased mitochondrial density
  Increased lactate threshold
  Lower heart rate and blood pressure at a fixed submaximal work rate
  Lower myocardial oxygen demand at a fixed submaximal work rate
  Lower minute ventilation at a fixed submaximal work rate

Decreased risk of the following:
  Mortality from all causes
  Coronary artery disease
  Cancer (colon, perhaps breast and prostate)
  Hypertension
  Non-insulin-dependent diabetes mellitus
  Osteoporosis
  Anxiety
  Depression

Improved blood lipid profile
  Decreased triglycerides
  Increased high-density lipoprotein cholesterol
  Decreased postprandial lipemia

Improved immune function

Improved glucose tolerance and insulin sensitivity

Improved body composition

Enhanced sense of well-being

Many of the health benefits accrue from physical activities that may have relatively little effect on increasing cardiorespiratory fitness (2, 8–10).

muscles. Flexibility training should be promoted to improve range of motion and joint mobility. Enhanced flexibility may also improve performance in some sports, especially those requiring obvious flexibility components, such as gymnastics and wrestling.

Following a flexibility enhancement program, both long- and short-term adaptations exist. Immediately following the completion of a stretching program, the muscle's core temperature is increased. There is an increase in the blood flow to the working muscles, which positively alters the body's blood distribution to cope with the increasing demands placed on the musculature. Consequently, the body's ability to deliver hemoglobin (hence oxygen) to the working muscle is enhanced. There is also an increase in the interactions of the muscle's actin and myosin filaments, which increases the speed and force of each muscular contraction, thereby improving performance. Relaxation of the antagonist muscles is promoted. This reduces the resistance to movement and decreases the risk of muscle and tendon injuries, such as in strains and sprains. As muscle tension is reduced, the body becomes more relaxed and coordinated. This in turn promotes increased joint movement and enhances range of motion (61).

For long-term adaptation, the range of motion of the joint is increased, resulting in a decrease in muscle soreness. Furthermore, an inverse relationship has been demonstrated between neuromuscular tension and musculotendon extendibility. Improving flexibility reduces the likelihood of strains, tears, and tightness that may result in muscular pain, spasm, and cramping. Flexibility training also lengthens the fascia, which supports and stabilizes the muscles, organs, and most body tissues. From the physiological standpoint, this flexibility-enhancing effect may be traced to an inhibition of the spinal cord neurons by the Golgi tendon organs following an overly aggressive short-term application of a given flexibility-enhancing modality.

SUMMARY

This chapter was designed to introduce the Personal Trainer to the discipline of exercise physiology. Many concepts are not discussed in this chapter for reasons of length, not because they are unimportant. Emphasis is placed on cardiovascular physiology, pulmonary physiology, and muscle function because that is what the Personal Trainer works with every day. However, endocrine function and other body functions are also important so it is suggested that as you come across new issues with your clients, you seek out additional references that can assist you in understanding the function of the human being under conditions of physical stress.

REFERENCES

1. Robergs RA, Roberts SO. Exercise Physiology: Exercise, Performance and Clinical Applications. St. Louis: Mosby-Yearbook, 1997.
2. McArdle WD, Katch FI, Katch VL. Essentials of Exercise Physiology. 2nd ed. Baltimore: Lippincott Williams & Wilkins, 1999.
3. Marieb EN. Human Anatomy and Physiology. 3rd ed. Redwood City, CA: Benjamin/Cummings, 1998.
4. Williams PL, Warwick R, Dyson M, Bannister LH, eds. Gray's Anatomy. 38th ed. London: Churchill Livingstone, 1995.
5. McArdle WD, Katch FI, Katch VL. Exercise Physiology, Energy, Nutrition, and Human Performance. 4th ed. Baltimore: Williams & Wilkins, 1996.
6. Hall-Craggs ECB. Anatomy as a Basis for Clinical Medicine. Baltimore: Williams & Wilkins, 1995.
7. Armstrong RB. Muscle fiber recruitment patterns and their metabolic correlates. In: Horton ES, Terjunk RL, eds. Exercise, Nutrition and Energy Metabolism. New York: Macmillan, 1988.
8. Karvonen, MJ, et al. The effects of training on heart rate: a longitudinal study. Ann Med Exp Biol Fenn 1957;35:307.
9. Spence AP, Reading MA: Basic Human Anatomy. 3rd ed. Redwood, CA: Benjamin/Cummings, 1991.
10. White JR. EKG changes using carotid artery for heart rate monitoring. Med Sci Sports 1977;9:88.
11. Gardner GW, Danks DI, Scharfsienin L. Use of carotid pulse for heart rate monitoring. Med Sci Sports 1979;11:111.
12. Dehn MM, Mullins CB. Physiologic effects and importance of exercise in patients with coronary artery disease. J Cardiovasc Med 1977;2:365–387.
13. Mitchell JH, Blomqvist G. Maximal oxygen uptake. N Engl J Med 1971;284:1018–1022.
14. Rowell IB. Circulation. Med Sci Sports 1969;1:15–22.
15. Zobi EG, Talmers FN, Christensen RC, et al. Effect of exercise on the cerebral circulation and metabolism. J Appl Physiol 1965;20:1289–1293.
16. Naughton J, Haider R. Methods of exercise testing. In: Naughton JP, Hellerstein HK, Mohler IC, eds. Exercise Testing and Exercise Training in Coronary Heart Disease. New York: Academic Press, 1973:79.
17. ACSM. ACSM's Guidelines for Exercise Testing and Prescription. 6th ed. Baltimore: Lippincott Williams & Wilkins, 2000:104.
18. Foss ML, Keteyian SJ. Fox's Physiological Basis for Exercise and Sport. 6th ed. Boston: WCB McGraw-Hill, 1998:238.
19. Comess KA, Fenster PE. Clinical implications of the blood pressure response to exercise. Cardiology 198168:233–244.
20. Buskirk E, Taylor HL. Maximal oxygen intake and its relation to body composition, with special reference to chronic physical activity and obesity. J Appl Physiol 1957;2:72–78.
21. Berger AJ. Control of breathing. In: Murray JF, Nadel JA, eds. Textbook of Respiratory Medicine, vol 1. 2nd ed. Philadelphia: WB Saunders, 1994:199–218.
22. Light RW. Pleural Diseases. 2nd ed. Philadelphia: Lea & Febiger, 1990:1–7.
23. Davis JA, Vodak P, Wilmore JH, et al. Anaerobic threshold and maximal aerobic power for three modes of exercise. J Appl Physiol 41:544–550, 1976.
24. Beck KC, Johnson BD. Pulmonary adaptations to dynamic exercise. In: Durstine JL, ed. Resource Manual for Guidelines for Exercise Testing and Prescription. 2nd ed. Baltimore: Williams & Wilkins, 1993.
25. McArdle WD, Katch FI, Katch VL. Exercise Physiology, Energy, Nutrition, and Human Performance. 4th ed. Baltimore: Williams & Wilkins, 1996.
26. Graham T. Mechanisms of blood lactate increase during exercise. Physiologist 1984;27:299.
27. Senior A. ATP synthesis by oxidative phosphorylation. Physiol Rev 1988;68:177.
28. Newsholme E. The control of fuel utilization by muscle during exercise and starvation. Diabetes 1979;28(Suppl 1):1.
29. Gaesser G, Brooks C. Metabolic bases of excess post-exercise oxygen consumption: a review. Med Sci Sports Exerc 1984;16:29.
30. Noth J. Motor units. In: Komi PV, ed. Strength and Power in Sport. Oxford, UK: Blackwell Scientific, 1992:21–28.

31. Fleck SJ, Kraemer WJ. Designing Resistance Training Programs. 2nd ed. Champaign, IL: Human Kinetics, 1997.

32. Knapik JJ, Mawdsley RH, Ramos NU. Angular specificity and test mode specificity of isometric and isokinetic strength training. J Orthop Sports Phys Ther 1983;5:58.

33. Gardner G. Specificity of strength changes of the exercised and nonexercised limb following isometric training. Res Q 1963;34:98.

34. DiNubile NA. Strength training. Clin Sports Med 1991;10:33.

35. Byrnes W. Muscle soreness following resistance exercise with and without eccentric contractions. Res Q 1985;56:283.

36. Stanish WD, Rubinovich RM, Curwin S. Eccentric exercise in chronic tendinitis. Clin Orthop 1986;208:65.

37. Coyle E, et al. Specificity of power improvements through slow and fast isokinetic training. J Appl Physiol 1981;51:1437.

38. Coggan AR, Spina RJ, King DS, et al. Skeletal muscle adaptations to endurance training in 60- to 70-yr-old men and women. J Appl Physiol 1992;72:1780–1786.

39. Jacobs I, Esbjornsson M, Slyvan C, et al. Sprint training effects on muscle myoglobin, enzymes, fiber types, and blood lactate. Med Sci Sports Exerc 1987;19:368–374.

40. Brooke MH, Kaiser KK. Muscle fiber types: how many and what kind? Arch Neurol 1970;23:369–379.

41. Fox EL, Bowers RW, Foss ML. The Physiological Basis of Physical Education and Athletics. 4th ed. Dubuque, IA: WC Brown, 1989:106–107.

42. Burke F, Cerny F, Costill D, Fink W. Characteristics of skeletal muscle in competitive cyclists. Med Sci Sports Exerc 1977;9:109–112.

43. Vrbova G. Influence of activity on some characteristic properties of slow and fast mammalian muscles. Exerc Sport Sci Rev 1979;7:181–213.

44. Komi PV, Karlsson J. Skeletal muscle fiber types, enzyme activities and physical performance in young males and females. Acta Physiol Scand 1978;103:210.

45. Faulkner J, Claflin D, McCully K. Power output of fast and slow fibers from human skeletal muscles. In: Jones N, McCartney N, McComas A, eds. Human Muscle Power. Champaign, IL: Human Kinetics, 1986:81–90.

46. Carola R, Harley JP, Noback CR. Human Anatomy and Physiology. New York: McGraw-Hill, 1990.

47. Noth J: Motor units. In: Komi PV, ed. Strength and Power in Sport. Oxford, UK: Blackwell Scientific 1992:21–28.

48. ACSM. ACSM's Resources Manual for Guidelines for Exercise Testing and Prescription. 4th ed. Baltimore, MD: Williams and Wilkins, 2001.

49. Tesch PA. Short- and long-term histochemical and biochemical adaptations in muscle. In: Komi P, ed. Strength and Power in Sports: The Encyclopaedia of Sports Medicine. Oxford: Blackwell Scientific, 1992:239–248.

50. Jackson C, Dickinson A. Adaptations of skeletal muscle to strength or endurance training. In: Grana W, Lombardo J, Sharkey B, Stone J, eds. Advances in Sports Medicine and Fitness. Chicago: Year Book Medical, 1988:45–49.

51. Fletcher GF, Balady G, Blair SN, et al. Statement on exercise: benefits and recommendations for physical activity programs for all Americans. Circulation 1996;94:857–862.

52. Blair SN, Kohl HW III, Paffenbarger RS, et al. Physical fitness and all-cause mortality: a prospective study of healthy men and women. JAMA 1989;262:2395–2401.

53. Blair SN, Kampert JB, Kohl HW III, et al. Influences of cardiorespiratory fitness and other precursors on cardiovascular disease and all-cause mortality in men and women. JAMA 1996;276:205–210.

54. Pate RR, Pratt M, Blair SN, et al. Physical activity and public health: a recommendation from the Centers for Disease Control and Prevention and the American College of Sports Medicine. JAMA 1995;273:402–407.

55. Frick M, Elovainio R, Somer T. The mechanism of bradycardia evoked by physical training. Cardiologia 1967;51:46–54.

56. Astrand PO, Rodahl K. Textbook of Work Physiology: Physiological Bases of Exercise. 4th ed. New York: McGraw-Hill, 1986.

57. Rerych, SK, Sholz PM, Sabiston DC, et al. Effects of exercise training on left ventricular function in normal subjects: a longitudinal study by radionuclide angiography. Am J Cardiol 1980;45:244–252.

58. Ades PA, Waldmann ML, Polk DM, et al. Referral patterns and exercise response in the rehabilitation of female coronary patients aged ≥62 years. Am J Cardiol 1992;69:1422–1425.

59. Franklin BA, Bonzheim K, Berg T. Gender differences in rehabilitation. In: Julian DG, Wenger NK, eds. Women and Heart Disease. London: Martin Dunitz, 1997:151–171.

60. Franklin B, Buskirk E, Hodgson J, et al. Effects of physical conditioning on cardiorespiratory function, body composition and serum lipids in relatively normal-weight and obese middle-aged women. Int J Obes 1979;3:97–109.

61. de Swardt A. Flexibility for cross country. Track Field Coaches Rev 1995;95(2):28–29.

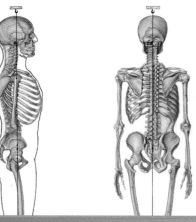

Anatomy, Kinesiology, and Biomechanics

John Mayer, D.C., Ph.D., Research Director, U.S. Spine & Sport Foundation, La Jolla, California

Chapter Outline

Objectives

- Provide an overview of anatomical structures of the musculoskeletal system
- Explain the underlying biomechanical and kinesiological principles of musculoskeletal movement
- Identify the key terms used to describe body position and movement
- Describe the specific structures, movement patterns, range of motion, muscles, and common injuries for each major joint of the body

A major goal of exercise training is to improve cardiovascular and musculoskeletal fitness. The physiological adaptation of muscle to exercise training is visualized through improvements in muscle strength, endurance, flexibility, and resistance to injury (1). The objective of this chapter is to gain an understanding of musculoskeletal functional anatomy of the major joint structures during exercise movements, with emphasis on body alignment, biomechanics, and kinesiological principles. A thorough understanding of these principles is essential for the Personal Trainer to design safe, effective, and efficient exercise training programs to improve musculoskeletal fitness.

BIOMECHANICS AND KINESIOLOGY

Personal Trainers teach clients how to perform exercise movements and how to use exercise or rehabilitation equipment. The disciplines primarily involved in describing and understanding human movement are biomechanics and kinesiology. Biomechanics is the study of the motion and causes of motion of living things, using a branch of physics known as mechanics (2). The study of biomechanics is essential for Personal Trainers because it forms the basis for documenting human motion (kinematics) and understanding the causes of that motion (kinetics).

Kinesiology is the study of human movement and specifically evaluates muscles, joints, and skeletal structures and their involvement in movement (3). Kinesiology is primarily based on three fields of science—biomechanics, musculoskeletal anatomy, and neuromuscular physiology. Kinesiology includes the study of gait, posture and body alignment, ergonomics, sports and exercise movements, and activities of daily living and work. A variety of healthcare practitioners use biomechanical and kinesiological principles, including personal trainers, exercise physiologists, athletic trainers, physicians, physical educators, occupational therapists, physical therapists, chiropractors, and ergonomists (4).

DESCRIBING BODY POSITION AND JOINT MOVEMENT

Anatomical Position

Anatomical position is the universally accepted reference position used to describe regions and spatial relationships of the human body and to refer to body positions (e.g., joint motions) (5). In the anatomical position, the body is erect with feet together and the upper limbs hanging at the sides, palms of the hands facing forward, thumbs facing away from the body, and fingers extended *(Fig. 7.1)*. Other common terms to describe anatomical spatial relationships and positions are shown in Table 7.1 (4).

Planes of Motion and Axes of Rotation

Another useful tool used to describe anatomical motions is the body planes, or planes of motion. There are three basic imaginary planes that pass through the body *(Fig. 7.2)*. The sagittal plane divides the body or structure into the right and left sides. The frontal plane (also called the coronal plane) divides the body or structure into anterior and posterior portions. The transverse plane (also called the cross-sectional, axial, or horizontal plane) divides the body or structure into superior and inferior sections (5). Activities of daily living, exercise, and sport usually involve movement in more than one plane at a given joint structure. If movement occurs in a plane, it must rotate about an axis that has a 90°

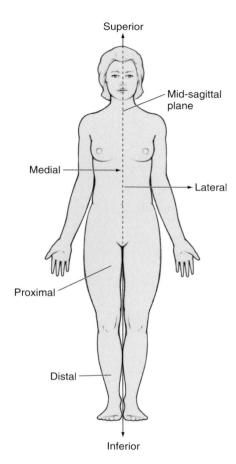

Superior

Mid-sagittal plane

Medial

Lateral

Proximal

Distal

Inferior

FIGURE 7.1. Anatomical position: Body is erect with the feet together, upper limbs hanging at the sides, palms of the hands facing anteriorly, thumbs facing laterally, and fingers extended. Typically, all anatomical references to the body are relative to this position. (Reprinted with permission from ACSM's Resource Manual for Guidelines for Exercise Testing and Prescription. 5th ed. Baltimore: Lippincott Williams & Wilkins, 2006.)

relationship to that plane. Thus, movement in the sagittal plane rotates about an axis with a frontal arrangement; movement in the frontal plane rotates about an axis with a sagittal arrangement; and movement in the transverse plane rotates about an axis with a vertical arrangement (3).

Center of Gravity, Line of Gravity, and Postural Alignment

An object's center of gravity is a theoretical point where the weight force of the object can be considered to act. Center of gravity depends on body position and changes with movement. While standing in a neutral position, the body's center of gravity is approximately at the second sacral segment (2). The kinematics (variation in height and horizontal distance) of the center of gravity relative to the base of support (2) are often studied to examine balance exhibited by the performer. In a sit–to–stand movement, for example, the center of gravity is shifted over the base of support when there is a transition from primarily horizontal motion to a vertical or lifting motion *(Fig. 7.3)*.

The line of gravity of the body is an imaginary vertical line passing through the center of gravity and is typically assessed while the subject is standing (5). The line of gravity helps define proper body alignment and posture using various superficial landmarks from the head, upper extremity, trunk, and lower extremity regions as guides. From the sagittal view, the line of gravity should be slightly posterior to the apex of the coronal suture, through the mastoid process, through the midcervical vertebral bodies, through the shoulder joint, through the midlumbar vertebral bodies, slightly posterior to the axis of the hip joint, slightly anterior to the axis of the knee joint, and slightly anterior to the lateral malleolus. In the frontal plane, the line of gravity should pass through the midline of the body; and bilateral structures such as the mastoid, shoulder, iliac crest, knee, and ankles should be in the same horizontal plane (5) *(Fig. 7.4)*. Personal Trainers should consider the ideal line of gravity when describing postural abnormalities.

Table 7.1 DEFINITIONS OF ANATOMICAL LOCATIONS AND POSITIONS

Term	Definition
Anterior	The front of the body; ventral
Posterior	The back of the body; dorsal
Superficial	Located close to or on the body surface
Deep	Below the surface
Proximal	Closer to any reference point
Distal	Farther from any reference point
Superior	Toward the head; higher (cephalic)
Inferior	Away from the head; lower (caudal)
Medial	Toward the midline of the body
Lateral	Away from the midline of the body; to the side
Ipsilateral	On the same side
Contralateral	On the opposite side
Unilateral	One side
Bilateral	Both sides
Prone	Lying face down
Supine	Lying face up
Valgus	Distal segment of a joint deviates laterally
Varus	Distal segment of a joint deviates medially
Arm	The region of the shoulder to elbow
Forearm	The region of the elbow to the wrist
Thigh	The region of the hip to the knee
Leg	The region of the knee to the ankle

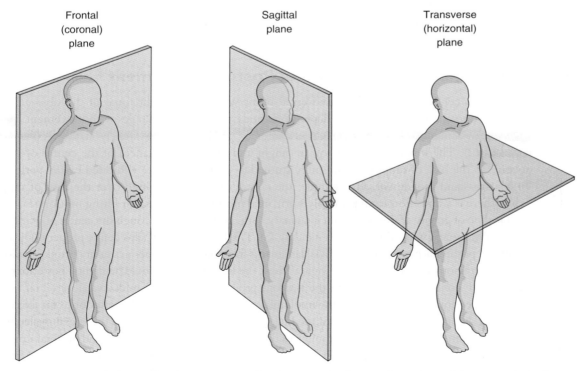

Frontal (coronal) plane   Sagittal plane   Transverse (horizontal) plane

FIGURE 7.2. Anatomical planes of the body. (Reprinted with permission from Cohen BJ, Wood DL. Memmler's The Human Body in Health and Disease. 9th ed. Philadelphia: Lippincott Williams & Wilkins, 2000.)

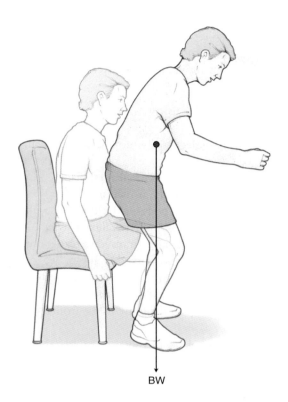

FIGURE 7.3. The initial phase of the sit-to-stand movement involves trunk lean and horizontal weight shift to position the center of gravity over the new base of support (feet). The movement of the center of gravity in several directions is often used to study balance. BW, body weight. (From ACSM's Resource Manual for Guidelines for Exercise Testing and Prescription. 5th ed. Baltimore: Lippincott Williams & Wilkins, 2006.)

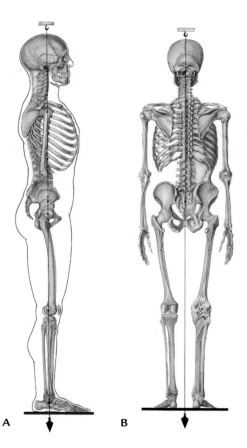

FIGURE 7.4. Line of gravity of the skeletal system. **A.** Lateral view. **B.** Posterior view. (Asset provided by Anatomical Chart Co.)

Joint Movement

Joint movement is often described by its spatial movement pattern in relation to the body, typically in terms of anatomical position. Terms used to describe joint movement are listed below (5) and discussed in detail for the major joints in the next section:

- ➤ Flexion: Movement resulting in a decrease of the joint angle, usually moving anterior in the sagittal plane
- ➤ Extension: Movement resulting in an increase of the joint angle, usually moving posterior in the sagittal plane
- ➤ Abduction: Movement away from the midline of the body, usually in the frontal plane
- ➤ Adduction: Movement toward the midline of the body, usually in the frontal plane
- ➤ Horizontal abduction: Movement away from the midline of the body in the transverse plane, usually used to describe horizontal humerus movement when the shoulder is flexed at 90°
- ➤ Horizontal adduction: Movement toward the midline of the body in the transverse plane, usually used to describe horizontal humerus movement when the shoulder is flexed at 90°
- ➤ Internal (medial) rotation: Rotation in the transverse plane toward the midline of the body
- ➤ External rotation: Rotation in the transverse plane away from the midline of the body
- ➤ Lateral flexion (right or left): Movement away from the midline of the body in the frontal plane, usually used to describe neck and trunk movement
- ➤ Rotation (right or left): Right or left rotation in the transverse plane, usually used to describe neck and trunk movement
- ➤ Elevation: Movement of the shoulder superiorly in the frontal plane
- ➤ Depression: Movement of the shoulder inferiorly in the frontal plane
- ➤ Retraction: Movement of the scapula toward the spine in the transverse plane
- ➤ Protraction: Movement of the scapula away from the spine in the transverse plane
- ➤ Upward rotation: Superior and lateral movement of the inferior border of the scapula in the frontal plane
- ➤ Downward rotation: Inferior and medial movement of the inferior border of the scapula in the frontal plane
- ➤ Circumduction: A compound circular movement involving flexion, extension, abduction, and adduction
- ➤ Radial deviation: Abduction of the wrist in the frontal plane
- ➤ Ulnar deviation: Adduction of the wrist in the frontal plane
- ➤ Opposition: Diagonal movement of thumb across the palmar surface of the hand to make contact with the fifth digit
- ➤ Eversion: Abducting the ankle
- ➤ Inversion: Adducting the ankle
- ➤ Dorsiflexion: Flexing the ankle so that the foot moves anteriorly in the sagittal plane
- ➤ Plantarflexion: Extending the ankle so that the foot moves posteriorly in the sagittal plane
- ➤ Pronation (foot/ankle): Rolling the foot inward
- ➤ Supination (foot/ankle): Rolling the foot outward

MUSCULOSKELETAL ANATOMY

The three primary anatomical structures of the musculoskeletal system that are of interest to the Personal Trainer are bones, joints, and muscles. Mechanically, the interaction of the bones, joints, and muscles determines the range of motion of a joint, the specific movement allowed, and the force produced. This section provides an overview of these structures. For in-depth study, the reader is referred to a variety of excellent sources (6–10).

Skeletal System

The skeletal system consists of cartilage, periosteum, and bone (osseous) tissue. The bones of the skeletal system support soft tissue, protect internal organs, act as important sources of nutrients and blood constituents, and serve as rigid levers for movement. There are 206 bones in the human body, 177 of which engage in voluntary movement. The skull, vertebral column, sternum, and ribs are considered the axial skeleton; the remaining bones, in particular those of the upper and lower limbs, are considered the appendicular skeleton (11). The major bones of the body are illustrated in Figure 7.5.

The structure of a bone can be explained using a typical long bone such as the humerus (the long bone of the upper arm). The main portion of a long bone or shaft is called the "diaphysis" *(Fig. 7.6)*. The ends of the bone are called the "epiphyses." The epiphyses are covered by articular cartilage. Cartilage is a resilient, semirigid form of connective tissue that reduces the friction and absorbs some of the shock in synovial joints. The region of mature bone where the diaphysis joins the epiphyses is called the "metaphysis." In an immature bone, this region includes the epiphyseal plate, also called the "growth plate." The medullary cavity, or marrow cavity, is the space inside the diaphysis. Lining the marrow cavity is the endosteum, which contains cells necessary for bone development. The periosteum is a membrane around the surface of bones that are not covered with articular cartilage. The periosteum is composed of two layers, an outer fibrous layer and an inner highly vascular layer that contains cells for the creation of new bone. The periosteum serves as point attachment for ligaments and tendons and is critical for bone growth, repair, and nutrition (2).

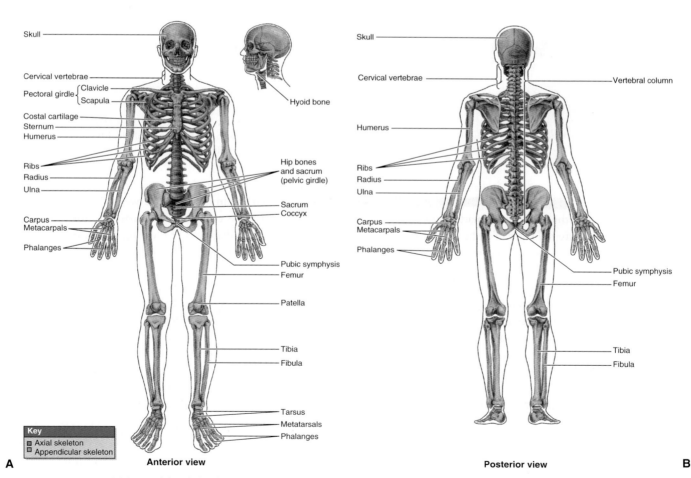

FIGURE 7.5. Divisions of the skeletal system (From Moore KL, Dalley AF II. Clinical Oriented Anatomy. 4th ed. Baltimore: Lippincott Williams & Wilkins, 1999.)

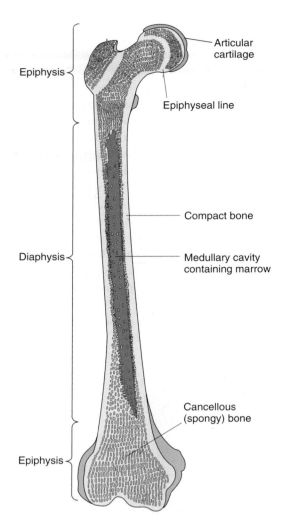

FIGURE 7.6. Bone anatomy. (From Willis MC. Medical Terminology: A Programmed Learning Approach to the Language of Health Care. Baltimore: Lippincott Williams & Wilkins, 2002.)

There are two types of bones: compact and spongy (2). The main difference between the two types is the amount of matter and space they contain. Compact bone contains few spaces and forms the external layer of all bones of the body and a large portion of the diaphysis of the long bones, where it provides support for bearing weight. In contrast, spongy bone is characterized as being much less dense. It consists of a three-dimensional lattice composed of beams or struts of bone called "trabeculae." Open spaces are present between the trabeculae, unlike in compact bone. The trabeculae are oriented to provide strength against the stresses normally encountered by the bone. In some bones, the space within these trabeculae is filled with red bone marrow, which produces blood (2).

Bones are also classified according to their shape. Long bones contain a shaft or body with a medullary canal (e.g., femur, tibia, humerus, ulna, and radius). Short bones are relatively small and thick (e.g., carpals and tarsals). Flat bones are plate-like (e.g., sternum, scapulae, ribs, and pelvis). Irregular bones are oddly shaped (e.g., vertebrae, sacrum, and coccyx). Finally, sesamoid bones are found within tendons and joint capsules and are shaped like sesame seeds (e.g., patella) (3).

Articular System

Joints are the articulations between bones, and along with bones and ligaments, they constitute the articular system. Ligaments are tough, fibrous connective tissues anchoring bone to bone. Joints are classified as synarthrodial, amphiarthrodial, or diarthrodial (synovial) (2). Synarthrodial joints (e.g., sutures of the skull) do not move appreciably. Amphiarthrodial joints move slightly and are held together by ligaments (syndesmosis; e.g., inferior tibiofibular joint) or fibrocartilage (synchondrosis; e.g., pubic symphysis). Synarthrodial and amphiarthrodial joints do not contain an articular cavity, synovial membrane, or synovial fluid (2).

SYNOVIAL JOINTS

The most common type of joint in the human body is the synovial joint. Synovial joints contain a fibrous articular capsule and an inner synovial membrane that enclose the joint cavity. Figure 7.7 illustrates a synovial joint's unique capsular arrangement. There are five distinct features of a synovial joint (2):

1. It is enclosed by a fibrous joint capsule.
2. The joint capsule encloses the joint cavity.
3. The joint capsule is lined with synovial membrane.
4. Synovial fluid lines the inner surface of the capsule.
5. The articulating surfaces of the bones are covered with hyaline cartilage, which helps absorbs shock and reduced friction.

The synovial membrane produces synovial fluid, which provides constant lubrication during movement to minimize the wearing effects of friction on the cartilaginous covering of the articulating bones (2). Ligaments sometimes reinforce synovial joints. These ligaments are either separate structures or a thickening of the outer layer of the joint capsule. The collagen fibers of ligaments are typically arranged to counteract multidimensional stresses. Some synovial joints have other structures such as articular disks (e.g., meniscus of the knee). There are six major types of synovial joints classified by the shape of the articulating surface or type of movement allowed. Table 7.2 summarizes the joint classifications and examples in the human body. Table 7.3 summarizes the motions of the major joints and the planes in which they occur.

Synovial joints are typically perfused by numerous arterial branches and are innervated by branches of the nerves supplying the adjacent muscle and overlying skin. Proprioceptive feedback is an

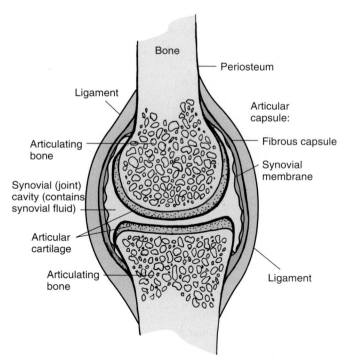

FIGURE 7.7. A synovial joint. (From Oatis CA. Kinesiology. The Mechanics and Pathomechanics of Human Movement. Baltimore: Lippincott Williams & Wilkins, 2003.)

Table 7.2 CLASSIFICATION OF JOINTS IN THE HUMAN BODY

Joint Classification	Features and Examples
Fibrous	
Suture	Tight union unique to the skull
Syndesmosis	Interosseous membrane between bone (e.g., the union along the shafts of the radius and ulna, tibia and fibula)
Gomphosis	Unique joint at the tooth socket
Cartilaginous	
Primary (synchondroses; hyaline cartilaginous)	Usually temporary to permit bone growth and typically fuse; some do not (e.g., at the sternum and rib [costal cartilage])
Secondary (symphyses; fibrocartilaginous)	Strong, slightly movable joints (e.g., intervertebral disks, pubic symphysis)
Synovial	
Plane (arthrodial)	Gliding and sliding movements (e.g., acromioclavicular joint)
Hinge (ginglymus)	Uniaxial movements (e.g., elbow, knee extension and flexion)
Ellipsoidal (condyloid)	Biaxial joint (e.g., radiocarpal extension, flexion at the wrist)
Saddle (sellar)	Unique joint that permits movements in all planes, including opposition (e.g., the carpometacarpal joint of the thumb)
Ball-and-socket (enarthrodial)	Multiaxial joints that permit movements in all directions (e.g., hip and shoulder joints)
Pivot (trochoidal)	Uniaxial joints that permit rotation (e.g., humeroradial joint)

Table 7.3 MAJOR JOINT MOTIONS AND PLANES OF MOTION

Major Joints	Type of Joints	Joint Movements	Planes
Scapulothoracic	Not a true joint	Elevation–depression	Frontal
		Upward–downward rotation	Frontal
		Protraction–retraction	Transverse
Glenohumeral	Synovial: ball-and-socket	Flexion–extension	Sagittal
		Abduction–adduction	Frontal
		Internal–external rotation	Transverse
		Horizontal abduction–adduction	Transverse
		circumduction	Multiple
Elbow	Synovial: hinge	Flexion–extension	Sagittal
Proximal radioulnar	Synovial: pivot	Pronation–supination	Transverse
Wrist	Synovial: ellipsoidal	Flexion–extension	Sagittal
		Abduction–adduction	Frontal
Metacarpophalangeal	Synovial: ellipsoidal	Flexion–extension	Sagittal
		Abduction–adduction	Frontal
Proximal and distal interphalangeal	Synovial: hinge	Flexion–extension	Sagittal
Intervertebral	Cartilaginous	Flexion–extension	Sagittal
		Lateral flexion	Frontal
		Rotation	Transverse
Hip	Synovial: ball-and-socket	Flexion–extension	Sagittal
		Abduction–adduction	Frontal
		Internal–external rotation	Transverse
		Circumduction	Multiple
Knee	Synovial: hinge	Flexion–extension	Sagittal
Ankle: talocrural	Synovial: hinge	Dorsiflexion–plantar flexion	Sagittal
Ankle: subtalar	Synovial: gliding	Inversion–eversion	Frontal

important joint sensation, as is pain, owing to the high density of sensory fibers in the joint capsule. This feedback has obvious importance in regulating human movement and preventing injury (2).

JOINT MOVEMENTS AND RANGE OF MOTION

Joint movement is a combination of rolling, sliding, and spinning of the joint surfaces (4). "Open chain" movements occur when the distal segment of a joint moves in space. An example of an open chain movement for the knee joint is leg extension exercise on a machine. "Closed chain" movements occur when the distal segment of the joint is fixed in space. An example of a closed chain movement for the knee joint is standing barbell squats. A joint is in a "closed pack" position when there is both maximal congruency of the joint surfaces and maximal tautness of the joint capsule and ligaments (4). A joint is in an "open pack" (loose) position when there is the least joint congruency and the joint capsule and ligaments are most loose. Movement at one joint may influence the extent of movement at adjacent joints because a number of muscles and other soft tissue structures cross multiple joints. For example, finger flexion decreases in the presence of wrist flexion because muscles that flex both the wrist and fingers cross multiple joints (4).

The degree of movement within a joint is called the range of motion (ROM). ROM can be active (the range that can be reached by voluntary movement from contraction of skeletal muscle) or passive (the ROM that can be achieved by external means). Joints with excessive ROM are called "hypermobile," and joints with restricted ROM are called "hypomobile" (4). Joint ROM is quantified using goniometers or inclinometers, and each joint has normal ROM values for reference purposes (5). ROM measures at baseline help guide the exercise prescription, and ROM measures at follow-up help document progress.

JOINT STABILITY

The stability of a joint is its resistance to displacement. All joints do not have the same degree of stability, and in general, ROM is gained at the expense of stability. Five factors account for joint stability (4):

1. Ligaments check normal movement and resist extensive movement.
2. Muscles and tendons that span a joint also enhance stability, particularly when the bony structure contributes little stability (e.g., shoulder).
3. Fascia also helps joint stability (e.g., iliotibial band of the tensor fasciae latae).
4. Atmospheric pressure pushes on the outside of joint with greater force than outward pushing force within the joint cavity (the suction created by this pressure is an important factor in aiding joint stability).
5. The bony structure of a joint is an important contributor to joint stability (e.g., limitation of elbow extension by the olecranon process of the ulna) (4).

Muscular System

Bones provide support and leverage to the body, but without muscles we would not be able to move. There are three types of muscles: skeletal, cardiac, and smooth muscle. Skeletal muscle is primarily attached to bones and is under voluntary control. Skeletal muscle is responsible for moving the skeletal system and stabilizing the body (e.g., maintaining posture). There are more than 600 skeletal muscles in the human body (3), approximately 100 of which are primary movement muscles with which Personal Trainers should be familiar (4). The superficial muscles of the body are shown in Figures 7.8 and 7.9.

Skeletal muscles are anchored to the skeleton by tendons. In most cases, tendons are dense cords of connective tissue that attach a muscle to the periosteum of the bone. The collagen fibers of tendons are in parallel arrangement, which makes the tendon suited for unidirectional stress. When

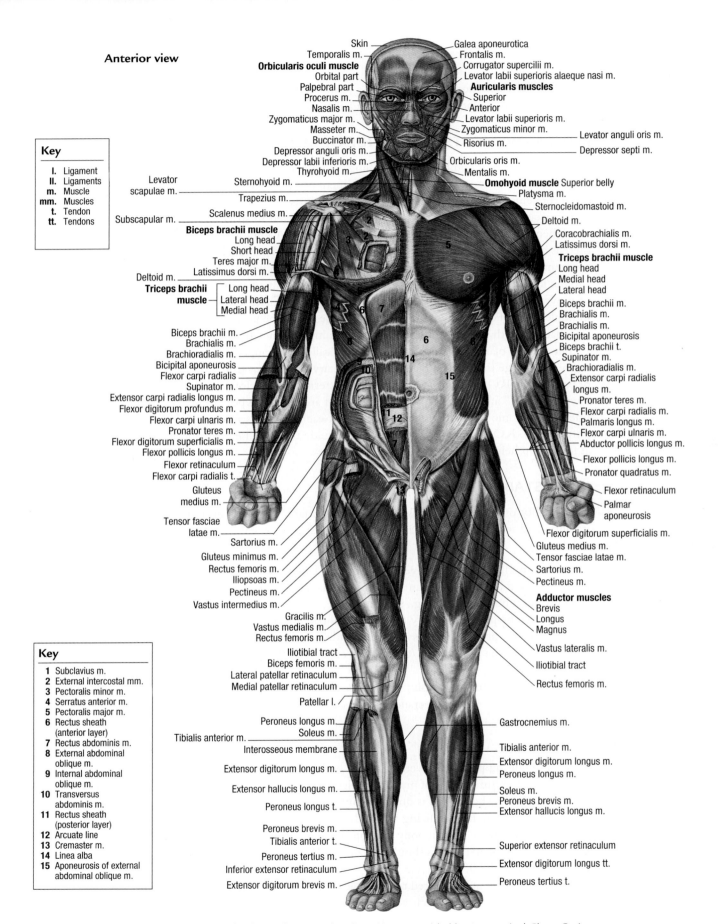

Anterior view

Skin
Temporalis m.
Orbicularis oculi muscle
Orbital part
Palpebral part
Procerus m.
Nasalis m.
Zygomaticus major m.
Masseter m.
Buccinator m.
Depressor anguli oris m.
Depressor labii inferioris m.
Thyrohyoid m.

Galea aponeurotica
Frontalis m.
Corrugator supercilii m.
Levator labii superioris alaeque nasi m.
Auricularis muscles
Superior
Anterior
Levator labii superioris m.
Zygomaticus minor m.
Risorius m.
Orbicularis oris m.
Mentalis m.

Levator anguli oris m.
Depressor septi m.

Levator
scapulae m.
Sternohyoid m.
Trapezius m.
Scalenus medius m.
Subscapular m.
Biceps brachii muscle
Long head
Short head
Teres major m.
Latissimus dorsi m.
Deltoid m.
Triceps brachii muscle
Long head
Lateral head
Medial head

Omohyoid muscle Superior belly
Platysma m.
Sternocleidomastoid m.
Deltoid m.
Coracobrachialis m.
Latissimus dorsi m.
Triceps brachii muscle
Long head
Medial head
Lateral head
Biceps brachii m.
Brachialis m.
Brachialis m.
Bicipital aponeurosis
Biceps brachii t.
Supinator m.
Brachioradialis m.
Extensor carpi radialis
longus m.
Pronator teres m.
Flexor carpi radialis m.
Palmaris longus m.
Flexor carpi ulnaris m.
Abductor pollicis longus m.
Flexor pollicis longus m.
Pronator quadratus m.
Flexor retinaculum
Palmar
aponeurosis

Biceps brachii m.
Brachialis m.
Brachioradialis m.
Bicipital aponeurosis
Flexor carpi radialis
Supinator m.
Extensor carpi radialis longus m.
Flexor digitorum profundus m.
Flexor carpi ulnaris m.
Pronator teres m.
Flexor digitorum superficialis m.
Flexor pollicis longus m.
Flexor retinaculum
Flexor carpi radialis t.
Gluteus
medius m.
Tensor fasciae
latae m.
Sartorius m.
Gluteus minimus m.
Rectus femoris m.
Iliopsoas m.
Pectineus m.
Vastus intermedius m.
Gracilis m.
Vastus medialis m.
Rectus femoris m.
Iliotibial tract
Biceps femoris m.
Lateral patellar retinaculum
Medial patellar retinaculum
Patellar l.
Peroneus longus m.
Tibialis anterior m.
Soleus m.
Interosseous membrane
Extensor digitorum longus m.
Extensor hallucis longus m.
Peroneus longus t.
Peroneus brevis m.
Tibialis anterior t.
Peroneus tertius m.
Inferior extensor retinaculum
Extensor digitorum brevis m.

Flexor digitorum superficialis m.
Gluteus medius m.
Tensor fasciae latae m.
Sartorius m.
Pectineus m.
Adductor muscles
Brevis
Longus
Magnus
Vastus lateralis m.
Iliotibial tract
Rectus femoris m.

Gastrocnemius m.
Tibialis anterior m.
Extensor digitorum longus m.
Peroneus longus m.
Soleus m.
Peroneus brevis m.
Extensor hallucis longus m.
Superior extensor retinaculum
Extensor digitorum longus tt.
Peroneus tertius t.

Key

I.	Ligament
II.	Ligaments
m.	Muscle
mm.	Muscles
t.	Tendon
tt.	Tendons

Key

1 Subclavius m.
2 External intercostal mm.
3 Pectoralis minor m.
4 Serratus anterior m.
5 Pectoralis major m.
6 Rectus sheath
  (anterior layer)
7 Rectus abdominis m.
8 External abdominal
  oblique m.
9 Internal abdominal
  oblique m.
10 Transversus
  abdominis m.
11 Rectus sheath
  (posterior layer)
12 Arcuate line
13 Cremaster m.
14 Linea alba
15 Aponeurosis of external
  abdominal oblique m.

FIGURE 7.8. Superficial muscles—anterior view. (Asset provided by Anatomical Chart Co.)

Posterior view

Skin

Galea aponeurotica

Superior auricular m.
Occipitalis m.
Posterior auricular m.
Trapezius m.
Sternocleidomastoid m.

Occipitalis minor m.
Semispinalis capitis m.
Splenius capitis m.

Levator scapulae m.

Key

l.	Ligament
ll.	Ligaments
m.	Muscle
mm.	Muscles
t.	Tendon
tt.	Tendons

Omohyoid muscle, Inferior belly
Supraspinatus m.
Infraspinatus m.
Teres minor m.
Deltoid m.
Teres major m.
Triceps brachii muscle
Long head
Lateral head

Deltoid m.

Infraspinatus m.
(covered by fascia)
Teres major m.

Triceps brachii muscle
Lateral head
Long head

Brachialis m.
Extensor carpi radialis
longus m.
Flexor digitorum
profundus m.
Flexor carpi ulnaris m.
Anconeus m.
Extensor carpi radialis
brevis m.
Supinator m.
Extensor pollicis longus m.
Abductor pollicis longus m.
Extensor pollicis brevis m.
Extensor indicis m.

Brachioradialis m.
Extensor carpi radialis longus m.
Anconeus m.
Extensor digitorum m.
Extensor carpi ulnaris m.
Extensor carpi radialis brevis m.
Abductor pollicis longus m.
Extensor pollicis brevis m.
Extensor retinaculum
Dorsal
interosseous m.

Flexor
carpi
ulnaris
m.

Adductor muscles
Minimus
Magnus
Vastus lateralis m.

Biceps femoris muscle
Short head
Long head

Vastus lateralis m.

Adductor magnus m.
Gracilis m.
Iliotibial tract
Vastus lateralis m.
Biceps femoris m.

Semitendinosus m.
Semimembranosus m.
Plantaris m.
Gastrocnemius muscle
Lateral head
Medial head

Gastrocnemius muscle
Lateral head
Medial head
Popliteus m.
Plantaris m.

Sartorius
m.

Gastrocnemius m.

Soleus m.
Peroneus muscles
Longus
Brevis
Flexor digitorum longus mm.
Flexor hallucis longus m.
Calcaneal t.
Peroneus tendons
Brevis
Longus

Soleus
mm.

Peroneus longus m.
Aponeurosis of soleus m.
Tibialis posterior m.
Flexor digitorum longus mm.
Peroneus brevis m.
Tibialis posterior t.
Flexor hallucis longus m.
Superior peroneal retinaculum
Inferior peroneal retinaculum
Flexor retinaculum

Key

1 Trapezius m.
2 Spine of C7
3 Rhomboid major m.
4 Latissimus dorsi m.
5 Spine of T12
6 Thoracolumbar fascia
7 External abdominal oblique m.
8 Internal abdominal oblique m.
9 Splenius cervicis m.
10 Serratus posterior superior m.
11 Rhomboid minor m.
12 Erector spinae mm.
13 Spinalis thoracis m.
14 Longissimus thoracis m.
15 Iliocostalis lumborum m.
16 Serratus anterior m.
17 Serratus posterior inferior m.
18 External intercostal m.
19 12th rib
20 Thoracolumbar fascia (removed)
21 Gluteus medius m.
22 Tensor fasciae latae m.
23 Gluteus maximus m.
24 Greater trochanter
25 Iliac crest
26 Gluteus minimus m.
27 Piriformis m.
28 Superior gemellus m.
29 Obturator internus m.
30 Sacrotuberal l.
31 Inferior gemellus m.
32 Obturator externus m.
33 Quadratus femoris m.

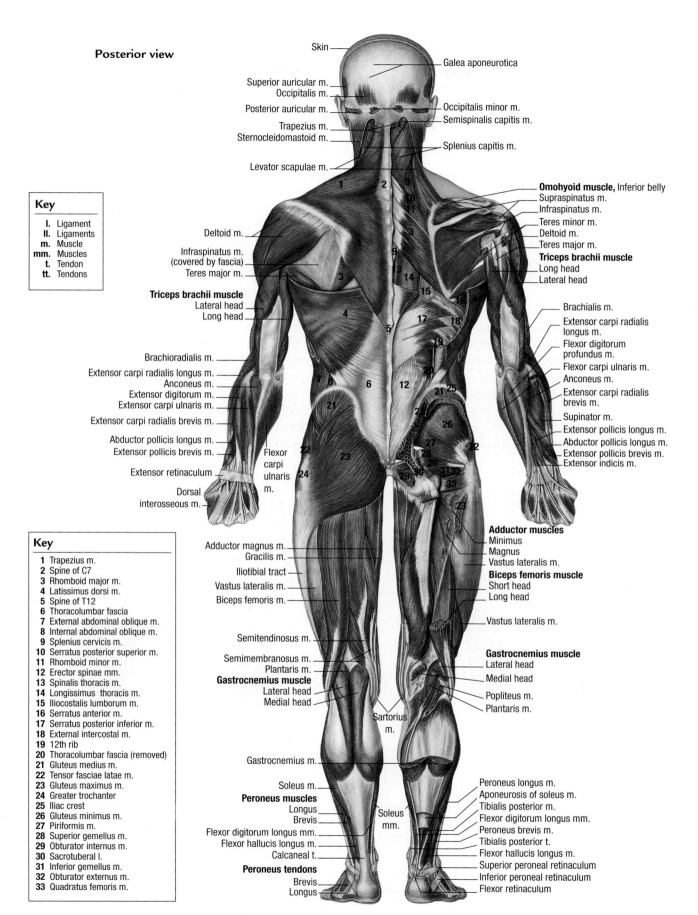

FIGURE 7.9. Superficial muscles—posterior view. (Asset provided by Anatomical Chart Co.)

the tendon is flat and broad, it is called an "aponeurosis." Tendons and aponeuroses provide the mechanical link between skeletal muscle and bone. Bursae are often positioned between tendons and bony prominences to allow the tendons to slide easily across the bones (2).

CLASSIFICATION OF SKELETAL MUSCLES

Skeletal muscles can be classified according to their muscle fiber architecture (i.e., the arrangement of muscle fiber relative to the line of pull of the muscle) *(Fig. 7.10)*. Muscles typically have either a parallel or a pennate arrangement. In parallel muscle, the muscle fibers run in line with the pull of the muscle. Fusiform muscles have a parallel arrangement and are spindle shaped, tapering at each end (e.g., brachioradialis of the arm). Longitudinal muscles are strap-like, with parallel fibers (e.g., sartorius of the thigh). Quadrate muscles are four-sided, are usually flat, and consist of parallel fibers (e.g., rhomboids of the upper back). Fan-shaped or triangular muscles contain fibers that radiate from a narrow attachment at one end to a broad attachment at the other (e.g., pectoralis major of the chest) (3).

In pennate muscle, the fibers run obliquely or at an angle to the line of pull. Pennate muscles can be classified as unipennate (fibers only on one side of the tendon; e.g., vastus lateralis of the thigh), bipennate (fibers on both sides of a centrally positioned tendon; e.g., rectus femoris of the thigh), or multipennate (two or more fasciculi attaching obliquely and combined into one muscle; e.g., middle deltoid of the shoulder) (3).

The number of joints they act upon can also describe muscles. For example, a muscle that causes movement at one joint is uniarticular (e.g., brachialis of the arm). Muscles that cross more than one joint are referred to as biarticular (having actions at two joints; e.g., hamstring muscles of the thigh,

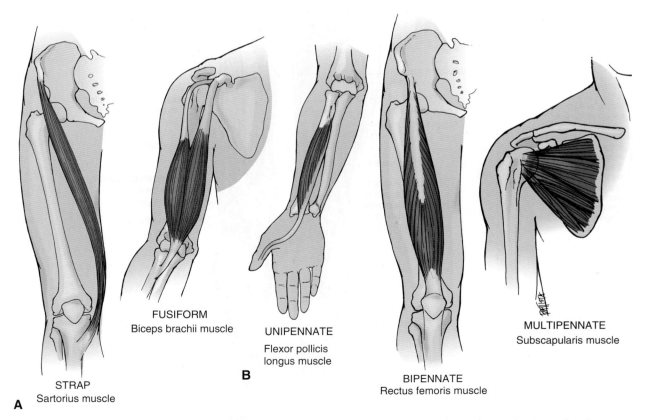

FUSIFORM
Biceps brachii muscle

UNIPENNATE
Flexor pollicis longus muscle

MULTIPENNATE
Subscapularis muscle

B

STRAP
Sartorius muscle

BIPENNATE
Rectus femoris muscle

A

FIGURE 7.10. Skeletal muscle architecture **(A)** and shape **(B)**. (From Oatis CA. Kinesiology. The Mechanics and Pathomechanics of Human Movement. Baltimore: Lippincott Williams & Wilkins, 2003.)

biceps brachii of the arm) or multiarticular (e.g., erector spinae of the back). The main advantage of bi- and multiarticular muscles is that only one muscle is needed to generate tension in two or more joints. This is more efficient and conserves energy. In many instances, the length of the muscle stays within 100% to 130% of the resting length. As one side of the muscle shortens, the other side stretches, maintaining a near constant length. This property of bi- and multiarticular muscles enhances tension production (4).

HOW MUSCLES PRODUCE MOVEMENT

Skeletal muscles produce force that is transferred to the tendons, which in turn pull on the bones and other structures, such as the skin. Most muscles cross a joint, so when a muscle contracts, it pulls one of the articulating bones toward the other. Usually, both articulating bones do not move equally; one of the articulating bones remains relatively stationary. The attachment that is usually more stationary and proximal (especially in the extremities) is called the "origin." The muscle attachment that moves the most and is usually located more distally is called the "insertion" (4).

Levers. Mechanically, to produce movement, the muscles, joints, and bones work as a system of levers. The bone acts as the lever, the joint functions as the center of rotation (COR), and the muscles produce the force or effort (F) to move the lever. The resistance (R), or the force that opposes the movement of the lever, could be the weight of the body part or, as in a case of lifting weights, the external resistance provided by the weights. Levers are classified into three types according to the position of the fulcrum and the forces of effort and resistance *(Fig. 7.11)*. Third-class levers are the most common type of levers in the human body and are designed for ROM and speed of movement (2).

Muscle Actions. Muscle action is the neuromuscular activation that leads to the production of force and contributes to the movement or the stabilization of the musculoskeletal system (12). Muscle can perform three basic actions: isometric, concentric, and eccentric. In an isometric (static) action, the muscle generates force in the absence of joint movement or change in muscle length, such as holding a dumbbell in a biceps curl without movement. In a dynamic action, the muscle length changes and movement occurs. Concentric and eccentric actions are dynamic muscle actions. A concentric action occurs when the muscle force being generated exceeds the resistance and the muscle shortens, such as the upward phase of a biceps curl. An eccentric action occurs when the force generated by the muscle is less than the resistance being encountered. This results in the lengthening of an active muscle. Eccentric actions are often used when muscles have to slow down body parts or oppose external resistances (4). The downward phase of a biceps curl, for example, requires eccentric action of the biceps muscle.

Muscle Roles. Movements of the human body generally require several muscles working together rather than a single muscle doing all the work. Keep in mind that muscles cannot push, they can only pull; therefore, most skeletal muscles are arranged in opposing pairs such as flexor–extensor, internal–external rotator, and abductor–adductor. Muscles can be classified according to their roles during movement (3). When a muscle or group of muscles is responsible for the action or movement, it is called a "prime mover" or "agonist." For example, during a biceps curl, the prime movers are the elbow flexors, which include the biceps, brachialis, and brachioradialis muscles. The opposing group of muscles is called the antagonist (e.g., the triceps and anconeus muscles in biceps curl). Antagonists relax to permit the primary movement and contract to act as a brake at the completion of the movement. In addition, most movements also involve other muscles called "synergists." The role of synergists is to prevent unwanted movement, which helps the prime movers perform more efficiently. Synergists can also act as fixators or stabilizers. In this role, the muscles stabilize a portion of the body against a force (3). For example, the scapular muscles (e.g., rhomboids, serratus anterior, and trapezius) must provide a stable base of support for the upper extremity muscles during the throwing motion. Co-contraction is the simultaneous contraction of the agonist and antagonist. Co-contraction of the abdominal and lumbar muscles, for example, helps stabilize the lower trunk during trunk movements (13).

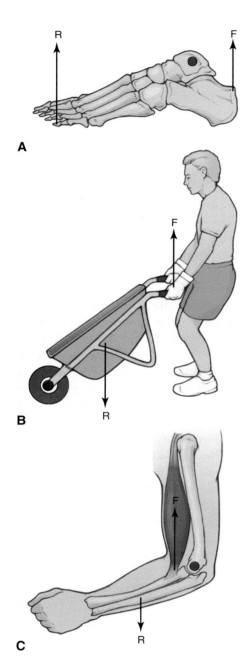

FIGURE 7.11. Examples of lever systems, where *F* is the exerted force, *R* is the reaction force, and the *red dot* is the center of rotation. **A.** First-class lever. **B.** Second-class lever. **C.** Third-class lever. Most musculoskeletal joints behave as third class levers. (From ACSM's Resource Manual for Guidelines for Exercise Testing and Prescription. 5th ed. Baltimore: Lippincott Williams & Wilkins, 2006.)

Factors Influencing Muscle Force Production and Movement Patterns. Muscles exert forces on the skeleton to create motion, stabilize a particular posture, or decrease the stress in bones created by other forces. Muscles create tensile forces that pull on all attachments and create torques about joints. The torques change as the joint moves through the ROM because the moment arms change as joints rotate, and muscle force production is related to muscle length and velocity. Therefore, the torque a muscle can produce is a complex phenomenon that is a combination of tension variations attributable to contractile conditions and geometric/moment arm changes for muscles. Further, the factors that determine the movement patterns created about a joint by muscle action are multifaceted (4). Some of these factors are described in the next section.

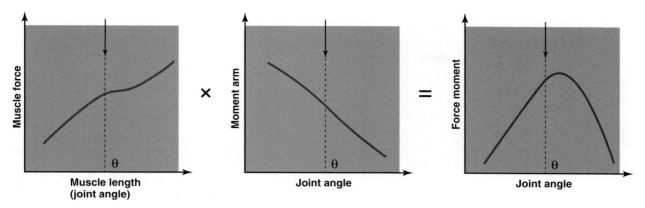

FIGURE 7.12. The joint moment-angle curve represents the strength curves of muscle groups. The shape of these curves is a combination of muscular properties (similar to the length–tension relationship) and muscle moment arms. (Adapted with permission from Zatsiorsky V. Science and Practice of Strength Training. Champaign, IL: Human Kinetics, 1995.)

Clinicians and researchers often assess muscle strength using measurements from dynamometers. A dynamometer is a machine that measures force or torque. Some dynamometers are designed to assess muscle force isometrically at various points throughout the ROM, while others assess force isokinetically in the ROM at constant speeds of shortening or lengthening (14). The torque-angle or moment-angle curves created by these machines illustrate the strength curves of muscle groups integrating the many mechanical factors affecting muscle force *(Fig. 7.12)*. Extensive normative data are available for most joints of the body, and these data are usually normalized to body mass and categorized for a variety of variables, such as age, gender, and sport (15).

Muscle Size and Architecture. The force a muscle can exert is proportional to its physiological cross-sectional area. Muscle fiber architecture also affects force generation, velocity of shortening, and ROM (2). For example, muscles composed of long muscle fibers tend to have parallel arrangements and demonstrate greater ROM and velocity of shortening than pennate muscles. In contrast, pennate muscles are composed of large numbers of short fibers, providing a larger cross-sectional area capable of generating greater force production, but less ROM, than muscles with parallel fiber architecture (2).

Line of Pull and Angle of Attachment. Joint movement produced by contracting muscle is determined by the type of joint the muscle spans and the relation of muscle's line of pull to the joint (4). For example, the pectoralis major acts as both a flexor and adductor of the glenohumeral (shoulder) joint. When the shoulder is abducted, the line of pull of the pectoralis major changes so that it contributes to shoulder adduction and horizontal adduction to a greater extent. While line of pull affects the direction of movement, the angle of attachment helps determine the magnitude of tension produced by the muscle. The angle of attachment often changes throughout the ROM. With a 90° angle of attachment, the muscle is efficient in producing joint motion. With a very shallow angle of attachment, most of the muscle tension will produce force along the bone. Shallow angle of attachments generally help joint stability (4).

Force–Velocity and Length–Tension Relationships. The amount of force a muscle can create depends on excitation and mechanical factors related to contraction velocity and muscle length. The force–velocity relationship dictates that the magnitude of force that a muscle can exert depends on the rate of length change or muscle velocity (16) *(Fig. 7.13)*. As the velocity of muscle contraction increases, the force the muscle exerts decreases. The length–tension relationship indicates that the magnitude of force that a muscle can produce varies with its length (17) (see Fig. 7.12). At intermediate lengths, muscles produce the greatest force. Less force is created in shortened (active insufficiency) and lengthened (passive insufficiency) conditions. Passive insufficiency can be offset by increases in passive tension, since the elastic force of stretched connective tissue and muscle proteins generates tension that can be used to create subsequent motion.

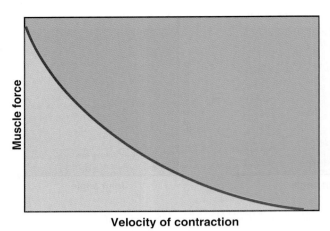

FIGURE 7.13. The force–velocity relationship of skeletal muscle illustrates skeletal muscle force potential for the rate of change of muscle length (velocity), so all three muscle actions can be visualized on the graph. (From Oatis CA. Kinesiology—The Mechanics and Pathomechanics of Human Movement. Baltimore: Lippincott Williams & Wilkins, 2004.)

Influence of Gravity. Movement can occur in the same direction as gravitational forces (downward), opposing gravity (upward), or perpendicular to gravity (horizontal). Lifting and lowering motions are heavily influenced by gravity, while horizontal motion is not affected by gravity. Lifting a weight against gravity is the concentric contraction of an agonist, while slowly lowering a weight against gravity is an eccentric contraction of same muscle (4).

Neural Factors. Neural factors also play a role in force generation of muscles. By increasing the number of fibers recruited and synchronizing the firing motor neurons, muscles can exert more force (2). Also, motor learning, including practice of exercise movements and development of skills, can alter force production and movement patterns.

SPECIFIC JOINT STRUCTURES

Muscle actions produce force that causes joint movement during exercise. Personal Trainers need a solid working knowledge of the functional anatomy and kinesiology of major joint structures. Tables 7.4 and 7.5 summarize the major joint movements, muscles that produce those movements, normal ROM values, and example resistance exercises for the muscles. This knowledge is the basis for the development of exercise programs to be used in training (18). In this section, we describe the structure and function of each of the major joints of the body in four steps:

1. Structure: What are the initial considerations of the joint's structure (e.g., bones, muscles, tendons, ligaments, cartilage, bursae) and ability to move?
2. Movements: What movements occur at the joint? What are the normal ROMs for each movement?
3. Muscles: What specific muscles are being used to create the movements? How are the muscles being used (e.g., agonist, synergist, stabilizer)?
4. Injuries: What common injuries occur to the joint structure?

Upper Extremity

SHOULDER

The shoulder complex is a multi-joint structure that provides the link between the thoracic cage and upper extremity. The shoulder has a high degree of mobility and, as a result, the shoulder region is very unstable. Since the bony structures of the shoulder provide relatively little support, much of the responsibility of stabilizing this region falls on the soft tissues—the muscles, ligaments, and joint capsules. The shoulder is more likely to be injured than the hip, another ball-and-socket joint (19).

Bones. The bones of the shoulder region include the humerus, scapula, and clavicle *(Fig. 7.14)*. The humerus is a long bone and is the major bone of the arm. The humeral head is rounded and

Table 7.4 MAJOR UPPER EXTREMITY JOINTS: MOVEMENTS, RANGE OF MOTION, MUSCLES, AND EXAMPLE RESISTANCE EXERCISES

Joint	Movement	Range of Motion (°)	Major Agonist Muscles	Examples of Resistance Exercises
Scapulothoracic	Fixation		Serratus anterior, pectoralis minor, trapezius, levator scapulae, rhomboids	Push-up, parallel bar dip, upright row, shoulder shrug, seated row
	Upward rotation		Trapezius	
	Downward rotation		Rhomboids, pectoralis minor, levator scapulae	
	Elevation		Rhomboids, levator scapulae, trapezius	Shoulder shrug
	Depression		Pectoralis minor, trapezius	
	Protraction		Serratus anterior, pectoralis minor	Supine dumbbell serratus press, push-up
	Retraction		Rhomboids, trapezius	Seated row
Glenohumeral (shoulder)	Flexion	90–100	Anterior deltoid, pectoralis major (clavicular head)	Dumbbell front raise, incline bench press
	Extension	40–60	Latissimus dorsi, teres major, pectoralis major (sternocostal head)	Dumbbell pullover, chin-up
	Abduction	90–95	Middle deltoid, supraspinatus	Dumbbell lateral raise, dumbbell press
	Adduction	0	Latissimus dorsi, teres major, pectoralis major	Lat pulldown, seated row, cable crossover, flat bench dumbbell fly
	Horizontal abduction	45		Prone reverse dumbbell fly, reverse cable fly
	Horizontal adduction	135		Flat bench chest fly, pec dec, cable crossover
	Internal rotation	70–90	Latissimus dorsi, teres major, subscapularis, pectoralis major, anterior deltoid	Lat pulldown, bent over row, dumbbell row, rotator cuff exercises, dumbbell press, parallel bar dip, front raises
	External rotation	70–90	Supraspinatus, infraspinatus, teres minor, posterior deltoid	Ext. rotator cuff exercises— dumbbell side-lying, cable in, rotator cuff exercises—dumbbell side-lying, cable
Elbow	Flexion	145–150	Biceps brachii, brachialis, brachioradialis	Dumbbell curl, preacher curl, hammer curl
	Extension	0	Triceps brachii, anconeus	Dip, pulley triceps extension, close grip bench press, pushdowns, dumbbell kickback
Radioulnar	Supination	80–90	Biceps brachii, supinator	Dumbbell curl (with supination)
	Pronation	70–90	Pronator quadratus, pronator teres	Dumbbell pronation
Wrist	Flexion	70–90	Flexor carpi radialis and ulnaris, palmaris longus, flexor digitorum superficialis	Dumbbell wrist curl
	Extension	65–85	Extensor carpi radialis longus, brevis, and ulnaris, extensor digitorum longus	Dumbbell reverse wrist curl
	Adduction	25–40	Flexor and extensor carpi ulnaris	Wrist curl, reverse wrist curl
	Abduction	15–25	Extensor carpi radialis longus and brevis, flexor carpi radialis	Wrist curl, reverse wrist curl

Table 7.5 **MAJOR SPINE AND LOWER EXTREMITY JOINTS: MOVEMENTS, RANGE OF MOTION, MUSCLES, AND EXAMPLE RESISTANCE EXERCISES**

Joint	Movement	Range of Motion (°)	Major Agonist Muscles	Examples of Resistance Exercises
Cervical spine	Flexion	50	Sternocleidomastoid, anterior scalene, longus capitis/coli	Machine neck flexion
	Extension	60	Suboccipitals, splenius capitis/cervicus, erector spinae	Machine neck extension
	Lateral flexion	45	Unilateral contraction of flexor–extensor muscles above	Machine neck lateral flexion
	Rotation	80	Unilateral contraction of flexor–extensor muscles above	Machine neck rotation
Lumbar spine	Flexion	60	Rectus abdominis, internal/external oblique abdominus	Crunch, leg raise, machine crunch high pulley crunch
	Extension	25	Erector spinae, multifidus	Roman chair, machine trunk extension, dead lift, squat, good morning
	Lateral flexion	25	Quadratus lumborum, internal/external oblique abdominals	Roman chair side bend, dumbbell side bend, hanging leg raise
	Rotation		Internal/external oblique abdominals, intrinsic spinal rotators, multifidus	Broomstick twist, machine trunk rotation
Hip	Flexion	130	Iliopsoas, rectus femoris, sartorius pectineus, tensor fascia latae	Leg raise, sit-up, machine crunch
	Extension	30	Gluteus maximus, hamstrings	Squat, leg press, lunge, machine leg extension
	Abduction	35	lensor fascia latae, sartorius, gluteus medius & minimus	Cable or machine hip abduction
	Adduction	30	Adductor longus, brevis, and magnus, gracilis, pectineus, gluteus maximus	Power squats, cable or machine hip adduction,
	Internal rotation	45	Semitendinosus, semimembranosus, gluteus medius & minimus, tensor fascia latae, gracilis	lunge
	External rotation	50	Biceps femoris, sartorius, adductor longus, brevis, and magnus, gluteus maximus	
Knee	Flexion	140	Hamstrings, gracilis, sartorius, popliteus, gastrocnemius	Leg curl (standing, seated, prone)
	Extension	0–10	Quadriceps femoris	Lunge, squats, machine leg extension
	Internal rotation	30	Sartorius, gracilis, semimembranosus, semitendinosus	
	External rotation	45	Biceps femoris	
Ankle: talocrural	Dorsiflexion	15–20	Tibialis anterior, extensor digitorum longus, extensor hallucis longus	Ankle dorsiflexion resistance band
	Plantar flexion	50	Gastrocnemius, soleus, tibialis posterior, flexor digitorum longus, flexor hallucis longus	Standing/seated calf raise, donkey calf raise
Ankle: subtalar	Eversion	5–15	Peroneus longus and brevis	Elastic band eversion

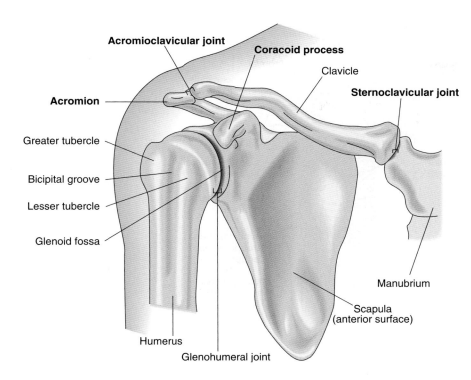

FIGURE 7.14. Bones and articulations of the shoulder region—anterior view. (From Bickley LS, Szilagyi P. Bates' Guide to Physical Examination and History Taking. 8th ed. Philadelphia: Lippincott Williams & Wilkins, 2003.)

articulates with the glenoid fossa of the scapula. The greater and lesser tubercles of the humerus are attachment sites for many of the muscles that act on the shoulder. The scapula is a large triangular bone that rests on the posterior thoracic cage between the second and seventh rib in the normal position. The scapula lies in the scaption plane, that is, obliquely at 30° to the frontal plane. The glenoid fossa of the scapula faces anterolaterally. The acromion process is located at the superior aspect of the scapula and articulates with the clavicle. The clavicle runs obliquely at 60° to the scapula and provides the link between the upper extremity and the axial skeleton. The clavicle provides protection for the neurovascular bundle called the "brachial plexus," supports the weight of the humerus, and helps to maintain the position of the scapula and humerus (11).

Ligaments and Bursae. The ligaments and bursae of the shoulder region are shown in Figure 7.15, and some of these structures are discussed below. The coracohumeral ligament (anterior and posterior fibers) spans the bicipital groove of the humerus and provides anteroinferior stability to the glenohumeral joint. The glenohumeral ligament (anterior, middle, and anteroinferior bands) provides stability to the shoulder joint in most planes of movement. The coracoacromial ligament, located superior to the glenohumeral joint, protects the muscles, tendons, nerves, and blood supply of the region. The acromioclavicular ligament is the major ligament that provides stability to the acromioclavicular joint. The coracoclavicular ligament (trapezoid and conoid bands) prevents superior dislocation of the acromioclavicular joint. The sternoclavicular ligaments (anterior and posterior) help strengthen the capsule of the sternoclavicular joint. The costoclavicular ligament connects the first rib and clavicle; and the interclavicular ligament connects the two clavicles and manubrium. The subdeltoid bursa, which lies between the supraspinatus and deltoid tendons and the acromion, allows gliding and cushioning of these structures, especially upon shoulder abduction (4).

Joints. The shoulder region is a complex of four joints: the glenohumeral (shoulder), acromioclavicular, sternoclavicular, and scapulothoracic joints (see Fig. 7.14). The glenohumeral joint is a ball-and-socket joint and is the most freely moveable joint in the body. It consists of the articulation of the spherical head of the humerus with the small, shallow, and somewhat pear-shaped glenoid fossa of the scapula. The glenoid labrum (which is composed of fibrocartilage) of the scapula deepens the fossa and cushions against impact of the humeral head in forceful movements (4) *(Fig. 7.16).*

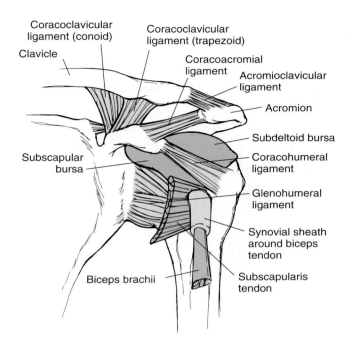

FIGURE 7.15. Ligaments and bursae of the shoulder region—anterior view. (From Hendrickson T. Massage for Orthopaedic Conditions. Baltimore: Lippincott Williams & Wilkins, 2002.)

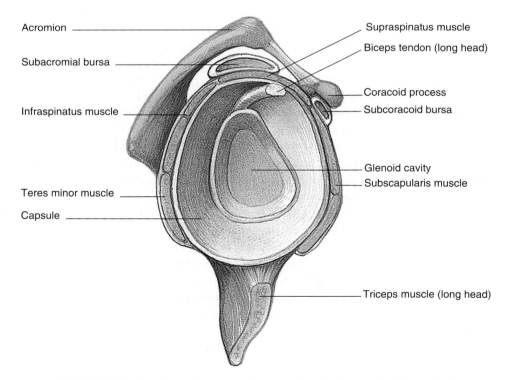

FIGURE 7.16. Shoulder joint socket. (Asset provided by Anatomical Chart Co.)

The acromioclavicular joint is a plane synovial joint of the articulation of the acromion and the distal end of the clavicle. The acromioclavicular joint moves in three planes simultaneously with scapulothoracic motion. The sternoclavicular joint, the articulation of the proximal clavicle with the sternum and cartilage of the first rib, is also a plane synovial joint. The sternoclavicular joint moves in synchronization with the other three joints of the shoulder region and, importantly, provides the only bony connection between the humerus and the axial skeleton (3).

The scapulothoracic joint is not a true joint, but a physiological joint. It is formed by the articulation of the scapula with the thoracic cage. In the kinematic chain, any movement of the scapulothoracic joint results in movement of the acromioclavicular, sternoclavicular, and glenohumeral joints. The scapulothoracic joint provides mobility and stability for the orientation of the glenoid fossa and the humeral head for arm movements in all planes (2).

Movements. Because the glenohumeral joint is a ball-and-socket joint, it is capable of motion in three planes: abduction–adduction in the frontal plane, flexion–extension in the sagittal plane, and internal–external rotation and horizontal abduction–adduction in the transverse plane. Further, the multiplanar movement of circumduction is possible at the glenohumeral joint (3). Glenohumeral movements are demonstrated in Figure 7.17, and normal ROM values are listed in Table 7.4.

The center of rotation of the glenohumeral joint occurs at the humeral head within the glenoid fossa. At 0–50° of abduction, the lower portion of the humeral head is in contact with the glenoid fossa, while at 50–90° of abduction, the upper portion of humeral head is in contact with the glenoid fossa. Since shear force creates friction across surfaces, the rolling of the humeral head within the glenoid reduces stress on the joint (4).

The scapulothoracic joint is also capable of motion in three planes. These motions include upward–downward rotation, retraction–protraction, elevation–depression, anterior–posterior tilting, and winging (4). Scapulothoracic joint movements are shown in Figure 7.18.

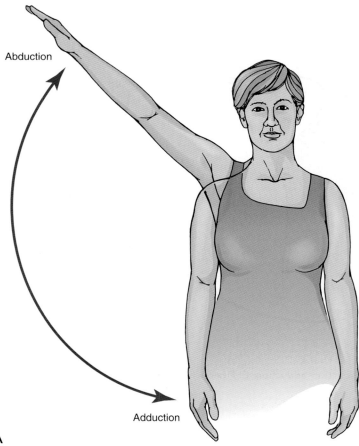

Abduction

Adduction

A

FIGURE 7.17. Movements of the shoulder. **A.** Abduction-adduction.

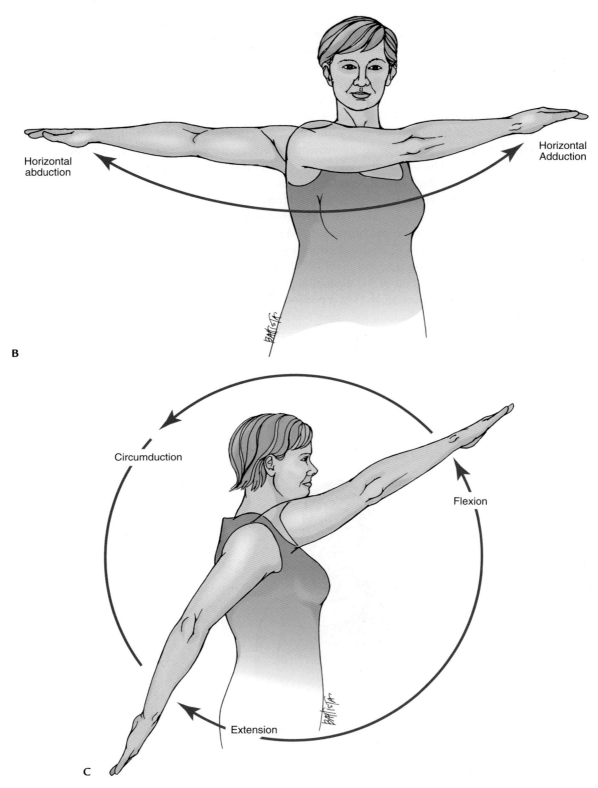

B

C

FIGURE 7.17. *(Continued)* **B.** Horizontal abduction–adduction. **C.** Flexion–extension and circumduction.

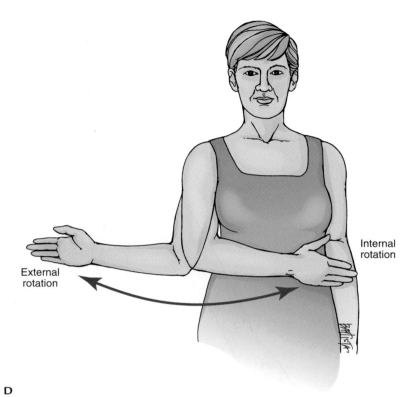

FIGURE 7.17. *(Continued)* **D.** Internal–external rotation.

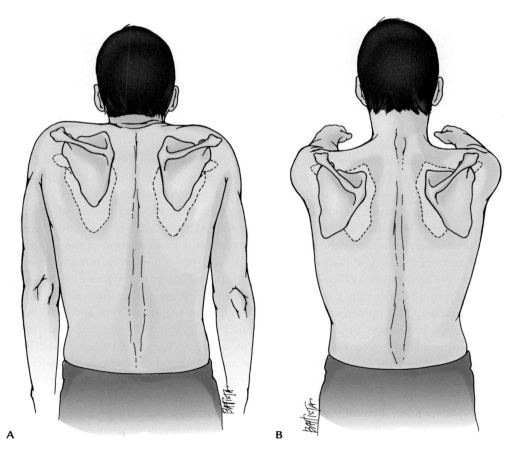

FIGURE 7.18. Movements of the scapulothoracic joint. **A.** Elevation–depression. **B.** Protraction–retraction.

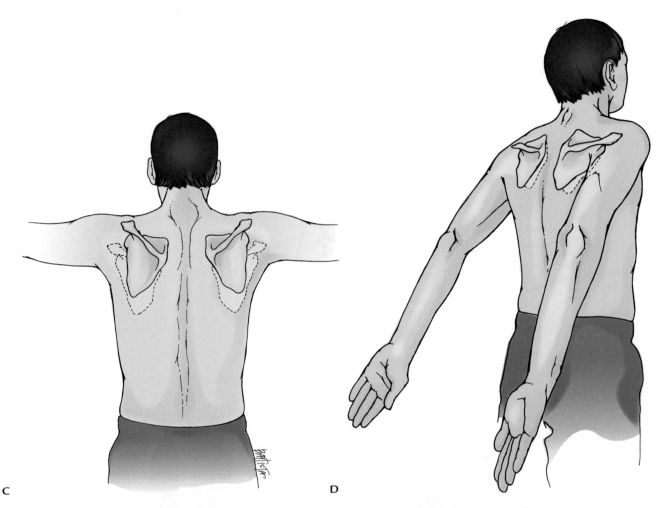

C   D

FIGURE 7.18. *(Continued)* **C.** Internal–external-rotation. **D.** Anterior–posterior tilt.

Scapulohumeral Rhythm. Full abduction of the arm requires the simultaneous movement of the glenohumeral and scapulothoracic joints. This dual movement is called "scapulohumeral rhythm" *(Fig. 7.19)*. Scapulohumeral rhythm allows a greater abduction ROM, maintains optimal length–tension relationships of the glenohumeral muscles, and prevents impingement between the greater tubercle of the humerus and the acromion. At about 120° of abduction, the greater tubercle of the humerus hits the lateral edge of the acromion. Lateral rotation of the scapula in the frontal plane causes the glenoid fossa of the scapula to face upward, making further elevation of the arm above the head possible (20). Overall, for every three degrees of abduction of the arm, two degrees of abduction occurs at the glenohumeral joint and one degree of rotation occurs at the scapula (21).

Muscles. The numerous muscles of the shoulder region are typically characterized as either shoulder joint muscles or shoulder girdle muscles. The shoulder joint and shoulder girdle muscles work together to perform upper extremity movements. The shoulder joint muscles directly move the arm, while the shoulder girdle muscles mainly stabilize the scapula on the thoracic cage and are particularly important in maintaining proper posture (3). The muscles of the shoulder region are shown in Figures 7.20 and 7.21.

Shoulder Joint. The anterior muscles of the shoulder joint are the pectoralis major, subscapularis, coracobrachialis, and biceps brachii. The posterior muscles of the shoulder joint are the infraspinatus and teres minor. The superior muscles are the deltoid and supraspinatus, and the inferior muscles

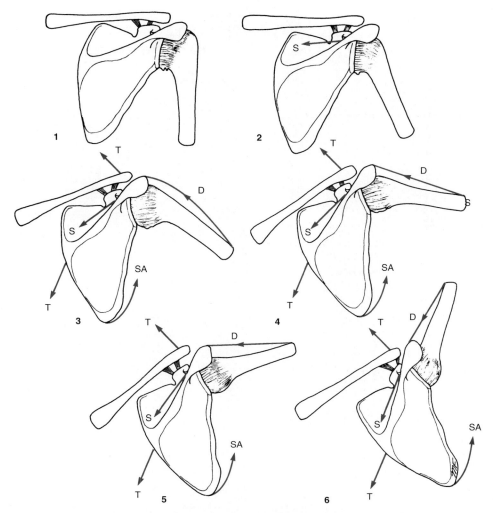

FIGURE 7.19. Scapulohumeral rhythm: Movements of shoulder abduction and scapular rotation, and the muscles that produce these movements at various stages of abduction. For every 3° of abduction of the arm, 2° of shoulder abduction and 1° of scapular rotation occur. *S,* supraspinatus; *D,* deltoid; *T,* trapezius; *SA,* serratus anterior. (From Snell RS. Clinical Anatomy. 7th ed. Baltimore: Lippincott Williams & Wilkins, 2003.)

include the latissimus dorsi, teres major, and long head of the triceps brachii. The pectoralis major is a large and powerful muscle that is a prime mover in adduction, horizontal adduction, and internal rotation of the humerus. The pectoralis major is triangular, originating along the medial clavicle and sternum and attaching to the greater tubercle of the humerus. The clavicular portion of the muscle primarily flexes the humerus, while the sternocostal portion extends the humerus from a flexed position (4). The coracobrachialis, a small muscle, assists with shoulder flexion and adduction. The biceps brachii is a two-joint, two-head muscle that crosses the shoulder and elbow. At the shoulder, the biceps brachii assists with horizontal adduction, flexion, and internal rotation (4). Its primary functions and anatomical considerations are discussed in the elbow section of this chapter.

The deltoid muscle has three heads: anterior, middle, and posterior. Each head inserts at the deltoid tuberosity on the lateral humerus. The anterior deltoid originates from the anterolateral aspect of the clavicle. It is chiefly responsible for shoulder flexion, horizontal adduction, and internal rotation of the glenohumeral joint. The middle deltoid originates from the lateral aspect of the acromion and is a powerful abductor of the glenohumeral joint. The posterior deltoid originates from the inferior aspect of the scapular spine, and its actions of glenohumeral extension, horizontal

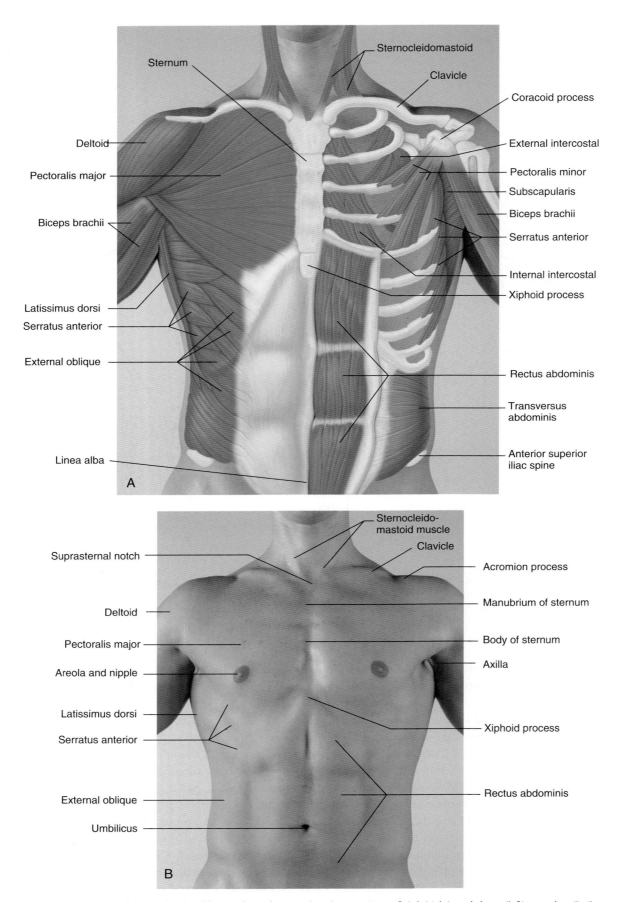

FIGURE 7.20. Muscles of the neck, shoulder, and trunk—anterior view. **A.** Superficial *(right)* and deep *(left)* muscles. **B.** Surface landmarks. (From Premkumar K. The Massage Connection Anatomy and Physiology. Baltimore: Lippincott Williams & Wilkins, 2004.)

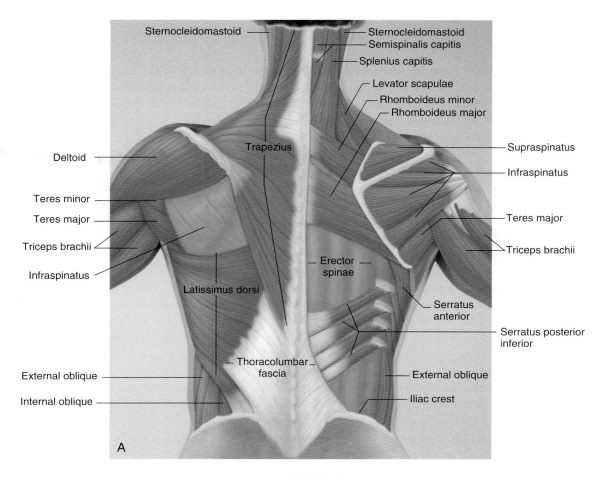

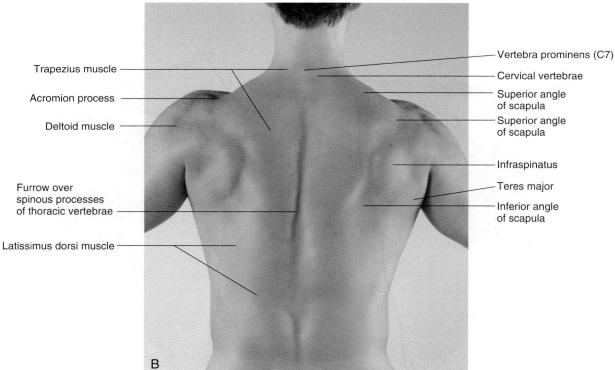

FIGURE 7.21. Muscles of the neck, shoulder, and trunk—posterior view. **A.** Superficial *(right)* and deep *(left)* muscles. **B.** Surface landmarks. (From Premkumar K. The Massage Connection Anatomy and Physiology. Baltimore: Lippincott Williams & Wilkins, 2004.)

abduction, and external rotation oppose those of the anterior deltoid (5). The anterior and posterior deltoids should be approximately the same size. However, in most individuals, the anterior deltoid is much more developed than the posterior deltoid. This imbalance can cause postural abnormalities (shoulder forward and internally rotated) and may be related to shoulder problems such as impingement syndrome (4).

The rotator cuff muscles include the supraspinatus, infraspinatus, teres minor, and subscapularis, which are often remembered by the acronym "SITS" *(Fig. 7.22)*. The rotator cuff muscles originate from the scapula and insert at the greater or lesser tubercle of the humerus (22). The supraspinatus primarily abducts the glenohumeral joint; the infraspinatus and teres minor externally rotate the glenohumeral joint, with assistance from the supraspinatus; and the subscapularis internally rotates the glenohumeral joint. The infraspinatus, teres minor, and subscapularis depress the humerus as well. The supraspinatus is active when maintaining normal posture (4).

The rotator cuff muscles are important stabilizers of the glenohumeral joint and aid in glenohumeral positional control (22). These muscles act like a strong ligament, holding the humeral head tightly in the glenoid fossa during arm movements initiated by the larger shoulder muscles. The rotator cuff stabilizes the shoulder through four mechanisms: *(a)* passive muscle tension, *(b)* contraction of the muscles causing compression of the articular surface, *(c)* joint motion that results in secondary tightening of the ligamentous restraints, and *(d)* the barrier effect of contracted muscle (23).

The latissimus dorsi is a large fan-shaped muscle that originates from the iliac crest and the posterior sacrum (via thoracolumbar fascia), lower six thoracic vertebrae, and lower three ribs. It inserts at the intertrabecular groove of the humerus. The latissimus dorsi is a strong extensor, internal rotator, and adductor of the glenohumeral joint. The angle of pull of the latissimus dorsi increases when the arm is abducted to 30–90°. The teres major muscle has actions similar to those of the latissimus dorsi. The triceps brachii is typically known as an elbow muscle, but its long head acts to extends the shoulder, as well (5).

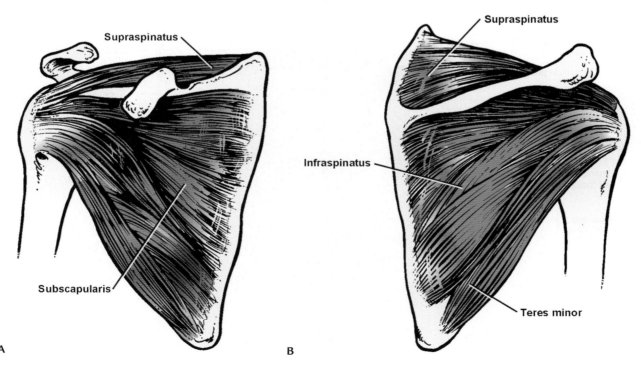

FIGURE 7.22. Rotator cuff muscles. **A.** Anterior view. **B.** Posterior view. (From Koval KJ, Zuckerman JD. Atlas of Orthopaedic Surgery: A Multimedial Reference. Philadelphia: Lippincott Williams & Wilkins, 2004.)

Shoulder Girdle. The muscles of the anterior shoulder girdle include the pectoralis minor, serratus anterior, and subclavius. The pectoralis minor originates from the anterior aspects of the third to fifth ribs and inserts at the coracoid process of the scapula. Contraction of the pectoralis minor causes protraction, downward rotation, and depression of the scapula. The pectoralis minor has a lifting effect on the ribs during forceful inspiration and postural control. The serratus anterior contains several bands that originate from the upper nine ribs laterally and insert on the anterior aspect of the medial border of the scapula. The serratus anterior protracts the scapula and is active in reaching and pushing. Winging of the scapula results from serratus anterior dysfunction, possibly related to long thoracic nerve problems. The subclavius is a small muscle that protects and stabilizes the sternoclavicular joint (5).

The posterior shoulder muscles are the levator scapulae, rhomboid (major and minor), and trapezius. The levator scapulae originates from the transverse processes of the upper four cervical vertebrae, runs obliquely, and inserts at the medial border of the scapular spine. The levator scapulae produces elevation and downward rotation of scapula, and also acts on the neck. The rhomboids originate from the spinous processes of the last cervical and upper five thoracic vertebrae and insert along the entire length of the medial border of the scapula. Rhomboid action results in scapular retraction, downward rotation, and slight elevation. Along with the trapezius, proper rhomboid activity is necessary for good posture (i.e., squeezing shoulder blades together) (4).

The trapezius muscle is a large triangular muscle and one of the largest muscles of the shoulder region. It contains three distinct regions: the upper, middle, and lower fibers. The origin of the trapezius covers a broad area from the base of the occiput to the spinous process of the twelfth thoracic vertebra; and its insertion runs from the lateral clavicle, medial border of the acromion, and scapular spine. Contraction of the upper trapezius causes scapular elevation; the middle trapezius causes scapular elevation, upward rotation, and retraction; and the lower trapezius causes scapular depression, retraction, and upward rotation (5).

Injuries. Impingement syndrome is probably the most common non–traumatic cause of shoulder pain (24). Impingement syndrome results from approximation of the acromion and greater tubercle of humerus, which causes entrapment of the rotator cuff tendons (22). Shoulder impingement may also be associated with subacromial bursitis, biceps tendonitis, and degenerative tears of the rotator cuff tendons (19). A primary factor of impingement syndrome is muscular imbalance at the shoulder exacerbated by external rotator cuff muscle weakness and highly trained internal rotator muscles (particularly the prime movers) (24). This imbalance can lead to postural abnormalities, such as anterior shoulder carriage with excessive internal rotation (shoulder rounded forward), adaptive shortening and fibrosis of the internal rotators, and inflamed rotator cuff tendons. The progressive loss of external rotation, due to fibrosis or adaptive shortening of the internal rotators, is the most common factor in chronic rotator cuff disorders. Some of the predisposing factors for impingement syndrome include biomechanically unsound exercises and sports activities (e.g., swimming), lifting weights with poor form, and training the same area of the body too often (overtraining anterior deltoids, pectoralis major, and latissimus dorsi) (24). Treatment for impingement syndrome is heavily focused on retraining proper exercise and posture. This includes strengthening and improving the function of the external rotators, stretching the internal rotators, and eliminating the training errors that started the dysfunction in the first place (24). All too often, however, a person who suffers from impingement syndrome is noncompliant with appropriate rehabilitation, and the condition becomes chronic, leading to permanent degenerative changes and dysfunction.

Thoracic outlet syndrome is another condition of the shoulder that can be related to faulty biomechanics, poor posture, and shoulder muscle imbalance (25). Thoracic outlet syndrome is compression of the neurovascular bundle (brachial plexus) in the shoulder region and results in symptoms of pain, numbness, and tingling in the upper extremity, usually ulnar distribution or C8 dermatome (fourth and fifth digits of the hand). The three sites of compression in thoracic outlet syndrome occur between the first rib and anterior scalene muscle, pectoralis minor muscle, or clavicle (25). Treatment for thoracic outlet syndrome includes correcting faulty biomechanics, strengthening the rotator cuff, and stretching the shoulder internal rotators and scalenes. As with impingement syndrome, complete recovery may take several months or longer.

The shoulder is also susceptible to traumatic injuries, such as joint separation or dislocation and tearing of tendons, ligaments, or joint capsules. Glenohumeral joint dislocation usually occurs anteriorly because of capsular tears (4). The mechanism of glenohumeral joint dislocation is typically excessive abduction, external rotation, and extension of the shoulder. Stabilizing the shoulder after suspected glenohumeral joint dislocation is important to prevent any further damage, particularly to the neurological structures. Acromioclavicular joint separation is classically due to a direct blow to the shoulder or fall on an outstretched arm (19). Signs and symptoms of acromioclavicular joint separation include elevation of the distal clavicle and sharp pain in the joint. Rotator cuff tendon tears (particularly of the supraspinatus muscle) can be caused by forceful throwing (e.g., baseball) and improper weight-lifting techniques (19).

ELBOW

The elbow is an important joint involved in lifting and carrying, throwing, swinging, and most upper extremity exercise movements. The elbow is commonly injured and is the second most injured joint from overuse or repetitive motion (26, 27).

Bones. The elbow consists of the humerus, radius, and ulna bones. The humeroulnar joint is the articulation of the distal humerus with the proximal ulna; the humeroradial joint is the articulation of the distal humerus with the proximal radius; and the radioulnar joint is the articulation of the proximal radius with the proximal ulna (3) *(Fig. 7.23).*

With the arms held at the side of the body and the palms of the hand facing anteriorly, the forearm and hands are usually held slightly away from the body. This is due to the carrying angle of the elbow, which is normally 5–15° in males and 20–25° in females. Carrying angle allows the forearm to swing free of the side of the hips during walking and provides a mechanical advantage when carrying objects (4).

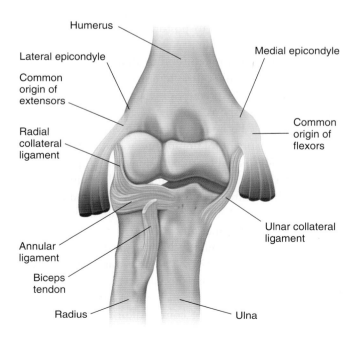

FIGURE 7.23. Bones and ligaments of the elbow joint—anterior view. (From Premkumar K. The Massage Connection Anatomy and Physiology. Baltimore: Lippincott Williams & Wilkins, 2004.)

Ligaments. Three major ligaments stabilize the elbow: the ulnar (medial) collateral ligament, which connects the humerus with the ulna; the radial (lateral) collateral, which connects the humerus with the radius; and the annular ligament, which connects the radius with the ulna. The collateral ligaments provide support for stresses in the frontal plane, the medial collateral for valgus forces, and the lateral collateral for varus forces. The annular ligament provides stability for the radius, securing it to the ulna (3) (see Fig. 7.23).

Joints. The elbow joint complex is a compound synovial joint that consists of two joints: the humeroulnar and humeroradial joints. The distal humerus articulates with both the proximal ulna and proximal radius, and the two joints are enclosed by one capsule. On the lateral side of the elbow, the capitulum of the humerus articulates with the head of the radius to form the humeroradial joint; medially, the trochlea of the humerus articulates with the trochlear notch of the ulna to form the humeroulnar joint. The proximal radioulnar joint, whose joint capsule is continuous with that of the humeroulnar and humeroradial joints, is the articulation of the medial aspect of the proximal radius with the radial notch of the ulna (3) (see Fig. 7.23).

Movements. Both the humeroulnar and humeroradial are hinge joints that flex and extend the elbow in the sagittal plane *(Fig. 7.24).* The normal ROM for flexion–extension is 145–150°, with the fully flexed position (elbow bent) represented by 145–150° and the fully extended position (arm straight with forearm) represented by 0°. During sagittal movement of the elbow, the trochlear notch of the humerus slides into the trochlear groove of the ulna. Upon full flexion, the coronoid process of the ulna approximates the coronoid fossa of the humerus. At full extension, the olecranon process of the ulna hits the olecranon fossa of the humerus, which adds to the stability of the elbow in full extension. The proximal radioulnar joint is a pivot joint, which permits axial rotation of the radius during supination and pronation of the elbow. Normal ROM for supination (forearm rotated laterally—palms facing anteriorly) is 80–90°; normal ROM for pronation (forearm rotated medially—palms facing posteriorly) is 80–90° (3).

Muscles

Anterior. The anterior muscles of the elbow mainly flex and pronate the elbow and include the biceps brachii, brachialis, brachioradialis, pronator teres, and pronator quadratus *(Fig. 7.25).* The three muscles that flex the elbow are the biceps brachii, brachialis, and brachioradialis (5). The biceps brachii is a two-head, two-joint muscle that acts on both the shoulder and elbow. Its long head

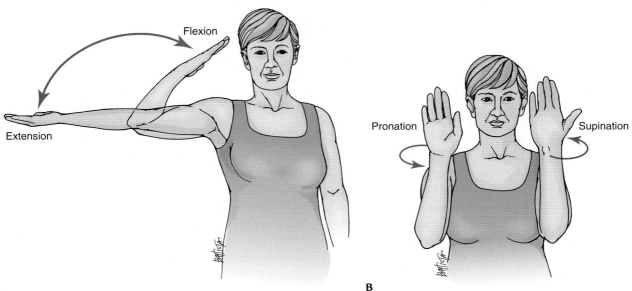

A   B

FIGURE 7.24. Movements of the elbow. **A.** Flexion-extension, **B.** Pronation-supination.

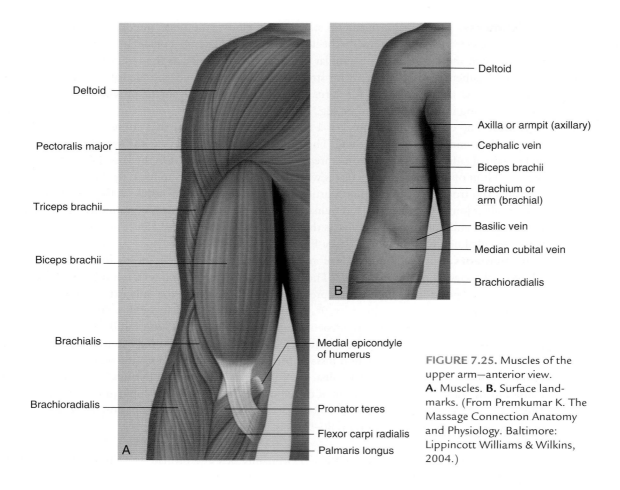

FIGURE 7.25. Muscles of the upper arm—anterior view. **A.** Muscles. **B.** Surface landmarks. (From Premkumar K. The Massage Connection Anatomy and Physiology. Baltimore: Lippincott Williams & Wilkins, 2004.)

originates from the glenoid fossa at the shoulder, and the short head originates from the upper humerus, with both heads inserting at the styloid process of the radius. The biceps brachii is a strong flexor and supinator of the elbow and is most active in supination. To optimally train the biceps brachii, exercise movements should include both elbow flexion and forearm supination (e.g., dumbbell biceps curl). The brachialis is considered the elbow flexor workhorse (4). Hammer curls, with the forearms maintained in a neutral position, are ideal to develop the brachialis and brachioradialis. As their names suggest, the pronator quadratus and pronator teres pronate the forearm. The pronator quadratus is the stronger of the two.

Posterior. The posterior muscles of the elbow primarily extend and supinate the elbow and include the triceps brachii, anconeus, and supinator *(Fig. 7.26).* The triceps brachii is a three-head, two-joint (long head) muscle that acts on the elbow and shoulder. Its long head originates from the glenoid fossa at the shoulder, while the medial and lateral heads originate from the upper humerus. All three heads insert at the olecranon of the ulna. The triceps brachii is the main elbow extensor, getting trivial assistance from the anconeus. The anconeus, a small muscle, also adds stability to the posterior elbow (5).

Injuries. Because of its use in most upper extremity daily living, exercise, and sport activities, the elbow is frequently injured from chronic overuse or repetitive motion (19). Tendonitis is evident in a variety of muscular insertion points at the elbow. Tennis elbow (lateral epicondylitis), which creates lateral elbow pain, is the most widespread overuse injury of the adult elbow (26, 27). It is usually caused by eccentric overload of the forearm extensor muscles (e.g., gripping a racquet too tightly, wrong grip size, faulty backhand technique, excessive racquet weight) (28). Golfer's elbow (medial epicondylitis), which produces medial elbow pain, is often caused by repeated valgus stresses

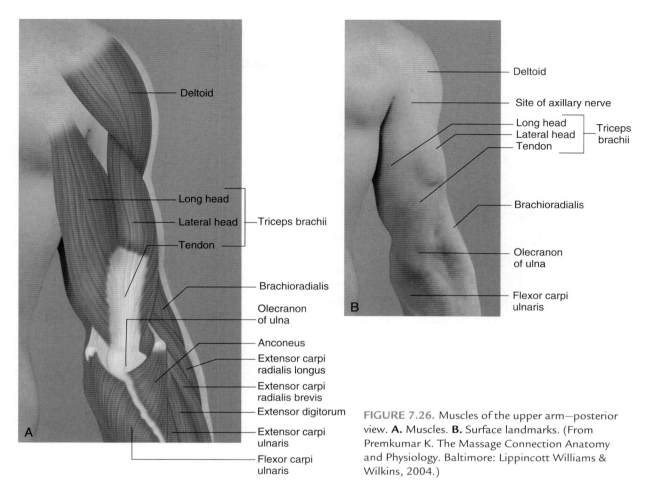

FIGURE 7.26. Muscles of the upper arm—posterior view. **A.** Muscles. **B.** Surface landmarks. (From Premkumar K. The Massage Connection Anatomy and Physiology. Baltimore: Lippincott Williams & Wilkins, 2004.)

placed on the arm during throwing or swinging of racquets or clubs. Triceps tendonitis, which produces pain over the olecranon, is caused by repetitive posterior stresses during elbow extension. Resistance and flexibility exercises for elbow flexion, extension, pronation, and supination are often incorporated to prevent and treat these injuries. Medial collateral ligament sprain often results from repetitive microtrauma and excessive valgus force (19).

The elbow is also the site for traumatic injuries. Olecranon bursitis, which typically produces a large red swelling over the posterior elbow, usually results from a fall directly on the elbow. Ulnar dislocation typically results from violent hyperextension or varus or valgus forces. Ulnar dislocation, which is most common in individuals under 20 years of age, results in obvious elbow deformity and may present with neurological symptoms into the hand (fifth digit) because of entrapment of the ulnar nerve at the elbow (19).

WRIST, HAND, AND FINGERS

The wrist, hand, and fingers are required for most daily living, work, and sports activities, including tasks such as gripping, lifting, writing, typing, eating, and throwing. Since adequate wrist and hand function is necessary for these activities, injuries to the wrist and hand are often disabling. This section focuses mainly on the functional anatomy of the wrist. The reader is referred to other sources (6–10) for the functional anatomy of the intrinsic hand and fingers.

Bones. The wrist, hand, and fingers consist of 29 bones: the distal ulna, distal radius, eight carpals, five metacarpals, and 14 phalanges (11) *(Fig. 7.27)*. The carpals are small oddly shaped bones arranged in two rows. The proximal row from lateral to medial includes the scaphoid (navicular),

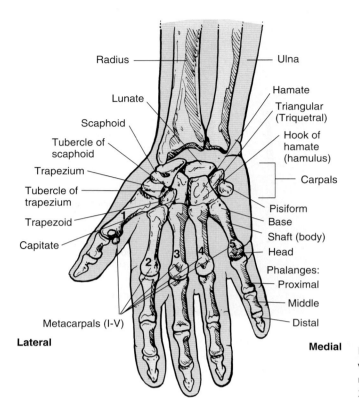

Radius

Ulna

Lunate

Hamate

Scaphoid

Triangular
(Triquetral)

Tubercle of
scaphoid

Hook of
hamate
(hamulus)

Trapezium

Carpals

Tubercle of
trapezium

Pisiform

Trapezoid

Base

Shaft (body)

Capitate

Head

Phalanges:

Proximal

Middle

Metacarpals (I-V)

Distal

Lateral

Medial

FIGURE 7.27. Bones of the wrist and hand—anterior view. (From Anderson M, Hall SJ. Sports Injury Management. 2nd ed. Baltimore: Lippincott Williams & Wilkins, 2000.)

lunate, triquetrum, and pisiform. The distal row from lateral to medial includes the trapezium, trapezoid, capitate, and hamate. There is one metacarpal per digit, which connects the carpals to the phalanges. Each digit has three phalanges, except the thumb, which has two (11).

Ligaments. The volar radiocarpal, dorsal radiocarpal, radial collateral, and ulnar collateral ligaments support the radioulnar joint. The radiocarpal ligaments provide stability in the sagittal plane, while the collateral ligaments provide stability in the frontal plane (11). There are numerous other ligaments that stabilize the wrist, hand, and fingers, many of which have clinical implications for health professionals other than Personal Trainers.

Joints. The primary wrist joint (radiocarpal joint) is a condyloid (ellipsoidal) joint consisting of the articulation of the distal radius with three proximal carpal bones: scaphoid, lunate, and triquetrum. The joint surface of the radius is concave, allowing the convex carpals to approximate it. The proximal and distal carpal bones form the complex mid-carpal joint. The distal radioulnar joint, a pivot joint, is situated medial to the radiocarpal joint and allows forearm supination and pronation (11).

Movements. The wrist allows approximately 70–90° of flexion and 65–85° of extension in the sagittal plane, and 15–25° of abduction (radial deviation) and 25–40° of adduction (ulnar deviation) in the frontal plane *(Fig. 7.28)*. Flexion–extension and abduction–adduction movements occur mainly at the radiocarpal joint. However, gliding motions at the midcarpal joint, which are facilitated by ligaments, allow full ROM in both planes. Circumduction of the wrist is also possible through the compound action of the radioulnar and midcarpal joints. The closed pack position of the wrist joint is full extension, while the open pack position is 0° of extension with slight adduction (4).

Muscles

Anterior. The wrist flexor muscles, which are located on the anteromedial aspect of the wrist and originate from the medial epicondyle of the humerus, include the flexor carpi radialis, flexor carpi ulnaris, and palmaris longus *(Fig. 7.29)*. In addition to the flexor activity, the flexor carpi radialis abducts the wrist, and the flexor carpi ulnaris adducts the wrist, as well (5).

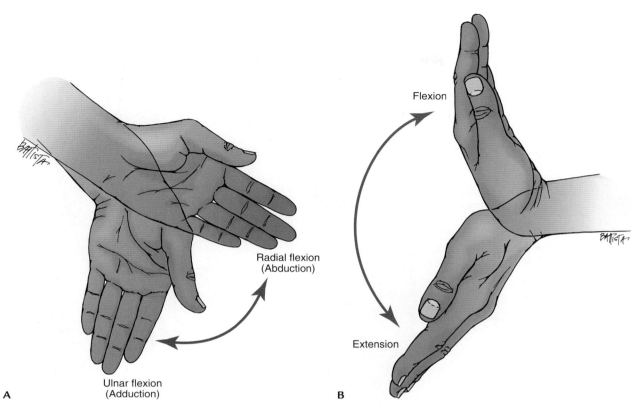

A

Radial flexion
(Abduction)

Ulnar flexion
(Adduction)

B

Flexion

Extension

FIGURE 7.28. Movements of the wrist. **A.** Abduction–adduction. **B.** Flexion–extension.

Posterior. The wrist extensor muscles, which are located on the posterolateral aspect of the wrist and originate at or near the lateral epicondyle of the humerus, include the extensor carpi radialis longus and brevis and the extensor carpi ulnaris *(Fig. 7.30)*. In addition to their extensor activity, the extensor carpi radialis longus abducts the wrist and the extensor carpi ulnaris adducts the wrist as well (5).

Injuries. Dislocations, fractures, and sprains are commonly at the wrist following falls. Falling on an outstretched arm with the wrist extended may cause lunate bone dislocation (usually anteriorly) or scaphoid bone fracture. Colles and Smith fractures are serious fractures affecting both the distal ulna and radius, which many times require fixation with rigid screws and plates to restore function (29). Wrist ligament sprains are frequently caused by axial loading of the palm during a fall on an outstretched arm (19).

Carpal tunnel syndrome is a widespread cumulative trauma disorder that is caused by median nerve entrapment at the anterior wrist (25). It usually results from repeated microtrauma to the carpal tunnel and flexor retinaculum due to prolonged manual work with the wrist in a flexed position (e.g., in individuals who work with computer keyboards, assembly line workers, cyclists). Its symptoms include pain, numbness, tingling, and weakness in thumb, index, and middle finger (median nerve distribution). Carpal tunnel syndrome usually requires physical rehabilitation, surgery, or ergonomic correction to restore function.

Lower Extremity

PELVIS AND HIP

The pelvis and hip region provides the link between the axial skeleton (trunk) and lower extremities. This region assists with motion, stability, and shock absorption and helps to distribute body weight evenly to the lower extremities (4).

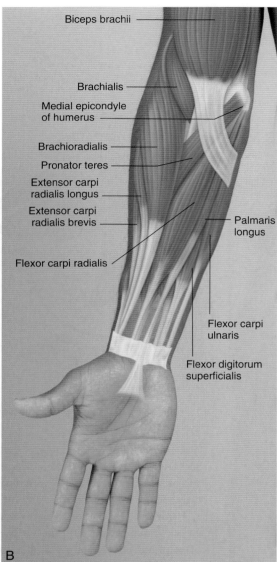

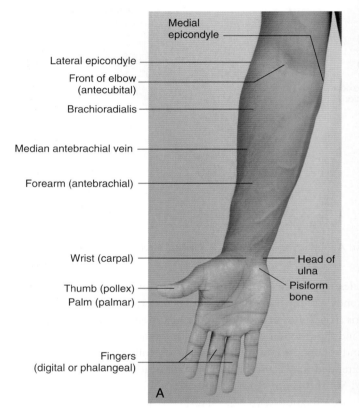

FIGURE 7.29. Muscles of the forearm—anterior view. **A.** Muscles. **B.** Surface landmarks. (From Premkumar K. The Massage Connection Anatomy and Physiology. Baltimore: Lippincott Williams & Wilkins, 2004.)

Bones. The bones of the pelvis and hip region are the sacrum, pelvis, and two femurs. The pelvis bones include the ilium (largest pelvic bone), ischium, and pubis on each side, which typically fuse by the end of puberty. The two sides of the pelvis join anteriorly at the pubis symphysis and posteriorly at the sacroiliac joints. The pelvis of females is usually wider than that of males, which contributes to the increased "Q angle" of the knee in females (4). The anterior superior iliac spine (ASIS) of the ilium is a bony protuberance that provides an attachment point for several muscles of the anterior thigh. The sacrum articulates with the pelvis on each side, forming the sacroiliac joints, and the pelvis articulates with each femur, forming the hip joints (11) *(Fig. 7.31)*.

Ligaments. The anterior, posterior, and interosseus ligaments bind the sacroiliac joint. The highly mobile hip joint is stabilized by several ligaments and a strong, dense joint capsule (3). The transverse acetabular ligament is a sturdy band that bridges the acetabular notch and completes the acetabular ring of the hip joint. The teres femoris ligament ties the head of the femur to the lower

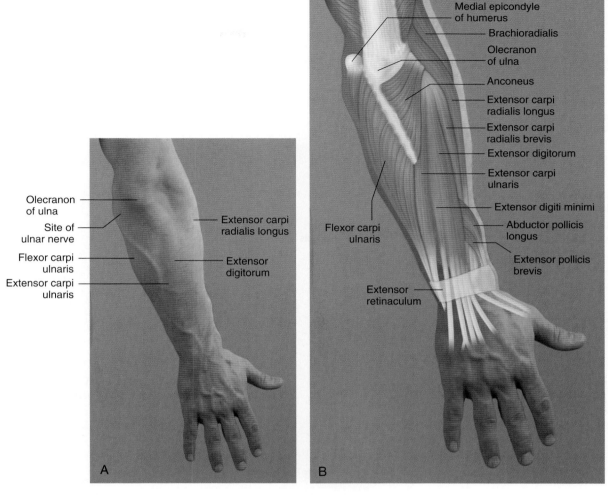

FIGURE 7.30. Muscles of the forearm—posterior view. **A.** Muscles. **B.** Surface landmarks. (From Premkumar K. The Massage Connection Anatomy and Physiology. Baltimore: Lippincott Williams & Wilkins, 2004.)

acetabulum of the pelvis, providing reinforcement from within the joint. The iliofemoral ligament ("Y" ligament) is an extraordinarily strong band that checks hip extension and rotation. The pubofemoral ligament prevents excessive abduction. The ischiofemoral ligament is triangular and limits hip rotation and adduction in the flexed position (3) *(Fig. 7.32)*.

Joints. The pubic symphysis connects each side of the pelvic girdle anteriorly and is an amphiarthrodial joint. The sacroiliac joint connects the sacrum to the ilium and is sometimes described as a gliding joint. These joints are capable of relatively little movement (3).

The hip joint is a ball-and-socket enarthrodial joint and is one of the most mobile joints in the body. The hip joint is formed by the articulation of the proximal femur (femoral head) with the acetabulum of the pelvis. The femoral head is covered with hyaline cartilage, except at the fovea capitis, and the acetabulum is lined with hyaline cartilage as well. The acetabular labrum is a fibrocartilaginous structure that adds depth to the joint and serves as a cushion for the femoral head (4) *(Fig. 7.33)*.

Movements. The pelvic girdle allows movement in three planes. These movements are shown in Figure 7.34. Movement at the pelvis during normal activities usually involves simultaneous motion of the hip and lumbar spine (3). In the sagittal plane, the pelvis is capable of anterior–posterior tilt. With anterior pelvic tilt, the pubic symphysis moves inferiorly, the lumbar spine

Anterior view

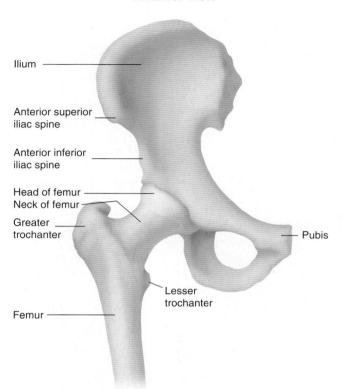

Ilium

Anterior superior iliac spine

Anterior inferior iliac spine

Head of femur
Neck of femur
Greater trochanter

Pubis

Lesser trochanter

Femur

FIGURE 7.31. Bones of the pelvis and hip region—anterior view. (Asset provided by Anatomical Chart Co.)

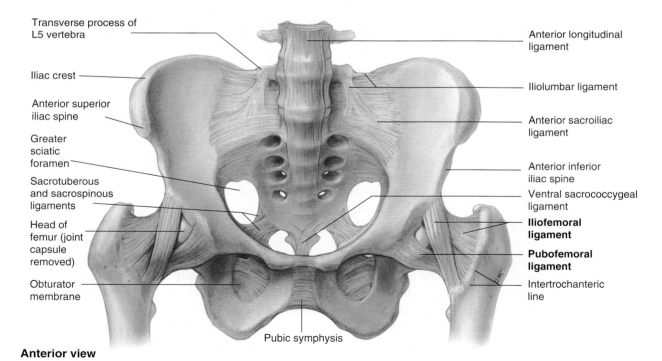

Transverse process of L5 vertebra

Iliac crest

Anterior superior iliac spine

Greater sciatic foramen

Sacrotuberous and sacrospinous ligaments

Head of femur (joint capsule removed)

Obturator membrane

Pubic symphysis

Anterior longitudinal ligament

Iliolumbar ligament

Anterior sacroiliac ligament

Anterior inferior iliac spine

Ventral sacrococcygeal ligament

Iliofemoral ligament

Pubofemoral ligament

Intertrochanteric line

Anterior view

FIGURE 7.32. Ligaments of the pelvis and hip regions—anterior view. (From Moore KL, Dalley AF II. Clinical Oriented Anatomy. 4th ed. Baltimore: Lippincott Williams & Wilkins, 1999.)

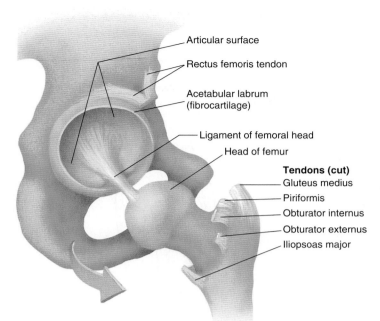

Articular surface

Rectus femoris tendon

Acetabular labrum
(fibrocartilage)

Ligament of femoral head

Head of femur

Tendons (cut)
Gluteus medius
Piriformis
Obturator internus
Obturator externus
Iliopsoas major

FIGURE 7.33. Acetabulum of the hip joint. (Asset provided by Anatomical Chart Co.)

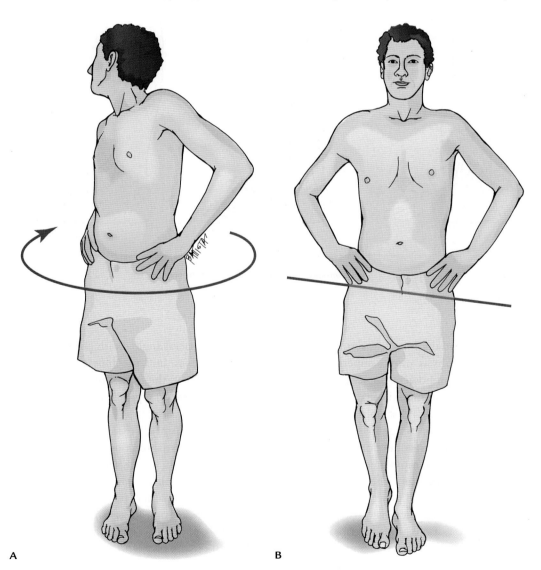

A

B

FIGURE 7.34. Movements of the pelvis. **A.** Rotation. **B.** Frontal (lateral) tilt.

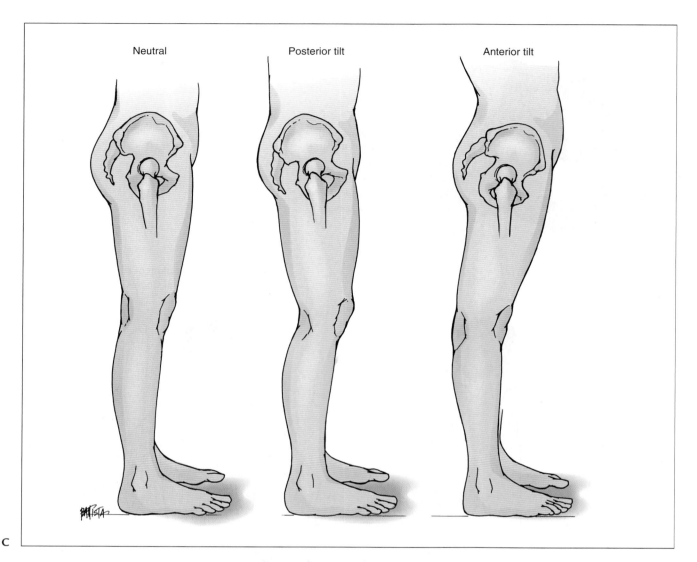

Neutral Posterior tilt Anterior tilt

C

FIGURE 7.34. *(Continued)* **C.** Sagittal (anterior–posterior) tilt.

extends, and the hips flex, resulting in an increased lumbosacral angle. With posterior pelvic tilt, the pubic symphysis moves superiorly, the lumbar spine flexes, and the hips extend, resulting in a decreased lumbosacral angle. Lateral tilt of the pelvis occurs in the frontal plane, and rotation of the pelvis occurs in the axial plane. Locomotion (walking or running) typically involves small oscillations of the pelvis in all three planes (3).

The highly mobile hip joint allows movement in three planes: flexion–extension in the sagittal plane, abduction–adduction in the frontal plane, internal–external rotation in the axial plane, and the combined plane movement of circumduction (3). Hip movements are shown in Figure 7.35.

Pelvic Muscles. The muscles of the pelvis include the muscles that act on the lumbar spine, lower trunk, and hip, which are discussed elsewhere in this chapter. In general, anterior pelvic tilt results from contraction of the hip flexors and lumbar extensors. Posterior pelvic tilt results from contraction of the hip extensors and lumbar flexors. Lateral tilt results from contraction of the lateral lumbar muscles (e.g., quadratus lumborum) and hip abductor–adductor muscles, and axial rotation occurs through the action of the hip and spinal rotator muscles (4).

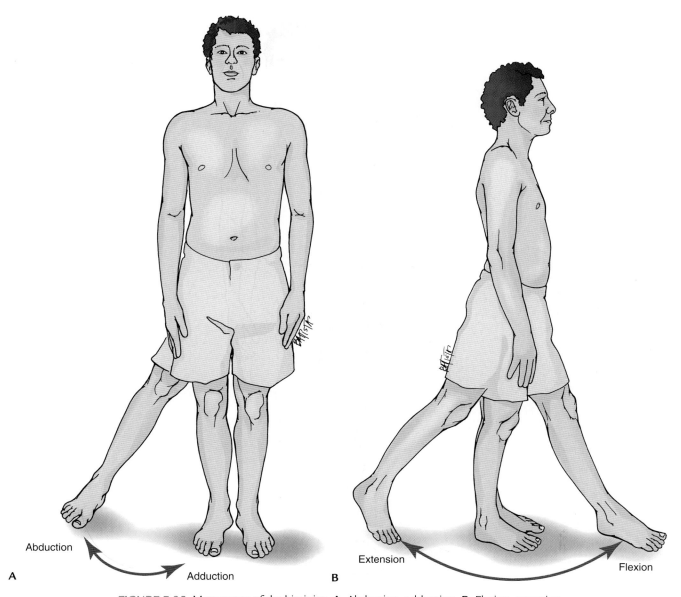

FIGURE 7.35. Movements of the hip joint. **A.** Abduction–adduction. **B.** Flexion–extension.

Hip Muscles. The muscles that act on the hip are shown in Figures 7.36 through 7.39.

Anterior. The anterior muscles of the hip region include the iliopsoas, pectineus, rectus femoris, sartorius, and tensor fasciae latae. The iliopsoas muscle group, which consists of the psoas major, psoas minor, and iliacus muscles, is a strong hip flexor. The pectineus is a small muscle that attaches the anterior pubis to the medial side of the proximal femur. It assists in hip flexion, adduction, and internal rotation. The rectus femoris is a large two-joint muscle that flexes the hip and extends the knee. The rectus femoris originates from the ASIS and inserts at the tibial tuberosity via the patellar ligament. The sartorius is the longest muscle in the body, originating from the ASIS and inserting at the medial tibial condyle. The sartorius flexes, abducts, and externally rotates the hip. The tensor fasciae latae originates from the anterior iliac crest of the ilium and inserts at the anterolateral tibial condyle via a long band of fascia—the iliotibial band. The tensor fasciae latae abducts and flexes the hip and stabilizes the hip against external rotation when the hip is flexed (5).

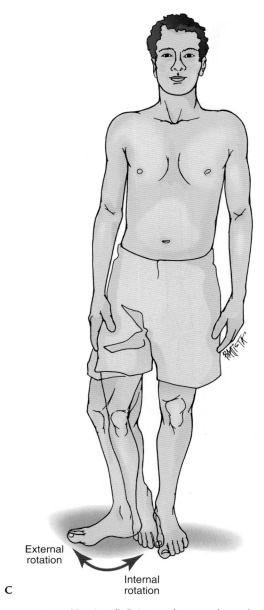

External
rotation

Internal
rotation

C

FIGURE 7.35. *(Continued)* **C.** Internal–external rotation.

Posterior. The posterior muscles of the hip include the hamstrings (biceps femoris, semimembranosus, and semitendinosus); gluteus maximus, medius, and minimus; adductor magnus, longus, and brevis; gracilis; and the six deep external rotators (piriformis, gemellus superior and inferior, obturator internus and externus, and quadratus femoris). The biceps femoris is a two-joint muscle that extends the hip and flexes the knee. It originates from the ischial tuberosity (long head) and proximal femur (short head) and inserts at the lateral tibial condyle and fibular head. The semitendinosus and semimembranosus are also two-joint muscles and act to extend and internally rotate the hip and flex and internally rotate the knee. The gluteus maximus, which forms the bulk of the buttock region, originates from the ilium and inserts at the lateral side of the greater trochanter of the femur. It is a powerful hip extensor, and its lower fibers assist in hip adduction. The gluteus medius and minimus lie deep to the gluteus maximus and assist in hip adduction and internal rotation. These muscles help

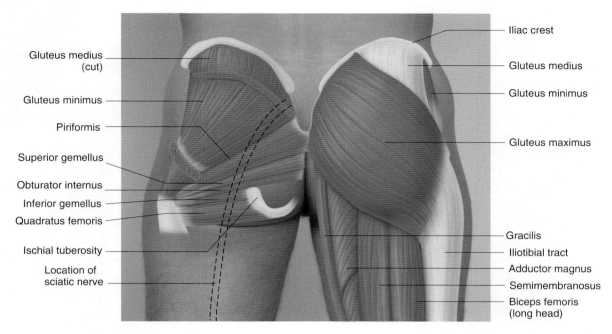

FIGURE 7.36. Superficial *(right)* and deep *(left)* muscles of the hip and pelvis—posterior view. (From Premkumar K. The Massage Connection Anatomy and Physiology. Baltimore: Lippincott Williams & Wilkins, 2004.)

the hip keep the correct abducted position during locomotion (3). The adductors (magnus, longus, and brevis) and gracilis primarily act to adduct the hip. The gracilis is a two-joint muscle that flexes the knee as well. These muscles originate from various points on the pubis and insert at the medial aspect of the femur and tibia (gracilis) (5).

Injuries. The hip and pelvis have a strong structural make-up, so traumatic sports injuries at these locations are relatively infrequent compared with other joints (19). However, the soft tissues of the thigh are often injured in sports (19), and the hip and pelvis are sites of several chronic overuse disorders.

Traumatic injuries of the pelvis and hip include dislocation, fracture, contusion, and muscle strain. Hip dislocation results from violent twisting of the hip or jamming the knee into the dashboard of a car. Some 85% of hip dislocations are posterior. Hip fractures (fractures of the femoral neck) are common in older adults with osteoporosis and can cause permanent disability. Contusions (crush injuries of muscle against bone) are common in the region. Iliac crest contusion ("hip pointer") is caused by direct blow to the pelvis region. Quadriceps contusion ("charley horse") and tearing can result in permanent muscle abnormality called "myositis ossificans" in which bone tissue is deposited within the muscle (19). Hamstring muscle strains and tears are often caused by sudden changes in direction and speed, with underlying factors of muscular imbalance, fatigue, and a deconditioned athlete (19). Hamstring injuries are frequent in preseason or early season activities.

Chronic and overuse injuries to the region include arthritis, bursitis, and tendonitis. Degenerative arthritis of the hip results from abnormal articular cartilage wear from either too much or too little resistance. Avascular necrosis of the hip is caused by the lack of proper blood flow to the femoral head and typically results in severe hip degeneration. Trochanteric bursitis involves irritation of the bursa between the iliotibial band and greater trochanter of the femur. Chronic bursitis in this region can lead to "snapping hip syndrome" (19). Iliotibial band friction syndrome is a chronic overuse injury that causes pain along the lateral aspect of the thigh. Piriformis syndrome is a myofascial disorder that can be caused by faulty lower extremity

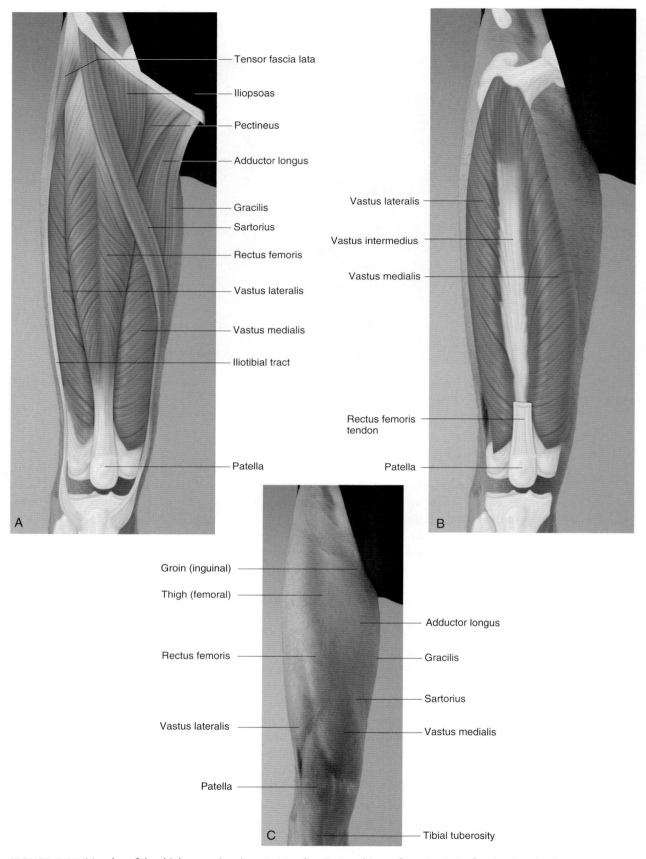

FIGURE 7.37. Muscles of the thigh—anterior view. **A.** Muscles. **B.** Quadriceps femoris. **C.** Surface landmarks. (From Premkumar K. The Massage Connection Anatomy and Physiology. Baltimore: Lippincott Williams & Wilkins, 2004.)

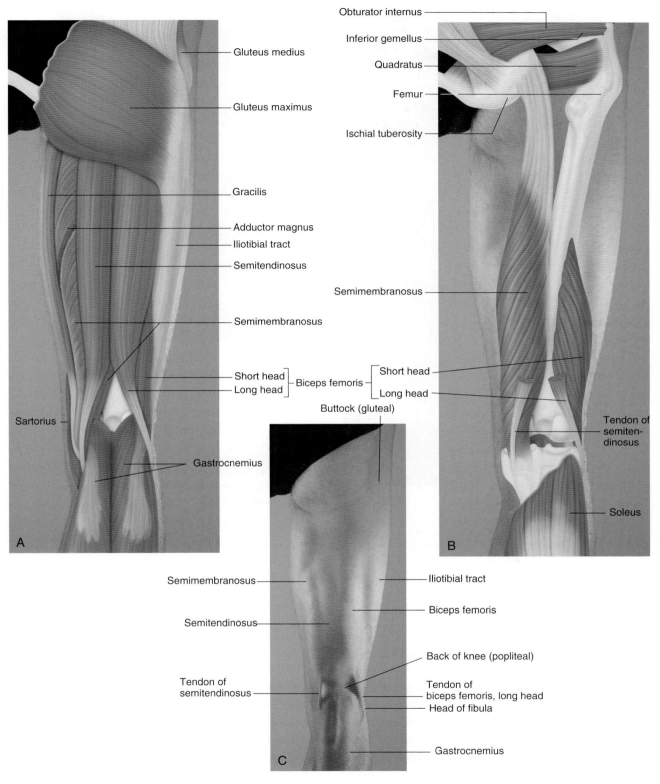

FIGURE 7.38. Muscles of the thigh—posterior view. **A.** Superficial muscles. **B.** Deep muscles. **C.** Surface landmarks. (From Premkumar K. The Massage Connection Anatomy and Physiology. Baltimore: Lippincott Williams & Wilkins, 2004.)

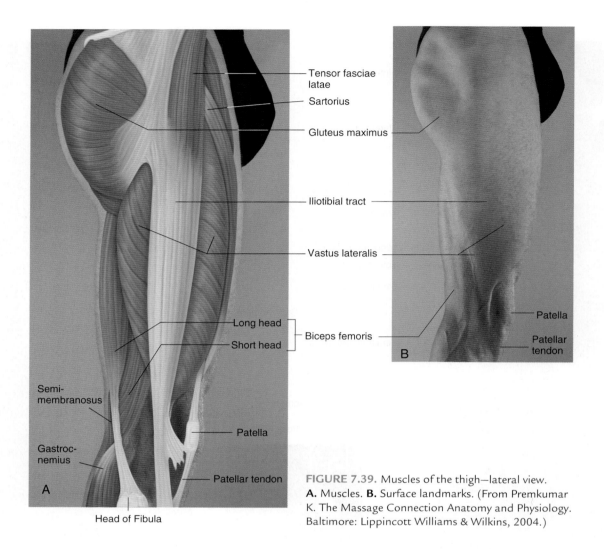

FIGURE 7.39. Muscles of the thigh—lateral view. **A.** Muscles. **B.** Surface landmarks. (From Premkumar K. The Massage Connection Anatomy and Physiology. Baltimore: Lippincott Williams & Wilkins, 2004.)

biomechanics. The hypertonic piriformis muscle may compress the sciatic nerve, since the nerve courses through the muscle. This results in pain and neurological symptoms of the posterior aspect of the lower extremity ("sciatica") (25).

KNEE

The knee joint is the largest joint in the body. Since the knee joint bears the load of the upper body and trunk and is crucial for locomotion, it is frequently subject to overuse and traumatic injuries (3).

Bones. The knee joint consists of the distal femur, proximal tibia, and patella *(Fig. 7.40)*. The tibia is the major weight-bearing bone of the leg. The proximal fibula, which serves as attachment sites for several knee structures, is usually not considered part of the knee joint (3). The patella (kneecap) is a triangular sesamoid bone that is located within the patellar tendon of the quadriceps muscle group. The patella protects the anterior knee (19) and creates an improved angle of pull for the quadriceps muscles, which results in a mechanical advantage during knee extension (3).

Ligaments. There are two major pairs of ligaments in the knee: the cruciate and collateral ligaments (see Fig. 7.40). The cruciate ligaments cross within the knee between the femur and tibia and are important in maintaining anterior–posterior and rotational stability at the knee. The anterior cruciate ligament is slightly longer and thinner than the posterior ligament (4).

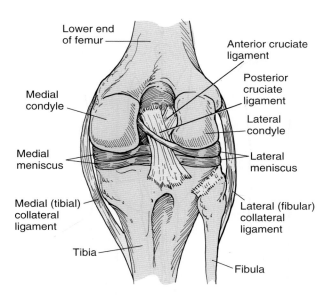

Lower end of femur

Anterior cruciate ligament

Posterior cruciate ligament

Medial condyle

Lateral condyle

Medial meniscus

Lateral meniscus

Medial (tibial) collateral ligament

Lateral (fibular) collateral ligament

Tibia

Fibula

FIGURE 7.40. Bones, ligaments, and menisci of the knee region—anterior view—with the knee flexed and patella removed. (From Cipriano J. Photographic Manual of Regional Orthopaedic and Neurological Tests. 2nd ed. Baltimore: Lippincott Williams & Wilkins, 1991.)

The collateral ligaments connect the femur with the lower leg bones—the medial collateral with the tibia and the lateral collateral with the fibula. The collateral ligaments aid in lateral stability of the knee, counteracting valgus and varus forces. The medial collateral ligament attaches to the medial meniscus of the knee, but the lateral collateral ligament does not attach to the lateral meniscus (4).

Menisci. The knee is equipped with fibrocartilage disks (menisci) that are attached to the tibial plateaus and knee joint capsule (4) (see Fig. 7.40). The menisci improve congruency of the joint surfaces (allowing better distribution of joint pressure), add stability, aid in shock absorption, provide joint lubrication, aid in load bearing, add anterior–posterior stability, and protect articular cartilage. The medial meniscus is larger, thinner, and more "C" shaped than the lateral meniscus (4).

Joints. The knee consists of the tibiofemoral and patellofemoral joints (see Fig. 7.40). The proximal tibiofibular joint, although an important attachment site for knee structures, is typically not considered a knee joint (3). The tibiofemoral joint is the primary joint of the knee and is often considered a hinge joint. The tibiofemoral joint is formed by the articulation of the medial and lateral femoral condyles with the medial and lateral tibial plateaus. The medial femoral condyle typically extends more distally than the lateral condyle, giving the knee a slight valgus arrangement (3).

The patellofemoral joint is an arthrodial joint formed by the posterior aspect of the patella and patellofemoral groove between the condyles of the femur. The "Q angle" is the angle formed from the line connecting ASIS to the center of the patella and the line connecting the center of the patella to the tibial tuberosity (4) *(Fig. 7.41)*. The Q angle determines the line of pull of the patella at the patellofemoral joint. A normal Q angle is 18° in females and 13° in males. A Q angle that is below normal (negative) results in a genu varum position of the knee (bow-legged), while a Q angle that is above normal results in a genu valgum position (knock-kneed) (4).

Movements. The major movements at the tibiofemoral joint are flexion and extension in the sagittal plane *(Fig. 7.42)*. The knee has a normal ROM in the sagittal plane of 140°, with 0° representing full extension (knee straight) and 140° representing full flexion (knee bent). When the knee is flexed, the tibiofemoral joint is also capable of internal and external rotation in the transverse plane. Approximately 30° of internal rotation and 45° of external rotation can be achieved at the knee (4). During the final few degrees of extension, the tibia externally rotates on the femur, which brings the knee into a closed packed, or locked, position. This phenomenon is known as the "screwing home" mechanism (19).

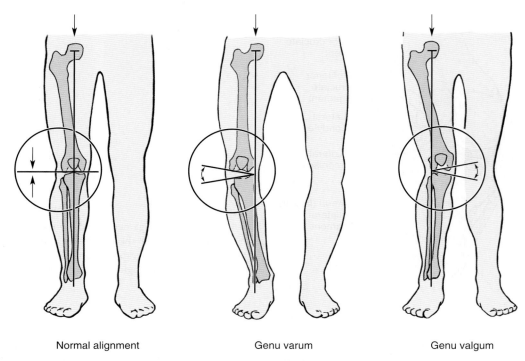

Normal alignment   Genu varum   Genu valgum

FIGURE 7.41. Q angle of the knee: normal alignment, genu varum, and genu valgum. (From Moore KL, Dalley AF II. Clinical Oriented Anatomy. 4th ed. Baltimore: Lippincott Williams & Wilkins, 1999.)

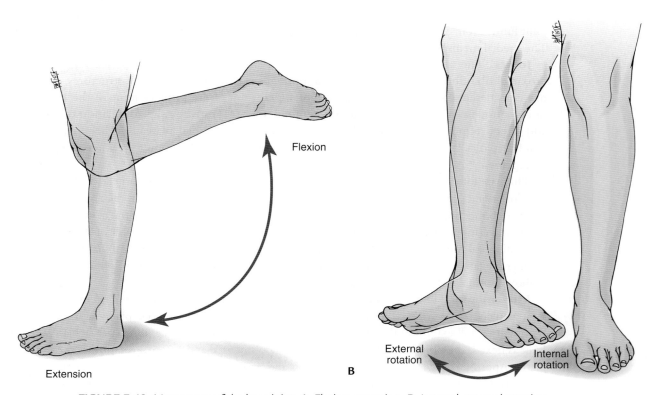

FIGURE 7.42. Movements of the knee joint. **A.** Flexion–extension. **B.** Internal–external rotation.

Muscles

Anterior. Large and powerful thigh muscles cross the knee joint, several of which are two-joint muscles acting on the hip joint, as well. The quadriceps muscles (i.e., rectus femoris, vastus lateralis, vastus intermedius, and vastus medialis) are anterior knee muscles and act to extend the knee joint (see Fig. 7.37). The quadriceps muscles insert into the superior aspect of the patella and patellar tendon to the tibial tuberosity. The rectus femoris is a large, two-joint muscle that originates from the anterior superior iliac spine. The rectus femoris flexes the hip in addition to extending the knee. The three vasti muscles originate from the proximal femur. The vastus lateralis and vastus medialis are pennate muscles that pull on the patella at oblique angles (5). The vastus medialis obliquus (VMO), which primarily contracts during the last 10–20° of knee extension, is a group of muscle fibers at the distal portion of the vastus medialis. Contraction of the VMO counterbalances the stronger vastus lateralis, which helps to maintain a proper line of pull for the patella and aids in knee stability (3).

Posterior. The muscles of the posterior knee joint are the hamstrings (biceps femoris, semitendinosus, and semimembranosus), sartorius, gracilis, popliteus, and gastrocnemius (see Fig. 7.38). The biceps femoris (lateral hamstrings) muscle contains a long head (which originates from the ischial tuberosity and is a two-joint muscle) and short head (which originates from the mid-femur). The biceps femoris inserts into the lateral condyle of the tibia and head of the fibula. It acts to flex and externally rotate the knee and extend and externally rotate the hip. The gracilis muscle functions similarly to the biceps femoris (5). The semimembranosus and semitendinosus (medial hamstrings) are two-joint muscles that act to flex and internally rotate the knee and extend and internally rotate the hip. The sartorius muscle is the longest muscle in the body. It originates from the ASIS and acts on both the knee and hip joints. The tendons of the sartorius, gracilis, and semimembranosus join together to form the pes anserinus, which inserts to the anteromedial aspect of the proximal tibia just inferior to the tibial tuberosity. The gastrocnemius muscle is a two-head and two-joint muscle that acts to flex the knee and plantar flex the ankle (5). The gastrocnemius is discussed in detail in the ankle section of this chapter.

Injuries. As mentioned above, the knee is a frequently injured joint, with its ligaments, menisci, and patellofemoral joint vulnerable to acute and repetitive use damage. Most knee injuries require exercise training for rehabilitation, and some require surgery as well. Predisposing factors to knee injury include (11, 19, 25):

➤ Lower extremity malalignment (e.g., Q angle abnormalities, flat feet)
➤ Limb length discrepancy
➤ Muscular imbalance and weakness
➤ Inflexibility
➤ Previous injury
➤ Inadequate proprioception
➤ Joint instability
➤ Playing surface and equipment problems
➤ Slight predominance in females (particularly for patellofemoral problems)

Ligamentous sprains and tears are common in the knee, particularly in athletes. Because of its structure and insertion points, the anterior cruciate ligament is more frequently injured than the posterior cruciate ligament. Classically, the anterior cruciate ligament is injured when external rotation of the tibia is coupled with a valgus force on the knee (e.g., direct force from the lateral side of the knee, planting the foot and twisting the knee) (19).

The menisci are also frequently injured, particularly in athletes. The medial meniscus is more frequently torn than the lateral meniscus, due in part to its connection to the medial collateral ligament. The menisci are poorly innervated and relatively avascular, thus they are not very pain sensitive and are slow to heal following injury. The "terrible triad" is a traumatic sports injury in which the anterior cruciate ligament, medial collateral ligament, and medial meniscus are damaged simultaneously (4).

Patellofemoral pain syndrome is a common disorder in young athletes (particularly females) that produces anterior knee pain. Often, patellofemoral pain syndrome is caused by an off-center line of pull of the patella, which irritates the joint surfaces and retinaculum of the knee (30). An off-center pull of the patella can result from insufficiency of the VMO and the resultant muscular imbalance during knee extension (31) and from excessive varus and valgus stresses from Q angles outside of the normal range of 13–18°.

ANKLE AND FOOT

The ankle and foot are responsible for weight-bearing and ambulation. Proper function and mechanics of the ankle and foot are essential for most sports activities and performance of activities of daily living. Slight abnormalities in the feet and ankles (e.g., muscular imbalance, proprioceptive dysfunction, and structural changes) are transmitted via the kinetic chain to most joints superior to them in the body (4). Thus, knee, hip, low back, neck, shoulder, and body alignment and postural problems can at times be traced to dysfunctional ankles and feet. This section focuses on ankle functional anatomy. For the functional anatomy of the intrinsic foot, the reader is referred to other sources (6–10).

Bones. The foot has 26 articulating bones contained in three functional units of the foot: the anterior (forefoot), middle (midfoot), and posterior (hindfoot) *(Fig. 7.43)*. The forefoot contains the five metatarsals (one for each digit) and 14 phalanges (toes). The midfoot contains the five tarsal bones: the navicular, cuboid, and three cuneiforms. The hindfoot contains the talus and calcaneus bones. The dome of the talus articulates with the distal tibia and fibula and provides the link between the leg and foot. The talus sits on the calcaneus. Most of the calcaneus represents the posterior projection of the heel. The calcaneus provides important attachment sites for the ankle plantar flexor muscles. The ankle mortise is formed by the distal tibia (tibial dome), the medial malleolus of the tibia, and the lateral malleolus of the fibula (25).

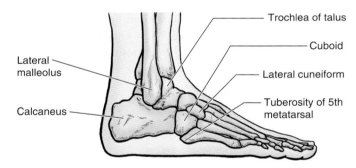

A Lateral foot

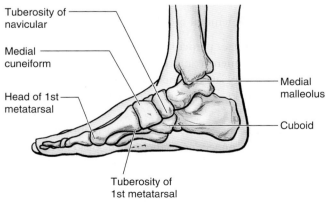

B Medial foot

FIGURE 7.43. Bones of the ankle and foot regions. **A.** Lateral view. **B.** Medial view. (From Moore KL, Dalley AF II. Clinical Oriented Anatomy. 4th ed. Baltimore: Lippincott Williams & Wilkins, 1999.)

Ligaments. There are approximately 100 ligaments in the ankle and foot region *(Fig. 7.44)*. On the lateral side of the ankle, the major ligaments include the anterior and posterior talofibular and the calcaneofibular ligaments. The deltoid ligament complex is on the medial ankle and includes the calcaneofibular, anterior and posterior talotibial, and tibionavicular ligaments. The plantar calcaneonavicular ligament (spring ligament) helps support the talus (11).

There are two arches on the plantar aspect of the foot that give the foot its shape and distribute body weight from the talus to the foot during various load-bearing conditions (19). The various ligaments and bones primarily support the arches, with muscles providing secondary support. The longitudinal arch extends from the calcaneal tuberosity to the five metatarsals, while the transverse arch extends crosswise from medial to lateral in the midtarsal region. The plantar fascia, or plantar aponeurosis, is a strong fibrous rod that provides support for the longitudinal arch. The plantar fascia is an extension of the Achilles' tendon of the plantar flexor muscles. During weight-bearing phase of gait, the plantar fascia acts like a spring to store mechanical energy that is then released during foot push-off (3).

Joints. The ankle contains two joints: the talocrural and subtalar joints (see Fig. 7.43). The talocrural joint is a uniaxial modified hinge joint formed by the articulation of the ankle mortise and the dome of the talus. The subtalar joint is a gliding joint consisting of the articulation of the talus and calcaneus. The distal tibiofibular joint is a fibrous syndesmosis joint in the ankle region, which is located between the inferior ends of the tibia and fibula. There are several joints in the foot and toes, including the midtarsal, tarsometatarsal, intermetatarsal, metatarsophalangeal, and interphalangeal joints (11).

Movements. The talocrural joint allows approximately 15–20° of dorsiflexion and 50° of plantar flexion in the sagittal plane. The subtalar joint allows approximately 20–30° of inversion and 5–15° of eversion in the frontal plane. The midtarsal and tarsometatarsal joints permit gliding

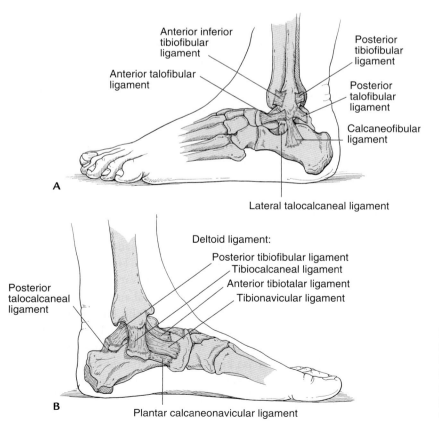

FIGURE 7.44. Ligaments of the ankle and foot regions. **A.** Lateral view. **B.** Medial view. (From Cipriano J. Photographic Manual of Regional Orthopaedic and Neurological Tests. 2nd ed. Baltimore: Lippincott Williams & Wilkins, 1991.)

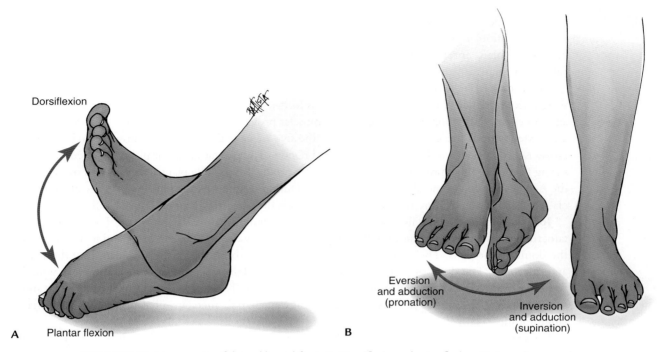

FIGURE 7.45. Movements of the ankle and foot. **A.** Dorsiflexion–plantar flexion. **B.** Inversion–eversion.

motion. The metatarsophalangeal and interphalangeal joints allow flexion and extension of the digits in the sagittal plane. Pronation and supination are combination movements at the ankle and foot. Pronation is a combination of talocrural dorsiflexion, subtalar eversion, and forefoot abduction. Supination is a combination of talocrural plantar flexion, subtalar inversion, and forefoot adduction (3) *(Fig. 7.45)*.

Muscles. The major muscles that act on the ankle and foot are located in the leg, and these muscles are typically grouped by their compartmental location—anterior, lateral, superficial posterior, and deep posterior (3).

Anterior and Lateral. The anterior muscles, tibialis anterior, peroneus tertius, extensor digitorum longus, and extensor hallucis longus, are ankle dorsiflexors *(Fig. 7.46)*. The tibialis anterior is also an ankle inverter, while the peroneus tertius and extensor digitorum longus are ankle everters. The extensor hallucis longus acts to extend the big toe. The lateral muscles, peroneus longus and brevis, are ankle everters and assist with dorsiflexion, as well (5) *(Fig. 7.47)*.

Superficial and Deep Posterior. The superficial posterior muscles, gastrocnemius, soleus, and plantaris are ankle plantar flexors *(Fig. 7.48)*. The gastrocnemius is a two-head and two-joint muscle, which is a powerful plantar flexor of the ankle as well as a flexor of the knee. The gastrocnemius has relatively more fast twitch fibers than the soleus. Thus, the gastrocnemius is used more during dynamic, higher force activities, and the soleus is more active during postural and static contractions (4). Since the gastrocnemius crosses the knee and ankle, the position of the knee during plantar flexion resistance exercise affects the activity of the gastrocnemius. At 90° of knee flexion, the gastrocnemius experiences passive insufficiency and thus is less active than when the knee is straight (0° of flexion). In other words, during calf raise exercise keep the knees straight to emphasize the gastrocnemius and bend the knees to emphasize the soleus. The deep posterior muscles—flexor digitorum longus, flexor hallices longus, tibialis posterior, and popliteus—are ankle plantar flexors (except for the popliteus) and inverters (3).

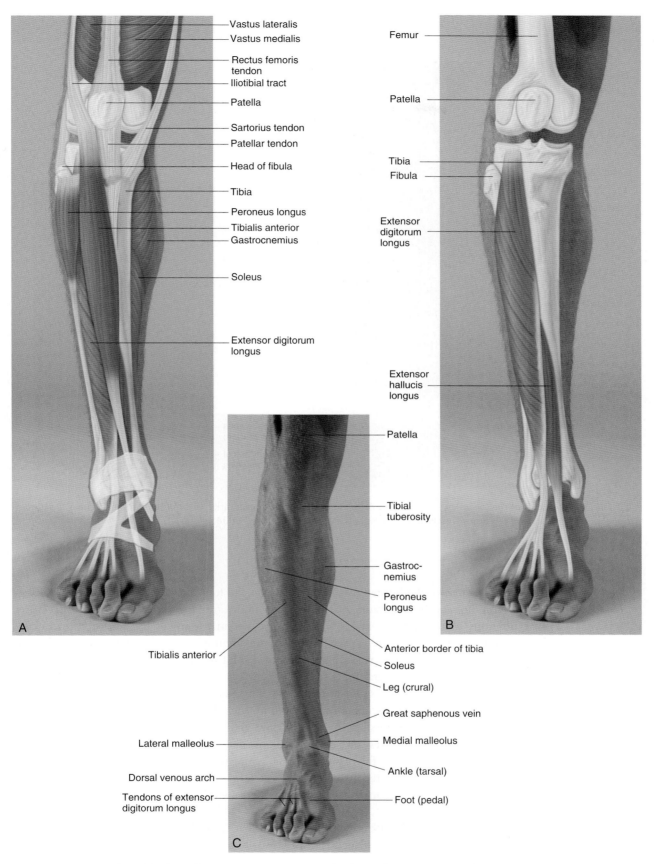

FIGURE 7.46. Muscles of the lower leg—anterior view. **A.** Superficial muscles. **B.** Deep muscles. **C.** Surface landmarks. (From Premkumar K. The Massage Connection Anatomy and Physiology. Baltimore: Lippincott Williams & Wilkins, 2004.)

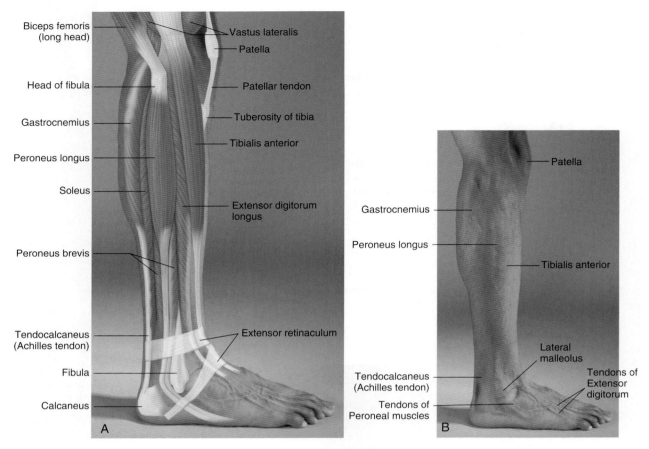

FIGURE 7.47. Muscles of the lower leg—lateral view. **A.** Muscles. **B.** Surface landmarks. (From Premkumar K. The Massage Connection Anatomy and Physiology. Baltimore: Lippincott Williams & Wilkins, 2004.)

Injuries. Because of the burden placed on the ankle and foot during activities such as walking, running, jumping, and lifting, traumatic and overuse injuries frequently occur to these structures (19). Numerous acute muscular strains and cramps occur in the lower leg and foot, and many ligament sprains occur in this region as well. Ankle sprains are more common on the lateral side than on the medial side because there is less bony stability and ligamentous strength on the lateral side. The mechanism of injury for lateral ankle sprains is excessive inversion (rolling out of the ankle), as occurs when landing on someone's foot after jumping in basketball. The anterior talofibular ligament is the most frequently sprained ligament in inversion injuries (19).

Achilles tendon rupture is possibly the most serious acute injury of the lower leg (19). Nearly 75% of Achilles tendon ruptures are seen in athletic males between 30 and 40 years of age. The typical mechanism is forceful plantar flexion while the knee is extended. These injuries almost always require surgical repair and extensive, long-term rehabilitation. Achilles tendon rupture is often a career-ending injury for athletes, especially if it occurs in the later stages of their careers (19).

Plantar fasciitis is a chronic inflammatory condition that typically results in pain at the calcaneal insertion of the plantar fascia (19). Plantar fasciitis is usually caused by chronic pulling on the plantar fascia, tight Achilles tendon, hyperpronation (flat feet or pes planus), or other factors that overload the fascia (e.g., obesity). Treatment for plantar fasciitis includes stretching and strengthening exercises for the posterior calf muscles, orthoses to correct hyperpronation, and physiotherapy

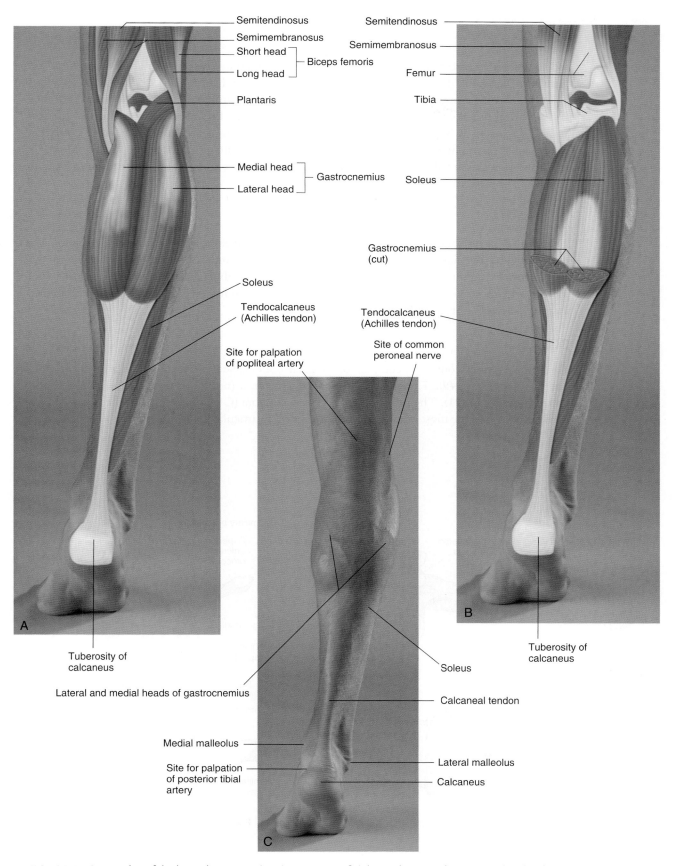

FIGURE 7.48. Muscles of the lower leg—Posterior view. **A.** Superficial muscles. **B.** Soleus. **C.** Surface landmarks. (From Premkumar K. The Massage Connection Anatomy and Physiology. Baltimore: Lippincott Williams & Wilkins, 2004.)

modalities and medication to reduce inflammation. Sometimes surgery is required to release the plantar fascia. Plantar fasciitis is often associated with calcaneal heel spurs (19).

Other chronic conditions of the foot and ankle include bunions, neuromas, Achilles tendonitis, and calcaneal bursitis. These conditions are frequently related to structural problems of the foot and ankle, such as hyperpronation or hypersupination (high arch or pes cavus). Unilateral hyperpronation or hypersupination may cause instability and proprioceptive difficulties at the ankle and postural imbalances and mechanical problems to proximal joint structures in the kinetic chain.

Spine

The spine is an intricate multi-joint structure that plays a crucial role in functional mechanics. The spine provides the link between the upper and lower extremities, protects the spinal cord, and enables trunk motion in three planes (19). Moreover, the rib cage of the thoracic spinal region protects the internal organs of the chest. Because of its intricacies, the spine is susceptible to injuries that may severely impair physical function.

BONES

The spinal column contains a complex of irregular bones called "vertebrae" that are stacked upon one another *(Fig. 7.49)*. There are 24 vertebrae: 7 cervical (neck), 12 thoracic (mid back), and 5 lumbar (low back) (11). The most superior cervical vertebra (C1) articulates with the occipital bone of the skull, while the most inferior lumbar vertebra (L5) articulates with the sacrum. The size of the

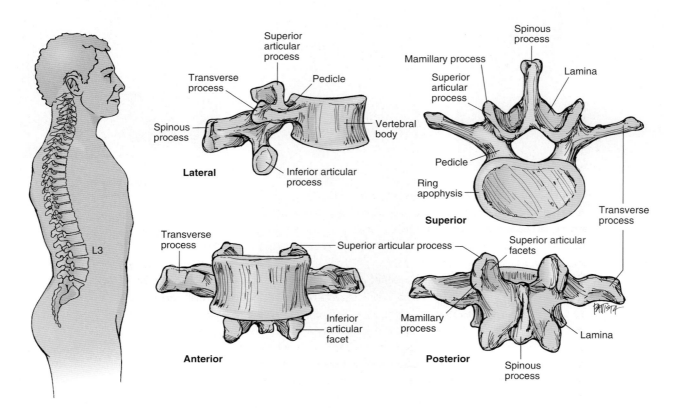

FIGURE 7.49. A typical lumbar vertebra (L3) in four views identifying the relevant landmarks. (From Oatis CA. Kinesiology. The Mechanics and Pathomechanics of Human Movement. Baltimore: Lippincott Williams & Wilkins, 2004.)

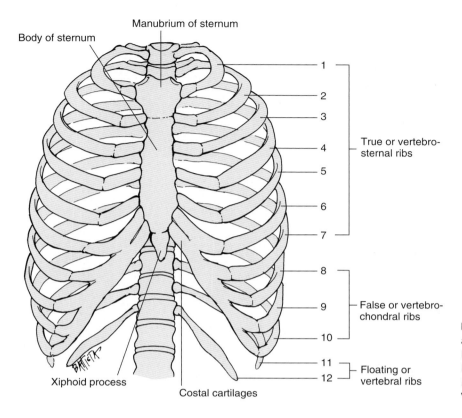

Body of sternum

Manubrium of sternum

1
2
3

True or vertebro-
sternal ribs

4
5
6
7

8

9 — False or vertebro-
chondral ribs

10

11 ┐ Floating or
12 ┘ vertebral ribs

Xiphoid process

Costal cartilages

FIGURE 7.50. The thoracic cage—anterior view. (From Oatis CA. Kinesiology. The Mechanics and Pathomechanics of Human Movement. Baltimore: Lippincott Williams & Wilkins, 2003.)

vertebrae increases from the cervical to the lumbar region because of an increase in load-bearing responsibilities. Each vertebra contains anterior and posterior elements. The anterior element, called the "vertebral body," is oval with flat superior and inferior surfaces for articulation with the adjacent vertebral bodies. The posterior element, or posterior arch, consists of pedicles and laminae, which join anteriorly at the body and posteriorly at the spinous process to form the vertebral foramen. The vertebral foramen provides a space for the spinal cord. The posterior arch also contains facets on each side and top and bottom for articulation with adjacent vertebrae. The spinous and transverse processes are bony protuberances that provide attachment points for the spinal musculature (11).

Ribs attach to each of the 12 thoracic vertebrae bilaterally and form the thoracic cage *(Fig. 7.50)*. The seven most superior pairs of ribs are considered true ribs and attach directly to the sternum. The five lower pairs of ribs are considered false ribs. Three pairs of false ribs attach indirectly to the sternum. Two most inferior pairs of false ribs do not attach to the sternum and are considered floating ribs (3).

The spinal column also contains a sacrum and coccyx, which are situated at the lower spine, immediately inferior to the fifth lumbar vertebra. The sacrum is a large triangular bone that acts as the transition point between the spine and pelvis. The coccyx is a series of small bones located at the distal sacrum (11).

In the sagittal plane, the spinal column normally is situated in four curves instead of a straight line *(Fig. 7.51)*. These curves give the spine mechanical advantage and improved load-bearing capabilities. When the convexity of the curve is posterior, the curve is known as kyphosis, and when the convexity of the curve is anterior, the curve is known as lordosis. The cervical and lumbar regions have lordosis, and the thoracic and sacral regions have kyphosis. Deviations in the sagittal plane are referred to as "hyperlordosis" or "hyperkyphosis." In the frontal plane, the spinal column should normally be positioned in the midline. Lateral deviation is referred to as "scoliosis" *(Fig. 7.52)* (4).

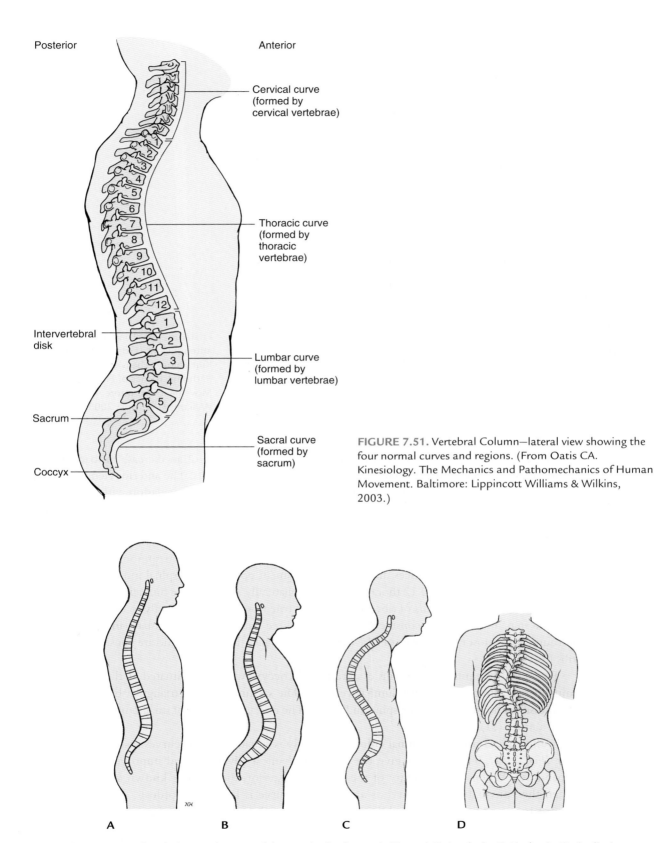

Posterior

Anterior

Cervical curve
(formed by
cervical vertebrae)

Thoracic curve
(formed by
thoracic
vertebrae)

Intervertebral
disk

Lumbar curve
(formed by
lumbar vertebrae)

Sacrum

Sacral curve
(formed by
sacrum)

Coccyx

FIGURE 7.51. Vertebral Column—lateral view showing the four normal curves and regions. (From Oatis CA. Kinesiology. The Mechanics and Pathomechanics of Human Movement. Baltimore: Lippincott Williams & Wilkins, 2003.)

A   B   C   D

FIGURE 7.52. Normal and abnormal curves of the vertebral column. **A.** Normal. **B.** Lordosis. **C.** Kyphosis. **D.** Scoliosis (Courtesy of Neil O. Hardy, Westpoint, CT.)

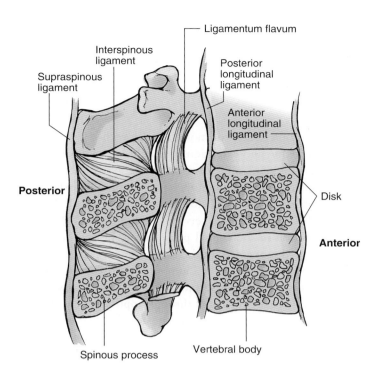

FIGURE 7.53. Ligaments and disks of the lumbar spine—mid-sagittal view. (From Oatis CA. Kinesiology. The Mechanics and Pathomechanics of Human Movement. Baltimore: Lippincott Williams & Wilkins, 2003.)

LIGAMENTS

The main supporting ligaments of the spinal column are the longitudinal ligaments, the anterior and posterior longitudinal ligaments, and the ligamentum flavum, which span from the upper cervical to lower lumbar region *(Fig. 7.53)*. The anterior and posterior longitudinal ligaments attach to the vertebral bodies, and the ligamentum flavum connects the posterior arches and forms the posterior border of the spinal canal. The interspinous and supraspinous ligaments attach to adjacent posterior arch structures (4).

INTERVERTEBRAL DISK

The intervertebral disks are important structures that provide load bearing, shock absorption, and stability to the vertebral column. The disks are located between the vertebral bodies and compose about 20–33% of the height of the vertebral column (2) (see Fig. 7.53). Each intervertebral motion segment contains a disk, except for the articulation between the first and second cervical vertebrae (the atlas and axis, respectively). The intervertebral disk consists of the nucleus pulposus, annulus fibrosis, and endplates. These structures are composed of various concentrations of water, collagen, and proteoglycans. The nucleus pulposus, located in the center of the disk, is gel-like and more liquid than the annulus. The nucleus dehydrates with age, which is one of the reasons why overall body height reduces with age (2). The annulus fibrosis, located at the periphery of the disk, is a more rigid structure and contains more collagen fibers than the nucleus. The oblique arrangement of the collagen fibers of the annulus helps the annulus resist tensile and compressive forces in various planes. However, the annulus is most susceptible to tearing with movements involving rotation and flexion under load. The vertebral endplates are thin layers of collagen that cover the inferior and superior aspects of the vertebral body and help anchor the disk to the vertebrae (13).

JOINTS

The spinal column consists of numerous motion segments (two adjacent vertebrae). Each motion segment of spine contains five articulations: one intervertebral joint and four facet joints. The intervertebral joint connects adjacent bodies, while the zygapophyseal joints connect adjacent facets (superior and inferior on each side). The lumbar zygapophyseal joints are angled to allow flexion and extension and restrict axial rotation. The cervical and thoracic zygapophyseal joints, on the other hand, are angled to accommodate axial rotation (4).

MOVEMENTS

The spine is capable of motion in all planes, and the extent of motion varies with region. In the cervical spine, the atlantooccipital joint allows flexion and extension and slight lateral flexion. The atlantoaxial joint allows primarily rotation. The remaining cervical joints allow flexion and extension, lateral flexion, and rotation. The thoracic joints allow moderate flexion, slight extension, moderate lateral flexion, and rotation. The lumbar joints allow flexion and extension, lateral flexion, and slight rotation (4) *(Fig. 7.54)*. Refer to Table 7.5 for normal cervical and lumbar ROM values.

Compound Trunk Extension. Trunk motion in the sagittal plane during normal activities, such as lifting and bending, requires the compound movement of the lumbar spine, pelvis, and hip joints (32). This action is called "compound trunk extension" or "lumbopelvic rhythm." From a position of full trunk flexion, the lumbar extensors (erector spinae and multifidus) and hip extensors (gluteals and hamstrings) work together to actively rotate the trunk through approximately 180° in the sagittal plane (25) *(Fig. 7.55)*. Lumbar movement accounts for approximately 72° of this motion, while hip and pelvis movement accounts for the remaining 108° (33). The relative contribution of individual muscle groups to force production during compound trunk extension is unknown, but it is assumed that the larger hip extensors generate most of the force (25).

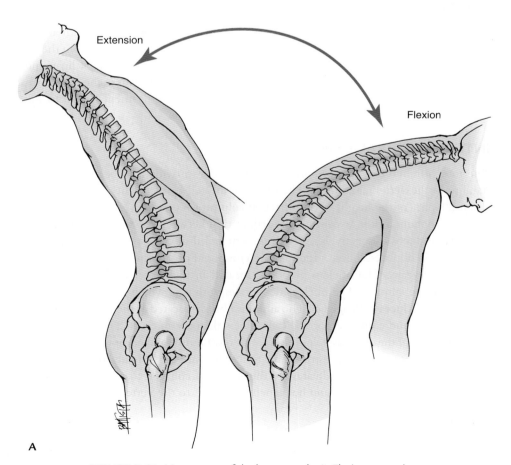

A

FIGURE 7.54. Movements of the lower trunk. **A.** Flexion–extension.

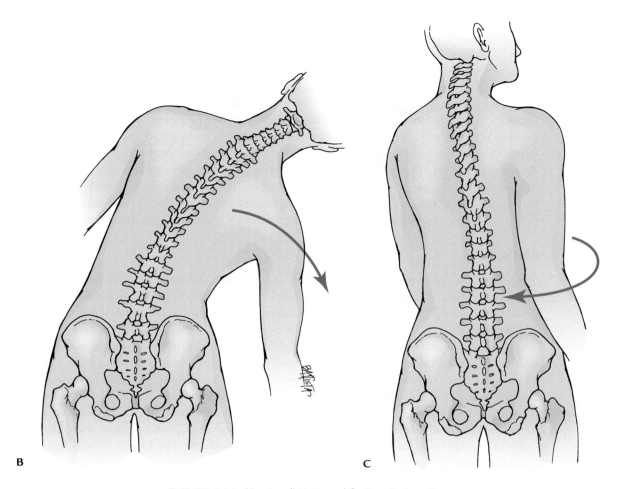

FIGURE 7.54. *(Continued)* **B.** Lateral flexion. **C.** Rotation.

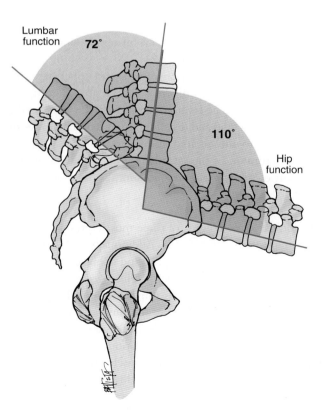

Lumbar
function

72°

110°

Hip
function

FIGURE 7.55. Compound trunk extension (lumbopelvic rhythm). Compound trunk extension involves the simultaneous movement of the lumbar spine (72°) and pelvis/hips (110°).

Since the pelvis remains free to move during activities of daily living such as lifting and bending, it is assumed that the small lumbar muscles play only a minor role in trunk extension torque production. Thus, they are considered to be the weak link in trunk extension movements (34). The rationale behind isolating the lumbar spine through pelvic stabilization mechanisms during exercise training is to force the lumbar muscles to be the primary trunk extensors, thereby providing the overload stimulus for strength gains (34). Dynamic progressive resistance exercise protocols on devices that stabilize the pelvis have produced unusually large gains (greater than 100%) in lumbar extension strength, even with training frequencies as low as one time per week (34). Clinically, patients with low back pain have displayed significant improvements in symptoms, disability, and psychosocial function following intensive exercise training with pelvic stabilization (35, 36).

MUSCLES

The spine and trunk muscles exist in pairs, one on each side of the body. In general, bilateral contraction results in movement in the sagittal plane. The anterior muscles flex the spine, while the posterior muscles extend the spine. Unilateral contraction results in lateral bend or axial rotation.

Cervical

Anterior. The major anterior muscles of the cervical region include the sternocleidomastoid, scalene (anterior, middle, and posterior), and longus (capitis and coli) muscles. On unilateral contraction, these muscles laterally flex and rotate the neck and head. On bilateral contraction, the anterior scalene, longus, and sternocleidomastoid muscles flex the neck and head. The scalenes attach proximally to the upper cervical transverse processes and distally to the upper two ribs. The sternocleidomastoid attaches proximally to the mastoid process of the occiput and distally to the sternum (medial head) and clavicle (lateral head) (see Fig. 7.20). The longus muscles run from the transverse processes of the upper cervical vertebrae to the anterior aspect of the superior cervical vertebrae (longus coli) or the base of the occiput (longus capitis) (5).

Posterior. The suboccipital muscles, which attach the upper cervical vertebrae to the occiput, extend the head when they contract bilaterally, and laterally bend and rotate the neck when they contract unilaterally. Similarly, the splenius (capitis and cervicis) and erector spinae (spinalis, longissimus, and iliocostalis) muscles extend the neck when they contract bilaterally, and laterally bend and rotate the neck when they contract unilaterally (5) (see Fig. 7.21).

Lateral. The lateral muscles of the neck and head include the levator scapulae and upper trapezius muscles, both of which laterally bend and rotate the neck on unilateral contraction. The upper trapezius extends the neck as well, on bilateral contraction. The levator scapulae attaches proximally to the transverse processes of the upper four cervical vertebrae and distally to the vertebral border of the scapula. The upper trapezius attaches proximally to the occiput and spinous processes of the cervical vertebrae and distally to the clavicle and acromion of the scapula (5). The levator scapulae and upper trapezius muscles also cause movement of the scapulothoracic joint, as discussed in the shoulder section of this chapter.

Lumbar

Posterior. The posterior musculature of the lumbar spine consists of three muscle groups, namely the erector spinae, multifidus muscles, and intrinsic rotators *(Fig. 7.56)*. Additionally, the latissimus dorsi, which is usually considered a muscle that acts on the shoulder, extends and stabilizes the lumbar spine through its attachment to the thoracolumbar fascia (13). The erector spinae group, which lies lateral and superficial to the multifidus, is divided into the iliocostalis lumborum and longissimus thoracis muscles (37). These muscles are separated from each other by the lumbar intramuscular aponeurosis, with the longissimus lying medially. The longissimus and iliocostalis are composed of several multisegmental fascicles, which allow for extension and posterior translation when the muscles are contracted bilaterally. The fascicular arrangement of the multifidus muscle suggests that the multifidus acts primarily as a sagittal rotator (extension without posterior translation) (38). Lateral flexion and axial rotation are possible for both the multifidus and erector spinae musculature during

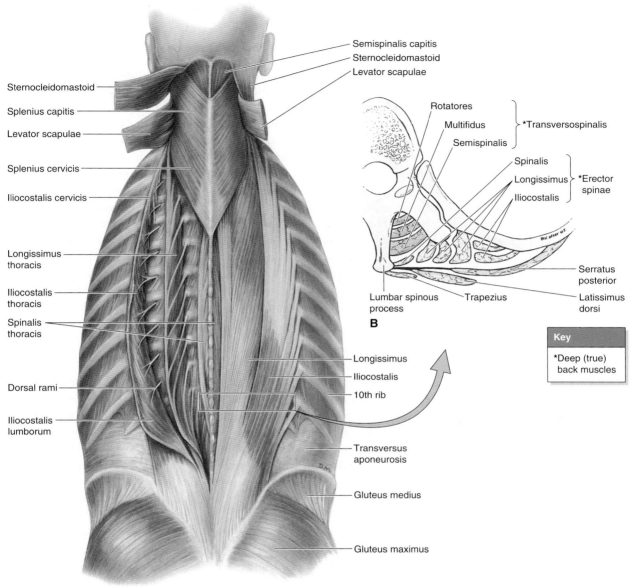

FIGURE 7.56. Deep muscles of the back. **A.** *Right,* the three columns of the erector spinae. *Left,* the spinalis is displayed by reflecting the longissimus and iliocostalis. **B.** Transverse section of the back showing arrangement of the erector spinae, multifidus, and rotator muscles. (From Moore KL, Dalley AF II. Clinical Oriented Anatomy. 4th ed. Baltimore: Lippincott Williams & Wilkins, 1999.)

unilateral contraction. The iliocostalis may be better suited to exert axial rotation on the lumbar vertebral motion segment than either the longissimus or multifidus muscles (37). Because of their anatomical and biomechanical properties, the posterior lumbar muscles are particularly adapted to maintain posture and stabilize the spine and trunk (37). The intrinsic rotators, rotatores and intertransversarii muscles, are primarily length transducers and position sensors for the vertebral segment (39).

Lateral. The lateral muscles of the lumbar spine include the quadratus lumborum and psoas (major and minor). The quadratus lumborum originates from the iliac crest and inserts at the twelfth rib and transverse process of the lower four lumbar vertebrae. The quadratus lumborum produces lateral bending of the lumbar spine with unilateral contraction and stabilizes the trunk with bilateral contraction. The psoas major muscle originates from the anterior surfaces of the transverse processes of all the lumbar vertebrae and inserts at the lesser trochanter of the femur. The psoas major flexes the trunk and the hip (5).

Anterior. The anterior muscles of the lumbar region consist of the abdominal group: the rectus abdominis, internal and external obliquus abdominis, and transversus abdominis (see Fig. 7.20). The rectus abdominus originates from the pubic bone and inserts at the fifth through seventh ribs and xiphoid process. The rectus abdominis exists as two vertical muscles separated by a connective tissue band, the linea alba. Horizontally, the rectus abdominis appears to be separated by three distinct lines. These lines represent areas of connective tissue that support the muscle in place of attachment to bones (3). The rectus abdominis is the primary trunk flexor, and through its attachment to the pubic bone, it also tilts the pelvis anteriorly. The internal and external obliquus abdominis muscles rotate the trunk on unilateral contraction and flex the trunk on bilateral contraction. The transversus abdominis runs horizontally, attaching medially to the linea alba via the abdominal aponeurosis and laterally to the thoracolumbar fascia, inguinal ligament, iliac crest, and the lower six ribs. Contraction of the transversus abdominis stabilizes the lumbar spine and increases intra–abdominal pressure, and aberrant firing patterns of the transversus abdominis appear to be related to low back pain (40).

To isolate the abdominal muscles during trunk flexion exercise, it is advisable to shorten the psoas and other hip flexor muscles (active insufficiency) by flexing the hips and knees (3). Thus, crunches with the hips and knees flexed may be more effective in conditioning the abdominals than straight knee sit-ups (5).

INJURIES

Cervical. The cervical region is the most mobile region of the spine, and relatively small cervical muscles are responsible for supporting the head. These factors make the cervical region vulnerable to instability and injury (19). The most dangerous injuries to the cervical region are traumatic fractures and dislocations that result in instability. The combination of axial compression and hyperflexion is a common mechanism for severe cervical injuries such as these (41). Diving into a shallow pool or a football player making a head-on tackle are examples of activities with these mechanisms. The most dire consequence of upper cervical dislocation or fracture is neural damage to the upper spinal cord, which may result in paralysis or death (19). Thus, any traumatic neck injury should be treated as a medical emergency (42).

Sprains and strains of the neck muscles and ligaments are frequently the result of violent hyperextension–hyperflexion from sudden acceleration–deceleration, such as a head-on car collision. This condition, commonly called "whiplash," can cause tears of the anterior and posterior structures of the cervical region, including the muscles (e.g., sternocleidomastoid, upper trapezius, and cervical paraspinals) and ligaments (25). After ruling out fracture, dislocation, instability, and disk herniation, treatment for whiplash usually includes passive modalities, stretches, and strengthening exercises for the neck.

Lumbar. Low back pain is one of the leading causes of disability and consistently ranks as one of the top reasons for visits to physicians. Low back pain affects 60–80% of the general population at some point during their lifetime, and 20–30% are suffering from this disorder at any given time (43, 44). Attaching a specific diagnosis to low back pain is difficult and elusive, since there often is no identifiable source of the pain or injury (45).

Some of the causes of low back pain include intervertebral disk herniation, facet joint inflammation, muscular strains, and ligamentous sprains. Injury to these structures can be traumatic, caused by events such as inappropriately lifting or falling, or degenerative, caused by a deconditioned lumbar spine, poor posture, prolonged mechanical loading, or poor body mechanics during work, home, or sports activities (19, 25). A common cause of lumbar disk herniation is forceful flexion and rotation of the lumbar spine. A protruded lumbar disk that encroaches on the lumbar nerve roots may result in lower extremity sensory and motor problems such as pain, numbness, and muscular weakness and atrophy. Bowel and bladder dysfunction are serious conditions that can result from herniated lumbar disks and require immediate medical treatment (19).

Restorative exercise designed to improve the structural integrity of the lower trunk is commonly used for the treatment of low back pain, and generally, the efficacy of this approach has been supported (46). Many types of exercises are used, including aerobic, flexibility, muscular strength and endurance, and core stability. The Personal Trainer should be particularly well-versed in low back exercise techniques, incorporating those needed when appropriate.

SUMMARY

This chapter provides an overview of musculoskeletal functional anatomy, biomechanics, and kinesiology of the major joint structures of the human body. These principles play a major role in nearly all aspects of the Personal Trainer's practice, including exercise testing, exercise prescription, and analysis of exercise movements. Thus, the Personal Trainer is urged to master these principles so that safe, effective, and efficient exercise training programs can be designed to improve musculoskeletal fitness.

REFERENCES

1. Graves J, Franklin B. Introduction. In: Graves J, Franklin B, eds. Resistance Training for Health and Rehabilitation. Champaign, IL: Human Kinetics, 2001.
2. Norkin C, Levangie P. Joint Structure & Function. Philadelphia: FA Davis, 1992.
3. Thompson C, Floyd R, eds. Manual of Structural Kinesiology. 14th ed. New York: McGraw-Hill, 2001.
4. Baldwin K. Kinesiology for Personal Fitness Trainers. New York: McGraw-Hill, 2003.
5. Kendall F, McCreary E. Muscles: Testing and Function. 4th ed. Philadelphia: Lippincott Williams & Wilkins, 1993.
6. Hall-Craggs E. Anatomy As the Basis for Clinical Medicine. 3rd ed. Baltimore: Williams & Wilkins, 1995.
7. Moore K, Agur A. Essentials of Clinical Anatomy. 2nd ed. Baltimore: Williams & Wilkins, 2002.
8. Moore K. Clinically Oriented Anatomy. 4th ed. Baltimore: Williams and Wilkins, 2004.
9. Olson T, Pawlina W. A.D.A.M. Student Atlas of Anatomy. Baltimore: Williams & Wilkins, 1996.
10. Agur A, Lee M, Anderson J. Grant's Atlas of Anatomy. 9th ed. Baltimore: Williams & Wilkins, 1991.
11. Rosse C, Clawson D. The Musculoskeletal System in Health and Disease. Hagerstown, MD: Harper & Row, 1980.
12. Knudson D, Morrison C. Qualitative Analysis of Human Movement. Champaign, IL: Human Kinetics, 2002.
13. McGill S. Low Back Disorders: Evidence-Based Prevention and Rehabilitation. Champaign, IL: Human Kinetics, 2002.
14. Nieman D, ed. Exercise Testing and Prescription: A Health-Related Approach. New York: McGraw-Hill, 2003.
15. Brown L. Isokinetics in Human Performance. Champaign, IL: Human Kinetics, 2000.
16. Hill A. The heat of shortening and the dynamic constants of muscle. Proc R Soc 1938;126:136–195.
17. Gordon A, Huxley A, Julian J. The variation in isometric tension with sarcomere length in vertebrate muscle fibers. J Physiol 1966;184:170–192.
18. DeLavier F. Strength Training Anatomy. Champaign, IL: Human Kinetics, 2001.
19. Anderson M, Hall S. Fundamentals of Sports Injury Management. Baltimore: Williams & Wilkins, 1997.
20. Oatis C. Kinesiology—The Mechanics and Pathomechanics of Human Movement. Baltimore: Lippincott Williams & Wilkins, 2004.
21. Snell R. Clinical Anatomy. 7th ed. Baltimore: Lippincott Williams & Wilkins, 2003.
22. Burkhead W. Rotator Cuff Disorders. Baltimore: Williams & Wilkins, 1996.
23. An K, Morrey B. Biomechanics of the shoulder. In: Matsen F, ed. The Shoulder. Philadelphia: WB Saunders, 1990.
24. Horrigan J, Robinson J. The 7-Minute Rotator Cuff Solution. Los Angeles: Health for Life, 1990.
25. Cailliet R. Soft Tissue Pain and Disability. 3rd ed. Philadelphia: FA Davis, 1996.
26. McCue F, Hussamy O. Hand and wrist injuries. In: Magee D, Quillen W, eds. Athletic Injuries and Rehabilitation. Philadelphia: WB Saunders, 1996.
27. Halikis M, Taleisnik J. Soft-tissue injuries of the wrist. In: Plancher KD, ed. Clinics in Sports Medicine. Philadelphia: WB Saunders, 1996.
28. Garrick J, Webb D. Sports Injuries: Diagnosis and Management. Philadelphia: WB Saunders, 1990.
29. Griggs S, Weiss A. Bony injuries of the wrist, forearm, and elbow. In: Plancher KD, ed. Clinics in Sports Medicine. Philadelphia: WB Saunders, 1996.
30. Westfall D, Worrell T. Anterior knee pain syndrome: role of the vastus medialis oblique. J Sports Rehabil 1992;1(4):317–325.
31. McGee D. Orthopedic Physical Assessment. Philadelphia: WB Saunders, 1987.
32. Mayer L, Greenberg B. Measurement of the strength of trunk muscles. J Bone Joint Surg 1942;4:842–856.
33. Pollock ML, Leggett SH, Graves JE, et al. Effect of resistance training on lumbar extension strength. Am J Sports Med 1989;17(5):624–629.
34. Graves JE, Webb DC, Pollock ML, et al. Pelvic stabilization during resistance training: its effect on the development of lumbar extension strength. Arch Phys Med Rehabil 1994;75(2):210–215.

35. Leggett S, Mooney V, Matheson L, et al. Restorative exercise for clinical low back pain: a prospective two-center study with 1-year follow-up. Spine 1999;24(9):889–898.

36. Mooney V, Kron M, Rummerfield P, Holmes B. The effect of workplace based strengthening on low back injury rates: a case study in the strip mining industry. J Occup Rehabil 1995;5:157–167.

37. Bogduk N, Twomey LT. Clinical Anatomy of the Lumbar Spine. New York: Churchill Livingstone, 1990.

38. MacIntosh J, Bogduk N. The attachments of the lumbar erector spinae. Spine 1991;16(7):783–792.

39. Nitz A, Peck D. Comparison of muscle spindle concentrations in large and small human epaxial muscles acting in parallel combinations. Am Surg 1986;52:273–277.

40. Richardson C, Jull G, Hodges P, Hides J. Therapeutic exercise for spinal segmental stabilization in low back pain. Edinburgh, Scotland: Churchill Livingstone, 1999.

41. Torg J, Vegso J, O'Neill MJ, Sennett B. The epidemiologic, pathologic, biomechanical and cinematographic analysis of football-induced cervical spine trauma. Am J Sports Med 1990;18(1):50–57.

42. Wiesenfarth J, Briner W. Neck injuries: urgent decisions and actions. Phys Sports Med 1996;24(1):35–41.

43. Frymoyer J. An overview of the incidences and cost of low back pain. Orthop Clin North Am 1991;22:263–271.

44. Deyo R, Tsui-Wu Y. Descriptive epidemiology of low back pain and its related medical care in the United States. Spine 1987;12:264–268.

45. Mooney V. Functional evaluation of the spine. Curr Opin Orthop 1994;5(11):54–57.

46. Liemohn W, ed. Exercise Prescription and the Back. New York: McGraw-Hill, 2001

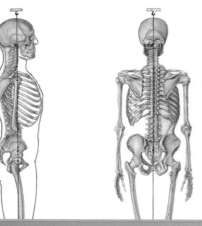

Motor Learning for the Personal Trainer

Howard Zelaznik, Ph.D., Professor, Department of Health and Kinesiology, College of Liberal Arts, Purdue University, West Lafayette, Indiana

CHAPTER 8

Objectives

- Help see the importance of motor learning principles to understand strength development
- Define motor learning
- Describe the measurement of motor learning
- Describe the nature of motor learning
- Present and discuss the most important principles of learning that we can apply to developing training regimens

Many Personal Trainers and their clients do not think about learning when they perform resistance or strength training movements. Strength training typically means working against a resistance, doing plenty of repetitions, and the possibility of feeling sore when finished. However, muscles are not the location for learning. The brain is the center of learning. Thus, in this chapter, the principles of movement learning (motor learning) are applied to resistance training movements and strength development.

STRENGTH DEVELOPMENT AND MOTOR LEARNING

When muscles contract, positively charged molecules enter the muscle cell and cause the muscle cell to depolarize, producing muscle contraction. The movement of these charged molecules produces an electrical potential, called a "voltage." By using a well-developed technique called "electromyography" (EMG), this voltage can be measured. Over the duration of the muscular contraction, the absolute value of the voltages can be summed up over the interval. This summed score is a measure of the total amount of electrical activity produced during the contraction. This is called the "integrated EMG." A linear relationship exists between the amount of force produced by a muscle and the amount of integrated EMG (*Fig. 8.1*). After strength training, and with no increase in muscle size, the same amount of muscular force requires less integrated EMG (represented by the *dashed line* in the figure). This relationship is based on the classic work of Moritani and DeVries (1).

How can less electrical activity produce the same amount of force? Each muscle is composed of approximately one-quarter million individual muscle fibers (2). Imagine that these fibers are like individual rowers on a very large boat. The boat will have maximal speed when all of the rowers are pulling at the same time, and all of the rowers are drawing at the same time. Practice is needed for rowers to move in synchrony. This practice is learning. Each rower is producing maximal performance, but when the team is not well practiced, much of the effort is lost because of this lack of synchrony. The same is true for muscle contraction.

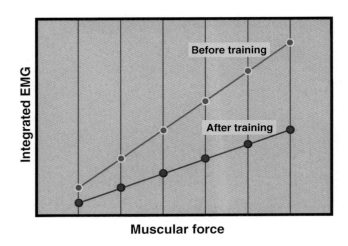

FIGURE 8.1. Displayed are two relations between muscular force and integrated EMG. The *solid line* displays the relation before training and the *dashed line* after practice. Notice that after training you need less integrated EMG for the same level of force produced before training. This is evidence for neural factors (learning) in strength development (idealized graph drawn based upon the result of Moritani and Devries (1)).

As a function of strength training, which is also considered practice (i.e., learning), the contraction of the individual muscle fibers becomes more tightly synchronized, and as such, more force is produced for the same amount of individual muscle fiber effort. In other words, the nervous system controlling muscle fibers becomes more efficient. Muscle fiber shortening becomes more synchronous, so that force buildup is more efficient. The central nervous system has also been trained during this period, resulting in more efficient muscle contraction. This adaptation is called "motor learning." In this chapter, some of the better documented principles of motor learning are discussed. Then, these principles are used to maximize the motor learning of resistance training programs and strength development. Clients must exercise with the proper load and repetitions to maximize the long-term physiological adaptation of muscle. When teaching resistance training movements, Personal Trainers design sessions for clients to practice and learn the proper motor patterns of each exercise. Furthermore, the Personal Trainer should be concerned about the learning of proper technique and posture (sometimes thought of as body alignment) associated with these exercises. Sometimes these two goals (the maximization of strength and the maximization of learning the proper technique) are at odds, creating a dilemma. Bad habits can be learned as well as good habits. A Personal Trainer cannot ignore the motor pattern requirements of a given resistance exercise and concentrate on strength and then hope to instill the correct pattern later. This may ensure a well-developed bad habit during the movements performance. This chapter provides no quick fix answers to this problem, but one hopes that an awareness will be raised that will allow the Personal Trainer to tailor the instruction to meet the goals and needs of clients.

MOTOR LEARNING DEFINED

Motor learning can be defined as the long-term adaptation of the central nervous system to the effects of practice. This definition by design does not include the structural changes in muscle and bone as an aspect of motor learning. For example, a Wimbledon Tennis Champion 50 years ago is now 75 years old. He cannot play tennis as well now as then. The muscles and perhaps the speed of the nervous system do not allow him to demonstrate what has been learned and remembered. On the other hand, an individual who has suffered a cerebral stroke will show decrements in performance that in fact can be thought of as a loss of learning. These individuals go through extensive training to re-learn skills that were once commonplace. The central nervous system is remarkable in its ability to regenerate, and as such, much retraining can occur. Therefore, the definition of learning can be reserved to central nervous system adaptations as a result of experience. These adaptations are relatively permanent and are resistant to loss. The definition of motor learning, as a relatively permanent change, requires that learning be assessed by applying a measure of relative permanence on a performance.

MEASUREMENT OF MOTOR LEARNING

Motor learning is best measured by examining the performance of a client after a period of no practice. This approach is called a "retention test." A retention test allows the Personal Trainer to see whether any improvements in performance as a result of practice are relatively permanent; in other words, is there evidence that the person exhibits a long-term adaptation? Students, clients, and athletes oftentimes will show improvements in performance during practice, under a teacher's, Personal Trainer's, or coach's watchful eye. However, they really have not yet developed long-term adaptation. Therefore, the next day, or the next hour, they do not perform as well as when originally instructed. It is important for the Personal Trainer not to confuse the temporary performance changes that occur and learning. The Personal Trainer provides guidance to the client. It may be that this guidance is the reason behind the immediate performance improvement rather than the client having acquired a long-term adaptation. There is a wealth of research evidence that helps demonstrate that clients can perform much better with guidance, but when the guidance is removed, performance deteriorates toward earlier levels.

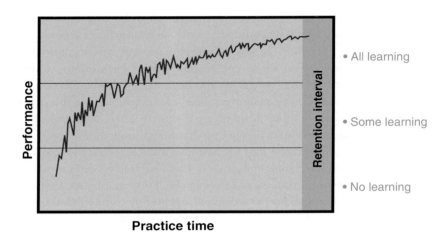

FIGURE 8.2. Idealized depiction of the power law of learning along with changes in performance variability with practice. Performance to the *right* of the retention interval depicts hypothetical results if all, some, or none of the improvements were due to learning.

The retention test can also be applied to examine whether the performance of the client during practice is the result of learning. In Figure 8.2, the performance of a hypothetical subject over a series of practice trials is presented. In the figure, performance appears to be improving with practice. Although performance is highly variable from one trial to the next, performance appears to be improving over time. The fluctuations between adjacent trials decrease as practice increases. These are the hallmark signs of learning. However, the Personal Trainer still has to test or evaluate for a relatively permanent change. Therefore, provide a period of no practice (perhaps 1 day) and then have the person come back and perform the task, without any guidance. If most of the improvement in performance was the result of learning, then performance would pick up where it left off. This is shown by the top signal (see Fig. 8.2) after the retention interval. If all of the improvement was temporary, and therefore not the result of learning, performance after the retention interval would be at the level at which the person first began the practice session. Finally, some of the performance improvement will be relatively permanent (and therefore learning), and some will be the result of the temporary effects of practice and/or instruction.

CHARACTERISTICS OF MOTOR LEARNING

"Highly skilled performers" show consistency in their capabilities to achieve a movement outcome or a required performance goal. Furthermore, skilled performers can continue to refine their movement patterns in the absence of a teacher, coach, or Personal Trainer. In other words, skilled performers can learn even though a teacher, coach, or Personal Trainer is not present. This type of learning is a very important characteristic of highly developed skill learning and in fact provides a powerful principle to which Personal Trainers should adhere. The goal of Personal Trainers is to make themselves not necessary after an appropriate amount of practice and instruction. In other words, the Personal Trainer provides clients with the proper evaluation and feedback to continue to improve and thus learn to train by themselves without supervision at the appropriate time.

It is the role of the Personal Trainer to determine which specific exercises and movement patterns clients may perform safely without the trainer being present. Effective evaluation of each exercise lets the trainer and the client measure performance during the session. They include activities such as the points of evaluation (see Chapter 3) that allow clients to test their progress toward stated objectives and to provide feedback for the Personal Trainer and client. As a result, both parties can better determine where to focus further practice, retraining, and solo workouts for the client.

Power Law of Learning

In most learning situations, clients make their biggest improvements at the early stages of practice, and then the gains in improvement negatively accelerate. This phenomenon has been characterized as the power law of learning. In Figure 8.2, the power law of performance improvement is also shown. The power law shows that the largest performance gains occur during the very early practice trials, and then the performance improvement rate decreases over practice time. In other words, after a rapid initial adaptation, changes in performance take more practice. For example, a client who shows a 50% improvement in performance over 3 months of practice will require at least 6 months to show an additional 50% improvement. A Personal Trainer must make certain that clients understand that the pace of change can slow as clients continue to practice, although they still will show some performance gains. This slower response might be one of the major reasons why adherence to exercise regimens is so poor. As an aside, this is a similar problem for adherence to diet regimens. The loss of weight is most rapid during the first week or two of caloric restriction. Personal Trainers must consider the loss of motivation when the rate of performance improvement decreases after the very large early gains in performance.

Stages of Learning

Learning can also be characterized in stages. A stage is a way to characterize a progression that can describe change. For example, the terms "infant," "toddler," "child," "teenager," and "adult" describe stages of human development. An infant who is 1 year old is not automatically a toddler, rather, the behavior of the child is less infant-like and more toddler-like. The demarcation line between stages is very ill defined. Even though stages are not discrete events, the Personal Trainer can understand skill learning by describing the client as passing through stages as practice continues.

In motor learning there are three major models of stages of learning (3–5). The early stage of learning is called the "cognitive stage." During this stage, the client attempts to "get the idea" of the movement (5). The Personal Trainer and the client use a lot of verbal and visual images to figure out the solution to the motor problem. At first, an exact solution is not needed, just some of the overarching strategies and patterns of movement. This is called a "heuristic strategy." The client tries to find a general solution. For skills that are very complex, such as pole-vaulting, for example, the Personal Trainer is crucial for helping an individual get into the right solution region. In these types of skills, a real partnership develops between the Personal Trainer and the client.

Simpler skills improvement in this stage of motor learning is rapid. The general nature of the solution is found quickly. The trick is to refine the solution. The refining process occurs during the second stage of motor learning, the associative stage. Most clients spend the rest of their practice and performance time in this stage. The goal during this stage of motor learning is to refine the general solution discovered earlier. Furthermore, it is during this stage that the client can recognize sensory information from muscles, vision, and joint receptors (collectively called "feedback") to evaluate the correctness of the movement. After a great amount of practice, clients can enter the autonomous stage. During this stage, performance is executed without attention or awareness.

This final stage (considered expert performance) seems to require many, many hours of practice (6). Most clients do not reach the expert level, but all can continue to show improvement with practice. Research on factory workers shows that even after 20 years on the job, performance still is improving (7). Researchers and practitioners know very little about the processes of learning for expert performers. Most of what practitioners know about motor learning and practice of motor skills is drawn from research with extremely moderate amounts of practice. This should not be a hindrance, as most Personal Trainers are concerned with helping clients who are often removed from expert performance.

Neurological Considerations

The central nervous system and in particular the motor cortex and the cerebellum are the prominent brain structures responsible for the learning and control of movements. Strokes and other trauma to these regions of the brain can leave an individual with moderate-to-severe motor impairments. However, the human brain has a tremendous capacity to relearn and retrain, so that even with moderate strokes, many people can regain good motor function. In terms of strength training, it is fair to say that when clients control movements, they are in fact controlling movements rather than controlling individual muscles. The classic example is examining a signature. Individuals can sign their names on a piece of paper, and the same pattern of motion is produced. This pattern is roughly the same in spatial and temporal terms. Even though the muscles used are different, there is little trouble with writing large, even though there has been a lot of practice in writing small.

Instructions to clients should be based in movement coordinates. For example, bend or straighten the elbow should be an instruction, compared with contracting the biceps muscle. When given the opportunity, clients appear to prefer thinking about movements relative to the coordinates of external space, the common x, y, and z three-dimensional coordinates, along with the coordinates of a local orientation system (roll, pitch, and yaw). Oftentimes it is better to provide an external reference point to make control easier. For example, it is much easier for a client to stand still with eyes closed than with eyes open, because the postural system can calibrate with an external system, even though in theory, joint and muscle receptor information, coupled with information from the vestibular (balance system in the inner ear) provides sufficient information and resolution for balance. However, without vision, it is hard to know the position of the head relative to the external environment.

What Is the Nature of Motor Skill Representation?

A fundamental question for movement scientists concerns the nature of the long-term adaptation called "motor learning." There are two major perspectives concerning this issue. The earliest proposal and one that is adhered to by many scientists and by many practitioners is known as the generalized motor program (8). In this framework, practice allows the individual to develop a representation in the brain of the spatial and temporal pattern of movement. This representation is abstract—in other words, the "language" of this representation is not muscle specific but rather geared toward the external coordinates and temporal aspects of movement. With practice, clients learn to scale this representation spatially and temporally so that movements of the same pattern can be produced large versus small, fast versus slow, and right limb versus left limb.

A more recent proposal about skill development suggests that the nature of skill is not privileged into one neuroanatomical structure. Rather, skill emerges from the nature of the central nervous system, the structural and functional aspects of muscles and bones, and the nature of the information provided (afforded) by the environment. This approach, often called "ecological psychology" (9), believes in finding the underlying regularities of coordination and searching for simple biophysical principles. Finally, this approach minimizes the role of a representation.

Regardless of which system turns out to be better supported by the evidence in the future, both perspectives, at the present time, allow for certain principles of learning and performance that a Personal Trainer can use.

GOALS OF TRAINING

Imagine a 52-year-old author of a book chapter who is beginning piano lessons. What is his goal? One goal is to learn to read music. A second goal is to develop some finger skills to be able to play the piano. Finally, a third goal is to appreciate piano music and perhaps music in general. In this example, the goal is not to play Chopin at Carnegie Hall. So the teacher (an accomplished pianist and music professor at a local college) instructs her student with the three goals in mind. Given these goals, exact fingering skills (or lack thereof) is not something about which she is very concerned. She is concerned about the student being able to read music and to understand the "timing" of music. Because the student's goal is to enjoy the piano, she adapts her teaching goals to fit the stated goals.

The same can be said about a client wanting to learn about strength training. His or her goal might be to gain additional functional strength, or perhaps the client knows that research has documented the loss of muscle strength and muscle mass with age and wants to work a little to prevent or slow the rate of loss. The client might not want or need to know the perfect technique. The Personal Trainer needs to evaluate the overall costs of focusing on perfect technique (maximizing learning, perhaps) versus the goals of the client to develop functional strength and improved fitness.

PRINCIPLES OF PRACTICE

Specificity of Practice Principle

Training produces benefits that are generalized as well as specific. Training produces improvements in the task that is being practiced. This benefit is maximal to the specific task being practiced. However, there are also benefits to tasks that are similar to the one being practiced. For example, if a client practices 30-lb (14-kg) biceps curls and the improvement in the form of that movement is measured, the client's performance will be better at the 30-lb (14-kg) weight than with 35 or 25 pounds (16 or 11 kg). Furthermore, if you then have that individual use the biceps muscle in a different task, there will not be 100% transfer. In other words, the client would have performed this new task better had he or she practiced it. This is known as specificity of practice. It is a very powerful determinant of learning. In fact, this principle is seen in the specificity of learning. Clients who practice a task without visual guidance will show decrements in performance when required to then practice with vision (10). Switching to vision would seem to be beneficial, as the client may have more information. Such is not the case, surprising as that may seem. Apparently, the client's movement pattern develops without visual guidance, and he or she is not capable of taking advantage of this new information. This specificity of practice principle is very important in structuring practice sessions, so that clients can continue to learn and perform well when exercising on their own and when not under the guidance of the Personal Trainer.

Knowledge of Results and Knowledge of Performance

Knowledge of results, although not used very much in actual sports, exercise, and therapy situations, has a long history of being studied in the motor learning laboratory. There is no reason to believe that the principles of knowledge of results administration will not apply to providing information to a client in an instructional setting. Knowledge of results is defined as information provided by an external agent (the Personal Trainer) about the outcome of a movement. In baseball, it is the umpire calling balls and strikes. In most rehabilitation and sports settings, the performer knows the outcome as part of the act of moving. Knowledge of results is redundant in many situations outside the laboratory situations. Teachers, coaches, and Personal Trainers most often provide what is termed "knowledge of performance." Knowledge of performance is information provided about the quality of movement in terms of whether the movement produced by the individual was accurate with respect to the goal of the required movement pattern. This type of information is readily provided when teaching a client a new exercise movement. The Personal Trainer emphasizes the proper movement and then provides knowledge of performance concerning the quality of the attempt relative to an ideal standard.

The term "feedback" is often used to describe knowledge of results and knowledge of performance. Although the term "feedback" is appropriate, knowledge of results and knowledge of performance are very precise in their meaning, and because of this, we will not use the term "feedback" in this chapter. Feedback is defined as sensory information that arises from the act of movement (11). Feedback is what a movement looks, feels, and sounds like.

Frequency of Knowledge of Results and Knowledge of Performance

Many researchers have shown that providing information often during early stages of learning is beneficial (12) because clients are still in the cognitive stage. Knowledge of results and knowledge of performance help the client discover the general idea of the task and the solution. Once clients have the general idea and are in the process of skill refinement, providing knowledge of results and/or knowledge of performance less than 100% of the time leads to better learning than providing knowledge of results or knowledge of performance every time. The reason is believed to be the benefits of forcing a client to rely upon the evaluation of sensory feedback rather than using the Personal Trainer as a "crutch." Forcing the performer to become independent produces the capabilities to evaluate the quality of performance and continuous improvement.

Precision and/or Amount of Information Provided

The mistake many Personal Trainers make is to provide too much information, particularly at an early stage of learning. Recall that in the early cognitive stage, clients are still trying to just get the idea of the movement. They attempt to discover a pattern of motion that solves the problem. Once discovered, the client then can work on refining that pattern.

Early in the learning process, clients use heuristics to figure out the most important aspects of the pattern. For example, when trying to teach a client to learn a tennis forehand, many instructors will force the beginner to swing very slowly. One big problem with beginning tennis players is that they wait too long to start swinging because they do not do well judging the ball. Second, swinging slowly forces the swing to come from the shoulder, a desirable biomechanical outcome, particularly for a beginner. Third, the player must have a good tight grip to swing slowly and impart enough force back to the ball. So, a very simple heuristic strategy (swinging slowly) will allow the player to perceptually learn to judge the ball and to begin to have the proper movement pattern. Notice that the instructor does not need to tell the person the proper pattern; he or she will discover the pattern based upon a simple instruction. The instructor now provides knowledge of results based upon the speed of the racket, not on the mechanics of movement. The mechanics fall out of the control of racket speed. Over time, the instructor can then work on increasing racket speed, once the pattern has been discovered.

Personal Trainers may provide too much information the first time they describe to a client how to perform a certain resistance training movement. Research clearly has shown that early in learning, too much information, or information that is too precise, will produce poorer learning than less information and less precision. Only when clients move out of the cognitive stage should more detailed information be provided. Personal Trainers should give learners a chance to find their pattern and thus the solution.

Blocked versus Random Practice Schedules

Although many of the details are still under debate, it seems safe to infer that to maximize learning of a variety of tasks, that those tasks should not be practiced individually in a large set (i.e., a block) of trials. In other words, people appear to need to practice various tasks in a mixed up or random order to maximize the benefits of learning (13). The benefits of a more loosely structured practice regimen are not seen during the initial practice bout. Rather, during initial practice, people do better when performing one task for a large set of trials before moving to the other task, rather than practicing one trial of task A, one of task C, one of D, one of B, and so on. However, if the Personal Trainer then provides an interval of no practice, the clients who practiced in the random order perform as well, if not better, than those who practiced under the blocked situations. This effect highlights the difference between the temporary effects of practice and the permanent adaptations called learning.

The benefits of random practice appear at odds with the methods necessary to develop strength. Resistance training movements require repetitions and practice. In other words, strength development requires blocked practice. However, to learn the appropriate motor skills of these strength tasks, random practice is recommended, creating a dilemma between block and random practice. An example may be to separate technique (i.e., learning) from physiological adaptations for strength. Clients can practice their technique under very light loads, and only practice one or three sets at a time, before moving on to another set of the same exercise at an increased resistance or load. Therefore, after the practice sets with the lower resistance levels have been completed, the client performs 10 repetitions at the higher resistance or load level to focus purely on the strength benefits. As the improvement in technique should occur rather quickly (power law of learning), and the client will be in the associative stage of learning, the Personal Trainer can then concentrate on the strength development portion of the work. Keep in mind that the Personal Trainer needs to be able to distinguish between when to work on technique (learning) solely versus strength. Recommendations on establishing practice sessions are reviewed in more detail in Chapter 5.

Variable versus Constant Practice

How should a client practice learning a particular pattern of motion for a set amount of weight? Traditionally, a Personal Trainer would set a weight that the client was strong enough to lift the required number of times. However, motor learning theory suggests that when people learn motor skills, they learn about the relative motions and the pattern (8). This generalized learning allows the client to perform new versions of similar tasks. A carpenter, for example, given a unique hammer does not need to learn a new hammering technique. Rather, through wielding the hammer, he or she picks up the relevant dynamics of the hammer and then can alter the already learned hammering pattern of motion to hammer with this new tool. How does one learn to produce these novel tasks? According to schema theory (8), an individual requires variable practice. Variable practice is defined as practice at a variety of tasks controlled by the same movement class, sometimes called a "generalized motor program." Therefore, a Personal Trainer may decide to teach a client a specific sequence or progression of exercise movements that requires a gradual increase of skills and abilities for learning a specific movement pattern. For example, a client may first be taught how to perform a back extension on a mat on the floor, which is in a fairly stable environment. After the client has practiced that movement for a period of 4 weeks, the Personal Trainer may then teach the client to perform the back extension while balancing on a stability ball. It is the same movement or motion but is more challenging for the client, requiring more neural demands.

Demonstrations

Early in the learning process, people benefit from demonstrations by expert performers. This area of research called "modeling" is now part of the domain of sport psychology research. Early work in the 1970s and 1980s clearly showed that a moving picture (i.e., demonstration) is very effective. Two things are crucial for a good demonstration. One, the demonstrator has to be credible. Second, the demonstrator has to provide critical, correct information and demonstration of the pattern of motion. Details on how to demonstrate a resistance training movement are presented in Chapter 5.

Stick figures, animated in real time, seem to work as well as a human demonstration. Work by Johansson (14) has shown that people do not need to see an entire person to ascertain the pattern of motion. In these studies, reflective markers are placed on individuals who are walking. The video of the individual is played back to a naïve subject. The naïve subject only sees these reflective points. Even though the visual display is of a stick figure, the naïve subject can determine that the person is walking, as well as the gender of the walker. The reason is that these point light displays provide the crucial information about relative motions to determine the action. This work has been extended to weight-lifting tasks. Shim and Carlton (15) have shown that individuals can judge the heaviness of an object by observing the point light description of a person lifting a load. These point light displays have been shown to be superior to full view human demonstrations, since the observer is not distracted by the irrelevant features and movements of the model.

SUMMARY

This chapter provides a few of the well-supported general principles of learning as it relates to practice. The major theme in this chapter concerns the difficulty of maximizing learning resistance-training movements along with maximizing strength development. Teachers as well as coaches and Personal Trainers should attempt to establish personal training sessions that allow clients to learn, practice, and eventually have the ability and confidence to train on their own.

REFERENCES

1. Moritani T, Devries HA. Neural factors versus hypertrophy in the time course of muscle strength gain. Am J Phys Med Rehabil 1979;58:115–130.
2. Klein CS, Marsh GD, Petrella RJ, Rice CL. Muscle fiber number in the biceps brachii muscle of young and old men. Muscle Nerve 2003;28:62–68.
3. Fitts PM, Posner MI. Human Performance. Belmont, CA: Brooks/Cole, 1967:167.
4. Adams JA. A closed loop theory of motor learning. J Motor Behav 1971;3:111–150.
5. Gentile A. A working model of skill acquisition with application to teaching. Quest 1972;17:3–23.
6. Ericsson K, Charness N. Expert performance: its structure and acquisition. In: Ceci SJ, Williams WM, eds. The nature–nurture debate: The essential readings. Essential Readings Dev Psychol 1999;199–255, 294.
7. Crossman E. A Theory of the Acquisition of Speed–Skill. Ergonomics 2. United Kingdom: Taylor & Francis, 1959:153–166.
8. Schmidt RA. A schema theory of discrete motor skill learning. Psychol Rev 1975;82:225–260.
9. Turvey MT. Coordination. Am Psychol 1990;45:938–953.
10. Proteau L, Cournoyer, J. Vision of the stylus in a manual aiming task: the effects of practice. Q J Exp Psychol 1990;42B: 811–828.
11. Schmidt RA. Motor Control and Learning: A Behavioral Emphasis. 2nd ed. Urbana, IL: Human Kinetics, 1988.
12. Winstein CJ, Schmidt RA. Reduced frequency of knowledge of results enhances motor skill learning. JEP: Learn Memory Cogn 1990;16:677–691.
13. Shea JB, Morgan RL. Contextual interference effects on the acquisition, retention, and transfer of a motor skill. JEP: Learn Memory Cogn 1979;5:179–187.
14. Johansson G. Visual perception of biological motion and a model for its analysis. Percep Psychophys 1973;14:201–211.
15. Shim J, Carlton LG. Perception of kinematic characteristics in the motion of lifted weight. J Motor Behav 1997;29:131–146.

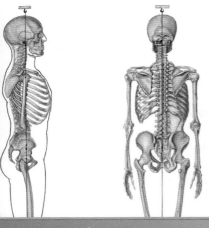

Pedagogy and the Client Learning Program

Terry Ferebee Eckmann, Ph.D., Associate Professor, Department of Teacher Education and Human Performance, Minot State University, Minot, North Dakota

Chapter Outline

- Explain the importance of pedagogical skills in personal training
- Define pedagogy, teaching, and learning
- Discuss the following learning theories: attribution theory, motivation theory, transfer theory, and goal theory
- Describe the eight elements of effective lesson design and discuss how they apply to the personal training session
- Explain how Personal Trainers can effectively apply understanding of brain research, learning styles, and multiple intelligences to program design
- Discuss how emotional intelligence can affect Personal Trainers
- Outline a framework for excellence in personal training

Pedagogical skills are essential for successful personal training. Effective Personal Trainers will have adequate knowledge of the four domains that make up a framework for teaching excellence: planning and preparation, the training environment, instruction, and professional responsibilities. This chapter provides an overview of application of learning theories and lesson design to personal training. An overview of brain research, learning styles, and multiple intelligences will provide Personal Trainers with ways to enhance program design.

PEDAGOGY AND TRAINING

Pedagogy is the science or profession of teaching. **Teaching** can be defined as the action of a person giving instruction or imparting skill or knowledge (1). Teaching is an action of someone who is assisting others in reaching their full potential.

The purpose/mission of a Personal Trainer is to help others achieve their health-related fitness goals. A Personal Trainer, much like a teacher, has the responsibility of helping others to learn and to behave in new and different ways. An effective teacher must have content knowledge along with an understanding of how to organize information, adapt to diverse learning styles, and effectively communicate (pedagogy). A teacher may have subject knowledge but not be able to teach. A Personal Trainer may have knowledge of exercise science and nutrition and not be able to effectively communicate information. Effective teachers use pedagogical techniques to convey information and teach skills. Personal Trainers will be more effective when they apply the pedagogical knowledge included in this chapter (i.e., effective teaching skills, professional communication skills, learning theory, learning styles, instructional design, and current brain research) to help their clients succeed.

There are many definitions of learning and although no one is universally accepted, all have commonalities. Moore (1) defines **learning** as a change in a student's capacity for performance as a result of experience. **Learning** is an enduring change in behavior or in the capacity to behave in a given fashion, which results from practice of other forms of experience (2). McCombs (3) defined **learning** as an individual process of constructing meaning from information and experience, filtered through each individual's unique perceptions, thoughts, and feelings. One common thread related to learning is change; learning changes thinking, perception, performance, and behavior. There continues to be an outpouring of scientific research on the brain and the processes of thinking and learning. By applying brain research and pedagogical knowledge and related skills to the personal training experience, Personal Trainers can better facilitate the process of learning to help clients reach their goals.

THE PERSONAL TRAINER'S ROLE AS AN EDUCATOR

To train clients to effectively perform exercises and change lifestyle behaviors, the Personal Trainer needs to have strong core knowledge of exercise science along with the pedagogical tools to enhance learning experiences. Experiences that are organized around personal training skills will increase the client's opportunity for success and ultimately the success of the Personal Trainer.

Clients employ Personal Trainers for a variety of reasons. To increase the likelihood of successful outcomes, the Personal Trainer and client must work together to set clear, specific goals. It is the Personal Trainer's job to help determine a plan of action. The Personal Trainer may need to educate the client in several areas to reach desired goals. For example, if a goal is weight management, the Personal Trainer may plan to educate the client on the process of change, basic nutrition, current weight management research, strategies for effective weight management, exercise technique for strength training, heart rate monitoring, and cardiovascular exercise options.

Knowledge does not necessarily lead to a change in behavior. After significant time with Personal Trainers, most clients will learn how to correctly perform exercises; however, they generally continue to use the services of those who provide new, safe, and effective exercises along with support that encourages adherence to the exercise program.

Moore (1) suggests that a teacher's many roles can be divided into three categories: instructional expert, manager, and counselor. The Personal Trainer must assume each of these roles as well. The Personal Trainer acting as an instructional expert must have extensive knowledge of exercise science based on the American College of Sports Medicine (ACSM) guidelines for exercise testing and prescription. The content of this knowledge base encompasses a variety of topic areas, including strength and cardiovascular training, nutrition, biomechanics, assessment of health-related fitness components as well as a solid background in the exercise sciences. Personal Trainers must also have knowledge of pedagogical skills to aid them in planning, guiding, and assessing client learning and progress. A Personal Trainer will need to apply knowledge of effective teaching and communication skills, learning theory, instructional design, learning styles, and brain research to be successful in the role of instructional expert.

The Personal Trainer must also be a manager who maintains business order. This involves ensuring that all administrative responsibilities, such as scheduling and financial accounting, are carried out.

The third role of counselor requires that Personal Trainers understand human behavior and learning so that they can work effectively with a variety of clients. This is an essential role of the Personal Trainer, whose biggest challenge is to help clients adhere to their exercise program and new lifestyle choices to reach their goals. Although it is essential that clients learn and manage key information to reach their personal goals, regular accountability, monitoring, and coaching is just as important.

By integrating a variety of pedagogical skills into the personal training process, the Personal Trainer can apply effective teaching and communication skills used by educators to personal training. Understanding learning theory, instructional design, learning styles, brain research, and effective communication skills can add an important dimension to personal training.

EFFECTIVE TEACHING SKILLS OF AN EDUCATOR/PERSONAL TRAINER

The Personal Trainer can use a framework for development of effective teaching skills first introduced by Danielson (4), with simple modifications, to serve as a guide for professional growth and development (Box 9.1).

Many of the components of professional practice for teachers can be adapted to develop a framework for effective personal training. Given the complexity of personal training, this framework can serve as a roadmap for novice Personal Trainers, providing them with a pathway to excellence. Experienced Personal Trainers can use this framework to reflect on their skills, mentor novice Personal Trainers, and continually adjust and focus their training efforts.

Box 9.1	Components of Professional Practice: A Framework for Excellence in Personal Training

Domain 1: Planning and Preparation
Domain 2: The Training Environment
Domain 3: Instruction/Training
Domain 4: Professional Responsibilities

DOMAIN 1: PLANNING AND PREPARATION

Component 1a: Demonstrating Knowledge of Pedagogical Skills

A Personal Trainer must have a solid understanding of the content knowledge to develop a safe and effective exercise prescription. A Personal Trainer cannot successfully teach what he or she does not know. Content knowledge is the foundation for the personal training experience. Knowledge of effective teaching (pedagogy) and communications skills must interconnect with content knowledge for training to be a successful experience for the client.

Component 1b: Demonstrating Knowledge of Clients

To maximize the training experience, Personal Trainers must have an understanding of their clients. The Personal Trainer will want to make an assessment of current health-related fitness components (e.g., muscle strength, endurance and flexibility, cardiovascular endurance, as well as anthropometric and health-related measures). This information will give the Personal Trainer and client measurable components to provide a basis for setting goals.

Prochaska's (5) Stages of Change Model can help the Personal Trainer better understand a client's readiness to change (for more details, see Chapter 10). A Personal Trainer may also benefit from a better understanding of a client's learning style and personality type. Understanding a client will help the Personal Trainer individualize a training program more effectively. Clients will vary greatly, and a "one exercise prescription fits all" approach to training will often lead to failure for both the client and the Personal Trainer.

Component 1c: Developing Client Goals

Developing goals for clients is a key component of successful programming for Personal Trainers. SMART goals with clear objectives will give the training experience direction and focus. All goals should be SMART:

Specific
Measurable
Attainable/**A**cceptable
Realistic/**R**elevant
Time anchored

Goals should be based on the client's level of health-related fitness and be determined by the client with professional guidance from the Personal Trainer. Personal Trainers should be aware of how to establish goals and know the difference between short-term and long-term goals.

Component 1d: Demonstrating Knowledge of Resources

Although Personal Trainers provide a diversity of services, it is essential to know when to refer clients to other healthcare practitioners when their needs are beyond the Personal Trainer's own expertise. Professional counselors, registered dietitians, physical therapists, and physicians should be called on for assessment and follow-up care when needed. Educational materials such as texts, websites, and exercise videos may also prove to be valuable resources for clients with special needs.

Component 1e: Developing an Organized and Effective Training Program

The training program should stem from the client's initial health fitness assessment and be based on SMART goals. The FITT formula (Frequency, Intensity, Time, Type) is a model that offers the Personal Trainer a guideline for exercise prescription that can be modified as needed to achieve goals. ACSM guidelines serve as an excellent foundation for the exercise prescription. Ongoing assessment and revision of SMART goals allows the Personal Trainer to apply the FITT formula to succeed.

Component 1f: Assessing Client Progress

Client progress should be measured regularly for the client to experience appropriate training improvements. The Personal Trainer should adjust frequency, intensity, and duration of activity as needed and discussed with the client. The type of activity must also be considered in this training assessment to maximize desired outcomes and avoid boredom. Regular assessment of the performance, anthropometric measures, and health outcomes will help the Personal Trainer make ongoing adjustments to the exercise prescription.

DOMAIN 2: THE TRAINING ENVIRONMENT

Component 2a: Creating an Environment of Respect and Rapport

Personal Trainers create a climate of respect and rapport with a client by the way they communicate. Covey's (6) principle of "Seek first to understand, and then to be understood" may be one of the most essential concepts for building respect and rapport with a client. A good rule of thumb is to treat others as you would like to be treated.

Component 2b: Establishing a Culture for Learning and Desire for Success

Actively involving clients in the SMART goal-setting process will help to establish a culture of learning and a desire for success. Teaching the client strategies to overcome barriers that prevent regular exercise and healthy lifestyle choices will also help to create a positive learning climate and feelings of empowerment. Personal Trainers may encounter clients who have acquired an attitude of learned helplessness. Those that may have failed repeatedly in achieving their health-fitness goals may have learned that failure is a result of their best efforts. An excellent resource for a client with this experience is the book *Learned Optimism* by Seligman (7). Seligman teaches the ABCDE approach to facing challenges:

> **A**dversity
> **B**eliefs
> **C**onsequence
> **D**ispute
> **E**nergize

When faced with **adversity** (e.g., a day in which a client with weight-loss goals deviates from the diet plan), the client attaches the experience to his or her **belief** system ("I am a failure . . . I will always be overweight because I have no willpower") and the **consequence** is a feeling of learned helplessness, which leads to giving up on an eating plan and exercise program. To change the consequence, the client can **dispute** the current belief ("I had a bad day and ate too much. Tomorrow I will get back on track, eat according to my plan, and resume my exercise program."). The result is an **energized** client who feels empowered to succeed.

Component 2c: Managing the Training Session

Effective Personal Trainers manage time and resources efficiently to get the most out of each training session. Application of lesson design can help a Personal Trainer focus the training while applying learning theory. Lesson design and learning theory are covered later in this chapter.

Component 2d: Managing Client Responsiveness

Responsibilities of both the Personal Trainer and client must be clear, with defined expectations. The Personal Trainer obviously has the major responsibility of managing the personal training experience, but without the client's cooperation, the training program is likely to be unsuccessful. Clients must be aware of the consequences of noncompliance, such as being late or canceling appointments. As well, Personal Trainers must focus on client behavior versus personality traits to improve adherence.

Component 2e: Planning Safe and Efficient Use of Physical Space

Personal Trainers work in a variety of settings. Whether training takes place in a client's home, a mobile gym, or privately owned or commercial training facility, the equipment must be well maintained and organized for a balanced and efficient workout. The physical space and equipment should be kept clean. Bright, motivational posters that inspire participation rather than falsely advertise "the perfect body" will create a more positive and encouraging environment. Mirrors can help Personal Trainers teach body alignment for safe and effective exercise technique.

DOMAIN 3: INSTRUCTION/TRAINING

Component 3a: Communicating Clearly and Accurately

Most communications specialists believe that communication is 7% verbal, 38% intonation or inflection, and 55% body language. It is not just the spoken word that communicates a message, but how the information is expressed (i.e., vocal inflection and body language). Eye contact and a pleasant smile are essential for building positive relationships.

Professional jargon can be confusing to clients with limited exercise experience. The Personal Trainer should ensure that concepts are clearly explained in simple, understandable terms. The first time in a club setting or exercise environment can be an overwhelming and intimidating experience for some. Introducing new material so it can be easily received and understood will increase the client's comfort level and opportunity to retain information. The use of professional terminology can gradually increase as the client's understanding of exercise principles increases.

Component 3b: Continually Checking for Understanding

In a personal training setting, understanding can be checked through observation of exercise movements/technique. It is essential for the client to perform exercises correctly. It is more difficult to unlearn old patterns than to correctly teach new ones. Specific questions should be directed to the client to ensure that there is adequate understanding of concepts taught. What the client perceives from instruction is not necessarily the message the Personal Trainer intends. Listening to what clients say about what is being taught can help ensure that they comprehend what the Personal Trainer is teaching.

Component 3c: Engaging Clients in Learning and Exercising

A client who actively seeks the services of a Personal Trainer is obviously interested in the training process. An engaged client is more likely to adhere to lifestyle changes. If clients are instructed to follow a training regimen that they are not comfortable with, do not understand, or do not have time for, retention is less likely. Clients need to be encouraged to express their feelings and provide input into the exercise program. If exercises are uncomfortable or exceed the time a client is comfortable spending, adherence and retention may be compromised. Personal Trainers should encourage questions and be open to discussion regarding training concepts.

Concept 3d: Providing Feedback to Clients

Feedback is information the Personal Trainer provides to the client regarding his or her participation and progress. Feedback should be immediate, specific, accurate, constructive, and meaningful. Feedback during training sessions may be specific to exercises performed. Feedback should also occur with ongoing assessment of health fitness-related measures.

Component 3e: Demonstrating Ability to Adapt to Changing Needs of the Client

Regular decision making is an essential aspect of the Personal Trainer's role. If a training program is not working, the Personal Trainer must be flexible and responsive to the client's needs. A Personal Trainer who is rigid and does not respond to unexpected barriers or challenges will not experience the same success as a Personal Trainer who can demonstrate flexibility and responsiveness.

DOMAIN 4: PROFESSIONAL RESPONSIBILITIES

Component 4a: Reflecting on Training

Ongoing reflection of the training session provides both Personal Trainer and client with valuable insight about program effectiveness. This reflection should also include the Personal Trainer's assessment of the client's attitude toward and enthusiasm for the training regimen. An effective Personal Trainer will regularly reflect on the client's progress to determine if the exercise prescription is working toward helping the client achieve defined goals.

Component 4b: Maintaining Accurate Records

Personal Trainers can use the FITT formula as a model for record keeping. Personal Trainers need to maintain a log of frequency, intensity, time (duration), and type of activity, including documentation of sets, reps, and load for strength training. Additionally, documenting assessment results will provide opportunities to objectively evaluate progress.

Component 4c: Communicating with the Client

Component 3a of the personal training framework provided a brief overview of key concepts of communication. Personal Trainers who become more aware of verbal and nonverbal messages will be more effective communicators. Personal Trainers who work in front of mirrors may find them an added tool for improving their own communication skills. Again, active listening and clear communication are key components to building a successful Personal Trainer–client relationship.

Component 4d: Contributing to the Organization and Community

Professionals who are generous with their knowledge and expertise can contribute in a variety of ways within their own communities. Professional Personal Trainers should invest in building relationships with colleagues in the fitness industry and be willing to share resources and information with those of lesser experience. Personal Trainers should be willing to reach out to the community to promote better health and fitness through events such as health walks, community health fairs, and other special fundraising events. Professional Personal Trainers may serve on committees working to promote specific health initiatives in the community. Active involvement in an organization and community is beneficial to everyone and provides networking opportunities for the professional that may be unavailable otherwise.

Component 4e: Growing and Developing Professionally

True professionals are lifelong learners, always striving to keep up to date on the latest research and literature while striving to master the skills of their profession. Attending workshops and conferences, reading professional journals, obtaining and maintaining credentials, and building professional networks are some ways the Personal Trainer can develop professionally. Personal Trainers who continue to grow and develop their content knowledge and pedagogical skills will be more energized and remain at the top of their profession.

Component 4f: Demonstrating Professionalism

Personal Trainers should possess an understanding of industry standards and demonstrate a commitment to being in compliance. Personal Trainers need to take a leadership role in promoting health and fitness.

REFLECTION ON LEVEL OF PERFORMANCE

Each component of this professional practice framework for teaching and personal training excellence can be used for reflection and assessment. Danielson (4) uses five levels of performance as a rating scale and guide for novices to continually improve performance. The five levels of performance are elementary, unsatisfactory, basic, proficient, and distinguished. Below is an example of how these five performance levels can be used as a guideline for growth when reflecting on or assessing Component 4e: Growing and Developing Professionalism:

Level 1. Elementary: Enhancement of content, knowledge, and pedagogical skills
Level 2. Unsatisfactory: Personal Trainer engages in professional development activities to enhance knowledge or skill
Level 3. Basic: Personal Trainer participates in professional activities to a limited extent when they are convenient
Level 4. Proficient: Personal Trainer seeks opportunities for professional development to enhance content knowledge and pedagogical skill
Level 5. Distinguished: Personal Trainer seeks out opportunities for professional development and makes a systematic attempt to conduct action research

PERSONAL ATTRIBUTES OF EFFECTIVE TEACHERS/ PERSONAL TRAINERS

As mentioned earlier, effective Personal Trainers need to be effective teachers. Cruickshank, Jenkins, and Metcalf (8) identified eight attributes that are characteristic of effective teachers:

1. Enthusiastic
2. Warm and humorous
3. Credible

4. Holding high expectations for success
5. Encouraging and supportive
6. Businesslike
7. Adaptable/flexible
8. Knowledgeable

Personal training is a relatively new profession with little research available that has investigated the personal attributes related to efficacy. Similarities between the professions of teaching and personal training suggest that eight personal attributes that characterize effective teachers can also be applied to Personal Trainers.

The personal characteristics of enthusiasm, credibility, warmth, and humor combine to serve as motivational forces for learning. Personal Trainers need to demonstrate personal attributes without compromising professionalism. They should attend to business and remain task-focused while being compassionate, flexible, and adaptive. A close look at the personal characteristics of effective teachers as identified by Barr (9) and more recently by Cruickshank et al. (8) supports emotional intelligence as an extremely important attribute for successful training. Barr (9) identified 12 characteristics important for successful teaching, which can be applied easily to personal training:

1. Resourcefulness: Originality, creativeness, initiative, imagination, adventurousness, progressiveness
2. Intelligence: Foresight, intellectual acuity, understanding, mental ability, intellectual capacity, common sense
3. Emotional Stability: Poise, self-control, steadfastness, sobriety, dignity, emotional maturity, stability
4. Considerateness: Appreciativeness, kindness, friendliness, courteousness, sympathy, tact, helpfulness, patience, politeness
5. Buoyancy: Optimism, enthusiasm, cheerfulness, sense of humor, pleasantness, expressiveness, wit, alertness
6. Objectivity: Fairness, impartiality, open-mindedness
7. Drive: Physical vigor, energy, ambition, industriousness, motivation, purposeful, quickness, endurance
8. Dominance: Self-confidence, forcefulness, decisiveness, self-reliance, self-assertiveness, determination
9. Attractiveness: Dress, neatness, cleanliness, posture, personal charm, appearance
10. Refinement: Good taste, morality, modesty, culture
11. Cooperativeness: Friendliness, generosity, adaptability, flexibility, trustfulness, unselfishness
12. Reliability: Accuracy, dependability, honesty, punctuality, responsibility, trustworthiness, consistency, sincerity

EMOTIONAL INTELLIGENCE AND THE PERSONAL TRAINER

Many of the personal attributes characteristic of effective teachers/Personal Trainers will be found within the framework of emotional intelligence. Salovey and Mayer (10) defined emotional intelligence as "the ability to monitor one's own and other's feelings and emotions, to discriminate among them, and to use this information to guide one's thinking and action." Goleman popularized the concept in his book *Emotional Intelligence* (11). Over the past decade, Goleman, with Hay/McBer Emotional Intelligence Services (www.eisglobal.com), have developed the Emotional Competency Inventory (ECI), a tool to measure emotional competencies in the workplace. An emotional competence is a learned capability, based on emotional intelligence, which results in outstanding performance at work (12). Emotional competencies are the personal and social skills that demonstrate emotional intelligence and lead to superior performance in the workplace. The ECI organizes these competencies into four clusters: self-awareness, self-management, social awareness, and relationship management (13).

Goleman's Four Cluster Emotional Competency Model

Self-awareness includes the competencies of self-assessment (i.e., knowing your personal strengths and weaknesses), emotional self-awareness (i.e., recognizing your emotions and their effects), and self-confidence (i.e., having a sense of self-worth and capabilities) (12).

Self-management includes achievement drive (i.e., striving to constantly improve and meet a standard of excellence), adaptability (i.e., having the flexibility to handle change), emotional self-control (i.e., keeping emotions and impulses in check), initiative (i.e., having the readiness to act on opportunities), and optimism (i.e., persisting in pursuing goals despite obstacles and setbacks).

Social awareness includes empathy (i.e., awareness and concern of the feelings of others), organizational awareness (i.e., consideration of the needs of the organization), and service orientation (i.e., understanding how to meet customer needs).

Relationship management includes conflict management, personal development, and influence on others through inspirational leadership and acting as a change catalyst to foster teamwork and collaboration. Strong relationship management skills will induce desirable responses in others.

Each of these competencies is independent of the others, making a unique contribution to performance on the job. Yet, each competency is interdependent, drawing to some extent on others. The emotional competencies are hierarchical, building on one another. For example, self-awareness is necessary to manage your goals to initiate or adapt to change (12).

REFLECTIVE TEACHING/TRAINING

Reflection on training includes the thinking that follows any training session. Professionals who learn to analyze and interpret events in ways to guide their own development can continually improve their training skills. Self-reflection is an important part of professional development. It is a way for a Personal Trainer to apply knowledge of content and pedagogical skills to a training experience and then determine what works and what does not. Reflection is a way to self-assess while at the same time assessing a training plan to make necessary modifications. Reflective Personal Trainers will ask themselves what worked and what did not, why am I doing what I am doing, what can I do differently to be more effective, and how can I improve.

Sometimes we do things because we have always done them in a certain way, a way we have observed or have been taught by a former teacher, coach, mentor, parent, friend, or significant other. The art of reflection can lead us in new directions by constantly asking why, while exploring other options. There are many ways to approach training, and reflective Personal Trainers will be less likely to get in a rut because they are always looking for ways to improve and accomplish goals.

LEARNING THEORIES

The following section provides an overview of theories that have been applied to influence learning. Motivation theory, attribution theory, transfer theory, retention theory, and goal theory can all be used by Personal Trainers to increase effectiveness. A definition of each theory and its application affords an overview of how learning theories can make a difference in personal training.

Motivation Theory

Motivation is a state of need or desire that influences a person to do something that will satisfy that need or desire. Personal Trainers must focus on creating circumstances that will affect the client's desire to learn, grow, and change. Hunter (14) identified six interrelating conditions or variables that Personal Trainers can use to motivate clients to learn. Motivation is greatest when there is a positive balance among all five conditions:

1. **Level of Concern.** Clients are more likely to be motivated to change if they are concerned about the consequences. Personal Trainers can influence the level of concern by how they instruct a client. For example, when teaching a "squat," a Personal Trainer can lower the level of concern by explaining to the client that the squat is a difficult movement that will require practice to perform it correctly. Conversely, the level of concern may be raised if the client perceives that there are high expectations of performance. There may be times when a Personal Trainer wishes to increase the level of concern to motivate a client by strategically posing additional challenges. As well, there may be times when a client is struggling or frustrated when the Personal Trainer may want to lower the level of concern by relieving stress with reassurance and/or interjecting humor.

2. **Feeling tone** is the atmosphere or climate of the training session that results from the Personal Trainer's attitude and training style. It can be pleasant, neutral, or unpleasant. A Personal Trainer who creates a positive feeling tone with a client will be more likely to achieve success. Emotion and learning are closely linked. While pleasant feeling tones will create an energized positive training environment, unpleasant feeling tones will very likely produce undesirable outcomes. The client experiencing an unpleasant feeling tone may associate the exercise experience with negative feelings. A Personal Trainer's words, vocal inflection, body language, and listening skills will all contribute to the creation of feeling tone.

3. **Interest** can be elevated when a Personal Trainer uses effective communication skills, explores the client's learning style, gears training toward that style, and introduces variety to the training regimen.

4. **Success** is the perceived level of accomplishment experienced by the client. The training experience must be challenging enough to elicit improvement, yet easy enough to provide a sense of accomplishment. To increase the likelihood of success, the Personal Trainer should carefully control the difficulty level of the training program to match the client's level of effort and ability.

5. **Knowledge of results** is the fifth element of motivation theory. Performing an exercise or completing a training session without knowing how well the exercises have been executed is not very stimulating or satisfying. Motivated clients will continually improve if they are aware of how well they are doing, what they need to do to improve, and how they can improve and do things better. Personal Trainers can provide knowledge of results by offering regular feedback that is immediate, specific, precise, and growth oriented and preserves the dignity of the client.

COMPONENTS OF VALUABLE FEEDBACK

Listed below is an example of feedback for a client performing a "squat" exercise:

1. Immediate: "Keeping your knees behind your toes. . . pull your hips back as if you were sitting in a chair. . . the imaginary headlights on your shoulders are scaling the wall in front of you. . . are you contracting your gluteal muscles?"
2. Specific: "You performed the squat using good body mechanics. Your knees were lined up with your ankles."
3. Precise: "Squats are one of the top exercises for the lower body. By contracting your gluteal muscles you will improve your execution of the squat and see better results."
4. Growth-oriented: "Since you were able to maintain proper body mechanics on the squat, we will be able to increase your workloads next session."
5. Preserves dignity: "It is not unusual for people to have difficulty performing the squat correctly. It may take some time before you're comfortable with the movement and master the technique."

6. Reward: Clients will experience intrinsic reward when they perform a task that is interesting, challenging, and exciting. An extrinsic reward is a tangible result of good performance that comes from an outside source. Personal Trainers using a training card that shows progress can provide extrinsic reward. The Personal Trainer's feedback is also an extrinsic reward that can increase levels of client motivation.

Attribution Theory

Attribution theory deals with the human need to explain why things happen in an attempt to gain control or increase predictability. Attribution theory serves as the foundation for our constant search for the causes of success and failure. Humans have a strong need to understand and explain what is going on in their world. Perceptions of causality, rather than reality, are critical because they influence self-confidence, self-control, and self-concept as well as expectations of the future and the motivation to work hard to achieve a goal. Many factors affect a person's level of effort. Perception of causality (or to what we attribute success) is one important stimulant to motivation, which ultimately influences level of effort. Clients will be more successful if they believe success depends more on their effort than on chance. Learned helplessness is the perception that no matter what the person does, he or she will fail.

CONTINUUMS OF CAUSALITY AND ATTRIBUTES OF SUCCESS AND FAILURE

There are **three continuums of causality:** locus of control, stability, and controllability. There are **four factors** to which we attribute success and failure: effort, task difficulty, native ability, and luck. There are **two types of explanations** as to why things happen: external attributions and internal attributions.

Locus of control can be internal (i.e., in my control) or external (i.e., not in my control). Feelings of self-esteem, shame, or guilt are based on one's perception of whether the cause is internal or external.

Stability is defined around expectations of outcomes of behavior. When success is attributed to stable causes, expectations of outcomes of future behaviors are consistent with outcomes from past experiences. Conversely, when success is attributed to unstable causes, no specific outcomes of behaviors are expected.

Controllability is the perception of the degree of influence a person has over a situation. A client will tend to be more focused and put forth more effort if he or she feels a high degree of control. Those who feel they have little or no control are more likely to develop learned helplessness. It is important to remember that specific situations may trigger different feelings or perceptions of causality based on a variety of beliefs, feelings, values, and experiences.

Cultural variances should also be considered. Different cultures attribute success and failure to actors of effort, task difficulty, innate or native ability, and luck. Attribution of these factors may vary for different tasks and in varied situations. Each factor can be applied to the three continuums of causality: locus of control, stability, and controllability. Typically effort and ability are internal factors and task difficulty and luck are external factors.

EXPLANATIONS OF WHY THINGS HAPPEN

People typically offer two types of explanations about why things happen. External attribution assigns causality to an outside agent or force (task difficulty or luck). Clients may blame overeating tendencies on the stress of their working environment or may say they cannot exercise because their spouse and/or children are too demanding of their time. Internal attribution assigns causality to factors within the person. Clients may indicate that they have no willpower and overeat whenever there is an opportunity. They may say that their feelings of guilt for taking time away from their family to exercise prevents them from being physically active.

The following section applies the variables of attribution theory as they interact with each other when combining the *three continuums* of locus, stability, and controllability with the *two types of explanations* and the *four factors of attribution*.

LOCUS OF CONTROL

Clients who attribute success or failure to an internal locus believe that they are responsible for what happens rather than being controlled by outside forces. Internal locus of control is the belief that inborn and learned abilities and effort are the cause of success or failure. The person who believes he or she is in control will feel proactive rather than reactive to the environment. Attribution of success to an internal locus leads to feelings of self-control and improved self-esteem. Attribution of failure to internal locus will result in shame or guilt.

If success or failure were attributable to an external locus of control, there is a perception that outside forces are responsible. The client attributes cause of success and failure to the factors of task difficulty and luck. Attribution of success to external locus leads to feelings of learned helplessness or powerlessness; a belief that one does not have control of what happens, outside factors control outcomes. Attribution of failure to an external locus may help clients believe that tasks are too hard and allow them to give themselves permission to expect less. Attributions of "not me" can be valid, as there are many things in life that are beyond our control. For example:

1. In an athletic contest, the winners explain their victory by their own skill, hard work, and preparation. The losers explain defeat on poor officiating, weather, bad luck, or other external circumstances.
2. Clients wanting to increase flexibility would explain success by their practice of yoga and stretching and would explain failure on the genetic aspects of their body that make it difficult for them to increase flexibility.
3. Personal Trainers explain their success with clients by the application of Personal Trainer knowledge of exercise science and pedagogy and their failure with clients on lack of client effort.

STABILITY

It is common to base expectations of the future on experiences of the past. Ability is often perceived as a stable force. This can lead to challenge in a personal training setting when working with clients who equate physical fitness to success in sport activity and have had unpleasant experiences in the sports arena. A client's perception of ability may make task difficulty a stable force. Clients may believe that because they are not good in sports, physical activity is too difficult for them. Clients may have feelings of being "uncoordinated." They see themselves as non–athletic and not able to succeed in an exercise program. Native or genetic ability is usually the only attribution that cannot be changed. Clients who believe that failure is inevitable may experience learned helplessness and believe there is no point in trying. For example:

1. A client who struggles with weight loss may think, "My mother is fat, my grandmother was fat, and I have always been fat. No matter how hard I try I will never reach an ideal weight and a healthy body composition." (Stable and due to genetics and native ability)
2. A client in a weight management program may get sidetracked because of personal misfortune or a death in the family and think "My efforts were changed when my brother died, I will get back on track." (Unstable due to luck)

CONTROLLABILITY

This aspect of causality is related to the client's feelings of control of the cause that will affect the outcome. The only causal attribution completely under personal control is effort. Only the client can determine how much effort he or she puts into any task. Abilities will improve as effort is applied, but clients do not have control of native ability, task difficulty, or luck.

Most clients will put forth effort if they believe it will directly influence the outcome. If clients believe that strength training will increase lean body mass and increase metabolism, they will be more likely to strength train on a regular basis. Clients who believe that they have a genetic predisposition to a high percentage of body fat and that exercise will do little to change that will be less likely to strength train on a regular basis.

Research completed on subjects believed to be high achievers revealed that successful people exert enormous efforts. Consequently, if personal training clients are to succeed, they must believe that when they expend effort, which is something they completely control, they will experience success. A client who believes that success or failure is the result of luck, native ability, or task difficulty will be less likely to put forth effort. It is perception of causality, not reality, that truly makes the difference. For example:

1. The client thinks, "I will always struggle with weight because of my genetic predisposition to a high percentage of body fat. I will settle for being 20 pounds over my ideal weight." (Not controllable due to genetics and native ability)
2. The client thinks, "If I write down my food intake and focus on smaller serving sizes I will eat less and achieve a negative caloric balance so that I will lose weight." (Controllable due to effort)

IMPLICATIONS OF ATTRIBUTION THEORY ON CLIENTS

Personal Trainers can help clients be more successful by applying attribution theory in their training practice. **Locus** of causality determines the client's belief about what he or she can achieve. If clients believe that personal success will be due in great part to their efforts, they will take pride when they are successful. Personal Trainer feedback to a client must focus on maximal efforts put forth by the client. Personal Trainers should "catch clients doing things right" and continually praise them. Personal Trainers should correct improper exercise or lifestyle choices with immediate and specific feedback.

Stability of causality prompts a client to believe that the future can be changed with effort. Personal Trainers must focus clients on believing that they can be successful if they put forth effort. It is also important to make clients accountable.

Controllability of causality creates the feeling of being commander of one's own fate and is a powerful determiner of emotional health. People who feel that they are controlled by outside forces will experience learned helplessness; the feeling that outcomes are outside their control. Personal Trainers should want clients to accept that much of what happens to their bodies is a result of exercise and positive lifestyle choices. The Personal Trainer should not accept less from clients than they are capable of doing. Feedback should be immediate, specific, precise, and growth oriented and should preserve the dignity of the client.

Transfer Theory

Transfer is the process of applying what is learned in one setting to other similar situations. "Positive transfer" occurs when prior learning experiences assist in the acquisition of new knowledge. For example, clients who have had positive experiences in physical education may be more likely to want to learn more about exercising. "Negative transfer," however, occurs when prior learning experiences interfere with the acquisition of new knowledge. For example, a client who has had negative experiences in physical education may be less interested in exercising and less likely to be physically active. There are four variables that raise the chances of transfer of learning: similarity, association, degree of original learning, and critical attributes.

Similarity of environments and emotions will facilitate transfer. Personal Trainers should want to help the client feel comfortable in the training atmosphere and with the training process. A client who can become comfortable in a gym setting under a Personal Trainer's supervision, will be more likely to exercise independently in similar settings. As well, a client who can become comfortable with certain exercises or with exercise equipment will be more likely to be comfortable as new exercises and/or equipment are introduced in their regimen. Personal Trainers will be most successful when they give verbal and written instruction, refer to diagrams and visual aids to define muscles and movement, and use strong visualization cues to go along with proper kinesthetic experiences. The more modalities used in training, the more effective the training experience will be for the client and the more likely positive transfer will occur.

Association occurs when two different learning experiences are associated with each other. For example, a Personal Trainer may train a client to do an abdominal crunch on a piece of selectorized equipment (sitting upright with resistance applied to the upper torso) and then have the client execute an abdominal crunch lying supine on a mat. Learning the exercise on the machine first may help the client feel the muscles and understand the concept of abdominal contraction. After the client has correctly learned the exercise on a mat, the Personal Trainer can add to this experience by having the client do an abdominal crunch on a stability ball.

Degree of original learning refers to how well information was taught and initially understood. Positive transfer is more likely to occur when original learning was thorough and reinforced. If a client is taught to perform an exercise properly and with appropriate practice, that experience will transfer and facilitate learning of new exercises.

Transfer of learning occurs when past learning has relevance and is applicable to a present situation. Identification of **critical attributes** that signal past learning and help to facilitate new learning can increase the likelihood of positive transfer. Teaching a client to perform a crunch correctly by engaging the rectus abdominus with cues such as "moving the ribs and hips closer together and pulling the navel toward the spine" provides critical attributes that will help the client learn and perform other exercises involving the rectus abdominus.

TIPS FOR POSITIVE TRANSFER

1. **Similarity:** Look for sources of possible similarity between learning situations. For example, a client is trained to use perceived exertion while walking on a treadmill during warm-up activity. The next session the client warms up on a bike using perceived exertion. The Personal Trainer encourages the client to tune into similarities in breathing, heart rate, core temperature, and feelings of muscle exertion while identifying perceived exertion levels.

2. **Association:** Pairing or associating new learning with something the student already knows. For example, a client has learned to correctly perform a modified plank pose to strengthen core muscles. The client is then asked what other exercises can be executed from this position. The client is trained to move into other exercise from this position (a modified push-up or full plank pose would be two associated exercises).

3. **Degree of original learning:** Making sure information is correct and understood before moving on to new information. For example, the client should be able to correctly perform an exercise before adding resistance with free weights or resistance tubing. Checks for understanding through observation and questions will be helpful in facilitating transfer using the variable of degree of original learning. It is also important for a Personal Trainer to know what "old learning" or "old beliefs" may be hindering new learning.

4. **Critical attributes:** Identifying essential and common elements to facilitate learning. For example, after a period of training the client should be able to identify all exercises that engage the oblique muscles by thinking about the critical attributes of where the muscles are, how they feel when engaged, the movement of rotation and flexion, and visualization of the rib coming closer to the opposite hip.

Retention Theory

Learning is the process by which new knowledge and skills are acquired. Memory is the process by which knowledge and skills for the future are retained. Retention refers to the process whereby long-term memory preserves information in such a way that it can locate, identify, and retrieve it for future use. According to Hunter (14), there are five factors that increase retention of information, which constantly operate simultaneously: meaning, degree of original learning, feeling tone, transfer, and practice:

1. **Meaning:** Material will be remembered longer if it is meaningful and if it is related to the learner's own life and experiences.
2. **Degree of original learning** refers to how well something was learned initially. New information should be learned well and reinforced before additional material is introduced. It is important to separate the significant information from the insignificant and concentrate time and effort on the information that matters. The Personal Trainer should expect to be challenged with correcting poorly learned behaviors and misconceptions.
3. **Feeling tone** will affect the learning process and the success of the training experience. We remember best the things that are associated with pleasant feelings.
4. **Transfer** is vital for retention. Positive transfer occurs whenever old learning assists new learning. Negative transfer occurs whenever old learning inhibits new learning.
5. **Practice** is successful if Personal Trainers involve four questions as they plan the practice:
   a. How much should a client learn and experience in one training session?
   b. How long should a client spend on learning an exercise or completing a training session?
   c. How often should a client train with the Personal Trainer?
   d. How will clients know how well they are doing (feedback)?

Goal Theory

Goal theory represents a relatively new concept of human motivation. A goal reflects a purpose and refers to quantity, quality, or rate of performance (2). Goal setting involves establishing a standard or objective to serve as the aim and direction of actions. In the case of personal training, goals should be set by the client and the Personal Trainer based on a thorough assessment of health fitness-related components and a medical/fitness history.

One of the central concepts of goal theory is goal orientation. A client hires a Personal Trainer to achieve personal health- and fitness-related goals. The training goals orient the client and focus attention on achievement of goals. The more intrinsically motivated clients are, the more likely they are to achieve their goals. The client's perception of personal ability to succeed is an important factor that the Personal Trainer must consider. Weight management clients who have lost and gained weight numerous times may feel learned helplessness and, although motivated, will struggle with the belief that they can succeed. Actively involving clients in writing goals, educating in regards to factors that will influence those goals (such as barriers to exercise and sticking to a nutrition plan), continual assessment of progress as related to goals, and encouragement will all play a significant role in perceived progress, leading to gains in achievement and overall success.

CURRICULUM AND INSTRUCTIONAL DESIGN

Curriculum is a systematic plan of instruction (1). Curriculum is what you plan to teach/train and instruction is how you teach the curriculum. A Personal Trainer will use the content of this book along with other resources to plan a training program (curriculum). The curriculum may include a series of strength and flexibility exercises, a variety of aerobic activities, and education about healthy living. The Personal Trainer will use learning theory, brain research, learning styles, effective teaching, and elements of lesson design to determine how he or she will train the client. The instructional design should address four basic questions:

1. Where are we going?
2. How will we get there?

3. How will we know we have arrived?
4. What will we do when we get there?

These questions of instructional design can be used to plan a single training session or a long-term training program. Each training session should have elements of effective lesson design (15).

Elements of Lesson Design

Hunter's research (15) has proved that effective teachers have a methodology to planning and presenting a lesson. She found that no matter what the teacher's style, grade level, or subject matter or the economic background of the students, a properly taught lesson contained eight elements that enhanced and maximized learning:

1. **The anticipatory set** (focus) is a short activity or prompt that focuses the client's attention before the training session begins. The anticipatory set should create a positive feeling tone and may be used to review the last training session or stimulate thinking about the upcoming training session.
2. **Objective or purpose** indicates what the client will accomplish as a result of the training session.
3. **Instructional input** is the verbal instruction the Personal Trainer will provide to the client.
4. **Modeling** involves instruction through demonstration.
5. **Guided practice** involves directing the client through the exercise through verbal and possibly physical commands.
6. **Checking for understanding** involves assessing the client's knowledge through observation and/or direct questioning.
7. **Independent practice** involves Personal Trainer observation without instruction or intervention.
8. **Closure** completes the training session. Closure may include an overview of the session along with a preview of what to expect at the next session.

PRINCIPLES OF EFFECTIVE INSTRUCTION/TRAINING

Hunter (16) outlines three basic instructional principles that will help Personal Trainers communicate verbal and written information more effectively:

1. **Determine basic information and organize it.** One must determine which information is essential to the client's understanding and then separate that information from more advanced information that can be presented later. The basic information must be organized so that it serves as a foundation for the more advanced information to follow. Organization of information facilitates understanding and retention.
2. **Present basic information in the simplest and clearest form.** Once information is organized, the Personal Trainer must present that information in a simple, clear, and understandable manner. The Personal Trainer should choose words that the client will understand and give clear examples whenever possible. Presenting material through the visual, auditory, and kinesthetic modalities will also help to facilitate clarity.
3. **Model the information or exercise.** Personal Trainers should model through demonstration. Whenever possible, a Personal Trainer should reinforce correct body alignment using visualization and physical manipulation.

LEARNING STYLES

There are a multitude of theories regarding learning styles. Styles are preferences that clients have that cause them to behave in predictable ways. Styles are all built on two major dimensions (17):

1. The manner in which clients take in, or perceive, stimuli (information)
2. The manner in which clients process, order, or make decisions about using stimuli (information)

Learning styles refer to individual differences in the way information is perceived, processed, and communicated. The most traditional way of defining learning styles is by the sensory channels or modalities through which we prefer to learn (i.e., visual, auditory, and/or tactile–kinesthetic). Most people use all modalities in learning but have a stronger preference or orientation to one or another.

Visual learners prefer demonstrations, diagrams, slides, posters, and specific written information. The visual learner tends to become distracted with verbal instruction as well as a disorganized environment.

Auditory learners prefer verbal instruction. They will be comfortable listening and talking and will tend to engage easily in conversation. The auditory learner may be distracted with a great deal of background noise in a learning environment.

Tactile–kinesthetic learners prefer being physically engaged in the learning process. The tactile learner may want to skip directions and begin an activity trying to "figure things out along the way." Tactile learners will prefer to write things down themselves and will remember best when they are documenting their own goals and progress. They will be somewhat distracted with a great deal of activity around them.

Internet Learning Style Inventories

There are a variety of learning style inventories available on the Internet. These inventories consist of simple checklists that can be easily administered and scored to assess the client's preferred style(s) of learning:

➤ http://www.engr.ncsu.edu/learningstyles/ilsweb.html
➤ Multiple Intelligence Inventory (http://www.ldrc.ca/projects/miinventory/miinventory.php)

Gardner's Multiple Intelligences (18)

Instead of viewing "smartness" in terms of scores on standardized tests, Gardner (18) defined intelligence as:

➤ The ability to solve problems that one encounters in real life
➤ The ability to generate new problems to solve
➤ The ability to make something or offer a service that is valued within one's culture

Gardner's *Frames of Mind* presents a theory of multiple intelligences (18). These intelligences are the tools we use for learning, problem solving, and creating throughout life. Knowledge of these intelligences may provide a better understanding of how a client thinks and learns, ultimately giving the Personal Trainer direction in structuring successful training programs.

Bodily–kinesthetic intelligence is evident in athletes, dancers, surgeons, and craftspeople. Individuals with high bodily–kinesthetic intelligence will acquire physical skills and movement patterns more easily and rapidly than those with lower kinesthetic intelligence.

Linguistic intelligence is the ability to think in words and to use language to express and appreciate complex meaning. Authors, journalists, poets, speakers, and newscasters often exhibit high degrees of linguistic intelligence. A client with high linguistic intelligence will appreciate and respond to verbal and written information.

Logical–mathematical intelligence is the ability to carry out complex mathematical operations. Those with high logical–mathematical intelligence have an ability to calculate, quantify, and consider propositions and hypotheses. Accountants, engineers, computer programmers, and scientists often demonstrate this dimension of intelligence. The logical–mathematical client will appreciate and respond to education detailing status, progress, and planning in quantifiable terms.

Interpersonal intelligence is the capacity to understand and interact effectively with others. Successful teachers, Personal Trainers, social workers, actors, and politicians will often demonstrate high interpersonal intelligence. People with high interpersonal intelligence also have high emotional intelligence, which allows them to understand the needs, feelings, and concerns of others. These skills are helpful in developing and influencing others, effectively leading, managing conflict, fostering teamwork, and collaborating to facilitate change. Successful Personal Trainers will typically have high interpersonal intelligence. Clients with high interpersonal intelligence will enjoy the process of personal training and be interested in building a relationship with the Personal Trainer.

Intrapersonal intelligence is the ability to construct an accurate perception of oneself. The emotional intelligence skills of self-awareness and self-regulation are closely aligned with this dimension of intelligence. Individuals with high intrapersonal intelligence are able to self-assess, are emotionally self-aware, and have high self-confidence. They understand personal strengths and weaknesses, are able to manage their lives effectively, and are able to adapt and be flexible to change. Achievement drive, initiative, and high levels of optimism are also characteristic of those with intrapersonal intelligence and high emotional intelligence. Psychologists, philosophers, and theologians are often individuals who demonstrate strong intrapersonal intelligence. Clients with high intrapersonal intelligence will usually be committed to their training goals and will work hard to achieve them. They will want to know what they can do personally to make the process of training more efficient and effective.

Musical intelligence is most evident in composers, conductors, musicians, music critics, and instrument makers. These individuals possess sensitivity to pitch, melody, rhythm, and tone. Providing music (with sensitivity to genre preferences) during a training session may positively influence and inspire a client with strong musical intelligence.

Naturalist intelligence is evident in farmers, botanists, hunters, ecologists, and landscapers. Naturalist intelligence consists of observing patterns in nature, understanding natural and man-made systems, as well as classifying objects. The naturalistic client will be most interested in the movement and the sequence of the activity in the training session.

Spatial intelligence is the capacity to think in three-dimensional ways and allows one to perceive external and internal imagery and to produce or decode graphic information. This dimension of intelligence involves sensitivity to color, line, shape, form, space, and the relationship between these elements. Pilots, sculptors, painters, architects, and artists typically have a great deal of spatial intelligence. This client may focus on physical attributes (body shape, size, proportion, and symmetry) as well as the physical environment of the training facilities.

BRAIN RESEARCH AND THE PERSONAL TRAINING CLIENT

The Brain and How It Learns

The 1990s are known as the decade of the brain, as more brain research was done in those 10 years than in the entire century before 1990. Brain research continues to improve our understanding of how learning occurs and is of great significance for the Personal Trainer.

Human beings perceive information through personal experiences, beliefs, and theories. If experiences and beliefs change, perceptions of information will also change. The human mind is structured to make sense of the data it perceives. Personal Trainers who apply learning theory and brain research can more effectively facilitate learning and create perceptions necessary for success.

About the Brain

The brain weighs a little over three pounds (1.4 kg) and is about the size of a small grapefruit that could fit in the palm of the hand. If you put your fists together, extend your thumbs and tip your hands inward, you have an approximation of the brain's size and position in the skull. The brain is always functioning, even when we are sleeping. According to Caine and Caine (19), the brain represents only 2% of our body weight, but it consumes 20% of our calories and uses one-fifth of the body's oxygen. The more we think, the more calories we burn.

The brain is thought to be "plastic" (continually changing) as we store learning and life experiences. The brain is sometimes compared with an overgrown jungle of 100 billion nerve cells, or neurons, which begin as round cell bodies that grow processes called axons and dendrites. Dendrites are the main way neurons get information. The more we use certain information the more dendrites connect to the neurons housing that information. The less we use certain information the fewer dendrites we have to the neurons housing the information. If we learn a skill and do not use it, the neurons will still house the information but most of the dendrites used to access the information will shrivel up and disappear. The information is still there but we need to find it and use it so we can quickly reconnect for easier access in the future.

The Grass Theory

The brain is somewhat like a computer (but with limitless memory). The neurons are like the computer files where we store information. If we do not use information for a long period of time we forget where it is stored. Once we find and use the information it becomes easier to access. Some scientists refer to that process as the "grass theory." If there is a large patch of tall green grass separating you from your destination and there is no defined route to take you there, it may take some time to find that place. After traveling across the patch of grass following the same path you will create a dirt pathway as you wear the grass down. This will result in easy access to your destination. If you learn a new movement it may feel uncomfortable at first, but after repeated practice you no longer have to think about what to do and how to do it. You have developed muscle memory (engrams), a pathway within your brain and from your brain to the muscle. We learn (20):

➤ 10% of what we read
➤ 20% of what we hear
➤ 30% of what we see
➤ 50% of what we see and hear
➤ 70% of what we discuss with others
➤ 80% of what we experience personally
➤ 95% of what we teach

IMPLICATIONS

The more senses we use in the learning environment, the higher the probability it will be remembered. According to Jensen (21), 99% of all sensory information is disregarded when it enters the brain. Personal Trainers using verbal, auditory, visual, and kinesthetic cues will observe better retention from their clients. Having the client demonstrate/recite what they have learned should also enhance the learning process and increase the likelihood of greater retention.

Primacy–Recency Theory

According to primacy-recency theory, individuals are likely to best retain information presented first in a learning session, followed by what is presented last, followed by what is presented within the lesson. Clients are most alert and ready to learn in the first 15 to 20 minutes of a presentation/session, after which there is a 5- to 10-minute recovery phase, which prepares the learner for increased attention and readiness to learn in the following 15 to 20 minutes. This phenomenon, also called "beginning–middle–end," emphasizes the importance of presenting key information at the beginning of each session. Additionally, learning will be more likely if the presenter focuses on a few key concepts and continues to reinforce.

IMPLICATIONS

When working with clients, the Personal Trainer should present what he or she most wants them to remember at the beginning of the session and at the end of the session. To capitalize on learning, Personal Trainers should tell clients what they are going to tell them during the session as an anticipatory set (introduction) and then provide that information throughout the training.

Mood and Learning

There is a growing body of knowledge supporting the belief that a leader's moods and behaviors influence the moods and behaviors of the clients. Emotions and moods are an open-loop system (11) feeding off the environment. Personal Trainers should appreciate the influence they have to promote an environment that motivates and energizes others.

IMPLICATIONS

Personal Trainers need to be positive throughout the training period. Clients that bring past negative experiences to the training may have to unlearn some negative self-talk. For example, a client who struggled with sport activities and was the one "nobody wanted on the team at recess" may have a fear of failure regarding physical activity in general.

SUMMARY

Effective teaching leads to a successful personal training business. Clients who succeed at reaching personal goals will tell others about their success. These clients will also perform better and most often look better. Successful clients are a walking and talking commercial for a Personal Trainer. A Personal Trainer is a teacher with the responsibility of helping clients to learn and to behave in different ways. Personal Trainers who apply a solid foundation of personal training and pedagogical skills based on ACSM guidelines can effectively lead clients through the change process to reach their goals.

REFERENCES

1. Moore K. Classroom Teaching Skills. 4th ed. Boston: McGraw-Hill, 1998.
2. Schunk D. Learning Theories. 4th ed. Columbus, OH: Pearson/Merrill Prentice Hall, 2004.
3. McCombs BL. Learner-centered Psychological Principles: Guidelines for School Redesign and Reform. Washington, DC: American Psychological Association, 1992.
4. Danielson C. Enhancing Professional Practice. Alexandria, VA: Association for Supervision and Curriculum Development, 1996.
5. Prochaska JO. How do people change, and how can we change to help many more people? In: Hubble MA, Duncan BL, Miller SD, eds. The Heart and Soul of Change: What Works in Therapy. Washington, DC: American Psychological Association, 1999:227–258.
6. Covey S. The Seven Habits of Highly Effective People. 1st ed. New York: Simon & Schuster, 1990.
7. Seligman M. Learned Optimism. 1st ed. New York: Pocket Books, 1990.
8. Cruickshank D, Jenkins DB, Metcalf K. The Act of Teaching. 3rd ed. Boston: McGraw-Hill, 2003.
9. Barr AS. Characteristics of Successful Teachers. Bloomington, IN: Phi Delta Kappa, 1958.
10. Salovey P, Mayer J. Emotional intelligence. Imagin Cogn Pers 1990;9(3):185–211.
11. Goleman D. Emotional Intelligence. New York: Bantam Books, 1995.
12. Goleman D. Working with Emotional Intelligence. New York: Bantam Books, 1998.
13. Sala F. Emotional Competence Inventory (ECI) Technical Manual. Boston: Hay/McBer, 2002.
14. Hunter M. Teach More, Faster! Thousand Oaks, CA: Corwin, 1967.
15. Hunter M. Mastery Teaching: Increasing Instructional Effectiveness in Elementary and Secondary Schools, Colleges, and Universities. Thousand Oaks, CA: Corwin Press, 1982.
16. Hunter R. Madeline Hunter's Mastery Teaching. Thousand Oaks, CA: Corwin Press, 2004.
17. Feden R, Vogel R. Methods of Teaching. Boston: McGraw-Hill, 2003.
18. Gardner H. Frames of Mind: The Theory of Multiple Intelligences. New York: Basic Books, 1983.
19. Caine R, Caine G. Making Connections: Teaching and the Human Brain. Alexandria, VA: Association for Supervision and Curriculum Development, 1991.
20. Glasser W. Schools without Failure. New York: Harper & Row, 1975.
21. Jensen E. Brain-based Learning. San Diego, CA: The Brain Store, 2000.

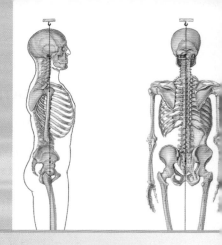

CHAPTER

10 Exercise Psychology, Motivation, and Behavior Change

Margaret Moore, B.S., M.B.A., Founder & CEO, Wellcoaches Corporation, Wellesley, Massachusetts

Frank Claps, M.Ed., Owner/Operator, Fitness For Any Body, Springfield Township, Bucks County, Pennsylvania

Gabrielle R. Highstein, RN, Ph.D., Instructor in Medicine, Washington University School of Medicine, Division of Health Behavior Research, St. Louis, Missouri

Kate Larsen, PCC, President, Certified Coach, Lifestyle Expert, Winning LifeStyles, Inc., Minneapolis, Minnesota

Lisa Todd Graddy, M.S.W., M.S., Licensed Mental Health Therapist, LCSW, Licensed Wellness Coach, Midway, Kentucky

Theresa J. Lavin, B.S., M.B.A., Licensed Wellness Coach, MGH Institute of Health Professions, Boston, Massachusetts

Chapter Outline

Objectives

- Define the Personal Trainer's role in the client's behavioral change process
- Introduce principles of behavior change theory that Personal Trainers can use to help clients master change
- Learn how the Personal Trainer–client relationship supports the change process and what elements are needed for an effective relationship
- Provide guidelines for helping clients develop fitness visions as a higher purpose for change as well as identifying and connecting to intrinsic motivators to change
- Learn how to help clients set behavioral goals that support behavioral change
- Offer a wide variety of approaches to helping clients overcome their obstacles along the path of change

PERSONAL TRAINER'S ROLE IN FACILITATING CLIENT CHANGE

Personal Trainers Help Clients Change

As a Personal Trainer, you are dedicated to your client's fitness success, combining a number of different roles: teacher and cheerleader, sometimes a sounding board, often a mentor, and, at times a challenger. Your clients come to you because they want your personal attention, knowledge, guidance, and accountability to help them safely and efficiently reach their fitness goals.

Helping clients establish fit lifestyles is really all about helping clients **change behaviors** and reach the stage wherein they are confident they can sustain fit lifestyles. Change is a challenging process, and it rarely proceeds swiftly and in a straight line to reach mastery of the change. Better understanding of the behavioral change process gives Personal Trainers approaches to help clients find and sustain their motivation, overcome their obstacles, and master their new fitness behaviors.

Clients Decide to Change

It is important to recognize that the **decision to change and the responsibility to change rests only with our clients.** Behavioral change is self-change. Our role as Personal Trainers is to facilitate and improve the success rate of the change process. Fortunately, the training relationship plays an important role in facilitating change, and the better the relationship, the higher the success rate.

The Personal Trainer–Client Relationship Is a Partnership

The Personal Trainer–client relationship is unique because the total focus is on *what your clients want to achieve* and how you can *help them* to reach their goals. While the bottom-line intention of personal training is to improve the client's health, fitness, and well-being, skilled Personal Trainers will also help their clients address the other aspects of their lives that are interfering with their ability to develop and maintain a fit lifestyle.

The relationship between Personal Trainer and client is a partnership to help clients go from where they are to where they want to be. It offers *a profound level of support and encouragement.* Your clients come to you because they want the benefits of regular exercise. To clients, having a Personal Trainer means employing a skilled professional who will help them find their way and stay on course. And, as you get to know your clients better and become more familiar with their strengths and weaknesses, their sources of pride, and their acts of self-sabotage, your ability to effect change increases:

Accountability

Personal training is very powerful because it provides a built-in structure of accountability. When people *share commitments to a plan and goals with someone they respect and who believes in them*, they are more *motivated* to keep those commitments. Accountability is extremely important in a Personal

Trainer–client relationship. To be effective, the accountability you establish must be free of judgment. It should encourage action and learning without placing blame or making clients feel shameful. Every challenge should be viewed as a learning opportunity, rather than as a failure.

As a Personal Trainer, your role in providing accountability is to:

➤ Guide and mentor your clients
➤ Focus on your clients' priorities and issues, building on their dreams and purpose
➤ Help your clients formulate short- and long-term plans
➤ Help turn goals into achievable action plans
➤ Listen and guide without judgment
➤ Hold your clients accountable for what they committed to do
➤ Ask probing questions so you can help clients understand themselves better
➤ Help your clients reach the stage wherein they can sustain a fit lifestyle and their new behaviors without you.

You help your clients master change by:

➤ Helping clients understand their readiness to change
➤ Encouraging realistic expectations and goals
➤ Helping your clients to recognize that changing behaviors is a process and that progress will come one step at a time
➤ Addressing all aspects of fitness
➤ Identifying solutions tailored to your clients' needs and wants
➤ Preparing your clients to take action, stay focused, and stay on track
➤ Offering honest input and feedback without criticism
➤ Guiding your clients on the road from "where they are" to "where they want to be"
➤ Celebrating your clients' small and large achievements to build positive momentum

THEORIES OF BEHAVIOR CHANGE

Identifying Stages of Readiness to Change

Prochaska and his team of researchers at the Cancer Prevention Research Center at the University of Rhode Island (1) developed the Transtheoretical Model of Behavior Change. It is presently the most widely used theoretical model of behavioral psychology in the fields of health and fitness. It grew out of Dr. Prochaska's frustration of trying to work with psychotherapy patients who were not yet ready to change their problem behaviors. Dr. Prochaska saw the need to recognize a patient's stage of readiness to change a behavior and to discover what processes of change worked best with people in different stages of change.

Personal Trainers can easily recognize this same type of frustration when they try to work with clients who have seemingly lost their interest, focus, and dedication to exercising and training. Many Personal Trainers make the mistake of taking it personally when their clients are no longer succeeding. This can lead to dissatisfaction for both the Personal Trainer and the client, who is probably feeling guilty at not meeting the Personal Trainer's expectations. In fact, the responsibility to change and stay on track remains with your clients. Personal Trainers cannot change clients. Clients change themselves. We can, however, teach clients about the change process and help them find ways to get back on track.

There are many possible explanations for why a client may have lapsed out of one stage into an earlier stage. A Personal Trainer needs to remember to always ask at every interaction about a client's present ability to dedicate themselves to the training program goals. In a long-term relationship, there are going to be times of dedication and times when the client is distracted from his or her training goals by other events of life. The Personal Trainer must recognize that change isn't often a straightforward process and *accept the person as he or she is at this moment.*

What Stage Is My Client in Today?

After more than 10 years of research, the stages of readiness to change were defined as (1):

➤ Precontemplation (PC) in which no change is being thought of:
  • Precontemplation can have two variants:
    • Precontemplation nonbelievers (PCNs): Those who are not thinking about doing the behavior because they do not believe that the behavior is important for them to do
    • Precontemplation believers (PCBs): Those who believe the behavior to be important but are too bogged down to even be able to think about doing the behavior now
➤ Contemplation (C), in which change is being thought about sometime in the next 6 months
➤ Preparation (P), in which change is being planned within the next 30 days and some type of approximate behavior is being attempted
➤ Action (A), in which the behavior that produces positive outcomes has been started within the last 6 months
➤ Maintenance (M), in which the behavior that produces positive outcomes has been being done for at least 6 months

Specific Behaviors and Stages of Change

Stage of change is a concept used with a specific behavior or a series of behaviors. For example, you cannot stage a person's readiness to manage his or her diabetes in general, but you can stage readiness to do a specific behavior, such as taking diabetes medications as prescribed or measuring blood sugar daily or having their eyes checked once a year. Patients can be in different stages for each of these behaviors. They could be in *I can't* for taking medications as prescribed, *I will* for measuring blood sugar daily, and *I still am* for having their eyes checked once a year.

For general wellness, we often stress regular exercise, good nutrition, and stress reduction. Regular exercise may be further subdivided into aerobic exercise, strength training, and flexibility. Good nutrition could be thought of as lowering fat, increasing fiber and water, or eating five servings of fruits and vegetables a day. Stress reduction could include deep breathing or progressive muscle relaxation. Clients can be in different stages of readiness for each of the specific behaviors they are attempting to change. *As a Personal Trainer you need to pay attention to readiness for each behavior.*

One of the first steps in translating this model from the research domain into the fitness arena was to put the psychological terms in more everyday language so that coach and client could more easily understand the concepts. The second step involves integrating the concepts of the model into training sessions. It is important that the Personal Trainer and client have a consensus on the stage of readiness for each fitness behavior (e.g., aerobic activity, strength training, flexibility). In each training session, it is a good idea to establish whether there has been any alteration in readiness for each type of behavior. Using the example shown in Figure 10.1 to create something similar may be helpful.

Strategies of Behavior Change

For each of the different behaviors that your client wants to work on, a different set of strategies matched to the client's present stage of readiness should be used. These strategies include:

➤ Decisional balance (2) (pros and cons of doing the behavior)
➤ Self-efficacy (3) (confidence in the face of challenging situations)
➤ Ten processes of change (1) (five cognitive/affective and five behavioral strategies)

Stage of readiness	Aerobic	Strength	Flexibility	Balance
PCN = I won't				
PCB = I can't				
C = I may				
P = I will				
A = I am				
M = I still am				

FIGURE 10.1. Sample readiness summary.

Decisional Balance (Weighing the PROS and CONS)

Decisional balance defines both the pros and cons of a behavior. The pros include benefits for one-self and for others, as well as self-approval and the approval of others. The cons include the costs for oneself and for others, as well as self-disapproval and the disapproval of others. *The bottom line is that for every client, the pros must outweigh the cons to start working on a specific fitness behavior and to stay on track to reach the maintenance stage.*

The pros function as a client's prime motivator and reason he or she is willing to make an effort to change. Clients need to think they are going to get something they **value** from making the effort to change the fitness behavior. The cons or barriers, on the other hand, need to be approached with openness, honesty, and no judgment. One sign of a good Personal Trainer–client relationship is that clients are comfortable in discussing and resolving their obstacles with a Personal Trainer. A Personal Trainer can help clients sort out which of their cons are real, which are excuses, and which can be overcome by a strong enough pro.

Fortunately, exercise science has tested and proved that there are many benefits or pros for regular exercise and for each type of exercise. However, each client will value different benefits, and you should not assume what they are! Sometimes clients have one single pro that is unique and very important to them that is all that they need to motivate them to exercise regularly. *Personal Trainers can provide clients with a list of proven benefits or pros of regular aerobic, strength-training, and flexibility exercise and ask clients to identify those that they value most.*

As an example, a client might personally prove to herself that if she exercises in the morning, she sleeps easily and well that night, and if she does not exercise, she does not sleep well or eas-ily. For this client, this is the single important pro that keeps her getting up at 5:00 AM every morning to work out. Even the con of getting up that early, especially in the cold and dark of the winter, has been outweighed by the payoff of a good night's sleep. Another useful exercise for clients, particularly for those whose commitment to change is wobbly, is to ask your clients to make a list of their pros and cons and determine whether the pros for change outweigh the cons for change *(Fig. 10.2)*.

Self-Efficacy (Confidence in Challenging Situations)

Within the transtheoretical model, self-efficacy is best described as confidence to do a specific be-havior in the face of challenging situations. Common challenging situations often include negative emotional situations (e.g., when angry, tired, or depressed), positive social situations (e.g., at parties

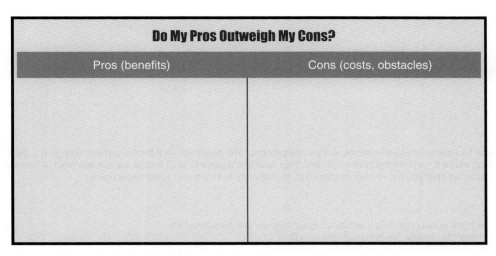

Do My Pros Outweigh My Cons?

Pros (benefits)	Cons (costs, obstacles)

FIGURE 10.2. Behavior: Aerobic workout three times per week at moderate intensity for 20 minutes.

with friends or family celebrations), and situations that disrupt a pattern (e.g., on vacations or when traveling). A Personal Trainer can help clients analyze the situations that trip them up:

➤ Who were you with?
➤ When did it happen?
➤ What were you feeling?
➤ What do you want to do about this situation?
➤ What could you do differently next time?

Once clients have thought what they could have done differently, you can help them develop a relapse prevention plan to be ready for the next time, which will inevitably come. *Not only do your clients need to identify pros they value and have their pros outweigh their cons, they also need workable strategies to overcome their cons.*

Figure 10.3 is a sample client handout called "Am I Ready to Change?" that you can provide to clients to help them understand the change process and to determine their readiness to change.

Cognitive (Thinking) or Affective (Feeling) Processes That Support Change

The five cognitive and affective processes of change include:

1. Consciousness raising (getting information)
2. Dramatic relief (being moved emotionally)
3. Self re-evaluation (self image)
4. Environmental re-evaluation (role modeling)
5. Social liberation (social norms)

These processes are of more use to people who have not yet begun to change (I won't, I can't, I may, and I will).

Getting Information. Getting information is necessary but not sufficient to induce behavioral change. For example, clear, scientific information about the positive effects of careful management of a health risk such as high blood pressure can constitute a good enough reason for someone to make the effort to adopt regular exercise. Another example may be a solid grasp of energy balance (e.g., calculating energy intake by daily calorie counting and approximating energy expenditure by logging minutes of daily exercise), which can motivate a client to successfully lose weight. A third

Am I ready to change?

— Research has shown that self-change is a staged process. We move from not thinking about changing a behavior, to thinking about it, to planning to change, and then testing out ways to do it before we actually start. A number of techniques can help you move from not thinking, to planning, to doing and to continue doing.

— When we think about changing a behavior, questions we ask ourselves are:
Why do I want to change the behavior (the *pros*)?
Why shouldn't I try to change this behavior (the *cons*)?
What would it take for me to overcome my cons and change the behavior (what's my strategy)?

— To move forward, we need to have our *pros* outweigh our *cons* and develop realistic strategies to overcome our *cons*.

— Behavioral scientists recognize 5 stages of readiness to change behavior:

- **Precontemplation:** I won't or I can't in the next 6 months

- **Contemplation:** I may in the next 6 months

- **Preparation:** I will in the next month

- **Action:** I'm doing it now

- **Maintenance:** I've been doing it for at least 6 months

— We want to help you determine how ready you are to change a behavior, so that we can best help you make that change. To help you understand your stage of readiness, we ask that you complete the short quiz below.

— Your Personal Trainer will discuss your answers with you, and make suggestions to help you move through the stages of change and reach your goals.

- The goal or behavior I want to work on first is:

- My reasons for wanting to accomplish this goal (same as change this behavior) are:

- The obstacles standing in the way of my changing this behavior are:

- My strategies to overcome my main obstacles are:

- The efforts I made toward changing this behavior in the last week are:

- My goal for next week with respect to this behavior is:

- My readiness to change this behavior is (write yes beside the level that best describes where you are):

| • I won't do it | • I can't do it | • I may do it | • I will do it | • I am doing it | • I am still doing it |

FIGURE 10.3. Client handout.

example may be teaching a client about the psychological benefits of exercise, including better mental clarity, more energy, and reduced stress, which can support the client's desire to change.

Being Moved Emotionally. This is a process that a Personal Trainer cannot typically deliver, but when it happens, it presents a great opportunity to support change. Many people had a strong emotional reaction to the movie "Super Size Me" (www.supersizeme.com). The extremely negative consequences to Morgan Spurlock from only eating at McDonald's for 30 days were shocking. The results of his liver function tests were extremely sobering; perhaps even enough to promote initiating immediate change in eating habits.

Self Image. A positive self-image that is aligned with the desired new behavior is essential. For example, the chance of getting someone who really believes that he or she is a "couch potato" to start to exercise is nil. This inconsistent self-image must be confronted for change to begin.

Role Modeling. This process touches on the fact that we care about how we are perceived by those around us, especially those who are important to us. For example, we want our children to be healthy so we make the effort to role model health behaviors even when we might not do it if no one was looking. Sometimes parents give up smoking only because they do not want their children to start smoking.

Social Norms. A support group like Weight Watchers best illustrates this process. In a support group, people who are all trying to start the same good health habit come together to meet. They not only share stories and strategies, but they also establish group norms and expectations. It can be tremendously helpful to interact with a group of like-minded people on a regular basis when you are trying to make a health behavior change.

Behavioral Processes That Support Change

The five behavioral processes include:

1. Self-liberation (making a commitment)
2. Stimulus control (reminders/cues)
3. Reinforcement management (rewards)
4. Helping relationship (social support)
5. Counterconditioning (substitution)

These processes are more useful when a person is in the stages of I will, I am, and I still am and is actively struggling with doing a new healthy behavior.

Making a Commitment. This is a valuable process for those in Preparation or I will. It entails making a formal commitment, perhaps having your clients write down exactly what they are going to do and when they will do it.

Cues. If your client makes a written commitment, it can be printed and posted in obvious places to serve as a reminder or cue to do the new healthy behavior. There is nothing sadder than to end the day having forgotten to do what one has made a commitment to do. Notes, beepers, alarm watches, and visual reminders such as a bag of workout clothes in the car can all function as cues to remind your client to exercise.

Rewards. This process points out the desirability of at least initially pairing the new healthy activity with something your client already enjoys and considers a pleasure or reward to do. If your client loves to "catch up on all the news" with her best friend, then she could schedule an exercise session at the local mall with her friend for a power walk with talk. Or your client could decide on a reward, including a "fun" outing or a spa activity, when he or she has accomplished something such as 4 weeks of regular exercise.

Social Support. This process is important at all stages of change. It represents all the help clients can get from both family and friends. Knowing that a friend is waiting for them to walk together will get them out the door when it is cold and they do not really feel like going. Changing eating habits can be much easier if the whole family is willing to cooperate. This process can also include clients protecting themselves from sabotage by family or friends who are threatened by the new healthier behavior and try to make doing the behavior difficult for them. Your possible advice to clients who feel they are being sabotaged is to suggest that they directly address the sabotaging person, point out in a relaxed, calm tone that his or her behavior is making things more difficult, and ask for his or her help to make things easier.

Substitution. This last process encourages people to substitute a new healthier activity for an old less healthy one. It can be called the "instead of" process. In the dietary area there are many low-fat or low-carbohydrate products that people can use instead of higher fat or higher carbohydrate items. In the exercise area, clients can think about taking the stairs instead of the elevator or biking to work instead of driving.

Applying the Theories of Behavior Change

As discussed earlier, Personal Trainers should understand that clients can be in different stages of readiness for each of the behaviors on which they are interested in working. Clients can also change the stage they are in quite rapidly. They can make progress or they can relapse back to an earlier stage. You must recognize the stage clients are presently in because as a Personal Trainer you are going to use strategies that are appropriate to their present stage of readiness for a particular behavior. **Decisional balance and the cognitive processes** are the most useful tools to use with people who have not yet started a behavior (i.e., I won't, I can't, I may, and I will). **Self-efficacy and the behavioral processes** are the most useful tools for those who have begun to change (i.e., I will, I am, and I still am).

Preparation (I will) is the stage that many people think they are in when they approach a Personal Trainer. Clients in Preparation have a need to both think and feel as well as experiment with doing the behavior. Potentially all of the cognitive and behavioral strategies could be appropriate.

By paying close attention to what your client says, you will know what stage your client is in and therefore what strategies will be most effective to move them into Action and Maintenance. If you use the wrong strategy, you run the risk of having your client disengage from the change process. When you push someone who is no longer on track, you risk imposing enough guilt that they will try to avoid contact with you. **All behavior change is self-change.** You must understand and respect what stage of readiness your clients are in and then use the right strategy to help keep them moving forward into Action and Maintenance. Figure 10.4 lists some behavioral change tips.

BUILDING A PERSONAL TRAINER–CLIENT RELATIONSHIP THAT FACILITATES CHANGE

Getting Started

With all the books, magazines, and Internet workouts available these days, why do you think clients hire a Personal Trainer to help them devise and maintain an exercise program? Well, chances are they've tried the other methods without success. And that's why they sought a Personal Trainer's "personal touch" as sometimes their last hope to make the changes necessary to establish a healthy lifestyle. And that's why the relationship a Personal Trainer builds will be as important as the workouts he or she prescribes to help these people avoid past failures and turn their lives around.

Building a relationship means building rapport. Rapport is the positive relationship between the Personal Trainer and client that facilitates change. Rapport is built on trust and mutual respect. Personal Trainers build rapport by:

➤ Being a partner in the client's change process
➤ Establishing credibility
➤ Being conscientious about confidentiality

Early stage behaviors: I won't, I can't, I will

Remember behavior change formula: To be ready to change, my pros must outweigh my cons, and I must have workable strategies to overcome my cons.

- Find valuable *pros*
- Share list of proven benefits
- Challenge clients to test and prove to themselves that a pro pays off for them

- Examine *cons*
- Which cons are real
- Which cons can be worked around

- Process exercise
- Talk about these strategies:

- Getting information
- Being moved emotionally
- Self image
- Being a role model
- Social norms

Later stage behaviors: I will, I am, and I still am

- Discover challenging situations
- Dialog about what situations could be problematic when they actually start the behavior
- Have person come up with strategies to cope before the situation actually arises

- Process exercise
- Talk about these strategies:

- Making a commitment
- Using cues
- Rewards
- Social support
- Substitution

FIGURE 10.4. Behavior tip sheet.

➤ Showing they care

➤ Being a good listener, allowing silence to help the client go deeper

➤ Asking powerful questions

➤ Communicating sincere empathy for clients' situations

➤ Offering genuine respect no matter how clumsy or out of shape the client may be

➤ Demonstrating that they accept clients "as they are"—without judgmental attitudes, impressions, or opinions

➤ Demonstrating that they understand

➤ Showing genuine interest in the client's life by asking questions—do not make assumptions

➤ Providing open and honest feedback

➤ Asking for open and honest feedback

➤ Engaging clients fully in planning and decision making

➤ Trusting that the client may know better what he or she needs than the Personal Trainer does

➤ Trusting one's intuition that is based on experience

As a Personal Trainer, your most important role is that of your client's partner in his or her change process toward a fit lifestyle. Building a partnership depends upon an excellent relationship that in turn depends on mastery of all of the following elements of a Personal Trainer–client relationship. *Personal Trainers form partnerships with their clients to help them move from where they are today to where they want to go. A powerful, effective Personal Trainer helps clients transform their lives and lifestyle choices.*

Establish Your Credibility

It is important to establish credibility with your clients at the beginning and during your training program. You can prepare a one-page biography and practice a 30-second, informal description of your education, experience, reasons for becoming a Personal Trainer, and commitment to helping your clients reach their best-ever level of fitness. If you have one, include a success story you can tell them about how you have helped a previous client in similar circumstances. If any confidential information or real names are used, be sure to get prior approval from your previous client before sharing his or her story. Sharing your passion and vision for yourself and your clients is encouraged.

Confidentiality

The training relationship is built on a foundation of confidentiality. Your clients' personal disclosure and discovery is the material with which you and your clients work. Some clients may initially be intimidated or uncomfortable about personal disclosure. You need to create a safe place by establishing a pattern of curiosity, non-judgment, encouragement, and continual acknowledgment and praise of your clients' honesty, effort, and progress.

Your clients may not feel comfortable talking to you in a crowded gym—especially if they feel out of place because of age or physical appearance. So you may need to find a quiet corner somewhere. Keep in mind, when in open areas of the gym or facility, even if the client is open about sharing, you need to keep your voice down and maintain a confidential nature to your conversation.

It is important that you encourage your clients to share the truth with you, because there is no consequence to truth sharing other than your clients' growth and learning. In the same respect, let your clients know that you will share the truth with them as well, by stating honestly what you see in them. By being honest and forthcoming, you are not judging your clients; you are, rather, helping them see themselves in a mirror. This process makes for an authentic and meaningful relationship.

One way to put a glitch in your relationship is to discuss other clients with your current client. Such disclosures may make your clients wonder what you say about them outside of their workouts and compromise their willingness to share important information with you.

Trust

Your clients' trust in you begins when they feel safe and confident that they can confide in you. The trust grows as you prove yourself trustworthy: delivering what you promise, being on time for sessions, and following through with all commitments you made to them.

Over time your clients will trust that you are on their side, believe in them, and are willing to be firm, honest, and direct for their own well-being. Trust is an empowering feeling for your clients and helps them to feel comfortable with making positive changes. *Trust can be defined as the willingness of your clients to be vulnerable based on their confidence in your benevolence, honesty, openness, reliability, and competence as a Personal Trainer.*

Being on Time

First of all, Personal Trainers earn their clients' trust through little things, like always being on time for a workout. Showing up on time makes a strong statement about a Personal Trainer's professionalism and indicates to your client that his or her time is important to you.

Meet Commitments

Personal Trainers also need to make sure to fulfill any commitments requested at previous sessions. If your client asks for information on a particular topic, it should be available the next session. Sometimes, too, sharing your own personal health and fitness information helps enhance the bonding process. But the information should be relevant to the client's health and fitness situation.

Accept Clients As They Are

You earn your clients' respect by giving your best to them, no matter what level of conditioning or coordination your client presents. Just because you're a world-class power lifter, bodybuilder, or runner doesn't mean your client can or wants to be. For many of your clients, the act of starting a fitness program deserves your sincere admiration.

Without being condescending or patronizing, be upbeat and energetic, praising the effort you see and encouraging improvement. The praise and encouragement should be based in reality and given within the scope of your personality. Going overboard or trying to be a cheerleader beyond your nature can appear phony to a client and obviously jeopardize the relationship.

Complete Focus

It is important that a Personal Trainer focuses entirely on the client during each session. All of a Personal Trainer's energy, thoughts, and actions should be directed toward the client, no matter what else (short of a five-alarm fire) is happening in the gym, studio, or fitness center. This complete focus lets clients know that their Personal Trainers care about them and, again, that they are important as individuals to their Personal Trainer.

One way to demonstrate this attention is for the Personal Trainer to turn his or her body to fully face the client during the session. Maintaining eye contact when speaking and listening also shows clients that what the Personal Trainer is saying to them and what they are saying is important. Body language and facial expression often tell the client more than what the Personal Trainer says.

Use Self-Disclosure Only When It Helps Your Client

The Personal Trainer/client relationship is not a two-way friendship in which both parties share information about themselves. Workout sessions are most certainly not the place for your private testimonial or confessional. *Prior to making a personal disclosure or discussing another client, stop, think, and make sure that your disclosure is in your client's best interest and supports his or her change process.*

Active Listening

One of the most important Personal Trainer–client relationship skills is called "active listening." Although some Personal Trainers are naturally better listeners, this is an important skill for all Personal Trainers to learn and develop. It is something you call upon in every training session and conversation with your client.

Essentially, aim to *listen until you don't exist—until the voices in your head are quiet.* Leave your own thoughts and concerns aside and focus completely on what you are hearing. Of utmost importance is that you allow your client to speak his or her mind without interrupting, keeping eye contact at all times. Think of how annoyed you get when others cut you off when you're trying to make a point.

Reflective Statements

A Personal Trainer who does not quite understand a client's point should restate it and have the client confirm whether or not it is correct. Even if the Personal Trainer is sure he or she understands, repeating it back assures the client that the Personal Trainer is listening, cares, and is trying to understand the client's perspective and concerns. So, a good technique to show you are listening, care, and want to understand is to wait until your client has made his or her point, then paraphrase (using your own words) or summarize (repeating your client's words) what you heard. *Repeating or summarizing what your client just said shows that you are listening carefully and trying to understand and encourages further dialogue.*

Listen for Facts AND Feelings

Sometimes your clients will communicate through actions rather than words, or their tone of speaking tells a story about their feelings. If you've maintained a complete focus on them, it becomes easier to interpret body language, voice inflection, and hesitation, for example, and tap into your intuition about what your client really means.

Although you can usually rely on *cognitive* listening (i.e., simply listening to the facts shared by your client), other times, you need to use your skills of *affective* listening (i.e., tapping into the emotions underlying the words you hear). For example, when you "hear" some anxiety, an appropriate response might be, "I have the feeling that you are upset about something. Can you share it with me?"

Ask Open-Ended Questions (Inquiry)

Don't be afraid to ask questions. This also shows you are listening and demonstrates your concern and desire to understand. Develop a pattern of being open, curious, and positive in a nonjudgmental way. A good rule is to ask open-ended questions—questions that cannot be answered with a simple yes or no, so start with "what" and not "do." Frame your questions so your client has to offer his or her views and opinions. This is a subtle way of empowering them. For example, instead of simply saying "Are you ready to work out?" you might try, "What are some of the concerns or questions you have about this workout?"

Show Interest in Your Client's Life

Although the early steps to develop trust are important, the process is ongoing. For that reason, begin each session by asking the client how his or her week went and demonstrating honest concern about his or her entire life, such as children or jobs. Often these are the barriers that impede consistent participation with you. For these kinds of clients, maintaining an on-going open dialogue is extremely important. They need to be able to discuss with you the psychological and physical barriers that seem to be cropping up again. You need to be empathetic without being judgmental. You must demonstrate to your client that you understand the family/work stresses he or she is going through. Remember that even though fitness is your "life" and profession, your clients have other priorities.

Holding Up the Mirror

There may also be times when you need to confront your clients about what you perceive as dwindling interest or efforts. You need to use all of the techniques listed earlier, beginning with questions such as "It sounds as though your commitment is waning. Am I reading this correctly? What seems to be the problem?" or "I have some concerns that you may find difficult to hear . . . may I share them with you?" In this situation, it is important—and empowering—to seek your client's permission before broaching the problem. If the answer is negative, move on.

But sometimes, through the process of inquiry, your client comes upon a resolution to the problem. Again, only a client-centered solution will result in greater commitment. Sometimes, also, a silent nod encourages the client to go further.

Provide and Encourage Open, Honest Feedback

If your relationship is going to help the client proceed, getting and giving feedback is most important. Although your clients may seem satisfied at first, don't assume continued success. Keep asking questions and fine-tuning the program. Again, the questions should be open-ended. Instead of "Are you satisfied?" try "What do you think is helping you?" and "What do you think is hindering you?" and "What was the most helpful thing that we did today?"

As you have gathered by now, excellent communication skills are important for the Personal Trainer–client relationship, and feedback is very important, along with listening and asking questions. Feedback used with the client should be non-threatening, objective, clarifying, and reflective, as well as supportive. Initially, clients look to the Personal Trainer as the one that they are doing the work for, thus praise or criticism is the means by which they assess their attempts. Feedback should reflect the client's efforts and phrased so as not to be misinterpreted.

Client Participation in Planning and Decisions

Understanding individual differences and levels of competency is extremely necessary when you design each individual's exercise program. It is also crucial to keep the client involved when planning the workout regimen. Remember that the client is the only one who can commit to and make change happen. You cannot dictate, only facilitate—help the client find his or her way out of the woods and onto the right path.

With people whose motivational level isn't as high as yours, involving them in their workout planning and individual workout sessions helps them to feel more part of the process. This creates more loyalty and increases the probability of lasting behavioral change. If your clients feel they had a part in the planning, they are more likely to be faithful to its implementation. In addition, this can create some early success, which can be built upon and referred back to in later sessions.

For many of your clients, their "self-efficacy," or belief that they can perform and benefit from exercise, is low. Early success helps reverse those feelings, paving the way for a successful long-term commitment. The greater the sense of ownership of the program that your clients gain, the greater will be their level of confidence and sense of control.

Encouraging client participation in the planning process can be a balancing act. You want them to be involved, but you, as an exercise professional, should be aware of potential outcomes of different workout regimens and intensities. Your honesty in explaining this to your clients will help *them* make the right choices and increase your worth in their eyes.

Much of this planning will require as much listening as explaining on your part. Many clients will not easily open up to you, especially early on when they don't know you very well and are in a situation filled with uncertainty and anxiety for them. If you want them to share their thoughts and feelings, good or bad, with you, you must develop good listening skills and be nonjudgmental, both verbally and nonverbally.

FITNESS VISIONS AND INTRINSIC MOTIVATORS

Sometimes it's easy to spot the clients who won't be with you very long. They come to you with vague, ill-defined goals, such as "want to feel better," "hope to get fit," "drop a few pounds," or something equally nebulous. Many times they've not really thought through what they want or why they want it, or they are there at someone else's (spouse's, doctor's) request. As a result, they never really buy into changing their behavior. Not surprisingly, they soon fade from your appointment schedule. Or you get the eager beaver, the guy or gal who jumps in with both feet, is tremendously motivated for the first few weeks, then slowly starts to regress, canceling sessions and coming up with excuses for reducing the routine when he or she does show up.

We all know the benefits exercise offers. So does most of the public—at least intellectually. Exercise decreases the risk of heart disease, stroke, and some cancers; it helps manage stress, improves depression, and can mitigate the effects of aging. So why can't these folks "just get it"—why do they keep failing at something as beneficial and seemingly simple as maintaining an exercise program?

Although it may be tempting to just grab these people by the lapels and try to shake some sense into them, professional propriety (not to mention the law) precludes that kind of treatment. But maybe the best "shake-up" is a psychological/emotional one you can lead them through before you ever hit the weights or treadmill. This may be the best time to try to get "inside the head" of these reluctant clients and help them find out what it is that makes them tick, what it is that they really want out of an exercise program, and what it is that will keep them coming back session after session. Short of hypnosis or intensive therapy, how does one go about this?

Help Your Client Create a Personal Fitness Vision

What you need to do is help each client to develop a "personal fitness vision," the picture of the person he or she wants to become relative to health and fitness, and then help uncover the "motivators," those intrinsic, deep-seated factors (similar to behavioral pros) that will help keep his or her interest level strong even when faced with obstacles and adversity. All of this has nothing to do with sets and reps; or minutes, seconds and heart rate. Yet it may be more important than any of those items in helping many of your clients change behaviors that have sabotaged previous efforts at starting or maintaining exercise programs.

The process of describing a fitness vision can be very difficult—even more so because it's probably not something your client anticipated when he or she signed up with you. You want to guide your clients on a trip to the future so they can describe the person they want to become as a result of working with you and listening to your advice on fitness. It is a picture in their minds of what they want themselves and their level of fitness to look like or what kind of person they want to be as it relates to fitness. It is important for each client to develop some conception of the person he or she wants to be with respect to fitness.

The vision can relate to:

1. Behavior (I will be a regular exerciser, sleep better, eat very little junk food)
2. Outcomes (I will be stronger, look younger, have more endurance, be able to play with my kids without getting tired)
3. Motivators (pros) (I want to be a role model for my children, I want to reduce my stress)
4. All of the above, such as:
   a. My fitness vision in the next 6 months is to reverse my trend of steady weight gain so that I can look better, younger, and wear stylish clothes
   b. My fitness vision in the next 3 months is to establish an exercise routine that will give me the energy to be more productive and a better parent and spouse
   c. My fitness vision is to establish an exercise program that will help me feel younger and lighter

Sometimes you have to probe more to help a client discover his or her vision. To stimulate the thought/introspection process, some key questions you can ask might be:

➤ What would you like your fitness level to be in 3 months, 1 year, and 2 years?
➤ What would your life be like if you can (or cannot) sustain an exercise program?
➤ What is the best-case scenario you might envision from participation in a fitness program?
➤ What do you think is the best possible outcome of consistent adherence to an exercise program?
➤ What things in life do you value most, and how are they connected to your fitness level?

Visualization

Your clients should have clear heads when trying to develop their visions. One way to help facilitate this is to help them visualize what they want to be:

➤ Find a quiet place and ask them to close their eyes.
➤ Take a deep breath from the lower stomach, and slowly let the breath out.
➤ Ask them to imagine themselves in a place where they feel comfortable, peaceful, strong, and confident.
➤ Ask "How do you feel about being there?"
➤ Then ask them to look into the future and pretend they have accomplished all their fitness goals.
➤ What does it feel like?
➤ How will you feel about yourself?
➤ How will others feel about you?
➤ Touch on the physical and emotional outcomes and rewards of exercise—weight loss, improved energy, reduced tension, stress management, mood elevation.

Some of the questions in the previous list may be relevant. Keep prodding until the answers are as *specific* and *personal* as possible. Then tell them to open their eyes and discuss with you what they saw. This will help you help each client form the vision. But remember, it has to be *their* vision, something *they* designed themselves and to which *they* feel personally committed. Have your clients write down their vision and give you a copy. Then you can return to it when you see enthusiasm waning.

Finding Your Client's Most Powerful Intrinsic Motivators

Even with a strongly desired fitness vision, clients are still apt to backslide and revert to old habits over time. That's why you must also help them uncover their motivators—those deep-seated values, concerns, and rewards that will help them maintain their fitness program even in the face of adversity. It is these "motivators" that you must call upon when you see your client begin to waver, to help him or her overcome any psychological or physical barrier. These motivators should be of specific and personal importance to clients—something valued enough to keep them on track when facing a difficult obstacle (e.g., "I value being a role model for my children more than sleeping in an extra 45 minutes or eating this piece of chocolate cake"). Typically, one or more of the client's behavioral "pros" is the same as his or her most powerful motivator(s).

It will be very tempting for a client to restate the well-publicized benefits of exercise; but only those that are specifically important and valuable to him or her will ensure compliance with an exercise program. Obviously, this is an on-going process, something you can use throughout your client's training program. Some examples might include:

➤ Feel more energetic or alert
➤ Feel more confident
➤ Improve my self-esteem

➤ Look better in my clothes
➤ Be a role model for my family
➤ Improve my overall coordination and strength
➤ Sleep better to improve my energy
➤ Improve my mood

This is often another area where clients need help navigating. To provide some guidance, again, ask such questions as:

➤ What are the top three values in your life?
➤ How is your fitness linked to these values?
➤ What part of your life is most important to you?
➤ How does your fitness fit in?
➤ What would you like more (less) of in your life? How is that linked to your fitness?
➤ What would your life be like if you do (not) achieve your goals? How would that feel?

At times, it may be helpful to return to the "pros and cons" and decisional balance for a fitness program and, for your more business-oriented clients, go over the cost-benefit ratio of consistent physical activity. The motivators that work the best are of the *internal* variety. Your clients must look within themselves for the reasons they want to change, why they want to improve their health and fitness and would value a fit lifestyle.

One possible internal motivator you might want to help them tap into is a feeling of competence and self-management—control of at least one part of their life. Job and family responsibilities often make people feel somewhat "frazzled" and out of control. In addition, many of the clients you see were not the greatest athletes growing up and feel inferior in a gym or fitness setting. So you may try to help them create a sense of competency with early successes.

Down the road, these early successes can be incorporated into a feeling of personal achievement that may be missing in other areas of their lives. This can be very powerful. These are defined as "intrinsic" motivators. There is no external reward involved here—it doesn't involve looking better, getting into that dress, or reducing dependence upon prescription drugs, for example. *Competence and personal control are deep-seated—and universal—motivators.*

Keep this in mind as you go through the workout program, making sure your clients experience some early success. This also may mitigate any fears of the "no pain/no gain" mentality inexperienced exercisers bring to the table. It may also overcome the anxiety felt by those who were never top athletes growing up. You may have to return to these motivators from time to time and remind clients of their early triumphs—especially since improvements tend to be less frequent or profound as one continues exercise and diet programs. Reminding your clients of the benefits they've already received may help see them through those times when their improvements seem to have hit a temporary plateau.

Sometimes, the vision and motivators need to be revised and refined as the process continues. Personal Trainers should be constantly asking clients to reconsider both during the course of their relationship. This is as important as changing workout routines to avoid or overcome plateaus and staleness. Motivators may change over time. For some clients, the actual act of physical activity—moving a heavy weight or deep breathing in a fast walk along a nature path—can prove to be an intrinsic motivator that you can develop and tap into.

Wanting to get in shape for loved ones, employees, etc., *external motivation,* will often result in frustration, feelings of guilt, and possibly resentment by the other person. Acceding to the wishes of a physician or spouse often leads to quitting the program. When clients confirm that their motivators are external, it is important to redirect them to internal, intrinsic motivators. The only chance for long-lasting change occurs when clients are doing something for theselves, not for another person and not for an external reward. On a long-term basis, external rewards just don't work.

The process of developing a fitness vision and intrinsic motivators may not be easy and may seem like another waste of time that keeps your client temporarily out of the gym. But if you want your client to continue coming back and if you want to reverse past failures, it is crucial for your clients to invest something of themselves into the process. This can help begin a process of self-monitoring and self-management that can lead to a long-term commitment to exercise and physical/mental fitness.

BEHAVIORAL GOAL SETTING

Why We Help Clients Set Behavioral Goals

Our main reasons for helping our clients set goals are:

➤ To help our clients establish new fitness behaviors (reach the maintenance stage of readiness to change), hence, fitness goals should be behavioral goals
➤ To allow us to measure success—Was my client successful? Was I successful as a Personal Trainer?
➤ To enable our clients to measure their progress against their initial baseline (something they can forget quickly and easily)

It is important to distinguish among behavioral goals, outcomes, and motivators. Goal setting is what our clients do (behaviors), not what happens when they do the behaviors (outcomes) or the reasons they want to do the behavior (motivators).

Have your clients include their intrinsic motivators and desired outcomes in their fitness visions and *avoid* goals that are really outcomes and/or motivators such as the examples below:

➤ Increase cardiovascular fitness (outcome) so that I don't get out of breath when climbing stairs (outcome and/or motivator)
➤ Lose weight (outcome) so that I look younger (outcome and/or motivator)

It is much *better* to link the outcomes and motivators with specific behavioral goals as in the examples below:

➤ I will do three 30-minute sessions of walking each week at a high intensity (behavioral goal) to improve my cardiovascular fitness (outcome and/or motivator) and feel more energetic (outcome and/or motivator).
➤ I will exercise 5 days a week for 30–40 minutes (behavioral goal) to lose weight (outcome and/or motivator) and look younger (outcome and/or motivator).

The Power of Accountability and Goals

As discussed earlier in this chapter, accountability is a very powerful tool in helping your clients to accomplish their goals. When they commit to certain goals and actions, they are accountable and want to honor their commitments.

Accountability is not the same as pestering or nagging. Your clients are committing to goals that you helped them design for themselves. To be accountable means that they commit to giving an account or description including what they did, what happened, what worked, what didn't work, and what they would do differently next time. You are holding your clients accountable for *their* plan and actions, not yours.

Some of your clients may associate goal setting with New Year's resolutions, which is often discouraging. Breaking down their goals into small, manageable steps can be a breakthrough. Your clients may be intimidated by looking at the mountain ahead rather than just focusing on the first foothill.

How to Set SMART Goals

As thoroughly reviewed in Chapter 13, help your clients develop goals that are **behavioral** goals and are:

Specific
Measurable
Attainable/**A**cceptable
Realistic/**R**elevant
Time-anchored

A SMART goal is one that the client is fully in charge of accomplishing through specific steps. Examples of SMART goals include:

➤ I will increase my exercise by walking three times a week for 15 minutes during the first week, and increasing by 5 minutes/session each week until I've reached 30 minutes/session by the 4th week.
➤ I will do a strength-training routine of five exercises (listed on my workout) using 12-pound (5.5-kg) dumbbells, and doing 12 reps with a 15-second rest between each exercise on Tuesday at 6:30 AM and Saturday at 10 AM.

Examples of poorly designed goals (*not* SMART goals):

➤ I am going to exercise more (no baseline, not specific or measurable)
➤ I am going to walk at a higher intensity (not specific or measurable)

Other keys to goal setting are:

➤ Never let your clients use the words "try" or "may" or "maybe" in their goals; "Do" is the correct action word.
➤ Define goals so that success and failure can be measured by yes or no, and the percentage of goal achievement is quantified as much as possible.
➤ The goals need to be reasonable ones at the time they are set. All of us can become better, if we set realistic goals.
➤ Remind your clients often that gradual change leads to permanent change.
➤ It is important for your clients to extend themselves a little beyond their comfort zone each week.

Setting Three-Month Behavioral Goals

In the workplace and at home, your clients have many plans and goals, and they are accountable to their bosses and families for achieving results. When it comes to their fitness, your clients are accountable only to themselves, which often isn't enough. Often your client's own self-care goals drop down on their priority lists. One responsibility of the Personal Trainer is to make sure this does not happen. The single most important element in helping your clients change their behaviors is to set realistic behavioral goals. Goal setting forces them to focus and mobilize their motivation around realistic and meaningful actions and outcomes. Developing a set of 3-month behavioral goals is a critical first step.

It is important for clients to develop a set of medium-term goals, and a 3-month time frame is sufficient for clients to start, learn, and possibly maintain a new set of behaviors. A 3-month time frame is also close enough to provide a sense of urgency for weekly goal setting. *Three-month behavioral goals are behaviors that your client commits to be doing consistently (which means that he or she has reached self-efficacy or is confident in the face of challenges) 3 months from now.* It is appropriate (at least every 4 weeks) to check progress toward 3-month goals. It may even be appropriate to change the 3-month goals if the goals are not challenging enough or are too difficult at this stage. When helping your clients define their 3-month behavioral goals, ask the following questions to help them determine for each goal:

➤ What do you want to do?
➤ What are your reasons for wanting to do it?
➤ What result are you looking for?
➤ For whom do you want to make the change (to be sure it's for yourself and not someone else)?
➤ Do you think you are being realistic?
➤ What's in the way?
➤ What's the real obstacle to achieving this goal?
➤ What strategies can you implement to overcome this obstacle?

By addressing the issues behind each goal, it will be easier for your clients to stick to their plans because they will remember, with your help, why they wanted to change in the first place. Understanding the reasons behind the goals is essential for keeping clients on track. If the client says, "I want to lose 10 pounds (4.5 kg)," the Personal Trainer asks, "Why do you want to lose 10 pounds (4.5 kg)?" Then once the reason is pinned down, the Personal Trainer asks, "Is this enough to get you to the finish line? Is this the reason that will keep you on track to make the change?" Once you get at the "why" that is really important to the client, make this a positive motivator. Create a picture that the client can recall later.

Setting Weekly Behavioral Goals

Setting SMART weekly behavioral goals is the basis for clients making small, manageable steps toward their 3-month behavioral goals. These are the list of specific behaviors to be done in the next week. A good guide for you is to help your clients set weekly behavioral goals to reach 60–80% of goal achievement each week. If their goal achievement is less than 60%, the goals are too ambitious, and if it is consistently 100%, the goal setting may not be ambitious enough to maintain your client's interest.

Tracking and Measuring Progress

Establishing a variety of baseline measurements is a necessary tool that can be used to:

➤ Track client progress over time
➤ Motivate your clients towards achieving their goals

It is important to have your clients use a variety of baseline measurements and tracking techniques with which they are comfortable. The following summarizes a range of baseline measurements and tracking techniques. Stress the importance of establishing these measurements during their initial sessions.

Subjective Self-Reporting

When clients include outcomes of a subjective nature in their fitness visions, such as energy levels, self-esteem, and level of well-being, it is helpful to assist them set a quantitative baseline and the desired outcome, and then monitor progress toward the desired outcome. For example, you can discuss with clients which of the following they wish to track. Develop a scale of 1 to 10 (10 being highest) on any of those that the client wishes to track. Take a baseline assessment on a scale of 1 to 10:

➤ Level of well-being (feeling better)
➤ Decreased stress

➤ Increased self-esteem
➤ Increased productivity
➤ Better sleep patterns
➤ Increased energy

Assessment of Goal Achievement

Assessment of goal achievement is central to your clients' process to change their behaviors. Assessment needs to be both objective and subjective. Some questions to pose to your clients are:

➤ Did you achieve your weekly or 3-month goal? Rate the achievement level, e.g., 100%, 75%, 50%, or 10%?
➤ Do you think the goal was appropriate?
➤ If you didn't reach 75% to 100%, is there something not working, or is the goal too ambitious?
➤ How is it going? Do you like what you are doing? Why or why not?
➤ Do you think it is time to set a new, more ambitious goal?
➤ Do you think this goal is too ambitious and needs to be scaled back?
➤ Any injuries, frustration, or guilt feelings?
➤ Are you feeling good and feeling good about yourself (self-esteem may be the best measure of success)?

OVERCOMING OBSTACLES

Recognize and Welcome Obstacles

Obstacles are something that impedes progress or achievement of goals. They are a necessary and welcome part of the change process! Obstacles are what make us human. Learning how to work through obstacles is what increases our emotional maturity and self-confidence in our ability to change. Obstacles can be our own inner thoughts and misguided perceptions, old self-defeating behaviors, unconscious choices, or environmental traps. The most important point in facing obstacles is being aware of them and recognizing them for the lessons that they are.

By welcoming and accepting obstacles, you can help your client tackle them effectively. Assuming that one will never face an obstacle is to assume that being human is being perfect. So, a client addressing the issue of obstacles up front with the Personal Trainer is, in reality, facing his or her own humanness. Then, when facing the obstacle—whether it is an old behavior or a sudden and immediate crisis—your client can summon up the personal resources or the new skills that he or she has been developing and apply them to the current situation.

Obstacles Are Learning Opportunities

Obstacles are indeed learning opportunities; they are challenges, barriers, and setbacks, but not failures. They provide the experience necessary for discovering how to tackle the problem. They give clients the testing ground to try out new behaviors in challenging situations.

In striving to overcome personal obstacles, clients build the self-confidence required to face any future hurdles, which in turn increases self-efficacy. Although it may taste bittersweet at the time, help clients understand that there are no failures, only lapses, and every lapse is an opportunity to learn more about what works, what doesn't work, and how difficult and precarious these new steps are. Lapses are part of being human and of changing ingrained habits. When clients lapse, help them understand the barrier without feeling overwhelmed by it. Say, "Let's figure out what we can learn from this so that we avoid having it happen again." Elicit your client's ideas on how to avoid recurrence, so he or she feels in charge again. If your client is "stuck" and can't see past the failure, come up with your own suggestions. For example, "Would it help if I send you an email reminder before your next yoga class so you know I'm counting on you to attend?"

If the lapse is even partly your fault (e.g., you pushed the client into an activity that he or she wasn't eager to do), take responsibility. Say lightly but sincerely, "This is my failure, not yours, and I learned from it not to push you into an activity that you're not excited about." By emphasizing what you and your client can learn from the lapse and how to change things to avoid it happening again, you act as a team, and you empower your client to get back on track. Help clients understand that lapses are part of the process and encourage them to get back on track.

Ambivalence and Backsliding

Ambivalence is the existence of coexisting and conflicting feelings that can inhibit attempts to change a behavior. It is a common attitude to have when attempting to change a behavior. This can occur after repeated attempts at behavioral change or it comes at the beginning when an individual's self-efficacy is low. Self-awareness and goal setting are powerful tools for dealing with ambivalence.

Backsliding or a lapse is a short-term regression to a previous behavior. However, such an obstacle can be a good learning situation, much like trial-and-error learning. This is an opportunity to gain more information about the attempt to change, and it is also a chance to explore different ways of changing. It is rare for the first attempt to be successful in changing old patterns of behavior. Personal Trainers need to reinforce this message with their clients and encourage them to use lapses as a good tool to explore themselves, thus increasing their self-awareness and self-efficacy.

Problem Solving

When obstacles have been identified by your client, an important skill to help your client develop is problem solving. Problem solving can be done together to determine solutions for your client's obstacles. Learning the process of problem solving is more important than learning a set of solutions for any one barrier; this way the client will know how to tackle barriers in the future. Problem solving, therefore, fosters independent thinking and self-confidence in one's abilities to remain physically active. Problem solving involves several different steps. The acronym IDEA has been developed to identify the four steps:

1. **I**dentifying the problem
2. **D**eveloping a list of solutions
3. **E**valuating the solutions
4. **A**nalyzing how well the plan worked

The first step involves identifying the problem. From the list of obstacles that your client has been able to identify, have your client pick one that is most pressing. In identifying the problem, it will be important to think through the problem fully to determine the key element or elements.

The second step is to develop a list of solutions. This is a brainstorming discussion in which the client thinks of any and all solutions while withholding any evaluation of them until later. This is a time to be creative. You may help clients with a few if they have trouble getting started. It is likely that you will need to remind your client that you do not evaluate the ideas at this stage. Have the client write down all of the solutions that are generated.

The third step is to evaluate solutions. Some solutions will be more realistic and address more of the details of the problems than others. You can work with your client to determine which of the solutions seem most appropriate. Whatever the solutions, work with your client to set goals and make a concrete plan about to implement the solution.

The final step is to analyze how well the plan worked. If a plan worked well, then praise the client for a job well done. Many times, however, the plan will not have worked as intended. It is important to emphasize that problem solving is a process that allows for learning and that it is not uncommon to need to fine-tune the solution.

In some cases, attempts to implement a solution elicit new details regarding the problem or new barriers. This information is critical to correctly identifying all of the important aspects of a problem and searching for a solution that addresses these aspects. Clients may be discouraged with their progress. It is important to emphasize the positive of what the client did accomplish, emphasize the importance of learning from what does not work, and work together to generate new solutions and plans.

Offer a Solution to Every Problem Your Client Presents

Clients need to count on you to be upbeat and solution oriented. Empathize with the severity of the problem ("I really understand how hard it is for you when . . .") but don't view it as insurmountable. It is best when clients come up with their own solutions. But when they don't, it is up to you to activate the brainstorming of solutions. Never offer a solution worded "You should . . ." or "Do this . . ." Instead, ask "What if you tried. . .?" or "How would this work for you?" Clients must feel in charge of choosing solutions that will work for them:

1. Continually help your client identify benefits from goals attained.
2. Help your client celebrate success.
3. Help your client find solutions to barriers of ingrained habits.
4. Convey to your client that a lapse is part of the process and encourage him or her to commit to getting back on track.

Be Firm When Appropriate

Firmness (truth telling or holding up the mirror) is appropriate when clients are spinning their wheels, getting stuck and not being honest about it, not cooperating, or not going with the program. If none of the recommended strategies have helped and it is clear that you are working harder to help your client overcome obstacles than your client is, it might be time for truth telling or "tough love."

To begin, admit to your client that you feel like you're spinning your wheels and you're getting frustrated. Tell the client that you need a firm commitment that he or she will take responsibility and move forward.

Next, ask your client in a non-threatening way to be honest about what is interfering. Listen to the response and help the client develop a new, more rigorous structure that he or she promises to stick to, such as emailing you daily after each workout.

You may need to say, "I've noticed that you've promised for the past four weeks that you'd walk twice a week, and you haven't walked at all. What is happening?" or "Shall we look at the impact of this on your other goals? You're frustrated that you're not losing the weight you wanted, and you know that aerobic exercise will help. To succeed you may need to renew your commitment to your walking goal. You might need to get up a half hour earlier and take that time to walk. May I challenge you to commit to that?"

You must already have a strong, trusting relationship before you try this method. Some clients are sensitive and need more nurturing than firmness. You can temper the firmness by saying, "Would you consider doing this. . ." instead of "I want you to do this . . ."

Help Your Client Find a Support System

Clients often make changes more easily if they have a support system in addition to their Personal Trainers. Encourage your clients to identify other people in their circle of friends, colleagues, and relatives who have similar goals and to set up a system of helping each other, whether it is emotional support, practical support, partnering, or just listening. Here are some ways that your clients can seek support:

➤ Exercising with someone
➤ Phoning someone daily, or several times a week

➤ Reporting progress regularly to someone
➤ Eating with someone and being supportive of health-supporting choices
➤ Sharing exercise goals
➤ Joining a gym with a friend or spouse
➤ Having your spouse watch the kids while you go for a walk

Your clients' behaviors can be changed if they view or track others with similar goals taking the necessary steps toward those goals. An overweight client who wants to start a walking program may find it easier to start if he or she sees other overweight people walking on a regular basis or has an email dialogue with another overweight person on the same path.

Focus Mainly on the Present and Future

You want to know about clients' past experiences, but encourage them to acknowledge the past, apply to the present what they have learned from the past, and then move forward without looking back. Whenever they fall into a pattern of letting past failures control their actions or decisions, point out what you observe and guide them to different strategies.

Many clients have experienced past trauma and failure in their lives. While you need to be compassionate, do not let clients dwell in the past. Help them figure out strategies for moving on and taking charge of their lives. Help them see what they have the power to control and how to take charge. Realize that clients who see themselves as victims or failures will have trouble doing this. Help your clients take very small steps to achieve success—this is imperative.

Help Your Clients Find Solutions to Obstacles Embedded in Their Lives

There are some obstacles to healthy living that your clients will not have control over. For example, their spouses may not be supportive or their hours at work can be long and stressful. Help your clients address these obstacles by helping them brainstorm solutions to barriers they see as difficult or impossible to penetrate.

Ask "What might get your spouse to support you better?" or "What are some strategies for finishing work early" or "How can you find ten or fifteen minutes during your long workday when you can fit in some exercise?" If your client responds, "Beats me!" (or the equivalent), offer some solutions, but not until you've given the client the chance to figure it out first. If the client can't come up with solutions, help by throwing ideas out for him or her to consider and build on. Be prepared with a variety of solutions to similar barriers.

Keep the solutions simple. The easier the solution, the better it is as a first step. For example, you might say, "You don't have to exercise for thirty minutes or more for it to be valuable. Would you be able to find ten minutes two or three times a day for now?" If the problem is more complex, such as an unsupportive spouse, help the client identify some new approaches to communicating with the spouse or to getting help from a relationship expert.

Identify Triggers

Clients may feel that their pattern of failure is ingrained or that their behavior is out of control. Their poor behavioral patterns may have triggers that are worth exploring. Triggers are specific incidents or situations that cause an individual to act. Cues from one's environment can cause an individual to act. If it is cold, one will put on more outer clothing or find a warm place. Triggers evolve into patterned behavior.

Triggers can be personal thoughts or emotional feelings as well as environmental cues. Triggers can be catalysts for positive or negative behavior, thus they can be used for positive change or evolve into obstacles. With these triggers, an individual can find the means to change behavior. The client can identify the problematic triggers that cause the unhealthy behavior and discuss with the Personal Trainer about how to approach them to modify the identified behavior. A Personal Trainer can help clients build self-confidence in learning how to handle the triggers to unhealthy behaviors that they desire to change.

Help clients look at the triggers and patterns. What triggers a bump in the road? How can they avoid those triggers? If the triggers are inevitable, what strategies or behaviors can they put in place to change the outcome? Keeping a journal is one helpful way for clients to examine their behavior and feelings and to see how one event or emotion may trigger another.

Remind Your Client of Prior Progress

Clients easily lose sight of prior progress when they have setbacks or don't reach their goals as quickly as they would like. Keep reminding them of past progress, large and small. For example, "But three months ago, you couldn't walk a mile! Give yourself a lot of credit!"

Negative Self-Talk

Negative self-talk is the conversation that plays in one's head, informing how one thinks, views and, ultimately, feels about one's self. Negative self-talk is often established in childhood or during past experiences. It can be described as a negative tape that has been installed in one's mind. These tapes are the thought process that individuals have acquired that is connected with their present self-concept and thus their self-esteem.

We do not need enemies; we have ourselves! We can be our own worst enemies at times because of this distorted self-image that we carry with us in our heads. So having a Personal Trainer help to acknowledge the negative self-talk and install new and positive tapes in one's thinking can be powerful. Some clients have had such negative tapes or negative self-talk for so long that they really do end up sabotaging every attempt at behavior change. So, watch for clients who have some deeply rooted negative self-concepts that will constantly interfere with behavioral change.

The arena of physical fitness, weight management, and body sculpting is a very challenging one for individuals with a poor self-concept. They already have low self-esteem because they do not have a perfect physique. So, in their thought system, they have already failed. This feeling of failure just reinforces their negative self-talk that they can never attain that perfect shape. Negative self-talk usually leads to fatalistic self-talk. So, as a Personal Trainer, ask clients about their self-image in the first interview.

For clients whose self-confidence is low, a Personal Trainer can help increase it by supplying the client with the realistic information that fitness is hard work but with a good support team, aided with scientifically sound information and with lots of trial and error experience, positive and permanent change is realistic.

Self-Sabotage

Don't wrestle with clients who are not meeting their goals week after week. Make sure first that the goals are realistic and based on the clients' expressed desires and that you have exhausted all sources of ideas, including this book.

Self-sabotage evolves from a combination of negative self-talk and low self-efficacy. Watch for mental health issues that may hurt their attempts to develop fitness behaviors and suggest that they get help from a physician and/or qualified mental health professional.

Whether their desire is to lose weight, establish an exercise routine, or stop smoking, ask pertinent questions about their prior attempts and their successes and failures. Help raise your clients' awareness of their patterns of behavior. Point this out to them and ask them to recognize it. This helps the Personal Trainer establish a non-threatening, trusting, and open communication in the beginning of the relationship.

Stay Positive and Avoid Being Judgmental

Personal and intrinsic thoughts are what is said inside one's head, and they have a profound effect on behavior. Overcoming negative thoughts and staying positive is both a challenge and a necessity to practice. Have the client run some personal negative statements by you and then rephrase the statements into positive ones. One of the most powerful tools a Personal Trainer can use in working with clients is to help reestablish positive self-talk.

Using positive affirmations when working with clients is a major boon to changing any negative self-concept. A simple tool to use is to have clients write a positive note after each workout about their efforts. They can keep a daily workout journal, noting after each workout how they felt about themselves that day. This gives them a record of their attempts, the Personal Trainer's comments, and a tool for reflection.

Time Management

One fact of life is that people make time for the things that they really want to do. Many clients will tell Personal Trainers that they don't have enough time to exercise regularly. What they're really saying, is that they value their other activities more than exercise. Personal Trainers can't give clients more time, but we can help clients connect with why they value being fit and the benefits of making exercise a higher priority (behavioral pros). We can also suggest that they choose activities of lower priority that they are willing to give up to make time for regular exercise. One of the benefits of helping clients develop fitness visions is that visions can help them link their values to regular exercise and then make exercise a higher priority.

Effective time management contributes to a more balanced lifestyle—a critical foundation for overcoming obstacles. Some skills to suggest to your clients to manage time effectively include:

1. Prioritize major tasks; it is helpful to write them out in a daily journal or scheduler.
2. Schedule self-care activities including exercise.
3. Identify activities that can be dropped.
4. Be realistic about what you can and cannot accomplish.
5. Learn to say "NO."
6. Take baby steps; don't tackle the overwhelming tasks, break big tasks into small ones.
7. Set goals and reward yourself.
8. Delegate tasks to others when appropriate.

Stress Management

Stress management is a major obstacle when trying to change behaviors. Stress management is also too large a topic for this chapter, and so this section highlights the areas of concern for the Personal Trainer.

Cumulative stress can produce high levels of anxiety and can damage health in the long run. Change is also stressful even when it is focused on better health and fitness, but change requires effort and conscious awareness. It may be helpful to notice how your clients typically react to stress in their environment. A review of their life events that occurred in the past year, as well as a review of significant life stressors that they have and have not resolved would aid a Personal Trainer in establishing how a client responds to stress. Some types of responses to stress to look for include:

➤ Negative or false expectations
➤ Negative mental imagery
➤ Negative self-talk
➤ Controlling behavior
➤ Perfectionist behavior
➤ Anger

A Personal Trainer can suggest that the client seek new skills for managing and thus lowering his or her stress level. There are two approaches for managing stress. Self-control is the responsibility of clients in changing their cognitive perception, which deals with their personal belief systems and attitudes. Situational control includes effective problem solving, assertiveness communication skills, effective conflict resolution skills, time management, and physical, emotional, social, and spiritual self-care.

Make the Training Program Interesting

It is important to keep the coaching sessions interesting by adding variety, changing approaches, or simply surprising your clients with emails that share insights and articles you've read that might interest them.

Welcome Feedback

Clients may be reluctant to give negative feedback about you or the coaching process, even if they feel something in your approach is holding them back. As coaches, we tend to assume that everything is going fine if the client doesn't tell us otherwise, and then boom, we may learn from a client evaluation that things are not fine. We need to know the problems in time to fix them on the spot. It may be uncomfortable to ask for feedback from clients, but it's an important part of the process.

Clients need to understand that your goal is to make the session as good as it can be for them and that you will not take criticism personally or defensively. Ask one or more of these questions during every session:

➤ "How can I make this work better for you?"
➤ "What can I add to your program so that you feel you're getting 100%?"
➤ 'What is your program missing that you'd like to include?"
➤ "What would you like me to do now to help you?"

If a client never offers criticism, don't assume it means that there is nothing you could do better. The client may simply feel uncomfortable talking to you about it, even though you've asked for this feedback. In this case, say "Please email me if you think of anything—anything at all that would make this program work better for you or for others. It's important to me to know this."

When you do receive some negative feedback, do not respond defensively. Thank your client for being honest and share the fact that you are striving to continue to grow and develop. Restate the criticism to be sure you understand it and either suggest a solution or promise to think about how to resolve the problem.

Examples:

Client #1: "I know I liked that circuit training program you gave me when I first started, but now I'm bored with it and I feel like I'm just coasting."

Personal Trainer: "You're bored with the circuit training program and you're not seeing progress any more. Thanks for letting me know that—shall we develop a new program to start next week?"

Client #2: "I feel like you're repeating things too much. I get them the first time. I'm paying for every minute, so I want to go faster."

Personal Trainer: "It sounds as though you don't need the amount of repetition I'm giving you and you feel we're going too slowly. Thank you. I appreciate knowing that. Many clients need a lot of repetition, but I shouldn't have assumed that you do. I am happy to speed things up! Will you promise to stop me if you need more explanation about anything!"

Figure 10.5 is a summary of a training program evaluation, which you can ask clients to complete.

Name of Personal Trainer: _____

Name of Client: _____

Program start date: _____

Please indicate your Personal Trainer's performance on a scale of 1 to 10.
(10 being excellent, 1 being poor). Please feel free to add any comments.

	Rating	Comments
Knowledge:		
Helpfulness:		
Understanding of your circumstances:		
Quality of advice:		
Quality of instruction:		
Motivation provided:		
Effectiveness of training methodology:		
Other comments:		
Areas for improvement:		
In what ways has training benefited you the most or changed you the most? If possible, describe before & after		
What goal is most important to you:		
Other comments:		

FIGURE 10.5. Training program evaluation.

Please comment on how training has benefited you in any of the following areas:

Appearance:

Motivation:

Energy:

Work performance/productivity:

Exercise habits:

Eating habits:

Sleep:

Stress management:

Self-esteem:

What are your Personal Trainer's best qualities?

How could your Personal Trainer improve?

How does your training experience differ from your expectations?

FIGURE 10.5. *Continued*

SUMMARY

This chapter outlines behavioral modifications of clients leading to behavioral change and then provides the motivation necessary for someone to make the necessary lifestyle changes that lead to a healthier person. The behavioral processes that lead to change are explored with some additional techniques to make those changes permanent. The chapter also provides a framework for Personal Trainers to first analyze the psychology of change, then to provide programs for permanent change in their clients' lifestyle.

REFERENCES

1. Prochaska JO, Norcross JC, DiClemente CC. Changing for Good. New York: William Morrow, 1994.
2. Janis I, Mann L. Decision Making: A Psychological Analysis of Conflict, Choice and Commitment. New York: Collier Macmillan, 1977.
3. Bandura A. Self-efficacy: Toward unifying theory of behavioral change. Psychol Rev 1977;84:191–215.

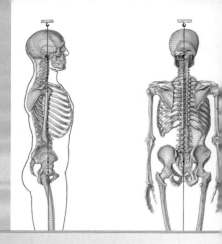

Dan Benardot, Ph.D., DHC, RD, LD, FACSM, Laboratory for Elite Athlete Performance, Division of Nutrition, School of Health Professions, College of Health and Human Services, Georgia State University, Atlanta, Georgia

Walter R. Thompson, Ph.D., FACSM, FAACVPR, Professor of Kinesiology and Health (College of Education), Professor of Nutrition (College of Health and Human Sciences), Department of Kinesiology and Health, Georgia State University, Atlanta, Georgia

Chapter Outline

Objectives

- **Understand the functions of the three energy substrates (carbohydrate, protein, and fat) in health and performance**
- **Know the interrelationships between vitamins and minerals in health and performance**
- **Understand the importance of hydration in maintaining health and achieving optimal performance**
- **Know the essential elements of energy balance as it relates to weight control, body composition, and performance**
- **Understand issues related to nutrient supplementation and strategies for discerning the circumstances under which specific supplements may be warranted**
- **Understand practical issues related to eating for performance, including eating on the road, the pre-competition meal, during-competition nourishment, and post-competition replenishment**

Nutrition and athletic performance are closely linked, making it impossible to experience success with a physical training program that has no parallel nutrition strategy. Personal Trainers who recommend the use of nutrition strategies for achieving an ideal weight or body composition without considering the impact of the strategy on physical performance may be counterproductive and may predispose clients to disease and injury.

An improvement in client conditioning cannot be realized by focusing only on time in the gym to increase flexibility and improve endurance or power. The adjunct nutritional strategies clients should follow before they get to the pool or gym, the foods they consume after they go home, and what they do to ensure an optimal flow of fluid and energy into their muscles are critical to improving power, sustaining concentration, and optimizing performance. Failure to consider nutrition as an integral component of the skills training and/or conditioning program will increase health risks and result in poor improvement rates. Well-nourished clients do better, recover more quickly from soreness and injuries, and derive more performance-improving benefits from long and strenuous training sessions. Unfortunately, Personal Trainers often fail to help clients match the dynamics of exercise with a supportive nutrition strategy.

A great deal of scientific information exists on the relationship between good nutrition and exercise performance, but the massive quantities of misinformation on nutrition makes it difficult for Personal Trainers to know when and what to eat before practice and competition; the foods that will best sustain energy levels; the best drinks and foods to consume before, during, and after exercise; how to balance an optimal energy intake with an ideal body composition; and how to make certain nutrient intake meets nutrient needs. These and other issues are covered in this chapter with the aim of helping the Personal Trainer to assist their clients in understanding the key nutritional strategies that are related to improving exercise performance.

SCOPE OF PRACTICE

In many places, the profession of dietetics is regulated by law. The practice of dietetics is typically performed by a registered dietitian who has the academic degree and proper certifications or licenses to provide public-specific meal plans or diet plans. The Personal Trainer must respect these professionals by always seeking out their assistance when governed by laws. Typically, Personal Trainers do not develop meal plans or specific diet plans for clients (that is the scope of practice for Registered Dietitians). However, Personal Trainers can, and should, recognize when it is appropriate to refer clients to a registered dietitian.

Although laws typically have been written to protect the scope of practice for dietitians, the specific scope of practice for Personal Trainers regarding nutrition is not as clear. However, it appears as though Personal Trainers can teach fundamentals of nutrition to clients (as outlined in this chapter) as well as assist with a weight loss program that would include both diet and exercise. Personal

Trainers should also be aware of, and be able to recognize, patterns of disordered eating and make the appropriate referral to a healthcare practitioner who has the experience necessary to treat these conditions. Personal Trainers are urged to investigate any and all laws pertaining to the practice of dietetics in their local area.

ESSENTIAL NUTRITION CONCEPTS

Nutrients give muscles the energy needed for work and provide the building materials for muscles, organs, and bones. Well-nourished clients are more likely to stay healthy, have better cardiovascular function, are more likely to grow normally and build needed muscle tissue, and will heal well if they are injured. For clients to be healthy and successful, they must consider nutritional needs as important as the skills training they may want to acquire.

Nutrients

There are six classes of nutrients: carbohydrates, proteins, fats, vitamins, minerals, and water. Clients should not think of any individual nutrient as more important than any other nutrient. Rather, the focus should be on nutrient balance, which is critical to good health and performance. With your help, clients should try to find the appropriate balance between all the nutrients, since too much or too little of any single nutrient increases the risk of health and/or performance problems. For example, too little iron intake would lead to poor endurance and a lower ability to burn fat, while too much protein could increase urine production and increase the risk of dehydration. The best strategy for maintaining a nutrient balance is to eat a wide variety of foods, regularly consume fresh fruits and vegetables, and avoid a monotonous intake of the same few foods day after day. Consumption of a wide variety of foods will ensure optimal nutrient exposure. No single food has all the nutrients a person needs to stay healthy, so eating a wide variety of foods helps people know that all the needed nutrients are available to them. An added benefit of eating a wide variety of foods is avoidance of nutrient toxicities that may result from an excess consumption of vitamins and/or minerals. Easily available and inexpensive nutrient supplements dramatically increase the possibility of nutrient toxicities. The common belief that, "if a little bit of a nutrient is good, then more must be better" is wrong. Providing more nutrients than the body can use does not provide a benefit, and it forces people into using valuable energy resources to excrete the surplus, with the additional risk of developing toxicity reactions.

There is a great deal of nutritional information on television and in popular magazines, making it difficult for people to make the right nutritional decisions. Most people wouldn't take the word of a car salesman about which car is best to buy, but they often believe people (particularly celebrities) who sell nutritional supplements despite the lack of credible scientific evidence for what they're selling. Part of the problem is that the "placebo effect" is at play with nutrition (i.e., if you believe that something will work, it will actually work, even though there may be no biological reason for the result). Personal Trainers should ask for evidence about whether nutritional products actually work, and when a claim is made, there should be immediate follow-up: "Show me the evidence." Scientific (peer-reviewed) journals are the best source of information. It should be clearly understood that one person's positive experience from taking a substance does not translate into a universal benefit. Claims that sound too good to be true probably are *not* true.

NUTRIENTS THAT PROVIDE ENERGY

Energy nutrients provide fuel for cellular work. Carbohydrates, proteins, and fats (Table 11.1) are considered energy nutrients because they all provide carbon (fuel) that can be burned (used for energy production). Energy nutrients allow us to do muscular work, transfer electrical energy between nerve cells, and help us maintain body temperature at 98.6° Fahrenheit (37°C). Energy is

Table 11.1	IDEAL ENERGY (CALORIE) DISTRIBUTION FOR ATHLETES AND FOR PHYSICALLY ACTIVE ADULTS (2)

65% from carbohydrate

15% from protein

20% from fat

measured in calories, which in nutrition are often referred to as kilocalories (kcal) because they represent 1000 times the calorie unit used in physics. So, for our purposes, the word "calories" is used synonymously with kilocalories, or kcal (1).

Exercise causes an increase in the *rate* at which energy is burned. This process is not 100% efficient, so 40% or less of the burned energy is converted to mechanical energy while more than 60% of the energy is lost as heat. This extra heat causes body temperature to rise, which makes the body increase its sweat rate as a means of cooling down body temperature. Therefore, the two essential components of sports nutrition that Personal Trainers should focus on are:

1. Finding ways to provide enough extra energy at the right time to satisfy the needs of physical activity
2. Finding ways to provide enough fluid at the right time to maintain body water and replace the fluid that was lost as sweat

Meeting Energy Needs for Optimal Weight and Body Composition

The relationship between weight and caloric intake is relatively simple: If you eat more calories than you burn (expend), you will store the excess calories, and body weight will rise. If you eat fewer calories than you burn, you will use some of your existing body tissues for needed energy, and body weight will drop. Consistently consuming too little energy will burn enough of your lean mass (muscles) that the *rate* at which you burn calories (called the "metabolic rate") will decrease. The end result of a lower metabolic rate is usually higher body weight (from more body fat) because you lose your ability to burn the calories you eat. Therefore, staying in an energy-balanced state or deviating from it only slightly is an important strategy for both body weight and body composition maintenance. Clients wishing to increase muscle mass should perform the exercises needed to enlarge muscle mass and slightly increase (by 300 to 500 calories) daily caloric intake. Clients wishing to decrease body fat should make only subtle decreases (no more than 300 calories) in daily caloric intake while maintaining a vigorous conditioning schedule to maintain muscle mass.

For your athletic competitors, lower weight results in lower resistance, and all sports have resistance associated with them. Skaters must overcome the resistance of a skate blade going over the ice, cyclists must cope with air resistance, power lifters have the resistance from weights, divers and gymnasts experience resistance as they tumble through the air. Sports performance is related to the ability of the athlete to overcome resistance (or drag) and the ability to sustain power output by overcoming this resistance on repeated bouts or long distances (3). While these two factors (overcoming resistance and sustaining power output) are clearly related to performance, they are perceived by many athletes to be in conflict—a fact that causes many athletes problems with meeting energy needs. Athletes often view their ability to overcome resistance or drag with their ability to carry lots of muscle and relatively little fat. As fat mass does little to contribute to sports performance and may contribute to drag, this makes lots of sense. However, the *strategy* that athletes often use to reduce fat mass and maximize muscle mass is to diet by dramatically lowering total energy intake. This dieting strategy is counterproductive because it restricts the intake of energy that is needed to sustain power output.

Herein lies the dilemma: How can your clients maximize their ability to sustain power output while, at the same time, reducing body fat percentage? A number of studies suggest that the answer may lie in consuming small but frequent meals to stay in better energy balance throughout the day. Energy balance has typically been assessed in 24-hour units. That is, if you consume 3000 calories during the day and you burn 3,000 calories during the day, you are in "energy balance." However, what happens *during* the day to achieve a state of energy balance makes a difference. If you spend most of the day in an energy-deficit state (i.e., you burned far more calories than you consumed) but then eat a huge meal at the end of the day to satisfy your energy needs, you might still be in energy balance. However, it appears that people who do this have different outcomes than those who stay close to an energy-balanced state throughout the day. Eating small but frequent meals has the following benefits (4–11):

➤ Maintenance of metabolic rate
➤ Lower body fat and lower weight on higher caloric intakes
➤ Better glucose tolerance and lower insulin response (making it more difficult to manufacture fats from the foods you eat)
➤ Lower stress hormone production
➤ Better maintenance of muscle mass
➤ Improved physical performance

Surveys have suggested that people (particularly athletes) tend to delay eating until the end of the day, and many experience severe energy deficits earlier in the day (particularly on days when they train hard and need the energy the most!). Problems with energy deficits include (12):

➤ Difficulty maintaining carbohydrate stores (this would impede endurance in high-intensity activities)
➤ Problems maintaining lean (muscle) mass
➤ Lower metabolic rate
➤ Difficulty meeting nutrient needs (foods carry both energy *and* other nutrients)
➤ Increased risk of injury (undernourished athletes may develop mental and muscular fatigue that, in some sports, would predispose them to injury)
➤ Missed opportunities to aid muscle recovery

Maintaining energy balance throughout the day by consuming small but frequent meals *during* the day is an excellent strategy for reducing these problems.

Carbohydrate

Carbohydrate is often referred to as if it is a single compound. In fact, carbohydrate comes in many different forms that have different nutritional outcomes. Some carbohydrates are digestible while others are not, some are considered "complex" while others are "simple," and some carbohydrates contain soluble fiber while others contain insoluble fiber. The basic carbohydrate for human nutrition is the simple sugar glucose, but our bodies make a complex carbohydrate called glycogen, which is the storage form of glucose (Tables 11.2–11.4).

Table 11.2 QUICK FACTS ABOUT CARBOHYDRATE	
Minimum intake	50 to 100 grams per day (200–400 calories) needed to avoid ketosis
Average U.S. intake	200 to 300 grams per day (800–1200 calories)
Recommended fiber intake	20 to 30 grams per day, or more
Average U.S. fiber intake	10 to 15 grams per day
Recommended intake of carbohydrate as percentage of total caloric intake	55% of total calories; up to 65% of total calories for athletes
Good sources of carbohydrate	Grains, legumes, seeds, pasta, fruits, vegetables

Table 11.3 SAMPLE OF GOOD HIGH-CARBOHYDRATE SNACKS

Apple	Fruit cup	Orange juice
Bagel	Fruit smoothie	Popcorn
Baked corn chips	Energy bar	Rice
Baked potato	Grapes	Saltine crackers
Banana	Mashed potatoes	Spaghetti
Beans toast	Mixed berries	Whole wheat

Table 11.4 COMMON SOURCES OF FOODS HIGH IN CARBOHYDRATE

Food	Calories from Carbohydrate (%)	Total Calories
Sugar (1 tbsp)	100	48
Pretzel sticks (10 small)	100	8
Maple syrup (1 tbsp)	100	64
Cranberry juice (1 cup)	100	152
Cola, regular (12 oz)	100	164
Apples (1 med)	100	84
Apricot juice (1 cup)	97	148
Sugar frosted flakes cereal (1 oz)	96	108
Raisins (1 cup)	94	489
Orange (1 raw)	94	64
Rice, white (1 cup)	93	216
Orange juice (1 cup)	93	112
Sweet potatoes (1 med)	93	120
Corn flakes cereal (1 oz)	92	104
Potato, baked (1 med)	91	224
Banana (1 raw)	89	121
Carrots (1 raw)	88	32
Potato, mashed with milk (1 cup)	86	173
Tomato sauce (1 cup)	86	84
Cantaloupe (1/2 melon)	84	105
Tomato (1 raw)	83	24
Green beans (1 cup)	83	48
Spaghetti (1 cup cooked)	82	157
Yogurt, low-fat fruit flavored (8 oz)	75	230
Bread, wheat (1 slice)	74	65
Bread, oatmeal (1 slice)	74	65
Beans (1 cup)	70	217
Broccoli (1 spear)	58	69

Adapted from USDA Nutrient Data Laboratory, Agricultural Research Service. USDA National Nutrient Database for Standard Reference Release 17. Washington, DC: Government Printing Office, 2004 (13).

CARBOHYDRATE FUNCTIONS

➤ *Provide energy* (4 calories per gram). Carbohydrate is the preferred fuel for the body, and it is an instantaneous energy source.
➤ *Protein sparing.* This is an often overlooked, yet very important, function of carbohydrates. Because carbohydrate (glucose) is a preferred fuel, providing enough carbohydrate to meet most energy needs preserves (i.e., "spares") protein from being broken down and used as a source of energy.
➤ *Oxidation of fat.* It has been said that "fats burn in a carbohydrate flame." That is, to burn fats efficiently and completely, some carbohydrate is needed.
➤ *Part of other compounds.* Carbohydrates are essential components of other compounds essential in human nutrition.
➤ *Stored energy.* Carbohydrates have two storage forms: glycogen and fat. The ideal storage form for carbohydrate is glycogen because it can be easily converted back to glucose and used for energy.

TYPES OF CARBOHYDRATE

➤ *Simple carbohydrates (sugars).* These are sugars that include glucose, fructose (typically found in fruits and vegetables), galactose (one of the sugars in milk), sucrose (table sugar), lactose (milk sugar), and maltose (grain sugar).
➤ *Polysaccharides.* These are carbohydrates that contain many molecules of connected sugars. Polysaccharides can be digestible (starch, dextrins, and glycogen) or indigestible (cellulose, hemicellulose, pectin, gums, and mucilages). Dietary fiber is carbohydrate that cannot be digested but is useful in the diet because it may lower fat and cholesterol absorption, improves blood sugar control, and may reduce the risk of colon cancer and heart disease.

Should the focus of your client's diet be carbohydrate, protein, or fat? Many studies show that *carbohydrates are the limiting energy substrate.* That is, when carbohydrates run out, people typically reach a point of exhaustion. For this reason, people should consume 55 to 65% of total calories from carbohydrates (2). Therefore, a person consuming a 3000-calorie diet should consume between 1650 and 1950 calories from carbohydrates. Expressed another way, athletes should consume between 6 and 10 grams of carbohydrate per kilogram of body weight. For a 75-kg (165-lb) person, that amounts to between 450 grams (1800 calories) to 750 grams (3000 calories) per day from carbohydrate alone.

Different activities have different carbohydrate requirements per unit of time. For instance, when walking at a brisk pace, 17% of the fuel comes from carbohydrate; when jogging at a medium pace, approximately 50% of the fuel comes from carbohydrate; and when running at a very fast pace, approximately 72% of the fuel comes from carbohydrate (14). However, because the length of time spent in these activities is usually much different (you can walk at a brisk pace much longer than you can run flat out), the **total** carbohydrate requirement may be similar when calculated over the total time invested in the activity.

You should consider that a single 30-second bout of high intensity activity could reduce muscle carbohydrate (glycogen) storage by more than 25%. By consuming a high carbohydrate diet and carbohydrate-containing sports beverages, you can improve energy reserves and enhance performance of repeated bouts of high-intensity activity.

The Glycemic Index

The **Glycemic Index** is a measure of how different consumed carbohydrate foods affect the blood sugar level. Foods are compared with the ingestion of glucose, which has an index value of 100. It is generally believed that focusing on foods with a lower glycemic index helps to maintain blood sugar, avoids an excessive insulin response that can encourage the manufacture of fat, and

Table 11.5 GLYCEMIC INDEX OF SOME COMMON FOODS (15)

High Glycemic Index (>85)	Medium Glycemic Index (60–85)	Low Glycemic Index (<60)
Glucose	All-bran cereal	Fructose
Sucrose	Banana	Apple
Maple syrup	Grapes	Applesauce
Corn syrup	Oatmeal	Cherries
Honey	Orange juice	Kidney beans
Bagel	Pasta	Navy beans
Candy	Rice	Chick-peas
Corn flakes	Whole grain rye bread	Lentils
Carrots	Yams	Dates
Crackers	Corn	Figs
Molasses	Baked beans	Peaches
Potatoes	Potato chips	Plums
Raisins		Ice cream
White bread		Milk
Whole wheat bread		Yogurt
Sodas (non-diet)		Tomato soup
Sports drinks		

keeps people feeling better longer. Although the glycemic index (Table 11.5) is a useful guide, you should be aware that different people have different responses to food. For instance, people who exercise regularly are much more tolerant of foods with a high glycemic index than are people who rarely exercise (15). Young people must meet the combined energy needs of growth, exercise, and tissue maintenance and so will have a higher requirement for calories per unit of body weight (and therefore carbohydrate) than will adult athletes. Athletes interested in lowering either weight or body fat levels should consider focusing on foods with a medium to low glycemic index.

Protein

Proteins are complex compounds that are made of different connected amino acids, which uniquely contain nitrogen. Body proteins are constantly changing, with new proteins being made and old ones broken down. Growth hormone, androgen, insulin, and thyroid hormone are **anabolic** hormones (i.e., they cause new protein to be manufactured). Cortisone, hydrocortisone, and thyroxin are **catabolic** hormones (i.e., they cause the breakdown of proteins).

Despite the fact that the protein requirement for competitive athletes is about double that for non-athletes (Table 11.6), most athletes consume far more protein than they need. The non-athlete (average) adult requirement for protein is 0.8 grams per kilogram of body weight, while the adult athlete requirement for protein is between 1.5 and 2.0 grams per kilogram of body weight. An athlete who weighs 180 lb (about 82 kg) would require between 123 and 164 grams of protein per day (16). At 4 calories per gram, this is between 492 and 656 calories from protein per day. Most athletes far exceed this amount of protein just from the foods they consume. Consider that the protein in a hamburger, a chicken fillet sandwich, and one cup of milk combined provides more than half the total daily protein requirement for a 180-lb (82-kg) athlete (Table 11.7).

Table 11.6	QUICK FACTS FOR PROTEIN
Recommended intakes	Infants: 2.2 grams per kg of body weight Children: 1.0–1.6 grams per kg of body weight Adults: 0.8 grams per kg of body weight Adult athletes: 1.5–2.0 grams per kg of body weight (endurance athletes have a slightly higher requirement than strength athletes) (16)
Recommended intake of protein	12–15% of total calories
Good sources of protein	Meat, poultry, fish, yogurt, eggs, milk; combinations of legumes (beans and dried peas) with cereal grains

PROTEIN FUNCTIONS

➤ *Enzyme and protein synthesis.* There are hundreds of unique tissues and enzymes that are proteins.

➤ *Transports nutrients to the right places.* Proteins make "smart" carriers, enabling nutrients to go to the right tissues.

➤ *A source of energy.* The carbon in protein provides the same amount of energy per unit of weight as carbohydrates (4 calories per gram).

➤ *Hormone production.* Hormones control many chemical activities in the body, and these are made of unique proteins. For instance, testosterone (male hormone) is an important tissue-building hormone.

➤ *Fluid balance.* Protein helps to control the fluid balance between the blood and surrounding tissues. This helps people maintain blood volume and sweat rates during physical activity.

➤ *Acid–base balance.* Proteins can make an acidic environment less acidic and an alkaline environment less alkaline. High-intensity activity can increase cellular acidity (through lactate buildup), which protein can help to buffer.

➤ *Growth and tissue maintenance.* Protein is needed to build and maintain tissue. This is one reason why the protein requirement for growing children can be double that of adults and slightly higher for athletes (17).

➤ *Synthesis of non-protein, nitrogen-containing compounds.* The compound phosphocreatine is a high-energy, nitrogen-containing compound that can quickly release energy over a short duration for quick-burst activities (Table 11.8).

PROTEIN QUALITY

Protein quality is determined by the presence (or absence) of essential amino acids. It is "essential" that we receive these amino acids from food because we are not capable of manufacturing them. Examples of foods containing protein with all the essential amino acids include meats, eggs, milk, cheese, and fish. Non-essential amino acids can be manufactured (synthesized), so it is not "essential" that we consume

Table 11.7	SAMPLE OF GOOD HIGH-PROTEIN SNACKS
Cheese	Tuna sandwich
Chicken	Hamburger
Cooked beef, lamb, or pork strips	Soy burger
Milk	Cottage cheese
Yogurt	Turkey sandwich

Table 11.8 SUPPLEMENTATION WITH CREATINE MONOHYDRATE

Research has shown that creatine monohydrate supplementation might improve performance in repeated high-intensity activities, particularly in athletes with marginal caloric intakes. **HOWEVER, CREATINE MONOHYDRATE SUPPLEMENTATION HAS NEVER BEEN TESTED FOR SAFETY. UNTIL THOSE TESTS ARE DONE, IT SHOULD NOT BE RECOMMENDED TO YOUR CLIENTS.** A safer strategy would be to ensure that people have adequate caloric and protein intakes.

foods that contain them. Most foods contain both non-essential and essential amino acids, but it is the presence of a comprehensive set of essential amino acids that makes a high-quality protein.

People frequently take protein supplements, but these often contain proteins with an incomplete set of essential amino acids, making the supplements low in quality. The best protein supplement would be a few pieces of steak or fish, or an egg. Vegetarians can ensure optimal protein quality by combining cereal grains (rice, wheat, oats) with legumes (dried beans or peas.) Vegetarians are clearly more at risk for inadequate protein intake because the best source of high-quality protein is foods of animal origin (i.e., meat and fish). However, with some good dietary planning, vegetarians can consume enough high-quality protein.

Protein is the focus of many diets (Table 11.9), but there is a tendency to consume too much of it. Studies have found that people do best with protein intakes that supply approximately 15% of total calories or between 1.5 and 2.0 grams of protein per kilogram of body weight. For a 75-kg (165-lb) person, that amounts to no more than 150 grams (600 calories) of protein per day (17). Studies have shown that athletes often have protein intakes of 3 or more grams of protein per kilogram of body weight per day (16). It is quite possible that the perceived benefit from this much protein is actually a calorie (not a protein) benefit. That is, we must supply an adequate amount of

Table 11.9 COMMON SOURCES OF FOODS HIGH IN PROTEIN

Food	Calories from Protein (%)	Total Calories
Tuna, canned in water (3 oz)	93	129
Shrimp, canned (3 oz)	87	97
Chicken, roasted, breast (3 oz)	80	185
Turkey, roasted light meat (3 oz)	79	127
Crab meat, canned (1 cup)	75	123
Chicken, roasted, drumstick (1.6 oz)	73	66
Clams, raw (3 oz)	72	61
Salmon, baked (3 oz)	65	129
Turkey, roasted dark meat (3 oz)	64	150
Beef steak, broiled (5 oz)	62	284
Halibut, broiled, with butter (3 oz)	60	134
Lamb, leg, roasted, lean (2.6 oz)	60	134
Salmon, canned (3 oz)	60	113
Pork, roasted (5 oz)	53	304
Cheese, cheddar (1 oz)	26	109
Peanut butter (1 tbsp)	19	104

Table 11.10	QUICK FACTS FOR FATS
Recommended intakes	Fat intake should provide between 10 and 30% of total calories
Essential fatty acid	Linoleic acid (and alpha-linoleic acid) is the essential fatty acid, and must be provided in consumed foods; this fatty acid is found in corn, sunflower, peanut, and soy oils
Carrier of vitamins	Fat is the carrier of the fat-soluble vitamins: vitamins A, D, E, and K
Calorie-dense nutrient	Fats provide more than twice the calories, per equal weight, of carbohydrate and protein (9 calories vs. 4 calories per gram)
Cholesterol–fat relationship	High fat intakes (not just high cholesterol intakes) result in higher circulating blood cholesterol levels
Food sources	Oil, butter, margarine, fatty meats, fried foods, prepared meats (sausage, bacon, salami), and "whole milk" dairy products

fuel to perform adequately, and the extra consumed protein may be helping people meet their *fuel* needs rather than their *protein* needs.

Protein isn't the best fuel for physical activity, but it is a fuel that helps meet energy needs. There is no question that energy needs must be satisfied before you can consider the best way to distribute carbohydrate, protein, and fat.

Fat

Many people hold the mistaken belief that higher fat intakes can enhance athletic performance. The generally accepted healthy limit for fat intake is no more than 30% of total daily calories. For someone consuming 2500 calories per day, this amounts to 750 calories per day as fat (about 83 grams of fat). Although this is considered the accepted healthy limit, people will do better with fat intakes that are no higher than 25% of daily calories. This level of intake will provide more room in the diet for needed carbohydrates (Tables 11.10 and 11.11).

FAT FUNCTIONS

➤ *Fats are a source of energy.* Fats provide 9 calories per gram (compared with 4 calories per gram from both carbohydrates and proteins).
➤ *Fat provides insulation from extreme temperatures.*
➤ *Cushion against concussive forces.* Fats protect organs against sudden concussive forces, such as a fall or a solid "hit" in football.
➤ *Satiety control.* Fats, because they stay in the stomach longer than other energy nutrients, make us feel fuller longer.
➤ *Fats give our food flavor.*
➤ *Fat carries essential nutrients.* Make sure your clients get the necessary fat-soluble vitamins (A, D, E, and K) and essential fatty acids, which are found in vegetable and cereal oils.

FAT CLASSIFICATIONS AND DEFINITIONS

➤ *Fats and oils:* Fats are solid at room temperature and usually contain a high proportion of saturated fatty acids; oils are liquid at room temperature and typically (there are notable exceptions) contain a high proportion of unsaturated fatty acids.
➤ *Triglycerides, diglycerides, and monoglycerides:* Triglycerides are the most common form of dietary fats and oils, while diglycerides and monoglycerides are less prevalent but still commonly present in the food supply.

Table 11.11   FAT AND CALORIE CONTENT OF COMMON FOODS

Food	Calories from Fat (%)	Total Calories
Butter (1 tbsp)	100	99
Margarine (1 tbsp)	100	99
Mayonnaise (1 tbsp)	100	99
Corn oil (1 tbsp)	100	126
Vegetable shortening (1 tbsp)	100	117
Olive oil (1 tbsp)	100	126
Blue cheese salad dressing (1 tbsp)	90	80
Cream cheese (1 oz)	88	102
1000 island salad dressing (1 tbsp)	87	62
Sour cream (1 tbsp)	87	31
Sausage, brown & serve (1 link)	85	53
Brazil nuts (1 oz)	84	203
Hazelnuts (1 cup)	83	780
Hot dog (1)	83	141
Cream, half & half (1 tbsp)	82	22
Bologna (2 slices)	80	180
Coconut, raw, shredded (1 cup)	80	303
Almonds, whole (1 oz)	74	183
Cheddar cheese (1 oz)	74	109
Feta cheese (1 oz)	73	74
Blue cheese (1 oz)	72	100
Avocado (1 whole)	65	371
Donuts, plain (1)	50	216
Milk, whole (1 cup)	49	148
Chicken, fried breast (1 breast)	46	354
Milk, 2% (1 cup)	36	125
Milk, 1% (1 cup)	25	107

➤ *Short-chain, medium-chain, and long-chain fatty acids:* The most common dietary fatty acids are long-chain, containing 14 or more carbon atoms. Medium–chain triglycerides (MCT oil) have received some attention recently as an effective supplement for increasing caloric intake in athletes. Although MCT oil may hold some promise in this area, it has not been adequately tested.

➤ *Polyunsaturated fatty acids:* These fatty acids have a tendency to lower blood cholesterol. The good thing about these fats is that they are typically associated with lots of vitamin E (found in vegetable and cereal oil, such as corn oil), which many people need.

➤ *Monounsaturated fatty acids:* These fatty acids tend to lower blood cholesterol while maintaining HDL (good) cholesterol (found in olive oil and canola oil).

➤ *Saturated fatty acids:* These fatty acids tend to increase serum cholesterol (found in meats and dairy products).

➤ *Low-density lipoproteins (LDL):* This is the major carrier of cholesterol and other lipids in the blood.

➤ *High-density lipoproteins (HDL):* These lipoproteins carry lipids away from storage and to the liver for metabolism and/or excretion. Because they are associated with removal of cholesterol, they are considered "good cholesterol."

For a 75-kg (165-lb) person consuming a 3000-calorie diet, approximately 600 to 750 calories would come from fat if fat contributed about 25% of total calories. Because fats provide 9 calories per gram, this amounts to between approximately 65 and 85 grams of fat per day. There has been a great deal of attention given to high-fat, high-protein, low-carbohydrate diets recently, but there is no evidence that these diets are useful for enhancing athletic performance. Cheuvront (18) described "The Zone" as a low-carbohydrate diet (both in relative and absolute terms). For instance, a male marathoner weighing 64 kg with 7.5% body fat would, following The Zone, have a 1734-calorie intake, while his predicted caloric requirement is more than 3200 calories. This is a calorically deficient diet by any standard. It is, therefore, quite true that people on The Zone would lose weight because it is an energy-deficient intake. However, your clients must meet energy requirements to sustain power output, so any severely energy deficient diet, such as The Zone (whether it is high fat, high protein, or high carbohydrate), is not recommended for optimizing athletic performance.

VITAMINS AND MINERALS

Vitamins are substances that help essential body reactions take place. The best strategy for ensuring an adequate intake of all the vitamins is to eat a wide variety of foods and consume lots of fresh fruits and vegetables daily. Some vitamins are water soluble, while others are fat soluble. See Tables 11.12 through 11.14 for a summary of major vitamins and minerals. Remember that nutrient balance is a key to optimal nutrition, so people should avoid single-nutrient supplementation unless this has been specifically recommended by a physician to treat an existing nutrient deficiency disease. If a nutrient supplement is warranted because of an obviously poor-quality food intake, people should try a multivitamin, multimineral supplement that provides no more than 100% of the Dietary Reference Intakes (DRI) for each nutrient. The scientific literature suggests that vitamin and mineral deficiencies are uncommon for most people. When deficiencies exist, they are most likely for vitamin B_6 and other B-complex vitamins, iron, and calcium, especially when caloric intake is too low to meet energy demands (19).

Water-Soluble Vitamins

Water-soluble vitamins, including the B vitamins and vitamin C, are vitamins for which we have limited storage capacity. These vitamins are typically associated with carbohydrate foods, such as fresh fruits, breads and cereals, and vegetables. The B vitamins are needed for the metabolism of carbohydrates, proteins, and fats and so are critical to the higher energy requirements of athletes. Luckily, good-quality foods that are high in carbohydrates are typically also foods that provide B vitamins (e.g., enriched breads, enriched cereals, pasta) (20).

Vitamin C is a water-soluble vitamin that is often the focus of supplements taken by most people. Although vitamin C is critical to good health, people should be reminded that the DRI for vitamin C is only 75–90 milligrams (mg), and that level is two standard deviations above the average human requirement. Most supplements contain between 250 and 500 mg of vitamin C or more, providing a good deal more than is needed. On top of the vitamin C intake from foods, which is typically well above the DRI for this vitamin, you can see how easy it is for people to get too much. Although the potential toxicity of vitamin C is relatively low, even an excess of this relatively non-toxic vitamin can increase the risk of kidney stones. People should be encouraged to have a balanced exposure to all the vitamins, a strategy that will help encourage good health and avoid problems associated with excess intake and deficiencies.

Table 11.12 **WATER-SOLUBLE VITAMINS**

Vitamin and Adult Requirement	Functions	Deficiency/Toxicity	Food Sources
Vitamin C (also called L-ascorbate) 75–90 mg/day	· Antioxidant · Collagen formation · Iron absorption · Carnitine synthesis · Norepinephrine synthesis **Athletic Performance: Conflicting study results; as antioxidant, may be useful in alleviating muscle soreness and in aiding muscle recovery**	Deficiency: Scurvy, bleeding gums, fatigue, muscle pain, easy bruising, depression, sudden death	Fresh fruits and vegetables, particularly high in citrus fruits and cherries
Thiamin (also called vitamin B$_1$) 1.1–1.2 mg/day	· Oxidation of carbohydrates · Nerve conduction **Athletic Performance: Conflicting study results**	Deficiency: beriberi (heart disease, weight loss, neurological failure)	Seeds, legumes, pork, enriched/fortified grains and cereals
Riboflavin (also called vitamin B$_2$) 1.1–1.3 mg/day	· Oxidation of carbohydrates and fats · Normal eye function · Healthy skin **Athletic performance: Low-level supplement may be desirable for athletes involved in low-intensity, high-endurance sports**	Deficiency: Swollen tongue, sensitivity to light, cracked lips, fatigue	Milk, liver, whole and enriched grains and cereals
Niacin 14–16 mg/day	· Oxidation of carbohydrates and fats · Electron transport (energy reactions) **Athletic Performance: Conflicting study results**	Deficiency: Pellagra (diarrhea, dermatitis, dementia)	Amino acid tryptophan (60:1 conversion ratio), and enriched grains and cereals
Vitamin B$_6$ (also called pyridoxine, pyridoxal, pyridoxamine) 1.3–1.5 mg/day	· Protein synthesis and breakdown · Conversion of tryptophan to niacin · Glycogen breakdown · Neurotransmitter synthesis **Athletic Performance: Supplement appears to improve performance when food intake is low; because vitamin is toxic if taken in high doses, best strategy is to consume adequate calories**	Deficiency: Neurological problems Toxicity: Sensory neuropathy (loss of sensation in the fingers)	Meat, fish, potatoes, sweet potatoes, bananas, vegetables

continued

Table 11.12 WATER-SOLUBLE VITAMINS (CONTINUED)

Vitamin and Adult Requirement	Functions	Deficiency/Toxicity	Food Sources
Pantothenic acid 5 mg/day	Energy reactions for carbohydrates, proteins, and fats Fatty acid synthesis **Athletic Performance: Studies inconclusive**	Deficiency: GI tract problems; fatigue	In almost every food (deficiency is very rare)
Biotin 30 micrograms (μg)/day	Carbon dioxide transfer (normal respiration)	Deficiency: Dermatitis, anorexia, and hair loss (deficiency is extremely rare)	Egg yolk, nuts, legumes, bacterial synthesis in the gut
Vitamin B$_{12}$ (also called cyanocobalamin) 2.4 μg/day	· Red blood cell formation · Folate use	Deficiency: Pernicious anemia, neurological degeneration, loss of mental function	Foods of animal origin and intestinal synthesis (pure vegetarians may be at risk for deficiency)
Folic acid (also called folate) 400 μg/day	· Synthesis of DNA · Cell division · Maturation of red blood cells	Deficiency: Neural tube defects in offspring of deficient women, megaloblastic anemia	Organ meats, green leafy vegetables, whole-grain foods (this may be the most common vitamin deficiency)

Adapted from Manore M, Thompson J. Sports Nutrition for Health and Performance. Champaign, IL: Human Kinetics, 2000; Williams MH. Nutrition for Health, Fitness & Sport. 6th ed. Boston: McGraw-Hill, 2002; and Benardot D. Nutrition for Serious Athletes: An Advanced Guide to Foods, Fluids, and Supplements for Training and Performance. Champaign, IL: Human Kinetics, 2000.

Table 11.13 FAT-SOLUBLE VITAMINS

Vitamin and Adult Requirement	Functions	Deficiency/Toxicity	Food Sources
Vitamin A (retinol) ~1000 retinol equivalents 700–900 μg/day (This vitamin is-potentially highly toxic taken in large amounts)	· Vision · Growth · Reproduction · Immune function · Healthy skin **Athletic Performance: No evidence that supplementation aids performance**	Deficiency: Night blindness, eye disease, growth failure, unhealthy skin, susceptibility to infections Toxicity: Headache, vomiting, hair loss, bone abnormalities, liver damage, death	Fish liver oils, liver, butter, vitamin A + D–added milk, egg yolk Pro-vitamin A (beta-carotene) in dark-green leafy vegetables, yellow vegetables and fruits, and fortified margarines
Vitamin D (ergocalciferol and cholecalciferol) Requirement difficult to establish because of variations in sunlight exposure 5 μg/day (This vitamin is extremely toxic taken in high amounts)	· Calcium absorption · Phosphorus absorption · Mineralization of bone **Athletic Performance: No studies**	Deficiency: Rickets in children, osteomalacia in adults, poor bone mineralization Toxicity (This is the most toxic of the vitamins): Renal damage, cardiovascular damage, high blood calcium, calcium deposits in soft tissues	Fish-liver oils, fortified (A & D) milk, skin synthesis with exposure to light; small amounts found in butter, liver, egg yolk, and canned salmon and sardines
Vitamin E (alpha-tocopherol) 15 mg/day	· Powerful antioxidant · Involved in immune function **Athletic Performance: Antioxidant properties may be useful in preventing oxidative damage and/or in muscle recovery**	Deficiency: Premature breakdown of red blood cells, anemia in infants, easy peroxidative damage of cells	Vegetable oils, green leafy vegetables, nuts, legumes (foods of animal origin are NOT good sources)
Vitamin K (phylloquinone K₁, menaquinone, menadione) 90–120 μg/day	Involved in blood clotting (referred to as the antihemorrhagic vitamin) **Athletic Performance: Athletes taking EPO could be at serious risk taking vitamin K supplements**	Deficiency: Longer clotting time	Green leafy vegetables and intestinal bacterial synthesis

Adapted from Manore M, Thompson J. Sports Nutrition for Health and Performance. Champaign, IL: Human Kinetics, 2000; Williams MH. Nutrition for Health, Fitness & Sport. 6th ed. Boston: McGraw-Hill, 2002; and Benardot D. Nutrition for Serious Athletes: An Advanced Guide to Foods, Fluids, and Supplements for Training and Performance. Champaign, IL: Human Kinetics, 2000.

Table 11.14 MINERALS

Minerals and Adult Requirement	Functions	Deficiency/Toxicity	Food Sources
Calcium 1,000 mg/day	· Structure of bones and teeth · Blood coagulation · Nerve impulse transmission · Muscle contraction · Acid–base control **Particularly critical in athletes to ensure adequate bone density to reduce the risk of stress fractures**	Deficiency: Reduced bone density, osteoporosis, stress fractures	Milk and other dairy foods, dark green leafy vegetables, canned fish (with bones), calcium-fortified orange juice
Phosphorus 700 mg/day	· Structure of bones and teeth · Component of ATP and other energy-yielding compounds · Part of many B vitamin coenzymes · Part of DNA and RNA · Acid–base control	Deficiency (rare) may occur with large, long-term intakes of magnesium-containing antacids	Meats, cereals, grains, and dairy products
Iron 700 mg/day	· Involved in oxygen transfer to cells (hemoglobin in blood; myoglobin in muscle) · In numerous oxidative enzymes **Commonly inadequate in athletes, resulting in poor performance and other health problems**	Deficiency: Microcytic anemia, leading to weakness, loss of energy, easy fatigue (this is the most common mineral deficiency)	Most absorbable iron: Meats, poultry, fish, egg yolk Less absorbable iron: Dark-green vegetables, legumes, peaches, apricots, prunes, raisins
Zinc 8–11 mg/day	· Immune system · Wound healing · In more than 70 enzymes involved in energy metabolism	Deficiency: Growth retardation, poor wound healing, frequent infections, muscle weakness	Seafood, organ meat, meat, wheat germ, yeast (most plant foods are not good sources)
Magnesium 320–420 mg/day	· Energy metabolism of carbohydrate and fat · Protein synthesis · Water balance · Muscle contractions	Deficiency: Muscle weakness	Available in many foods, but highest in meats, whole-grain cereals, seeds, and legumes

Adapted from Manore M, Thompson J. Sports Nutrition for Health and Performance. Champaign, IL: Human Kinetics, 2000; Williams MH. Nutrition for Health, Fitness & Sport. 6th ed. Boston: McGraw-Hill, 2002; and Benardot D. Nutrition for Serious Athletes: An Advanced Guide to Foods, Fluids, and Supplements for Training and Performance. Champaign, IL: Human Kinetics, 2000.

Fat-Soluble Vitamins

Fat-soluble vitamins are those vitamins that are delivered with fats and oils. For instance, milk is fortified with the fat-soluble vitamins A and D, which are in the fat component (cream) of the milk. Vegetable and cereal oils are excellent sources of vitamin E, an important antioxidant that can help protect cells from becoming damaged through oxidation. This is very important because physical activity increases the amount of oxygen pulled into cells, thereby increasing the risk for oxidative damage.

Supplements of vitamins A and D should be taken only under the advice of a physician because of their high potential toxicity.

MINERALS

Minerals are inorganic substances that are involved in water balance, nerve impulse stimulation, acid–base balance, and energy reactions (see Table 11.4). Iron and zinc are critically important for energy metabolism but are also among the nutrients of which people may not be consuming enough. This is particularly true of vegetarians, because the best source of these minerals is red meat.

The most common nutrient deficiency in most industrialized countries is a deficiency in iron. Because of the prevalence of this deficiency, people (especially females) should periodically have a blood test to determine iron status. This test should include an assessment of hemoglobin, hematocrit, and ferritin. An assessment of iron status is particularly important for vegetarians or people who are on weight loss diets.

FLUID AND HYDRATION

Water carries nutrients to cells and carries waste products away from cells. It serves as a body lubricant and, through sweat, helps to maintain body temperature. Lean tissue (muscles and organs) is more than 70% water, and about 60% of total body weight is water (17). A failure to supply sufficient water is more likely to cause quick death than a failure to supply any other single nutrient.

We lose water through breathing (breath is moist), through the skin (this happens even if there is no obvious "sweat"), and through urine, sweat, and feces. It is critically important to consume sufficient fluid to maintain body water stores, yet most people rarely stay optimally hydrated. In fact, many people commonly wait until they become extremely thirsty (indicating a state of dehydration) before they consume fluids. Weight stability before and after exercise is a good indication that water needs have been met during an exercise program. People who experience significant weight (i.e., water) loss during practice should learn how to drink more fluid to stabilize weight, since a 2% body weight loss is associated with reduced performance.

Meeting Fluid Needs

A key to athletic success is *avoidance* of a state of underhydration. This is not as easy as it may seem, because many people rely on "thirst" as the alarm bell for when to drink. Thirst, however, is a delayed sensation that does not occur until the person has already lost 1 to 2 liters of fluid. Because of this, people should learn to consume fluids on a fixed time interval rather than relying on thirst for when to drink. Staying optimally hydrated and fueled during exercise has multiple benefits, including (16):

➤ A less pronounced increase in heart rate
➤ A less pronounced increase in core body temperature
➤ Improvement in cardiac stroke volume and cardiac output
➤ Improvement in skin blood flow (enabling better sweat rates and improved cooling)
➤ Maintenance of better blood volume
➤ A reduction in net muscle glycogen usage (improving endurance)

Fluid intake recommendations are to (2, 21):

➤ Drink as much as needed to match sweat losses
➤ Not rely on thirst as a stimulus to drink (the thirst sensation will only occur after 1 to 2 liters—1 to 2% of body weight—has already been lost)
➤ Sweat rates are often 1 to 2 liters per hour, and it is difficult to consume and absorb enough fluid to match these losses
➤ Consumption of large volumes of fluid increases the risk of gastrointestinal distress, thereby affecting performance
➤ Ingestion of large volumes of dilute, low (or no) sodium fluid may increase the risk of hyponatremia
➤ If left on their own, athletes will often develop dehydration even when there are sufficient fluids nearby for them to consume
➤ To ensure better athlete compliance, fluids should be cool, should taste good, and should be readily available

Fluid Consumption Guidelines (22)

Before training and competition	• Drink adequate fluids the day before • Drink at least 2 cups (17–20 oz) of fluid 2 to 3 hours before exercise or competition
During training and competition	• Replace sweat losses • Drink 7–10 oz every 10 to 20 minutes
After training and competition	• Monitor fluid losses • Drink 3 cups (24 oz) for every 1 lb of weight lost through sweat (you should replace 150% of sweat losses because you are continuing to sweat) • Rehydrate within 2 hours post-exercise

The National Athletic Trainers' Association (NATA) guidelines are useful for avoiding dehydration, but the type of fluids consumed is also important for achieving optimal performance. In general, studies have shown that a 6% carbohydrate solution, such as that found in some sports beverages, is ideal from the standpoint of gastric emptying and intestinal absorption for reducing mental and physical fatigue during both stop-and-go sports and endurance sports, for encouraging drinking during physical activity, and for improving performance. Studies comparing a 6% carbohydrate solution with water and solutions with a higher carbohydrate concentration have consistently found that the 6% solution is best (2).

Water versus Sports Drinks

There are clear advantages for sports drinks over water for most exercising adults (22):

➤ Water provides no flavor or electrolytes, which cause people to want to drink. Beverages that cause people to *want* to drink help them stay well hydrated. Studies show that people drink 25% more sports drink than water, and young children will drink 90% more sports beverage than water (23, 24).
➤ Water has no energy while sports beverages contain carbohydrate. The carbohydrate helps to provide muscles with needed fuel to avoid early fatigue and poor performance.
➤ The sodium provided by sports beverages helps to maintain blood volume, a factor that is critical to maintaining sweat rates and performance. Sweat contains sodium that water alone does not replace (Table 11.15).

Table 11.15	**WARNING SIGNS OF DEHYDRATION, HEAT EXHAUSTION, AND HEAT STROKE: WHAT TO DO**
Dehydration with loss of energy & performance	Drink carbohydrate- and electrolyte-containing sports drinks; avoid beverages with carbonation, which can cause GI distress.
Dehydration with muscle cramps	Immediately stop exercising and massage the cramping muscle(s); consuming a sports beverage that contains sodium may help relieve the cramp.
Heat exhaustion with dizziness, light-headedness, and cold, clammy skin	Immediately replace fluids while in a cool, shaded area until the dizziness passes; stretching may improve circulation and prevent fainting; lying with the legs elevated will improve blood circulation to the head, thereby alleviating the dizziness.
Heat exhaustion with nausea/headaches	Rest in a cool place until the nausea passes; drinking fluids to rehydrate is critical; lying down may help relieve headaches.
Heat stroke with high body temperature and dry skin	Immediately get out of the heat and seek immediate medical treatment; feeling chilly with arms tingling and with goose bumps means skin circulation has shut down and heat stroke is imminent; this is an extremely serious condition that must be immediately treated.
Heat stroke with confusion or unconsciousness	Confusion strongly suggests, and unconsciousness confirms, heat stroke. This is a medical emergency that calls for fast cooling with ice baths or any other available means to lower body temperature.

Adapted from Casa DJ, Armstrong LE, Hillman SK, et al. National Athletic Trainers' Association position statement: fluid replacement for athletes. J Athl Train 2000;35(2):212–224.

DIETARY SUPPLEMENTS AND ERGOGENIC AIDS

Dietary supplements are concentrated sources of vitamins, minerals, and energy substrates that are taken to "supplement" the nutrients derived from foods. Ergogenic aids are substances that enhance a person's athletic ability, either through improvement in power or enhanced endurance. The terms "dietary supplements" and "ergogenic aids" often are used interchangeably, but they are not the same.

Dietary supplements may be used to conveniently intervene in a known dietary deficiency, while ergogenic aids are often taken for the sole purpose of improved performance whether or not there is a known deficiency. It is common, for instance, for people with iron deficiency anemia to be pre-scribed iron supplements to help them supplement the iron they are getting from the food they eat and build up their iron stores. The proven effectiveness for many nutritional supplements, in the face of a nutrient deficiency disorder, has been demonstrated in numerous clinical trials. However, there is no evidence that it is useful or warranted to take high doses of dietary supplements in the absence of a known nutrient deficiency. An example of the overuse of dietary supplements is protein and/or amino acids (the building blocks of protein). In fact, excess nutrients may cause toxicity or, at the very least, create the need to expel the excess nutrients. People wishing to take a nutrient supplement without the diagnosis of a specific nutrient deficiency should limit their intake to multivitamin, multimineral supplements that provide no more than 100% of the recommended daily allowances.

Ergogenic aids, on the other hand, have typically not been tested for either effectiveness or safety. There are two ergogenic aids that have been clearly shown to improve a person's capacity to perform better: carbohydrates and water. With the exception of these, there is little consistent evidence to suggest that other substances touted as having an "ergogenic benefit" actually do anything to improve performance (Table 11.16). When ergogenic aids do work, it is usually because they help meet energy or nutritional requirements as a result of poor eating behaviors. It is clearly healthier and less costly to eat better foods than to rely on substances that are often of unknown origin and unknown quality and untested for safety or effectiveness.

Table 11.16	A SAMPLE OF PRODUCTS COMMONLY SOLD AS ERGOGENIC AIDS
Supplement	**Facts**
Androstenedione	Advertised as useful for increasing muscular strength and size. It is a hormone that is used to synthesize the hormone testosterone. (Testosterone is a male anabolic steroid hormone that is known to aid in the development of muscle mass.) There may be negative side effects (increased body hair and cancer are established problems) similar to those of testosterone, but studies on efficacy and safety have not been published. *This substance is banned by the IOC, NCAA, USOC, NFL, and NHL.*
Caffeine	Advertised as useful for improving endurance by enabling more effective fat metabolism during exercise. It is a central nervous system stimulant but has a reduced dose effect (people adapt to it, so increasingly higher doses are needed to obtain an ergogenic benefit). In high doses, caffeine may have a diuretic effect, thereby increasing the chance for dehydration. While in the past caffeine was on the banned substance list by the IOC, it was removed from this list early in 2004.
Creatine	Creatine is synthesized from three amino acids and is part of phospho*creatine*, which is a fuel used anaerobically to initiate high-intensity activity. However, stored phosphocreatine suffices to support activity for only several seconds and must be resynthesized for use in similar subsequent activities. It is hypothesized that supplemental creatine aids in this resynthesis, and some studies have shown that creatine supplementation is effective in maintaining strength/power for repeated bouts of short-duration, high-intensity activities. However, creatine supplementation is associated with weight increases (from muscle or water or both), and studies have not evaluated its effectiveness in athletes who are known to be consuming sufficient energy. In addition, the safety of creatine supplementation has not been adequately studied.
Ephedrine	This is a central nervous stimulant that is sold over-the-counter as a decongestant. *Its use is banned by the NCAA and the IOC,* and it has undesirable side effects when taken in frequent and/or large doses. (The Food and Drug Administration (FDA) recommends a maximum of no more than 8 mg/dose provided three times daily for a maximum of 7 days when used as a decongestant.) The side effects associated with ephedrine include increased heart rate, increased blood pressure, and nervousness, all of which are associated with strokes, seizures, and heart attacks. Caffeine consumption appears to increase the effect of ephedrine. It is theorized that ephedrine improves athletic performance and reduces body weight. Its chemical similarity to amphetamine suggests that it may lower appetite and thus have an impact on weight, but there is no evidence that it improves athletic performance.
Ginseng	There are numerous claims for ginseng, ranging from a cure for all ills to improving energy to enhancing immune function. However, it has been difficult to do athletic performance studies with ginseng because concentrations of the active ingredient(s) vary widely within and between brands. Therefore, there is no good evidence to support supplemental ginseng as an ergogenic substance. Luckily, it also appears that ginseng consumption has little risk of producing negative side effects, with the possible exception of causing insomnia in some subjects.
L-Carnitine	This is a substance produced by the body and used to transport fat into cell mitochondria so it can be used as energy. It is theorized that taking carnitine supplements will increase the amount of fat that is moved into mitochondria, thereby increasing the total amount of fat burned and helping to reduce body fat levels. There is no solid evidence that supplementary carnitine has this effect.
Medium-chain triglycerides (MCT oil)	MCT oil is sold as a substance that can improve muscular development and increase the loss of body fat by increasing metabolic rate. While there is no evidence of these effects, MCT oil may be an effective means of increasing total caloric intake in athletes with high energy requirements who are having difficulty meeting energy needs. It is metabolized more like a carbohydrate than a fat, but is has a higher energy density than carbohydrates. Large intakes may be associated with gastrointestinal disturbances.

Table 11.16	A SAMPLE OF PRODUCTS COMMONLY SOLD AS ERGOGENIC AIDS *(CONTINUED)*
Omega-3 fatty acids (fish oils, canola oils)	It is hypothesized that omega-3 fatty acids stimulate the production of growth hormone (somatotrophin), thereby enhancing the potential for muscular development. It is well established that omega-3 fatty acids reduce red-cell stickiness, thereby reducing the chance for a blood clot leading to a heart attack. Omega-3 fatty acids are also associated with a reduced inflammatory response in tissues through the production of specific prostaglandins. One of these prostaglandins (E1) may be associated with the production of growth hormone. While supplemental intake of omega-3 fatty acids may not be warranted, there is sufficient evidence of some beneficial effects that athletes should consider consuming cold-water fish (salmon, tuna) twice weekly.
Pyruvic acid (pyruvate)	Pyruvate is produced from carbohydrates as a result of anaerobic metabolism and is a principle fuel leading into aerobic metabolism. It has been hypothesized, therefore, that supplemental pyruvate will enhance aerobic metabolism and promote fat loss. However, since carbohydrate intake adequately satisfies the entire need for pyruvate, it makes little sense that supplementation of pyruvate will improve performance.

Adapted from Manore M, Thompson J. Sports Nutrition for Health and Performance. Champaign, IL: Human Kinetics, 2000; Williams MH. Nutrition for Health, Fitness & Sport. 6th ed. Boston: McGraw-Hill, 2002; and Benardot D. Nutrition for Serious Athletes: An Advanced Guide to Foods, Fluids, and Supplements for Training and Performance. Champaign, IL: Human Kinetics, 2000.

PRACTICAL CONSIDERATIONS

One Day before a Competition

> Avoid high-fat foods such as fried food, chips, cake, and chocolate
> Eat a good breakfast (e.g., toast, oatmeal, cereal, milk, and fruit)
> Have sandwiches, rolls, pasta, or rice for lunch
> Have rice, pasta, noodles, or potatoes plus vegetables and lean meat, chicken, or fish for dinner and yogurt and fruit for dessert
> Eat a carbohydrate snack at dinner
> Drink an extra 16 oz (475 mL) of fluid throughout the day

Immediately before Exercise or Competition

The pre-exercise meal should focus on providing carbohydrates and fluids. Ideally, people should consume a high-carbohydrate, low-fat meal 3 hours before exercising or before competition. Light carbohydrate snacks (e.g., crackers) and carbohydrate-containing beverages can be consumed after the meal and before exercise, provided large amounts are not consumed at one time. There are several goals for the pre-exercise meal, including (20):

> Making certain that athletes obtain sufficient energy to see them through as much of the exercise bout as possible
> Preventing feelings of hunger (hungry people may be letting blood sugar get low, which is not a good way to start an exercise bout)
> Consuming enough fluids to begin exercise in a fully hydrated state
> Consuming only familiar foods
> Avoiding foods high in fiber or foods that cause gas (e.g., broccoli, cauliflower)
> Drinking 17 to 20 oz (500–600 mL) of fluid 2 to 3 hours before practice or competition
> Drinking an additional 7 to 10 oz (200–300 mL) of fluid 10 to 20 minutes before practice or competition

Table 11.17	PRACTICAL SUGGESTION FOR ASSESSING FLUID INTAKE DURING EXERCISE

Weigh an athlete before and after exercise. If the weight difference is more than 1 lb (0.45 kg), the person did not consume enough fluid during exercise to maintain an optimal hydration state.

During Exercise or Competition

There is evidence that people involved in stop-and-go sports of relatively short duration benefit from consumption of carbohydrate-containing drinks (see hydration recommendations on page 256). For long-duration activities that allow for consumption of solid foods (e.g., cycling, cross-country skiing), some people prefer to periodically consume bananas, breads, and other easy-to-digest carbohydrate foods (Table 11.17). If solid foods are consumed, there should still be ample consumption of carbohydrate-containing beverages. Drink 28 to 40 oz of fluid (sports beverages containing a 6 to 7% carbohydrate solution and electrolytes are preferred) per hour. This corresponds to about 7 to 10 oz (200–300 mL) every 10 to 15 minutes, but this amount may need to be adjusted on the basis of body size, sweat rate, exercise intensity, and environmental conditions. Two main goals are to avoid dehydration and to avoid the mental and muscular fatigue that can be caused by inadequate carbohydrate (20).

After Exercise or Competition

Muscles are receptive to replacing stored glycogen following exercise. Because of this, people should consume 200 to 400 calories from carbohydrates immediately following activity and then an additional 200 to 300 calories from carbohydrates within the next several hours. People who have difficulty eating foods immediately following exhaustive exercise should try high-carbohydrate liquid supplements (20). Some examples of high-carbohydrate foods are included in Table 11.18.

After exercise, people should drink at least 20 oz (600 mL) of fluid per pound of body weight that was lost during the exercise session (25). This should be consumed within 2 hours of finishing the practice or competition, with the goal of returning body weight to near pre-exercise weight before the next exercise bout.

Eating on the Road

Although it may take a little more effort to maintain a proper diet while traveling, it is well worth the effort. These suggestions should help your clients maintain a diet that will keep up your their

Table 11.18	EXAMPLES OF HIGH-CARBOHYDRATE FOODS

Food	Calories	Carbohydrate (%)
1 bagel	165	76
2 slices bread	135	81
1 Gatorade energy bar	250	75
1 cup plain pasta	215	81
3 cups popcorn	70	79
1 baked potato	100	88
1 apple	80	100
1 orange	65	100
1 cup vegetable juice	55	93

level. Try these strategies recommended by the Department of Nutritional Sciences, Cooperative Extension, of the University of Arizona (26):

Try to pack nutrient-dense foods for the trip. *Many foods can be packed easily in a gym bag or suitcase. By bringing your own food, you can eat familiar foods. This is especially important when traveling to a foreign country, where familiar foods may be harder to find. Foods such as sports bars, dried fruits, granola bars, bagels, and canned tuna are nutrient dense and travel easily.*

Upon arriving at your destination, make a trip to the local store to pick up some essentials. *Picking up some basic foods can allow some meals to be eaten in the hotel, especially if there is a microwave and refrigerator available. Some of these items may include fresh fruits and vegetables, applesauce, cheese, breads, and soups.*

If eating in hotel rooms or packing foods is an impossibility, it is still possible to eat for performance at restaurants. *Most restaurants have lower fat items from which to choose. In some cases finding these lower fat items may take some detective work, but in other instances the restaurant may have some healthier items already indicated on the menu. In either case, it is important to know what to look for. The following are some general guidelines.*

Breakfast
- *Order pancakes, French toast, muffins, toast, cereal, fruit, and juices. These are all higher in carbohydrate and lower in fat than traditional egg and bacon breakfasts.*
- *Request that toast, pancakes, etc. be served without butter or margarine. Use syrup or jam but no butter or margarine to keep carbohydrate high and fat to a minimum.*
- *Choose low-fat dairy products (e.g., skim or 1% milk, low-fat yogurt, low-fat cheese).*
- *Fresh fruit may be expensive or difficult to find. Carry fresh and/or dried fruits.*
- *Cold cereal can be a good breakfast or snack; carry boxes in the car or on the bus. Keep low-fat milk in cooler or purchase at convenience stores.*

Lunch
- *On sandwiches look for lower fat meats such as turkey and chicken. Remember that most of the fat in sandwiches is found in the spread. Prepare or order without the "mayo," "special sauce," or butter. Use ketchup or mustard instead.*
- *Choose foods that are broiled, baked, microwaved, steamed, or boiled rather than fried and try to avoid breaded items. Salad bars can be lifesavers, but watch the dressing, olives, fried croutons, nuts, and seeds— you could end up with more fat than any super-burger could hope to hold!*
- *Choose low-fat salad dressings. If low-fat dressings aren't available, pack your own.*
- *Baked potatoes should be ordered with butter and sauces "on the side." Add just enough to moisten the carbohydrate-rich potato.*
- *Soups and crackers can be good low-fat meals; stay away from cream soups.*
  Juices, low-fat milk, and low-fat milk shakes are a more nutritious choice than soda pop.

Dinner
- *Go to restaurants that offer high-carbohydrate foods such as pasta, baked potatoes, rice, breads, vegetables, salad bars, and fruits.*
- *Eat thick crust pizzas with low-fat toppings such as green peppers, mushrooms, Canadian bacon, and onions. Avoid fatty meats such as pepperoni or sausage, extra cheese, and olives.*
- *Eat breads without butter or margarine—use jelly instead. Ask for salads with dressing "on the side" so that you can add minimal amounts yourself. Ask for low-fat salad dressings.*

Snacks
- *Whole grain breads, muffins, bagels, tortillas, fruit, fruit breads, low-fat crackers, pretzels, unbuttered popcorn, oatmeal raisin cookies, fig bars, animal crackers, fruit juice, carrot sticks, cherry tomatoes, breakfast cereal, canned liquid meals, dried and fresh fruits*

Don't forget about fluids. To prevent dehydration you should keep well hydrated at all times, even on the road, by drinking frequently before, during, and after exercise.

- *Do not drown your thirst in calories! Drink plenty of water.*
- *In restaurants, including fast food ones, ask for water in addition to other beverages. Request that a pitcher of water be left at your table.*
- *You can buy bottled water or mineral water at grocery stores and convenience stores.*
- *Carry squeeze bottles of water, sports drinks, and fruit juices with you, especially on long airplane flights.*
- *Limit caffeinated or alcoholic beverages. Caffeine and alcohol are diuretics and cause fluid loss.*

ANSWERS TO FREQUENTLY ASKED NUTRITIONAL QUESTIONS

Should I Take Protein Supplements?

Protein supplements are popular in most sports, at most athletic levels—from beginners to elite athletes and regardless of the goals of the people taking them. Some people take protein supplements to lose weight, some to gain weight, some to gain muscle, some to make them stronger, and some to increase endurance. The fact is that humans are incapable of using protein for anabolic (tissue-building) purposes above the level of approximately 1.5 grams of protein per kilogram of body weight. Protein taken in excess of this amount is either burned as a source of energy (calories) or stored as fat. Neither of the latter two options are particularly good, since people rarely wish to put on additional fat weight, and getting rid of excess nitrogenous waste can make you dehydrated.

WHAT ABOUT CREATINE?

Creatine monohydrate supplements have been shown to help maintain power on repeated bouts of high-intensity activity. However, this benefit may be a result of an inadequate caloric intake in the tested subjects. As creatine monohydrate use has never been tested for safety (there is beginning evidence that taking supplements may alter the body's synthesis of creatine), it makes sense to avoid taking creatine but begin making certain that energy (calorie) consumption matches need. A good strategy for doing this is to eat small, frequent meals high in carbohydrates.

Should I Consume Sports Drinks or Does Water Work Just As Well?

Sports drinks contain carbohydrate and electrolytes that are useful in maintaining water and energy balance. Studies of endurance athletes, athletes in stop-and-go sports, and athletes in power sports all show that consumption of sports drinks during practice and competition does a better job of enhancing athletic performance than water alone.

Should I Stay Away from Caffeinated Beverages before a Workout?

People adapt to caffeine, so if you are accustomed to having a cup of coffee or a caffeine-containing cola there should be no problem with consuming it before a workout. You should never increase the consumption of a caffeinated food or beverage before exercise above a level to which you are accustomed. This would likely increase your heart rate and have a diuretic effect that could make you dehydrated.

Should I Skip Lunch if I'm Trying to Lower My Body Fat Level?

Skipping meals is one of the biggest reasons people have high body fat levels. If you are trying to lose body fat, your goal should be to maintain blood sugar levels through the consumption of small, frequent meals. Skipping a meal will cause you to produce excess insulin the next time you eat, which will make *more* fat than if you ate more frequently.

Will a High-Protein, Low-Carbohydrate Diet Help Me Lose Weight?

There is nothing in the literature to suggest that lowering carbohydrate intake is useful for improving exercise performance. On the contrary, inadequate carbohydrate intake is almost always associated with reduced performance. High-protein, low-carbohydrate diets are typically low-calorie diets—the reason for the weight loss. However, dramatic reductions in caloric intake almost always result in a rebounding of weight. The best strategy for weight loss is to consume a little less than is currently needed to maintain current weight (say, about 300 calories less) and to eat small, frequent meals to maintain blood sugar levels.

Should I Eat or Drink Anything during Exercise?

Maintaining a constant flow of carbohydrates to muscles and maintaining blood sugar during competition is an important strategy for success. Your clients should consider sipping on a sports beverage during competition to achieve this result. If there are long breaks during an exercise workout, then consuming a carbohydrate snack (e.g., crackers, bread) might be acceptable provided that fluid is also consumed.

I'm a Profuse Sweater and Occasionally Get Serious Cramps. Is There Anything I Should Be Doing to Avoid This Problem?

Cramps are typically associated with dehydration and sodium loss. Try making certain that sufficient sodium-containing fluids (i.e., sports beverages) are consumed during practice and competition. Unless you have a history of high blood pressure, you should also consider adding a small amount of salt to the food you eat, following with plenty of water.

How Can I Tell if I'm Dehydrated?

The easiest way to tell is that your urine will be dark, and there won't be very much of it. Light-colored or clear urine is a sign of adequate hydration, while dark urine suggests dehydration. It takes time to rehydrate, so avoiding dehydration is the appropriate strategy.

REFERENCES

1. McArdle W, Katch F, Katch V. Sports & Exercise Nutrition. Philadelphia: Lippincott Williams & Wilkins, 1999.
2. ACSM. Position statement: nutrition and athletic performance. Med Sci Sports Exerc 2000;32(12):2130–2145.
3. Lamb DR. Basic Principles for Improving Sport Performance. Barrington, IL: Gatorade Sports Science Institute, Sports Science Exchange. Publ no. 55. 1995:8(2).
4. Deutz B, Benardot D, Martin D, Cody M. Relationship between energy deficits and body composition in elite female gymnasts and runners. Med Sci Sports Exerc 2000;32(3):659–668.
5. Iwao S, Mori K, Sato Y. Effects of meal frequency on body composition during weight control in boxers. Scand J Med Sci Sports 1996;6(5):265–272.
6. Jenkins DJ, Wolever TM, Vuksan V, et al. Nibbling versus gorging: metabolic advantages of increased meal frequency. N Engl J Med 1989;321:929–934.
7. Luke A, Schoeller DA. Basal metabolic rate, fat-free mass, and body cell mass during energy restriction. Metabolism 1992; 41(4):450–456.
8. LeBlanc J, Mercier I, Nadeau A. Components of postprandial thermogenesis in relation to meal frequency in humans. Can J Physiol Pharmacol 1993;71(12):879–883.
9. Hawley JA, Burke LM. Meal frequency and physical performance. Br J Nutr 1997;77:S91–103.
10. Metzner HL, Lamphiear DE, Wheeler NC, Larkin FA. The relationship between frequency of eating and adiposity in adult men and women in the Tecumseh Community Health Study. Am J Clin Nutr 1977;30:712–715.
11. Zvolankova K. The frequency of meals: its relation to overweight, hyper-cholesterolaemia, and decreased glucose tolerance. Lancet 1964;614–615.
12. Benardot D, Martin DE, Thompson WR. Maintaining energy balance: a key for effective physical conditioning. Am J Med Sports 2002;4(1):25–30, 40.
13. USDA Nutrient Data Laboratory, Agricultural Research Service. USDA National Nutrient Database for Standard Reference Release 17. Washington, DC: Government Printing Office, 2004.
14. Romijn JA, Coyle EF, Sidossis LS, et al. Regulation of endogenous fat and carbohydrate metabolism in relation to exercise intensity and duration. Am J Physiol 1993;265(3):E380–391.

15. Rankin JW. Glycemic Index and Exercise Metabolism. Barrington, IL: Gatorade Sports Science Institute, Sports Science Exchange. Publ no. 64. 1997;10(1).

16. Manore M, Thompson J. Sports Nutrition for Health and Performance. Champaign, IL: Human Kinetics, 2000.

17. Williams MH. Nutrition for Health, Fitness & Sport. 6th ed. Boston: McGraw-Hill, 2002.

18. Cheuvront SN. The 'Zone' diet and athletic performance. Sports Med 1999;27:213–228.

19. Benardot D, Clarkson P, Coleman E, Manore M. Can vitamin supplements improve sports performance? GSSI Sports Science Exchange Roundtable. Publ no. 45, 2001;12(3).

20. Benardot D. Nutrition for Serious Athletes: An Advanced Guide to Foods, Fluids, and Supplements for Training and Performance. Champaign, IL: Human Kinetics, 2000.

21. Horswill CA. Effective fluid replacement. Int J Sports Nutr 1998;8:175–195.

22. Casa DJ, Armstrong LE, Hillman SK, et al. National Athletic Trainers' Association position statement: fluid replacement for athletes. J Athl Train 2000;35(2):212–224.

23. Gatorade Sports Science Institute. Fluids 2000: Sports Drinks vs. Water. Barrington, IL: Sports Science Center Topics, 2000.

24. Bar-Or O, Wilk B. Water and electrolyte replenishment in the exercising child. Int J Sport Nutr 1996;6(2):93–99.

25. Wilk B, Bar-Or O. Effect of drink flavor and NaCl on voluntary drinking and hydration in boys exercising in the heat. J Appl Physiol 1996;80:1112–1117.

26. Department of Nutritional Sciences, Cooperative Extension, The University of Arizona. Eating on the Road. Available at: http://ag.arizona.edu/nsc/new/sn/HP-eatonrd.htm. Accessed December, 2002.

Initial Client Consultation, Goals/Objectives, Screening, and Assessments

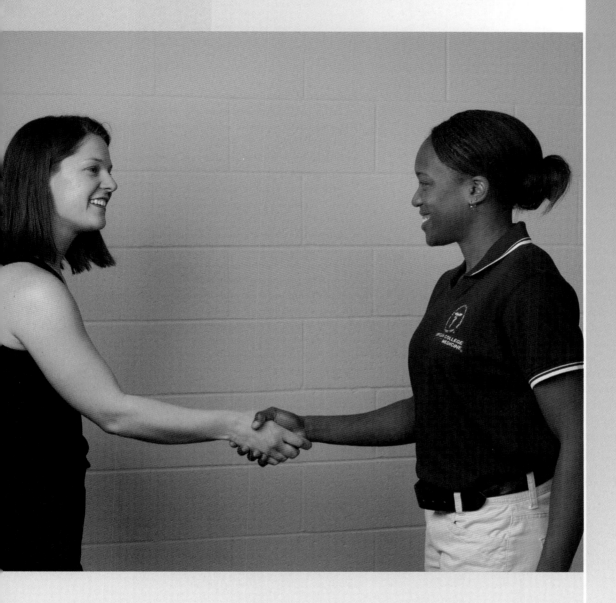

The Initial Client Consultation

Kenneth E. Baldwin, M.Ed., A.H. Ismail Center for Health, Exercise & Nutrition, Department of Health and Kinesiology, College of Liberal Arts, Purdue University, West Lafayette, Indiana

Chapter Outline

Objectives

- Use the potential client intake form to guide you through the initial client contact
- Understand the importance of the initial client consultation and how to structure the meeting
- Know the necessary steps to design and develop a client welcome packet
- Understand the communication skills needed to successfully conduct the initial client consultation
- Present and sell personal training services
- Know the basic requirements of on-going customer service

The initial client consultation is one of the cornerstones of a Personal Trainer's career. Along with the Personal Trainer's expertise in exercise and fitness, the initial client consultation provides the content for, and structures the relationship between, the client and the Personal Trainer. This chapter takes the reader through the objectives, preparation, content, and conduct of the initial client consultation and teaches the reader in detail how to create and organize a client welcome packet. Also critical to the initial client consultation are the Personal Trainer's communication skills. Based on the discussion in Chapter 5, this section describes in more detail communication techniques that facilitate the Personal Trainer's ability to obtain the client's commitment to a personal training program. The chapter focuses on the protocols that sustain the Personal Trainer's business and make the Personal Trainer's career a success.

THE INITIAL CLIENT CONTACT

Where do Personal Trainers find personal training clients? What type of people might the Personal Trainer be training? How do Personal Trainers set up an initial client meeting? What do they say? How do Personal Trainers get an individual to hire a Personal Trainer? These are all questions that prospective or current Personal Trainers need to answer. This chapter is structured to explain the initial client consultation process, which prepares Personal Trainers in the methods that help establish long-term client–Personal Trainer relationships.

The first stage to developing a strong client–Personal Trainer relationship begins at the point of initial contact. Through this initial process, the Personal Trainer begins to gather information about the potential client and has an opportunity to educate the individual about the approach the Personal Trainer takes in designing an exercise program. He or she is also laying the foundation of the potential client's relationship. He or she is able to see how the Personal Trainer will communicate, guide, and support the training process. Potential clients will want to hear the Personal Trainer's thoughts, experiences, and teaching methods used to educate and train current or past clients. The potential client will also observe the Personal Trainer's attention to detail, organizational abilities, and professional standards. The initial client contact allows the client and the Personal Trainer to ask and answer questions of each other. They, then, can determine if they will move forward to the next stage of the training process—setting up an initial client consultation.

Prepare for Personal Training Clients: Determine a Schedule

It is important to develop a set daily and weekly schedule before beginning the process of developing a client base. A schedule book is needed to function effectively. The Personal Trainer needs to establish specific times allocated to training clients, completing paperwork, and communicating with potential new clients. This also involves communication with the training facility where the training sessions take place to ensure that the facility will indeed be available for the times you anticipate training clients.

Demographics of Your Potential Clients

Before explaining the initial client consultation, the demographics of people who hire Personal Trainers provides a perspective on what type of clients are likely to seek personal training services. In 2004, IDEA—The Health and Fitness Association conducted a Personal Trainer Success survey of its personal training members, to which 157 responded (1). The experience levels of clients as established by respondents were beginning (41%), intermediate (43%), and advanced (23%). These experience levels were determined by those members surveyed, which included owners, personal training directors, fitness directors, general managers, and those with other areas of expertise. The average age of the clients as reported by respondents were 18 years of age and younger (8%), 18–34 years of age (16%), 35–44 years of age (26%), 45–54 years of age (30%), and 55 years of age and older (21%). The results suggest that most potential clients will be 45 years of age or older. These demographics may assist Personal Trainers to make more educated choices in the organization and marketing of their services to the appropriate demographic group.

Meeting Potential Clients

Personal Trainers will have opportunities to meet potential clients directly or to have potential personal training clients referred to them. Several examples are provided below:

1. Potential clients can be exposed to Personal Trainers working in a large health or fitness facility by observing them in an actual training session. Being active within a training facility will provide the Personal Trainer with opportunities to discuss personal training services with potential clients. It is important for Personal Trainers to always act professionally. Fitness club members often observe Personal Trainers to see how they handle and conduct themselves. Simply dressing well and conducting oneself professionally in the work environment can potentially provide many opportunities for members to ask questions related to fitness or the correct performance of specific exercise movements. At such moments a Personal Trainer needs to be prepared to offer advice and excellent customer service. Answering questions from members can turn into a potential client relationship.

2. New members could receive a complementary initial client consultation. This is a great practice because it gives the fledgling Personal Trainer opportunities to build a client base. Every new member a Personal Trainer meets represents a chance of gaining a new personal training client.

3. Potential clients or current members may contact the health club or facility to inquire about Personal Trainers and how to hire one. Usually a customer service representative or front desk staff person is fielding the potential client's inquiry and may refer the individual to either a personal training director or fitness manager to first screen the client. The director or manager will then refer the potential client to one of the appropriate Personal Trainers on staff to discuss the potential client's needs and schedule a first appointment.

4. Opportunities to make new client relationships can also come through referrals from the Personal Trainer's efforts to build a network within health and fitness-related fields that include, for example, physicians, physical therapists, registered dietitians, lawyers, accountants, fitness equipment stores, and chiropractors.

5. Referrals from existing clients satisfied with personal training services can be beneficial. Many successful Personal Trainers find this is the best way to attract and meet potential clients.

6. Phone inquiries directly forwarded to the Personal Trainer may come from a potential client.

7. Other times Personal Trainers may meet potential clients at professional events or business meetings such as charity functions, Chamber of Commerce meetings, facility-sponsored social events, health food stores, and restaurants.

However a potential client meets the Personal Trainer, the Personal Trainer must be prepared to ask the appropriate questions of the client and also be able to successfully represent himself or herself as a professional who is knowledgeable and caring.

The Potential Client Screening and the Potential Client Intake Form

A Personal Trainer must be prepared for the first meeting with the client. The client introduces himself or herself to the Personal Trainer at the training facility with questions about personal training services or simply calls the Personal Trainer on the phone asking for information.

Most often, the phone conversation will be the first opportunity to talk with a client. From this moment, the Personal Trainer begins to establish his or her professional standards. The best way to prepare for a phone inquiry is with a potential client intake form *(Fig. 12.1)*; therefore, always have the form and a pen readily available. A well-designed intake form can act as a script to guide the new or even seasoned Personal Trainer through a process of helpful questions to ask the potential client. Without an intake guide to assist the Personal Trainer during the question and answer process, important information may be missed. Writing down the answers a potential client gives you ensures accuracy and saves time. It is better to be organized and plan for a potential inquiry for services than to lose a client because of not being prepared. Screening potential clients begins here, at this initial first contact. Many of the Personal Trainer's and client's questions about whether this training relationship is right for the Personal Trainer and for the client can be answered quite quickly.

During this conversation, the Personal Trainer communicates a broad range of information, from his or her training approach to the costs of the personal training sessions. The initial client contact is the first screening process, and it determines whether or not it makes sense for both parties to move forward and schedule an initial client consultation. Important elements of the training sessions must be clearly communicated at this time, such as the location, cost, and times available. This avoids wasting the valuable time of both the potential client and the Personal Trainer with initial meetings that do not yield a training program because of time and/or cost constraints. These details need to be discussed openly in advance of the actual training session appointment. If the client cannot train at the time of the initial contact because of schedule restraints, a detailed potential client intake form will allow the Personal Trainer to follow up with the client at a later date. All forms should be kept for future reference.

THE POTENTIAL CLIENT INTAKE FORM

A well-designed potential client intake form should include the following information as well as space to write the information obtained and/or take notes:

➤ Date call received
➤ Potential client's name (first and last)
➤ Address. Where potential clients live might affect their ability to make their training sessions on time and/or train at the facility on a regular basis. Or, it may change the conversation to discuss whether the Personal Trainer might be offering home personal training services if the client cannot make scheduled appointments at the Personal Trainer's facility. In addition, the Personal Trainer then has the client's address for direct mail in case the client does not have email.
➤ Telephone numbers: home, work, and mobile. This is important in the event that the Personal Trainer cannot make the initial session because of an emergency or illness. The client must be notified under such circumstances, and the Personal Trainer should make an attempt to reschedule the session. *Note:* Personal Trainers should provide all their contact information to potential clients in case the client has a sudden change of plans and needs to reschedule the appointment.
➤ Email address. The Personal Trainer can either mail or email the medical health and history forms/questionnaires to the potential client to be completed before the scheduled meeting. This saves the 20 or 30 minutes it takes to fill in the forms during the first session. The first session can then focus fully on the initial client consultation. Other forms can be included with the medical history forms, including an introductory letter describing the initial client consultation along with what the client should wear during the assessments, directions to the facility, and general information about the personal training program.

Potential client intake form

Date call received: _____

Name: _____

Address: _____

Home phone: _____ Business phone: _____ Mobile phone: _____

Email: _____

Date call returned: Comments:

How did you find out about this personal training program? _____

History-background

- How long have you been considering getting into a regular exercise program? _____
- What prevented you from getting involved in the past? _____
- Do you have any physical limitations or medical conditions that must be considered? _____
- What are your current goals and objectives? _____
- How often are you planning on personal training per week and which days and times are best for you to work out? (provide days/times options) _____
- Physician/physical therapist name, contact numbers: _____

Personal trainer information

- Personal trainers background, history, and education/certification(s). _____
- Education-based personal training process, SET model, SET flowchart, SET session plan, points of evaluation, exercise training matrix, and exercise grading system. _____
- Current or past clients success stories, membership in professional organizations, press received, and personal training packages and prices. _____

Final reminders

- Date scheduled for initial client consultation: _____
- Email/mail documents to potential client: _____
- Physician clearance sent/received: _____

Comments: _____

FIGURE 12.1. Potential client intake form.

➤ How often per week does the client want to train? This will determine whether or not the Personal Trainer can fit the client into his or her schedule.

➤ What times during the day is the client available to train? This will determine whether the Personal Trainer can accommodate the potential client's schedule. If the Personal Trainer has no available time to train the potential client, the Personal Trainer can then recommend someone on his or her own staff or refer the individual to another ACSM Certified Personal Trainer[SM] working at another training facility. In addition, even if this was the Personal Trainer's first client, it puts the potential client on notice that the Personal Trainer may have a full schedule, which makes a positive impression on the potential client.

➤ Medical and health history. This information will determine whether the Personal Trainer needs to receive physician approval before he or she can conduct any future assessments on the potential client (2) (see Chapter 14).

➤ Physician's/physical therapist's name and contact number. Any acute or chronic diseases that the client may have (such as diabetes, heart disease, and/or high blood pressure) should be discussed, as well as any musculoskeletal conditions. If the client does have any health concerns, the Personal Trainer should ask for the client's allied health/medical professional's name and contact number so he or she can contact this professional to send the client's physician clearance forms.

➤ The medical release. It might also be necessary to discuss the client's condition with his or her health professional to decide whether the individual can be allowed to train. This process may involve legal constraints and often requires the client to sign a confidentiality waiver that allows communication to take place between the Personal Trainer and the physician (medical release).

➤ Initial client goals and objectives. This allows the Personal Trainer to see if this is a client he or she would be interested in training. For example, if the Personal Trainer's expertise lies in training college-bound athletes, the Personal Trainer will want to know in advance whether a prospective client matches this profile.

➤ Describe your objectives and the education–based personal training process. The Personal Trainer needs to provide information about his or her approach to personal training.

The type of information the Personal Trainer could provide to potential clients includes:

1. A brief description of his or her educational background and personal training experience to be used as a lead–in to discuss the training method
2. The details of the education–based personal training process and the approach that will be taken to design the client's exercise program
3. The assessment process and the importance of assessing posture and body alignment
4. An overview of the sequence and development of a personalized exercise program, describing how the potential client will be observed and evaluated for each exercise movement performed by implementing the points of evaluation, exercise training matrix, and exercise grading system
5. A demographic of current clients and/or clients that you have worked with in the past
6. Information on professional organizations
7. Any other pertinent information such as internships, special courses or workshops completed, awards or press received, and any articles written for publication

THE LAST PHASE OF THE POTENTIAL CLIENT CONVERSATION

The initial client contact over the telephone may take from 10 to 35 minutes, depending on the circumstance. Good listening skills are important. If the Personal Trainer senses that too much information is being provided and the individual is getting overwhelmed, ease up on how much is presented and end on a positive note by briefly reviewing how the potential client's needs and goals will be addressed.

THE DISCUSSION OF SESSION FEES

The final area of discussion should be the price charged for the initial client consultation, price per session, or price per session packages. It is common for facilities to charge for the initial client consultation at a higher rate than the actual session price. However, other facilities may also provide an initial complementary consultation for all new members that join the facility. Sessions are commonly 1 hour in length, and packages range anywhere from 5 to 10, 15, 20, 40, or 50 sessions. Some Personal Trainers and businesses have clients prepay for the entire personal training session package. Depending on the Personal Trainer's company policies for payment of individual sessions and packages, it is recommended that this information be presented to the client in detail beforehand. In addition, group personal training (2 to 4 clients) may be another service in which the client may be interested, so the Personal Trainer should be prepared to review price packages and information on this service. Any other company policies and fees should be disclosed to clients so they can make an informed decision about whether this is at least affordable for them and whether they would be able to agree to terms. It also allows the Personal Trainer to provide a pre-screening process to see it the potential client can pay for the services.

ENDING THE CONVERSATION

Lastly, the potential client who has been scheduled for an assessment should be reminded to:

➤ Bring all completed documents sent via email or mail (the health history and medical question-naire forms, learning style preference assessment, informed consent/medical history form, and any other business/contract forms)
➤ Dress appropriately for assessments
➤ Bring any signed physician medical clearances or other required documents necessary before beginning the assessment process
➤ Bring a water bottle
➤ Follow the guidelines as prescribed in the introductory letter

After all questions have been answered and both parties wish to move forward, the initial client consultation date and time should be established. The Personal Trainer should provide a brief overview of the format of their client consultation and the time required to review and perform assessments and conduct the meeting. Finish the conversation by saying "Thank you," using the client's name. This will help you learn it. Also, clarify what the client wants to be called (using the name several times at this point in the conversation helps you remember it and avoids the embarrassment of not knowing it for the first session). Thank the potential client again, using his or her name, and review the date(s), session time(s), and payment amount and/or billing method that you arranged. Finally, thank the potential client again by name.

FOLLOW-THROUGH WITH EMAILS AND DOCUMENTATION

The Personal Trainer should also forward via email or mail any documents and forms that the client can complete and review before the meeting. An alternative is to add all of the documents to the company website and send the website link to the client to download all the documents from the specified website. Either way, forwarding the documents before the initial meeting will allow the client an opportunity to review and complete the documents in a relaxed and comfortable setting. The Personal Trainer should also send an email or call 24 hours before the scheduled appointment as a reminder to the potential client.

The above preparation and planning of the initial client conversation gives the potential client a sense of the Personal Trainer's approach to the personal training process. The guidance and attention to detail that the client experiences in the first conversation indicates to him or her what to expect from you as a Personal Trainer. The next step in the process of building the client relationship is the initial client consultation, the next stage along the pathway of creating a long-term client–Personal Trainer relationship.

BUILDING A CLIENT–PERSONAL TRAINER RELATIONSHIP

The Initial Client Consultation

The next stage in building a strong client–Personal Trainer relationship is the initial client consultation. Potential clients will attend the initial meeting with different emotions, ranging through fear, anxiety, nervousness, and excitement (3). The Personal Trainer needs to be prepared to put the client at ease and make him or her comfortable (4). As communication begins to grow and the client feels more comfortable, the Personal Trainer begins to get to know the client and to put together a picture of the client's needs, desires, and expectations. The initial client consultation is a progressive process in which information is exchanged between the Personal Trainer and client to develop a mutually beneficial fitness and exercise training plan. This consists largely of clear and distinct goals and objectives based on the client's needs and abilities.

A Client-Focused Approach

By learning more about the client, the Personal Trainer will have a better insight into developing a successful exercise program focusing on the abilities and motivations of the client. The initial client consultation is therefore designed to focus on the needs of the client. This is the basis for establishing a caring and supportive environment in which the potential client feels comfortable discussing his or her personal medical history, health concerns, injuries, previous exercise experience, and other personal information (5). Incorporating individual learning preferences, motivational techniques, and communication skills discussed in earlier chapters will support the Personal Trainer when conducting the initial client consultation.

The client-focused initial client consultation addresses the following:

➤ The consultation area
➤ Making a good first impression
➤ Putting the client at ease
➤ What are clients looking for?
➤ Establishing the structure of your meeting

THE CONSULTATION AREA

The consultation and assessment area in the facility should be situated in a private, quiet area of the training room or in another area free of distractions. There should be no loud noise or music in the background, and a minimum of visual stimulation or activities that could distract or prevent the client from a focused conversation with the Personal Trainer. The area should be clean, organized, and professionally arranged. Comfortable seating for two to four people should be available. A desk or table wide enough to display all the forms and documents is also needed. The room or area should have good lighting and proper ventilation and be at a comfortable temperature for all parties. If it is not possible to have a separate room to conduct the initial consultation, a seat for clients that is facing the wall to prevent distractions is appropriate.

MAKING A GOOD FIRST IMPRESSION

If possible, the Personal Trainer should meet the potential client at the entrance of the training center with a friendly verbal greeting and a proper handshake *(Fig. 12.2)*. Dress should be appropriately modest, professional, and inoffensive to conservative tastes. Wearing scant clothing that is too

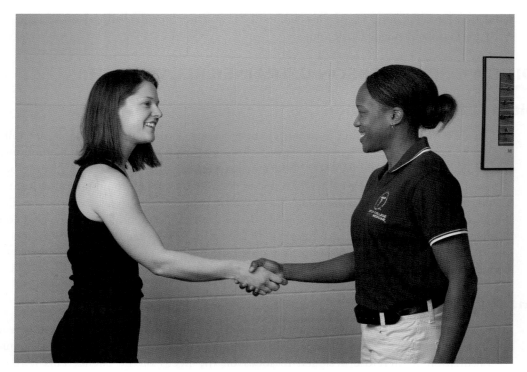

FIGURE 12.2. Making a good first impression.

revealing can cause the potential client and others around the Personal Trainer to feel uncomfortable or distracted. After the greeting, the Personal Trainer should provide a tour to potential clients who are not current members to familiarize them with the layout and surroundings. A brief tour can also provide some opportunities for relaxed conversation before beginning the initial client consultation.

PUTTING THE CLIENT AT EASE

Most new exercisers may be nervous and apprehensive at first until they have adjusted to the new surroundings of a health club or other facility. Some individuals need more time than others to feel comfortable in a new place. The Personal Trainer should be aware of each individual client's needs and be patient while their comfort level increases.

To support this process, the Personal Trainer should reassure the client that it is natural for it to take some time to get used to a new fitness setting. This lets the client know that the Personal Trainer understands the situation and can support clients through their apprehension. This also tells the client that the Personal Trainer will be patient with him or her as they learn exercise movements, which is often a concern causing client anxiety.

WHAT ARE CLIENTS LOOKING FOR?

Before the initial client process is discussed in further detail, the Personal Trainer should consider the things potential clients are looking for in a Personal Trainer. Personal Trainers should consider each of the following core principles when conducting an initial client consultation. Each of these factors can remind the Personal Trainer of core principles that might be addressed during the initial client consultation:

➤ Good, reliable service. The Personal Trainer should set a standard in the initial client consultation by providing the best service for clients and have it continue reliably throughout the client–Personal Trainer relationship.

➤ Individualized attention. Special populations may be in need of a Personal Trainer to design a specialized program for their condition. *Note:* A Personal Trainer should have the proper educational background and qualifications to train certain special populations, such as physically handicapped, geriatric, and post-rehabilitation clients.

➤ Professionalism. The Personal Trainer should dress, act, and conduct training sessions as a professional at all times.

➤ Education and knowledge. Well-studied and practiced skills teach clients what they are attempting to learn. These skills provide the Personal Trainer with the ability to safely train clients and develop new and creative exercise programs.

➤ Motivation and enthusiasm. The Personal Trainer is the primary influence on the client's motivation. The Personal Trainer's enthusiasm and passion for his or her job significantly motivates clients.

➤ Safe, supervised, and effective. The Personal Trainer should provide safe and effective exercise program designs that are well supervised and directed toward the client's needs.

➤ Achieving goals and objectives. Clients want to be assured that the design of the training program will lead them toward their goals and objectives.

➤ Empathetic listening and communication. Clients value Personal Trainers that listen to the their needs and goals and who encourage an engaging and interactive working relationship.

➤ Human interest. Clients want Personal Trainers who care about people and their welfare. Clients want to be treated with respect, supported in their goals, and guided in their learning of exercise and fitness.

➤ Good referrals. Clients often need referrals to good medical and/or healthcare. The Personal Trainer should maintain a close network of allied health and medical professionals on which the client can depend.

➤ High standards and high quality. Potential clients appreciate high standards and high quality in their Personal Trainers and training.

Review the Content and Sequence of the Initial Client Consultation

After the client has met the Personal Trainer and is adjusted to the setting, the Personal Trainer reviews the sequence and content of the initial client consultation. Even though the Personal Trainer has previously outlined the process in the initial client contact, it is recommended that a step-by-step review of the process be provided at this point. This is a good opportunity to present the sequential exercise program and the client welcome packet so the client can see the order and sequence in which assessments and information will be presented. The Personal Trainer should explain the assessment process. Clients who see the content and sequence of the initial client consultation in advance may feel more at ease with the process. In addition, clients can also express their concerns or feelings about performing a given part of the assessment. For example, clients might be uncomfortable with the prospect of a body-fat composition test that uses calipers because they are self-conscious about a weight problem. The Personal Trainer can then consider the client's feelings and not make this test essential or required in the initial client consultation. Box 12-1 contains an outline of the initial client consultation process that the Personal Trainer can share with the client.

Presenting the Client Welcome Packet

Before performing client assessments and reviewing health history documents, the Personal Trainer should present a professional client welcome packet (6). The welcome packet serves four purposes:

1. It provides the Personal Trainer with information organized within the folder that can be used as a script to present important information about the personal training and other areas.

Box 12.1	**"Today the session will involve a review of. . ."**

- The client welcome packet
- Completed documents, including health and medical history questionnaire, learning preference assessments, and current health level
- The client's and the Personal Trainer's starting goals and objectives
- The education-based personal training process
- Informed consent forms and other waivers of liability
- Various health and fitness assessments
- Performance of assessments
- The initial exercise plan and program structure based on the client's goals and assessment results
- The training center's policies, personal training agreements, and prices of the training packages
- After the review of this information, all required signatures should be obtained

2. It organizes the Personal Trainer's information in a presentable package for the client to learn about the Personal Trainer and their personal training approach.

3. The information is a deliverable press kit for media outlets to allow Personal Trainers to market themselves.

4. The welcome packet can be presented in business meetings to provide a history of the Personal Trainer and the company background.

Regardless of whether the Personal Trainer is working independently or in a personal training department within a facility, it is recommended that all of the staff or coworkers develop individualized welcome packets for potential clients. After the core materials are created for the welcome packet (see below), each Personal Trainer on staff can add his or her own personalized resume, business card, letters of recommendation, and any other materials pertinent to the Personal Trainer's profile. Individualized Personal Trainer welcome packets provide cohesion and uniformity in standards for all staff members. If the entire training center does not wish to create such packets, an individual Personal Trainer should not hesitate to prepare his or her own personalized welcome packet. The welcome packet gives the client information about the Personal Trainer and his or her training philosophy. The client welcome packet should include the following:

➤ Introductory letter
➤ Brochure
➤ Business card
➤ Personal Trainer's resume
➤ Copies of certification certificates
➤ Letters of recommendation (from clients; include client's before and after photos)
➤ Letters of recommendation (from health/medical professionals)
➤ Press clippings/media recognition you have received
➤ Fitness and training publications you have written
➤ Article(s) on health, wellness, or fitness
➤ ACSM Liability Insurance
➤ List of services (fitness and other related services)
➤ Client assessment/evaluation–related documents and forms

INTRODUCTORY LETTER

The introductory letter should provide a brief history about the company, business, or organization along with the core training principles and philosophy of the company or Personal Trainer

(Fig. 12.3). The letter may also address specialty programs and recognitions received by the company.

BROCHURE

Brochures are an excellent way to present information and inform the reader about the company for whom the Personal Trainer works and the personal training services provided. Brochures can be created not only for the client welcome packet but also for mailing to potential clients. Circulating enough brochures in a given community or neighborhood can market the Personal Trainer or facility to a potentially large client base at little expense. The brochure can also be put at designated locations such as:

➤ Waiting rooms or offices of physicians, dentists, physical therapists, registered dietitians, or chiropractors
➤ Local businesses (hair salons, massage therapists, or manicurists locations)
➤ Fitness clothing and equipment stores and/or departments
➤ Condominium and apartment complex management offices and/or training rooms
➤ Nutritional supplement stores

BUSINESS CARDS

Handing out business cards is standard practice for career professionals. An excellent place for a business card is in the inside pocket of the client welcome packets (see "Organizing the Client Welcome Packet" on page 279).

PERSONAL TRAINER'S RESUME

The Personal Trainer needs a professional resume that includes his or her education/certifications, achievements, employment history, memberships with professional organizations, goals and objectives, and a list of any publications written. An introduction at the top of the resume presenting the Personal Trainer's approach to personal training also is appropriate.

COPIES OF CERTIFICATIONS

A copy of the Personal Trainer's ACSM Certified Personal Trainer^{SM} Certification, current CPR Certification, and any other pertinent documents should be included in the packet.

LETTERS OF RECOMMENDATION (FROM CLIENTS)

If the Personal Trainer has a good working relationship with the client, the Personal Trainer can request a written recommendation from any client who has been successfully trained for longer than 6 to 8 weeks. Recommendations provide potential clients with insight into the history and background of the Personal Trainer's current or past clients. In addition, the Personal Trainer should ask clients for permission to include a client's before and after photos in the packet. This allows potential clients to see the results the Personal Trainer has been able to achieve and which populations the Personal Trainer has the most experience with or specialization in training.

LETTERS OF RECOMMENDATION (FROM HEALTH/MEDICAL PROFESSIONALS)

Personal Trainers who are building their business are advised to request letters of recommendation from allied health/fitness/medical professionals. Such recommendations show the potential client that fellow Personal Trainers and allied health and medical professionals advanced in the field respect the Personal Trainer.

Client introductory letter

(Company name or logo)

Dear New Client/Member,

Welcome to the personal training department at the _____ health and fitness facility, founded in 2001. The fitness facility has made it a priority to be a model of integrity and quality for personal training services in the local area. All of our personal training staff has received the ACSM Certified Personal Trainer℠ Certification and are CPR/AED certified. Our professional environment has allowed us the ability to accommodate personal training clients of different ages, medical conditions, and levels of experience. The qualified staff at the facility are prepared to work with you as a team and to develop formal communication with your health care provider (if necessary) to assist you in developing and maintaining a healthy lifestyle through our personal training services.

Personal training and membership are offered to the entire community and include a detailed medical history screening (incorporating an ACSM Risk Stratification Process), posture and body alignment analysis, body composition assessments, and other evaluations. Exercise programs are designed based upon the client's current health and fitness level taking into consideration the client's long-term goals and objectives. Our Personal Trainers will focus on developing a program that incorporates the client's current posture and alignment, learning preferences, abilities and experience.

We are delighted that you have chosen our facility to help you along the pathway to a healthier lifestyle. You will find a variety of information included in this packet about the services that are offered, along with a resume and letters of recommendation on your Personal Trainer. We have also included descriptive sample exercise plans implementing the Sequential Exercise Testing (SET) model, SET Session Plan, and SE Flowchart. Also included in the packet are reading materials on exercise, strength training, and motivation.

The facility staff wishes you the best of luck with your new personal training program. Please let us know if you have any questions, comments or concerns.

Sincerely,

_____

Fitness manager

FIGURE 12.3. Client introductory letter.

PUBLICATIONS AND PRESS CLIPPINGS/MEDIA RECOGNITION

Good-quality photocopies of any articles that the Personal Trainer has written for newspapers, magazines, journals, and newsletters also belong in the welcome packet. These articles help inform the client of the Personal Trainer's approach and demonstrate the Personal Trainer's ability to coherently express his or her knowledge of the fitness and training field. Clients will appreciate the fact that the Personal Trainer they may be hiring has been published. Also, if an article has been written about the Personal Trainer or business in a local newspaper or magazine, good-quality photocopies of such press clippings need to be included in the welcome packet.

SAMPLE EXERCISE TRAINING PROGRAM

Sample copies of an exercise training program can also be included in the welcome packet to provide clients with an overview of the exercise program's design and procedure. In addition, presenting these materials allows the Personal Trainer to introduce the client to the education-based personal training process. Other supplementary materials can be included, such as the points of evaluation, exercise grading system, and the exercise training matrix. These review materials give the client an opportunity to fully appreciate the details that would be involved in his or her personalized program design. Creating a complete picture for clients of how the program is designed involves them in the training process.

ARTICLE(S) ON HEALTH, WELLNESS, OR FITNESS

Personal Trainers can include helpful articles on health, wellness, and fitness in the welcome packet. These articles provide perspective and information on personal training that can motivate and educate a client on specific topics.

ACSM LIABILITY INSURANCE

Include a copy of the ACSM liability insurance document in the welcome packet. Presenting a copy to the client shows that the Personal Trainer is concerned with both self-protection and protecting the client.

LIST OF SERVICES

If the company offers services other than personal training, a list of all available services and programs is recommended in the welcome packet. This provides the client with easy access to the facility's other resources. Plus, the company has an opportunity to identify and market their other services.

CLIENT ASSESSMENT/EVALUATION-RELATED DOCUMENTS AND FORMS

Any documents that have not been previously emailed or mailed to the client need to be included in the welcome packet along with any other assessment forms that will allow the Personal Trainer to evaluate the client. An organized and prepared assessment form shows a professional approach and will save the Personal Trainer time.

Organizing the Client Welcome Packet

The welcome packet can be professionally created with the help of a graphic designer and printing company, or another less costly option is to purchase folders from a local office supply store. This is the least expensive way to create a packet. If folders are purchased separately, then labels are printed and placed on the cover of the folder. The labels should include information such as the business name, address, telephone number, email address, and the company website (if applicable).

Whichever option is chosen, a folder with two pockets for information and a slot for a business card works the best. One side of the folder can hold all of your professional information including the resume, certifications, and letters of recommendation. The introductory letter needs to be visible (placed on top) for clients to read right away. The other side of the folder can include the remainder of the information in an organized format.

Finally, after developing the format and arrangement of the welcome packet, it is easier to produce 25 to 50 client welcome packets at one time. Most Personal Trainers are surprised at how useful it is to hand a potential client this preplanned, ready, organized packet of information. Therefore, it is a good idea to make many welcome packets ahead of time rather than making them individually for each client that contacts you.

Summarize the Initial Client Consultation

The initial client contact has set up the initial client consultation. The initial client consultation is designed for the Personal Trainer to exhibit his or her education, expertise, organizational abilities, and communication skills. Successful and rewarding personal training sessions depend on the Personal Trainer's confident and open communication style during the initial client consultation and the training sessions as a whole. In summary, planning and organizing the initial consultation serves an important purpose and addresses important needs. The well-defined and well-executed initial client consultation:

➤ Establishes the foundation for a long-term client–Personal Trainer relationship
➤ Provides a visual "road map" that gives the client a sense of the preparation, direction, guidance, and support the Personal Trainer will provide to the client during the course of the relationship
➤ Establishes an open and receptive communication style between the client and Personal Trainer
➤ Provides Personal Trainers with the potential client's current and past medical, health, and fitness history
➤ Sets up procedures for client safety through the screening and ACSM risk stratification process
➤ Determines the client's goals and desires and brings out the client's expectations of a Personal Trainer
➤ Gathers additional information on the client's health and fitness level during the assessment performance (6)
➤ Defines the client's learning preferences through the Personal Trainer's assessment and observations
➤ Shows the Personal Trainer the client's current ability, skill level, and knowledge of exercise movements
➤ Educates the client on the details of the education-based personal training process
➤ Documents company policies and pricing structure for personal training sessions

THE ART OF COMMUNICATION AND PRESENTING YOUR SERVICES

Effective Communication Skills

An overview of communication is discussed in Chapter 5. This section addresses additional communication skills pertaining to interactive and engaging two-way communication with clients during the initial client consultation. Without sound communication, the client–Personal Trainer relationship will not develop well, and the training sessions may not be successful.

The Importance of Energy and Listening

Personal Trainers need to have potential clients open up and communicate during the initial client consultation. This requires effective communication, which respects the way in which the other person communicates and seeks to meet the speaker with his or her own speaking style. Personal

Trainers should listen to what potential clients have to say. They should give clients the time to discuss themselves, their needs, and their goals. Personal Trainers should observe how the potential client is talking and match the individual's energy level, speech rate, and voice tone. Learning to communicate effectively with new clients requires Personal Trainers to practice their sense of interpersonal awareness by sharpening observation and listening skills.

A Proactive Approach to Listening

A proactive approach to listening to a client's needs and goals means that the Personal Trainer focuses on clients and interacts with them by asking questions for clarification and verification. A potential client senses that the Personal Trainer is listening and will feel assured that the Personal Trainer is paying attention to their needs. An active listening approach provides clarification to the client's needs and expectations and also lets the client know that the Personal Trainer cares about them. Active listening includes the following:

➤ Repeating the information the client states
➤ Restating or rephrasing information
➤ Clarifying information
➤ Summarizing the conversation
➤ Concentrating on the ideas being communicated

Sending Positive Messages through Nonverbal Communications

Positive and effective communication with the client during the initial client consultation and the training sessions can also work through the use of nonverbal communication. Personal Trainers communicate not only through their verbal communication style but also through their nonverbal communication, such as eye contact, hand gestures, and postures. For example, imagine that a client is enthusiastically describing how he or she feels after the last training session while the Personal Trainer is leaning against the exercise machine, facing away from the client and looking off in another direction. How would this make the client feel? Another example would be when a client performs an exercise movement and then inquires if he or she is doing the movement correctly only to discover that the Personal Trainer is preoccupied with the television. How would this make the client feel?

The use of nonverbal communication is as important as active listening. The Personal Trainer should remind clients that he or she is engaged in what they are saying, not only through the use of verbal cues, but also through the use of body language, eye contact, posture, and body movements. This requires an effort on the part of the Personal Trainer to know how to communicate to others through nonverbal messages. One way to observe and evaluate non-verbal communication skills is by having a friend or family member record movements, posture, and body positioning while you conduct a simulated training session or an initial client consultation. The Personal Trainer can self-critique and find things that can be improved upon and then consciously work on them.

A good sense of non-verbal cues will also give the Personal Trainer increased sensitivity for a client's non-verbal messages. The Personal Trainer should notice the client's posture walking into the facility or office. Is the client slumped forward and fatigued when first entering the facility? Do your client's movements seem hesitant and confused when performing an exercise movement just taught to him or her? The client may not ask for assistance in words, but the body language may speak quite loudly. The Personal Trainer should learn to pay attention to a client's verbal and non-verbal patterns and be ready to address them effectively. Here is a summary of non-verbal communication patterns of which Personal Trainers need to be aware:

➤ Active posture and body movements. Body language consists of correct posture, crossed/ uncrossed arms and legs, sitting up/slouching, for example. It communicates basic attitude toward clients and needs to be positive and receptive.

➤ Nodding. A nod of the head in a "Yes" direction to the client lets him or her know that you understand and are actively listening.

➤ Facial expressions. A smile keeps contact with the client. A straight face, yawn, frown, raised eyebrow, or scrunched forehead tends to break down the communication contact.

➤ Eye contact. Direct eye contact strengthens communication. Distracted eyes, looking down at the floor or off to the side, weaken the contact.

➤ Hand movements. Hand movements communicate trust and confidence. When open and relaxed they affirm communication, and when tense or fidgety they break it down.

Learning to Ask Questions

Personal Trainers need to ask questions effectively to learn about the potential client's health history, goals, past exercise experience, and other important details. Open-ended questions are designed to extract a large amount of information that later can be narrowed in scope through close-ended questions. A strategy Personal Trainers may use is to ask open-ended questions in the beginning of the initial client consultation. For example, 2 years ago a potential client had rotator cuff surgery and subsequent rehabilitation. The Personal Trainer could ask an open-ended question such as "What kind of rehab program did the physical therapist design for you?" This will provide a generalized answer that can then be focused with a close-ended question, "What type of movements or exercises did the physical therapists have you perform, please describe or show them to me."

Close-ended questions are used to narrow the client's responses down to learn specific information. If the Personal Trainer asks the client close-ended questions back-to back, such as: "Was the rehab program effective?" or "How many days a week do you perform the rehab exercises?" the client can start to feel pressured. Since close-ended questions are narrow in focus, the Personal Trainer would most likely not want to ask too many close-ended questions in a row. Too many open-ended questions, however, will not yield enough specific information to give the Personal Trainer a clear picture of the client's history.

Selling and Recommending the Right Personal Training Package

Before reviewing the details of how to approach selling personal training to the client, the Personal Trainer should clearly define the right package for the client's needs. The design of the exercise program based on the client's goals and objectives determines the number of sessions a client needs to purchase. The Personal Trainer should recommend the appropriate training package based on the client's needs, goals, and objectives. Personal Trainers should let clients know as they go through the training process when sessions should be added or subtracted, based on the client's needs. For example, if an exercise-experienced client wants to learn some new exercise movements to supple- ment his or her current 4-day-a-week workout program, then the Personal Trainer probably does not need to train with the client more than once a week. However, a new client who is unfamiliar with exercise needs to learn from the beginning how to perform exercise movements accurately, safely, and correctly. To facilitate this learning as well as adapting to a new lifestyle habit of regular exercise, the client should most likely arrange for training sessions anywhere from 2 to 4 times per week for 4 to 16 weeks. This is the time it takes the average adult to begin to perfect and memorize the movement patterns and build the foundation for developing organized exercise sessions.

A problem occurs when the beginner exerciser purchases too few sessions and spaces them out so that they are too infrequent for the client to have the opportunity to memorize and perfect the movement patterns correctly. This results in a disappointed client who feels that the training is not providing the desired results. For this reason the Personal Trainer must be clear and "up front" with the client and specifically describe and advise the exercise program that the client needs to succeed. Once the client has learned the initial exercise training, and the client's body alignment has improved, the training sessions may be reduced, remain the same, or increase each week based on the client's goals and objectives. Thus the importance of clarity in the selling phase of the initial client consultation becomes apparent; it makes it possible for the client to see in advance why he or she needs a particular program to succeed.

Selling Personal Training Services

After the Personal Trainer has concluded reviewing the medical/health questionnaire and assessments and has presented an outline of the potential structure of the exercise program, the Personal Trainer may now ask the client for a firm commitment to schedule actual training sessions. The selling process by this point of the initial client consultation should be a positive one for both parties. Through developing an informative phone presentation during the initial client contact, and a thoughtful, caring, and educational approach to initial client consultation, the client's purchase of the personal training sessions will be the natural "next step" in the process of obtaining exercise and fitness training.

Another approach to the sale of training sessions is to review the personal training packages that the facility offers and to point out the most common package that is purchased by clients and why they like it. The price of personal training packages generally decreases with the volume of sessions purchased at one time. For example, package prices for individual 1-hour sessions might be something like this:

➤ 5 Sessions for $300, Package A
➤ 10 Sessions for $580, Package B
➤ 20 Sessions for $1100, Package C
➤ 40 Sessions for $2000, Package D

For example, the Personal Trainer can tell the client that most of his or her beginning training clients purchase package B and train 2 days per week. The Personal Trainer could ask, "Would you like to purchase that package?" or "How would you like to proceed?" This should be enough of a lead for the potential client to make a choice or decision on moving forward with purchasing a package of sessions.

Common objections to starting the program may arise from the potential client in the following areas because of money, time, procrastination, or other conflicts. The Personal Trainer should be prepared to respond and anticipate possible objections. The Personal Trainer should remember that pressuring a client into an exercise program to which he or she is not willing or is unable to commit could be a pitfall rather than a success story for both the client and the Personal Trainer. The Personal Trainer should maintain a positive attitude, relax, and listen to what the potential client has to say. The Personal Trainer should evaluate the objection and respond truthfully.

Obtaining Client Commitment

The Personal Trainer should remember that the client needs the help of a personal training professional and that this is the primary reason that the client has sought out personal training services. The Personal Trainer should focus the client's attention on the service, instruction, motivation, guidance, enthusiasm, safety, and education that he or she will receive from the personal training experience. The Personal Trainer should remind the client of the value of personal training, the increased sense of self-esteem, and the benefits of feeling healthier and being in better shape to actively enjoy life.

When the client commits, the Personal Trainer should not act surprised with the sale. The Personal Trainer should show appreciation by thanking the client. Then, the Personal Trainer should confirm the client's choice of the personal training package to be purchased. The Personal Trainer should have the client review and sign all required agreements or contracts. After the meeting, a thank you card or email to the new client is recommended. The Personal Trainer should make sure the card or email has the session date, time, location, and the Personal Trainer's full name on it. It can say that the Personal Trainer looks forward to working with him or her and then remind the new client to wear exercise clothes and to bring a towel and a water bottle. The card or email should close with the Personal Trainer saying that he or she looks forward to seeing the client at the first training session.

Finally, if a commitment is not obtained from the potential client, the Personal Trainer should maintain a positive perspective and remember that not everyone is going to seek services after an initial consultation. The Personal Trainer should maintain good manners and a positive attitude. He or she can recommend other sources clients can use to get fit and healthy. Perhaps in the future the potential client will refer friends or family members or decide to give personal training another chance. After the initial client consultation is over, the Personal Trainer should re-evaluate how the meeting went. Whether it ended in a client commitment or not, the Personal Trainer should spend some time to go over things and write down the positives and negatives that occurred in the consultation. He or she should work on the areas of communication skills or preparation that need improvement, practice the initial client consultation with friends and/or colleagues, and role-play several initial client consultations for practice in preparation for the next initial client consultation.

Customer Service and Professionalism

As the Personal Trainer builds a client base and business, retaining and maintaining clients is essential to continue as a successful Personal Trainer. Key areas to provide customer service include organization and reliability. As a Personal Trainer, you should demonstrate to clients that they can count on you by being a little early as well as on time for scheduled appointments and to respond quickly and courteously to phone calls and emails. A Personal Trainer should always use conservative language in phone calls and especially stay objective in email communications. He or she should listen to what clients are requesting and maintain effective interactive communication throughout the client–Personal Trainer relationship.

Value the Customer

The Personal Trainer should focus on exceptional service to clients. Here are more ideas for improving customer service:

1. Bring a copy of one current research or fitness-related article for your client.
2. Develop a monthly company newsletter or brief that can be emailed to clients, advisors, business associates, or colleagues.
3. Provide follow-up emails to clients after training sessions to ask them how they are feeling and to see how they are doing with the extra cardiovascular training recommended to them.
4. Provide fitness testing or reassessments every 6 to 8 weeks, if it applies to certain clients.
5. Send a follow-up card thanking clients for their patronage.
6. Send birthday and holiday cards to clients.
7. Respond to and solve customer complaints quickly:
   a. Determine the facts
   b. Offer a solution
   c. Follow through with action

SUMMARY

A strong client–Personal Trainer relationship begins with the initial contact the Personal Trainer makes with the client. The potential client intake form assists the Personal Trainer in conducting a focused and thorough information session. In this conversation, the Personal Trainer and the client have an opportunity to ask questions of each other and to decide whether or not to enter the next phase of the process—scheduling an initial client consultation. The initial client consultation provides the Personal Trainer with time to gather more information about the client through questions, assessments, and observations and to begin the design process of education-based personal training sessions. Clients have the opportunity to see how the Personal Trainer will communicate, guide, and support them through the training process and make a commitment to a training package. The client welcome package gives the Personal Trainer a compact and effective tool for communicating in detail his or her training profile to the client and facilitates the client's ability to choose to hire him or her. Communication techniques such as body language and open/closed questions also support having the Personal Trainer and the client come to an informed decision to proceed with the training program. The practice of responsible attention to the details of practical organization, reliable scheduling, and responsive communication ensure a solid operational base for the Personal Trainer as a career professional.

REFERENCES

1. Ryan P. Personal Trainer Survey. IDEA Personal Trainer Success 2004;1:2.
2. Brooks DS. Breaking in: you (yes, you!) can be a personal trainer. In: Bahrke MS, Crist R, Augspurger A, eds. The Complete Book of Personal Training. Champaign, IL: Human Kinetics, 2004.
3. Griffin JC. Getting to know our client: more than a history. In: Wilgren S, Mustain E, Graham M, eds. Client-Centered Exercise Prescription. Champaign, IL: Human Kinetics, 1998.
4. Grantham W, Patton R, York T, Winick M. Understanding your customer or member. In: Wikgren S, Rhoda J, Bott S, eds. Health Fitness Management. Champaign, IL: Human Kinetics, 1998.
5. Cantwell S. Essential corporate materials. In: Ryan P, ed. Policies That Work for Personal Trainers. San Diego: IDEA Press, 1997.
6. Nieman DC. Using screening results for risk stratification. In: Malinee V, Seely C, eds. Exercise Testing and Prescription. New York: McGraw-Hill, 2003.

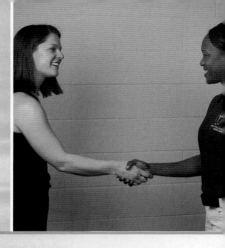

Tarra Hodge, Assistant Director Fitness/Wellness, Division of Recreational Sports, Purdue University, West Lafayette, Indiana

Chapter Outline

Objectives

- Define the difference between goals and objectives
- Learn how constructs of client psychology and behavioral change are incorporated into the goals-setting process
- Learn how to help clients set goals that initiate and maintain a learning environment
- Define goals and objectives of the Personal Trainer
- Provide guidelines for planning a client's program

Goal setting is a powerful strategy used for increasing participation in an exercise program. Goal setting is a technique that can be defined as a strategic approach to behavioral change, creating an opportunity to assess individual needs and develop an individualized plan of action in an attempt to achieve a desired outcome.

Personal Trainers should become familiar with the constructs of data gathering, client needs analysis, development of goals and objectives, exercise program development and implementation, and observation, evaluation, and feedback of exercise behaviors. The Personal Trainer can then determine programming strategies that can best be used to help engage individuals in the exercise training process. This chapter reviews the role of the Personal Trainer as a teacher and an educator of health, fitness, and exercise education and is based on the understanding that each component directly influences and/or is influenced by the client's goals and objectives.

Many personal training certification manuals do not take the learning process into consideration for exercise program design. By understanding the foundations of the learning process and goal setting and how to apply them in the context of an educator, the Personal Trainer can help identify for a client the best learning style approach to personal training.

GOALS AND OBJECTIVES: THE DIFFERENCE AND THE IMPORTANCE

Identifying goals and objectives is a major part of the Personal Trainer's role when developing logical and sequential exercise programs for clients. However, in many situations, Personal Trainers often use the words "goals" and "objectives" interchangeably, developing programs that do not facilitate an educationally based learning process. Understanding the purpose of goals and objectives, their differences, and how they should be applied within and throughout the personal training process is important to facilitating the role of a Personal Trainer as an educator.

The purpose of a **goal** is to provide meaning for something a person wants to achieve, influencing how a behavior is perceived and how a behavior will be performed (1). Personal Trainers can assume that exercise goals selected by a client hold purpose and meaning for them. However, Personal Trainers must also assume that simply identifying these goals does not guarantee that clients understand how to successfully engage in exercise behaviors to achieve these goals. For example: "I want to lose weight." This goal is a general statement of intent. Without a well-designed program in place, clients will approach the personal training session as a "training session" rather than as an educational process.

The Personal Trainer should identify specific actions to be taken to reach the established goals, creating the foundation for goal setting. **Objectives** identify measurable strategies that lead to achieving desired outcomes. Objectives are best described through statements of action that include specific information about what the client will be able to do, how well, how many, and to what degree (Table 13.1). For example, if a client wishes to lose weight, the Personal Trainer and the client together could establish the following objectives to be learned in a time period of 2 weeks:

➤ To demonstrate/identify portion sizes
➤ To demonstrate understanding of how to read a food label, and/or
➤ To demonstrate competency in identifying the five basic food groups

Table 13.1	EXAMPLES OF GOOD AND BAD OBJECTIVES
Objective	**Strength/Weaknesses/Comments**
To learn the major muscles of the body	This is a specific learning objective, including identifying specific characteristics that will aid in success of the ultimate goal
Lift weights	This objective is too vague and there are many components to doing this type of activity; the objective must be more specific, addressing what will be learned from the activity
To demonstrate proper knowledge of a lifting technique	This objective is very specific, identifying skills and knowledge about resistance training
To learn to monitor heart rate	This objective is also too general and does not narrow down the focus of the training enough for either learning or evaluation

CLIENT PSYCHOLOGY AND BEHAVIORAL CHANGE

Exercise is a process influenced by physical, psychological, social, and behavioral characteristics (2). In the past, health and fitness professionals have attempted to motivate people to exercise by adopting a health benefits/health risk approach. For example, if beliefs and attitudes toward the positive physical and mental outcomes of exercise were changed, clients would be more likely to adopt exercise as a habit, leading to increased adherence (3).

As change is typically viewed as an all-or-none event, individuals would be expected to modify their behavior through various intervention strategies proposed by health professionals. Translating a desire to change a health behavior, however, into actually changing that behavior is challenging for most. Though individuals may wish to eat healthier or be more physically fit, they may not have the knowledge, focus, or motivation to actually make those changes (4, 5). Just becoming aware of the consequences of specific behaviors, including sedentary lifestyles, high-fat diets, and/or smoking, does not facilitate engagement in healthier behaviors (6).

Behavior change programs recognize individual need to change, how people contemplate change, and what strategies are most effective in helping people make changes that will allow them to sustain exercise as a behavior. To help individuals adopt and maintain exercise as a lifestyle behavior, health professionals need to understand the attitudes, decisions, and actions involved in making that process successful.

A client's attitude toward exercise often is reflected by his or her perceived knowledge of, and/or ability to, successfully engage in the activity. **Self-efficacy** describes the confidence one has to perform specific behaviors in the face of challenging situations. It influences how people feel, the choices they make, the effort they put forth, and the persistence they distribute to the current behavior. For example, the perception/understanding of how to demonstrate the proper technique of an exercise (e.g., an abdominal crunch on a Swiss ball) will actually determine whether a client will be able to perform that exercise successfully. It influences the client's choices (decisions), effort, and persistence. The self-perception of performing that same exercise will also influence the client's ability to retain the knowledge and skill to perform that exercise on his or her own. It is important to remember that exercise is a series of logical progressions. An individual struggling with correctly performing a basic crunch on the floor will not be successful when performing a more advanced exercise (such as an abdominal crunch on a Swiss ball) and has probably never been properly educated on basic core exercises.

Self-efficacy beliefs largely determine how people feel, think, behave, and motivate themselves to carry out behaviors. Therefore, establishing a strong belief in competency in relation to exercise is highly important when determining success of the exercise program, especially in the beginning phases of activity (7). Identifying variables that may affect self-efficacy, as well as variables that may be affected by an individual's self-efficacy, should be considered when establishing objectives during the goal-setting process. Self-efficacy beliefs, in part, determine behavioral outcomes. They also demonstrate a strong correlation with individual levels of motivation.

MOTIVATIONAL FEEDBACK

Motivation refers to the forces acting either on or within oneself to initiate action toward a desired goal/behavior (8). Just as self-efficacy plays an important role in initiating exercise behaviors, motivation must play a similarly effective role in maintaining behaviors of exercise.

Initiating and/or maintaining a behavior is influenced by intrinsic and extrinsic sources of motivation. While intrinsically motivated behaviors are derived from an internal sense of satisfaction, extrinsically motivated behaviors are engaged in to achieve a goal or outcome. In more general terms, **intrinsic motivation** is a true desire to experience exercise with a sense of pleasure during its performance, with no incentive or reward other than the interest of the behavior itself (9). **Extrinsic motivation** implies that the desire to engage in a behavior is based on the expectation of an external reward. Although intrinsic and extrinsic motivation are defined independently of their influence to engage in a behavior, they are actually linked through the concept of internalization, or **self-determination** (9). For example, people often engage in exercise for enjoyment (intrinsic motivation) while also engaging in exercise for health reasons (extrinsic motivation). People who engage in a behavior and find it both intrinsically and extrinsically motivating often find the behavior to be self-fulfilling (9). It is therefore appropriate for the Personal Trainer to understand that exercise behaviors often are influenced by several motivating factors and often are associated with individual stages of readiness (7, 9, 10), as discussed in Chapter 10. This can help the Personal Trainer establish goal-setting strategies for the client that are unique and individualized to his or her learning style.

As learning typically takes place in the context of a relationship between the Personal Trainer and the client, how this interaction affects the development of the learning process is evaluated through the context of how the Personal Trainer provides feedback, how the feedback affects self-efficacy, and how self-efficacy affects one's actual performance. The client's level of motivation, competence, and adherence to the exercise activity is often determined by the positive or negative feedback given by the Personal Trainer (11).

Feedback is typically presented in two ways: *(a)* information based on the outcome of performance and/or *(b)* information pertaining to performance technique. Both forms of feedback can be intrinsically and extrinsically motivating to the client and should be positively reinforced immediately after the behavior is performed, to reflect established training objectives. This enhances self-competence to the exercise behavior, increasing the likelihood that it will be performed again (7).

For example, a Personal Trainer and the client may have established as a goal to demonstrate the proper form while performing a certain exercise. As the client is educated on the constructs of form, technique, breathing, cadence of movement, and muscle engagement, providing feedback on the performance progress and overall execution of the movement reinforces the pattern. In a more general sense, how clients identify the completion of, or progress toward, their goals and objective leads to self-evaluation of success or failure of their efforts.

Understanding a client's learning style is important to the development of learning objectives that focus on increasing self-competency and adherence to exercise. Behavioral change programs are facilitated through cognitive and behavioral processes of change that incorporate identified learning strategies into performance objectives. It is believed that incorporating cognitive learning strategies into initial learning objectives at the early stages of exercise may be important to enhancing motivation, competence, and adherence to exercise behaviors (5). An example might be to enhance awareness of kinesthetic senses to specific weight-training exercises through increased awareness of the body's positioning during the exercise, muscle and joint engagement, and balance of movement. As training continues, this cognitive behavior helps enhance the client's ability to self-maintain proper form and technique of an exercise independent of the Personal Trainer.

UNDERSTANDING THE ROLE OF REINFORCEMENT IN THE GOALS-SETTING PROCESS

The element of learning is an adaptation to change in relation to a behavior (12, 13). Behaviorism is based on the idea that we behave the way we do because of past consequences (reinforcement of the past). For example, the type of feedback may dramatically influence exercise adherence, or reinforcement, that a client is given from his or her Personal Trainer based on a given movement and when that feedback is given. This behavior (movement) is **operant** and reflects the target behavior that is intended to be repeated when reinforced. Operant behaviors should be clearly addressed in the objective statements of a client's session plan and reviewed with the client at the end of and prior to each training session. For example, objectives stating demonstration of proper form and technique in relation to resistance training exercises, such as seated chest press, seated row, and seated shoulder press, are specific and operant, identifying specifically what exercises are to be performed and reviewed. Because Personal Trainers are instrumental in developing and fostering a positive learning experience, understanding the context of behaviorism is a good way to evaluate how a Personal Trainer works with clients and responds to their actions (12–14).

CLIENT'S INITIAL GOALS AND OBJECTIVES: SHORT- AND LONG-TERM

As goals create the foundation of the training process, the development of goals plays an important role in identifying a purpose for participation in exercise behaviors and directing a focus to achieve desired exercise outcomes. Understanding the basic characteristics of goals and goal setting will help Personal Trainers better identify strategies that aid in the development of individualized exercise programs, establishing a link between motivation and overall success of desired changes.

Outcome, or long-term goals, are statements of intent that identify the desire to participate in a behavior (e.g., "I will eat a healthier diet"). Outcome goals are expressed in general terms that refer to long-range intended outcomes. To meet these long-term goals, it is important to identify **performance, or short-term, goals** that more specifically identify steps that point in the direction of long-term outcomes. An example of a short-term, or performance, goal for the above statement may be: "I will eat four servings of fruits and/or vegetables five days this week: Monday, Tuesday, Thursday, Friday, and Saturday." Because performance goals are more specific to identifying a timeline of activity to reaching outcome goals, they help reduce anxiety and help increase successful performance levels.

In the beginning of this chapter, goals and objectives are defined in general terms. Long-term and short-term goals (not unlike objectives) identify desired outcomes. However, the characteristic that distinguishes goals from objectives is the level of specificity. Process goals, which can also be termed "objectives," define specific learning outcomes (e.g., to demonstrate an understanding of food portion sizes within each of the five food groups). Process goals, whether cognitive, affective (attitude, personal, social), or behavioral, identify types of performances that clients are expected to demonstrate at the end of instruction. Understanding the purpose of process goals and how they contribute to desired long-term and short-term outcomes helps establish a foundation for successful programming by allowing the Personal Trainer to create a unique environment for learning (14).

Outcome, performance, and process goal-setting strategies have been shown to be most effective for improving performance and psychological skill development in exercise performance among individuals, especially when used together (14). Identifying desired outcomes (long-term) would help the Personal Trainer establish the best performance (short-term) goals to help the client attain

Table 13.2	EXAMPLES OF OUTCOME, PERFORMANCE, AND PROCESS GOALS	
Goal Type	**Example A**	**Example B**
Outcome	Improve body image in 6 months	Win a power-lifting event
Performance	Decrease body fat to 16% and increase muscle mass by 11 lb (5 kg)	Increase lifting totals by 10%
Process	Weight train: Mon, Wed, Fri (7 PM) Walk/run 20–45 minutes Tues, Thurs, Sat (6:00 AM) Implement specific dietary guidelines Monitor body composition monthly	Follow a structured periodized training program Monitor signs of overtraining Meet with a Personal Trainer three times per week Taper volume 1 week before event

a level of proficiency to reaching long-term outcomes. After outcome and performance goals have been identified, the Personal Trainer can establish process goals (learning objectives) that will identify specific skills to reach expected performance levels.

It is important to remember that success in achieving a goal behavior is based on the action plan (objective) that specifies what learners will be able to do, or perform, to be considered competent in those specific behaviors. Goal-setting strategies allow individuals to set goals in terms of successful outcomes based on personal performance measures and improvements in exercise technique (14). Table 13.2 demonstrates examples of outcome, performance, and process goals.

HOW TO HELP CLIENTS FORMULATE REALISTIC GOALS AND OBJECTIVES

Understanding the properties that make goals effective is critical to the success of actually writing adequate goals (15). Obtaining an accurate assessment of present skills, knowledge, abilities, and/or deficiencies to exercise is the first step of the goal-setting process.

The acronym SMART has long been used by behavioral psychologists to help individuals remember important characteristics of engaging in behaviors through goal setting, focusing on the overall process and outcome of a desired activity (14). SMART (Specific, Measurable, Attainable/Acceptable, Realistic/Relevant, and Time-anchored) goals and objectives describe each behavior and skill that will be taught throughout training sessions and must define each skill or behavior in ways that are positive and attainable to the client.

Specific goals provide enough detail to identify the action required to accomplish the goal. The variables of who, what, when, where, and how are typical goal-oriented questions to help make goals specific. Goals that are specific help individuals to focus on desired outcomes. Therefore, the more detailed the goals, the more likely they are to be achieved.

Good example: To eat at least three servings of vegetables a day
Poor example: To be healthier

Measurable goals identify what tasks are to be accomplished and when they have been reached. Measurable goals tell an individual if, and when, their goal has been achieved. For example, an individual will know if he or she ate one fruit and one vegetable a day, but not necessarily whether he or she became healthier from doing so. Therefore, it is important to identify how individual goals will be monitored (e.g., number of servings, body composition, change in blood pressure). The ability to see improvement in any measurement over time is an incentive for many to continue their training program.

Good example: To lose 15 pounds by February 1
Poor example: To lose weight

Attainable/Acceptable goals focus on activity that will produce results. These goals use words such as "I will . . . I am . . . I still am . . ." and help establish focus toward a specific goal, promoting action to the specific outcome.

> *Good example: To walk three times a week for 10 minutes*
> *Poor example: To get into shape*

Realistic/Relevant goals refer to practicality of reaching desired outcomes. These goals are goals that are challenging yet achievable. An individual who perceives a goal too far out of reach has a limited chance of ever reaching that goal.

> *Good example: To walk for 30 minutes at lunchtime*
> *Poor example: To run 20 miles a day*

Time-Anchored goals enable individuals to monitor progress at regular intervals. Goals that are too conservative often encounter quick results, allowing individuals to lose focus and motivation. Goals that are too aggressive, or drawn out, promote disengagement and increase the likelihood they will not be accomplished.

> *Good example: To lift weights 2 times a week for a month*
> *Poor example: To lift weights 2 times week*

NEEDS ASSESSMENT, GOALS, AND KSAs OF THE PERSONAL TRAINER

For training to be effective, efficient, and engaging, the focus of exercise programs must be based on the *needs* of the client. Chapter 3 identified the components of a needs analysis, and its relevance to establishing goals and objectives for the client should now be apparent.

For example, take a client whose right glenohumeral joint is assessed as 2 inches (5.08 cm) lower than the left and shows excessive internal rotation. Understanding that posture and body alignment is critical to the safety and overall effectiveness of a strength training program and identifying exercises to help correct glenohumeral posture should be incorporated into the exercise program before an emphasis on specific training of the upper thoracic region takes place. However, for many Personal Trainers, the evaluation of posture and body alignment and its application to exercise training often goes undetected because they have not been trained or educated properly.

As you become familiar with the knowledge, skills, and abilities (KSAs) of the Personal Trainer in the 7th edition of *ACSM's Guidelines for Exercise Testing and Prescription* (16), you will better recognize how the foundations of exercise are based on areas of human anatomy, exercise physiology, biomechanics, kinesiology, motor learning, exercise safety, and nutrition and how they apply to exercise involvement. Recognizing the KSAs of the Personal Trainer will help you identify constructs relative to exercise behaviors that can be applied to developing specific behavioral strategies (objectives) appropriate to helping clients achieve the knowledge, skills, and mastery of exercise movements. For example, in relation to the KSAs of the Personal Trainer, by recognizing the inconsistency in posture and body alignment of the client, you recognize its importance in exercise safety as well as the importance of correcting posture and body alignment to perform accurate and correct exercise movements of the shoulder region to produce visible results. Therefore, the Personal Trainer may focus on incorporating 4 weeks of posture and body alignment exercises for the glenohumeral joint into the goals and objectives of the client, emphasizing successful execution of each repetition.

Setting and Recording Client Goals and Objectives

A successful goal-setting program should provide a diversity of goals, including short-term and long-term goals, and be based on the scientific foundations of goal-setting research. Understanding the foundations of exercise behavior will allow Personal Trainers and their clients to set logical goals and objectives specific and unique to individual needs. As an example of a diversified goal-setting approach, think of a 28-year-old client who is a very talented swimmer. She has been competing in the 100-meter breaststroke and wishes to establish a self best time. The long-term goal should address her desired outcome and be stated in a way that is personally meaningful. Assuming this client has the talent and ability to achieve her performance goal if she optimizes her efforts and trains in a strategic manner, she should be able to improve her performance time, technique/performance of movement, and motivation. It is important to keep in mind that any individual will encounter motivational obstacles when striving for a challenging behavior; thus short-term goals must be incorporated into the context of a well-designed training program. The Personal Trainer should identify current levels and abilities of the client and incorporate strategies to improve those levels of abilities in the client's overall goals and objectives. On some training days, the client may focus on goals establishing breathing technique and mechanically efficient arm stroke. On other training days she may stress resistance training goals to enhance upper body strength/stamina. Still on other training days, she may concentrate on psychological goals with a positive focus.

Evaluating Client Goals and Objectives

When most Personal Trainers typically think of evaluating goals and objectives, they often think of the final evaluation, determining the client's overall success from the first training session to the last. However, just as clients are negatively affected by a lack of specificity in the detail of what they can expect to receive from personal training, they also are negatively affected by a lack of specificity in detail about how they perform. It is important to remember that evaluating cognitive and behavioral performance measures throughout each training session, exercise by exercise, repetition by repetition, helps demonstrate improvement of exercise performance, increasing self-efficacy, and motivation of behavior.

Understanding how goals and objectives are evaluated is critical to how goals and objectives are written. Goals and objectives can be evaluated and reinforced in two ways: through observation and through objective measurement.

Evaluating goals and objectives through observation is based on assessment of the individual knowledge, attitudes, and skills of the client. For example, if a client's goal is to demonstrate the proper technique of a seated shoulder press, the Personal Trainer may provide feedback relevant to the client's ability to execute the movement correctly. Evaluating clients through observation is usually done within the training session, reinforcing knowledge and skill of movement.

Assessing goals and objectives based on performance involves assessing and reassessing the progress of initial performance measurements to later performance measurements. This form of evaluation is typically applied toward short-term and long-term goals and usually requires a definitive time commitment to achieving its desired outcome. For example, a client sets a goal of losing 3% of body fat within 10–12 weeks. At the initial assessment, the client is measured at 28%. When she is re-assessed 3 weeks later she is measured at 25%. Objective measurements are highly motivational because they demonstrate visual evidence of progress, reinforcing positive outcomes of participating in related exercise behaviors.

Personal Trainer's Initial Goals and Objectives

It should now be evident that the role of the Personal Trainer as an educator is critical to the overall success of a training program. As any professional educator will tell you, success in teaching is based on creating a well-designed curriculum that identifies goals and objectives to helping students learn intended behaviors. Identifying educational goals and objectives in the learning environment allows the student (client) to focus on the task at hand and the Personal Trainer to focus on the task of teaching.

Chapter 5 emphasizes the role of the Personal Trainer as an educator and recognizes the skills and teaching methods necessary to successfully engage individuals in the learning process. Personal Trainers who are well educated in understanding the application of skills and teaching methods of personal training should be able to establish a vision of initial goals and objectives just through the first conversations with the client. At that time, they should also be able to identify the overall design of the training program and how its content will be selected, developed, implemented, observed, and evaluated. As the client goes through the needs assessment, the Personal Trainer will better be able to identify more specific goals and objectives that recognize learning and engagement strategies unique to that client.

The general points of learning and engagement for the client based on the foundations of exercise science, psychological and behavioral development, and motor learning are discussed in Chapter 3. Those statements present common points of exercise knowledge and skill that can be applied to the development of progressive teaching objectives unique to each client's ability and level of training. For example: A 55-year-old male wants to start a regular physical activity routine. He has never really lifted weights before but is intrigued by the benefits he may receive. After the screening and health and fitness assessment, the Personal Trainer notes that the client has exaggerated posture and body alignment. Therefore, the Personal Trainer may establish goals for the client to address the following:

➤ To demonstrate knowledge of anatomical location of the following muscles within 3 weeks of training: pectoralis major, latissimus dorsi, trapezius, deltoids, biceps, triceps, rectus abdominus, erector spinae, gluteus maximus, quadriceps, hamstring, soleus/gastrocnemius

➤ To demonstrate proper form and technique within 10 weeks for associated basic core exercises, including seated chest press, seated back row, shoulder/trapezius shrug, dumbbell lateral raise, internal/external rotation with exercise tubing, leg extension, seated leg curl, leg press, calf raise

➤ To improve posture and body alignment closer to the line of gravity after 10 sessions based on reassessment of posture and body alignment photos

Chapter 3 identifies a structured outline of a week-to-week training program designed to educate and foster progressive outcomes when training clients. The model defines suggested strategies for resistance training, cardiovascular training, and flexibility training, creating a positive environment for learning. By identifying the client's objective status, the model presents an opportunity for the Personal Trainer to introduce what will be done during each session, as well as to summarize what has been achieved after each session, enabling the client to reassess what has been learned and prepare for future meetings.

COMMUNICATION, FEEDBACK, AND CLIENT EVALUATION/ASSESSMENT

The importance of communication should not be overlooked when working with individuals in an exercise setting. It should be evident that good communication is fundamental to all forms of teaching and is an important aspect of teaching behavior. It is essential to exercise adherence that the Personal Trainer provide consistency in guidance and feedback on performance measures and progress of total goal achievement that is clear and measurable. Providing clear communication of goals, objectives, expectations, and evaluation of activity is an evolving process that enhances self-competency and self-efficacy of exercise behavior, increasing motivation and adherence to the exercise process (17). Creating a positive learning environment for increasing communication is an aspect of professionalism and key to becoming a good Personal Trainer. If communication is unclear at any point in the learning process, the educational experience of the client is diminished.

The effects of the goal-setting process on self-efficacy, motivation, provision of feedback, and the evaluation of performance measures is important to the total outcome of the client's learning experience. As each factor of the goal-setting process is directly affected by another, understanding the importance of involvement that the Personal Trainer has in developing goals and objectives is critical to the overall success of a client's training program.

12 STEPS TO EFFECTIVELY PLANNING YOUR CLIENT'S PROGRAM

Personal Trainers identify and design instructional content, materials, and methods necessary to develop educationally based training programs that help clients establish exercise as a lifestyle behavior. Understanding the goal-setting process and its contents as presented throughout this chapter will help the Personal Trainer guide individuals to identify realistic goals and objectives that establish a foundation for individualized exercise programming. The following steps represent an outline of how to help clients formulate realistic goals and objectives that will facilitate an evolving exercise process:

1. Determine the client's perceptions, attitude, and level of commitment to exercise.
2. Identify barriers to desired outcomes. Both the Personal Trainer and the client should recognize that absence of knowledge and skill of associated behaviors to the desired outcome could hinder achievement of performance. Evaluating the client's level of knowledge in the needs assessment will help set knowledge-based goals (e.g., learning the location and function of muscles in relation to specific resistance training exercises).
3. Establish a starting point. After the needs analysis, a Personal Trainer should be able to identify the client's "starting line." For instance, a client who has made numerous attempts to make exercise a regular habit but has failed to do so will not be able to start out as aggressively as someone who has been exercising but wants a more structured program.
4. Agree on and plan out long-term (outcome) goals.
5. Identify performance goals that will lead to long-term outcomes. If the goal is to run a 10K (6.2 miles) within 3 months and the client has never run before, the first performance goal might be to walk/run two or three times a week; the second performance goal might be to run three or four times a week, 1 to 2 miles a day; the third performance goal may be to run a 5K (3.2 miles); and the fourth goal may be to run a 10K.
6. Identify process goals (objectives) that will lead to performance and outcome goals. For example, a client who has established a goal to run a 10k within 3 months may have learning objectives that focus on establishing proper running form or foot strike, efficiently facilitating proper arm swing, or upper body mechanics when training, and/or establishing proper breathing technique while running.
7. Identify variables to make goals specific, measurable, action-based, realistic, and time-line (SMART). Goals that reflect these principles demonstrate practicality, relevance, and achievability to the client. Measurable and timely goals allow evaluation and recognition of achievement.
8. Ensure that goals are compatible with each other. Wanting to increase muscle mass and wanting to lose weight somewhat contradict each other in general statements because muscle weighs more than fat. If clients see goals conflicting, they compromise their chance for success.
9. Prioritize goals/objectives. The content of the exercise program should flow logically from one session to the next as well as from the beginning of the session to the end. Each new body of knowledge/skill should be built upon the preceding in order of importance. Determine that a client's goals coincide with your (the Personal Trainer's) expectations.
10. After setting goals, ensure that the client perceives they are attainable. If not, provide more specific strategies or adjust them.
11. As time goes on, evaluate goals and objectives to ensure continual progression of short-term goals toward overall desired outcomes. Goals can and should then be adjusted at regular intervals (e.g., every 2 weeks).
12. Revise and identify goals and objectives to initiate newer and more challenging tasks encouraging goal achievement.

SUMMARY

Goal setting is an important part of the exercise training process for both the client and the Personal Trainer. Setting goals that are specific, measurable, action-based, realistic, and time-lined helps encourage regular participation in exercise behavior. Understanding how to properly apply the goal-setting process to the actual training program helps motivate clients toward their established goals, minimizing delays and misconceptions and enhancing adherence to exercise behaviors.

REFERENCES

1. Lock EA, Latham GP. A Theory of Goal Setting and Task Performance. Englewood Cliffs, NJ: Prentice-Hall, 1990.
2. Sallis JF, Hovell MF, Hofstetter CR, et al. A multivariate study of determinants of vigorous exercise in a community sample. Prev Med 1989;18:20–34.
3. Wankel LM. Personal and situational factor affecting exercise involvement. The importance of enjoyment. Res Q Exerc Sport 1985;56(3):275–282.
4. Howley E, Franks D. Health and Fitness Instructors Book. Champaign, IL: Human Kinetics, 1997.
5. Prochaska J, Norcross J, Diclemente C. Changing for Good. New York: William Morrow, 1994.
6. Bandura A. Self-efficacy: Toward a unifying theory of behavioral change. Psychol Rev 1977;84:191–215.
7. Bandura A. Self-Efficacy: The Exercise of Control. New York: Freeman, 1997.
8. Encyclopedia Britannica, Encyclopedia Britannica Premium Service on the Internet at http://www.britannica.com/eb/article?tocId=9108744. Accessed March 22, 2005.
9. Deci EL, Ryan RM. Intrinsic Motivation and Self-Determination in Human Behavior. New York: Plenum Press, 1985.
10. Matsumoto H, Takenaka K. Motivational Profiles and Stages of Exercise Behavior Change. Int J Sport Health Sci 2004;2:89–96.
11. Escarti A, Guzman JF. Effects of feedback on self-efficacy, performance, and choice in an athletic task. J Appl Sports Psychol 1999;11:8–22.
12. Skinner BF. The Behavior of Organisms: An Experimental Analysis. New York: Appleton Century Crofts, 1938.
13. Skinner BF. Science and Human Behavior. New York: Macmillan, 1953.
14. Cox RH. Sport Psychology: Concepts and Applications. New York: McGraw-Hill, 2002.
15. Schunk DH. Self-Regulation through Goal Setting. ERIC Digest. Greensboro, NC: ERIC Clearinghouse on Counseling and Student Services (ERIC Document Reproduction Service No. ED462 671), 2001.
16. American College of Sports Medicine. ACSM's Guidelines for Graded Exercise Testing and Prescription. 7th ed. Baltimore: Lippincott Williams & Wilkins, 2005.
17. Lock EA, Bryan JF. The effects of goal-setting, rule learning, and knowledge of score on performance. Am J Psychol 1966;79:451–457.

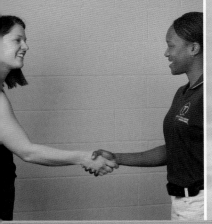

Screening and Risk Stratification

Cody Sipe, M.S., Director, A.H. Ismail Center for Health, Exercise & Nutrition, Purdue University, West Lafayette, Indiana

Chapter Outline

- **To communicate the importance of standardized screenings for clients**
- **To identify and describe appropriate screening components and processes**
- **To provide resources and templates for the screening process**

This chapter presents guidelines related to pre-participation health screening and risk that takes place during the initial client consultation. Other published guidelines, such as those from the American Heart Association (1, 2) and the American Association of Cardiovascular and Pulmonary Rehabilitation (3), provide additional guidance for exercise professionals and should be reviewed when establishing policies for pre-participation health screening and medical clearance.

WHY SCREEN?

Despite all of the health, fitness, and functional benefits that come from regular exercise participation, exercise can acutely and transiently increase a client's risk of sudden cardiac death (4, 5) and acute myocardial infarction (heart attack) (6, 7). It is important for the Personal Trainer to remember that exercise usually only provokes cardiovascular events in clients with pre-existing heart disease. Exercise typically does not promote cardiac events in clients with normal cardiovascular systems. However, many clients are unaware of their risk of cardiovascular disease or of how other health conditions may be affected by exercise training.

Purposes of Screening

To optimize safety during exercise participation, Personal Trainers should screen all new clients for risk factors and/or symptoms of cardiovascular, pulmonary, and metabolic diseases, as well as conditions (e.g., pregnancy, orthopedic injury) that may be aggravated by exercise. Even more specifically, the purposes of this pre-participation health screening include the following (8):

➤ Identification and exclusion of clients with medical contraindications to exercise
➤ Identification of clients at increased risk for disease because of age, symptoms, and/or risk factors who should undergo a medical evaluation and exercise testing before starting an exercise program
➤ Identification of clients with clinically significant disease who should participate in a medically supervised exercise program
➤ Identification of clients with other special needs
➤ Identification of the Personal Trainer best suited to work with the client based on the client's risk factors and/or medical conditions

In addition, the screening process begins the communication process between the Personal Trainer and the client's healthcare provider while providing opportunities for immediate client education.

THE SCREENING PROCESS

Since Personal Trainers work individually with clients, they are able to develop a more in-depth profile of a client than that typically performed by a client exercising independently outside a clinical program or by a typical health club. The process can be broken down into three distinct, but related, phases:

1. Risk stratification
2. Health history evaluation and related assessments
3. Medical clearance or referral

The screening process should be followed by a discussion of the results with the client, a description of any additional fitness assessments that he or she will perform, and completion of an informed consent. The Personal Trainer can adopt this process by following these steps:

Step 1: Determine the number of risk factors, based on Table 14.1, "Coronary Artery Disease Risk Factor Thresholds for Use with ACSM Risk Stratification," and the number of signs and symptoms, based on Table 14.2, "Major Signs or Symptoms Suggestive of Cardiovascular, Pulmonary, or Metabolic Disease."
Step 2: Determine whether the client is low, moderate, or high risk, based on Table 14.3, "ACSM Risk Stratification Categories."
Step 3: Determine if a medical evaluation or exercise testing is necessary based on Table 14.4, "ACSM Pre-Participation Screening Algorithm."
Step 4: Conduct a health history evaluation *(Figs. 14.1 and 14.2)*.
Step 5: Obtain a medical clearance if indicated by steps 3 or 4 *(Figs. 14.3 and 14.4)*.
Step 6: Complete an informed consent *(Fig. 14.5)*.
Step 7: Conduct appropriate assessments (see Chapter 15).
Step 8: Refer client to a physician or other healthcare provider if warranted.

Risk Stratification

The ACSM risk stratification process has been widely used to identify clients who should undergo a medical examination and exercise testing prior to beginning a moderate or vigorous exercise program. The process is based on the client's risk factors for cardiovascular, pulmonary, or metabolic disease; signs and symptoms suggestive of disease; and diagnoses of disease. It provides recommendations for both medical clearance and physician involvement in submaximal or maximal cardiovascular fitness testing.

This process is often not quite as straightforward as described here. Some Personal Trainers prefer to embed the ACSM risk stratification information into the health history evaluation so that they are not two separate pieces. There is certainly nothing wrong with doing this as long as the process to determine risk stratification is followed correctly. Potential musculoskeletal problems can also be assessed through the health history evaluation. Medical clearance should be obtained after the Personal Trainer has conducted both the risk stratification and a thorough health history interview with the client. This eliminates the aggravation of contacting the healthcare provider multiple times if medical clearance becomes necessary.

Self-administered questionnaires such as the Physical Activity Readiness Questionnaire (PAR-Q) (see Fig. 14.1) and the AHA/ACSM Health/Fitness Facility Pre-Participation Screening Questionnaire (2) have been used extensively as screening tools in both health/fitness facilities and unsupervised fitness facilities. The PAR-Q focuses on symptoms of heart disease while also identifying musculoskeletal problems that should be evaluated before participation. The one-page AHA/ACSM questionnaire is more extensive than the PAR-Q and uses history, symptoms, and risk factors to direct clients to either participate in an exercise program or contact their healthcare provider before participation. Although providing great value to independent exercisers or fitness facilities providing general supervision, they are not as useful for Personal Trainers, who require a more extensive health profile of their clients.

Personal Trainers who work in health clubs should not assume that since clients have been cleared for a membership based on either of these screening tools or based on more in-depth assessments collected previously, they do not require further evaluation or medical clearance. Personal Trainers should always confirm with clients that their risk stratification and health information is accurate and up-to-date before proceeding with exercise training. Signs and symptoms suggesting cardiovascular disease can appear suddenly, medication changes are frequent, and injuries may occur without warning. It is also possible that a client is seeking the assistance of a Personal Trainer because he or

Table 14.1	CORONARY ARTERY DISEASE RISK FACTOR THRESHOLDS FOR USE WITH ACSM RISK STRATIFICATION
Positive Risk Factors	**Defining Criteria**
Family history	Myocardial infarction, coronary revascularization, or sudden death before 55 years of age in father or other male first-degree relative, or before 65 years of age in mother or other female first-degree relative
Cigarette smoking	Current cigarette smoker or those who quit within the previous 6 months
Hypertension	Systolic blood pressure ≥140 mm Hg or diastolic ≥90 mm Hg, confirmed by measurements on at least two separate occasions, or on antihypertensive medication
Dyslipidemia	Low-density lipoprotein (LDL) cholesterol > 130 mg · dL^{-1} (3.4 mmol · L^{-1}) or high-density lipoprotein (HDL) cholesterol <40 mg · dL^{-1} (1.03 mmol · L^{-1}), or on lipid-lowering medication; if total serum cholesterol is all that is available, use >200 mg · dL^{-1} (5.2 mmol · L^{-1}) rather than LDL > 130 mg · dL^{-1}
Impaired fasting glucose	Fasting blood glucose ≥100 mg · dL^{-1} (5.6 mmol · L^{-1}) confirmed by measurements on at least two separate occasions
Obesity[a]	Body mass index >30 kg · m^{-2} or Waist girth >102 cm for men and >88 cm for women or Waist/hip ratio ≥0.95 for men and ≥0.86 for women
Sedentary lifestyle	Persons not participating in a regular exercise program or not meeting the minimal physical activity recommendations[b] from the U.S. Surgeon General's Report
Negative Risk Factor	**Defining Criteria**
High serum HDL cholesterol[c]	>60 mg · dL^{-1} (1.6 mmol · L^{-1})

Handwritten annotations: + 140 SBP, + 90 DSP; LDL 130+ BAD, HDL 60+; + BAD; 40 inches, 35 inches

Reprinted with permission from Guidelines for Exercise Testing and Prescription, 7th ed. Baltimore: Lippincott Williams & Wilkins, 2006:22.
Hypertension threshold based on National High Blood Pressure Education Program. The Seventh Report of the Joint National Committee on Prevention, Detection, Evaluation, and Treatment of High Blood Pressure (JNC7), 03-5233, 2003. Lipid thresholds based on National Cholesterol Education Program. Third Report of the National Cholesterol Education Program (NCEP) Expert Panel on Detection, Evaluation, and Treatment of High Blood Cholesterol in Adults (Adult Treatment Panel III). NIH Publ no. 02-5215, 2002. Impaired FG threshold based on Expert Committee on the Diagnosis and Classification of Diabetes Mellitus. Follow-up report on the diagnosis of diabetes mellitus. Diabetes Care 2003;26:3160–3167. Obesity thresholds based on Expert Panel on Detection, Evaluation, and Treatment of Overweight and Obesity in Adults. National Institutes of Health. Clinical guidelines on the identification, evaluation, and treatment of overweight and obesity in adults—the evidence report. Arch Intern Med 1998;158:1855–1867. Sedentary lifestyle thresholds based on United States Department of Health and Human Services. Physical activity and health: a report of the Surgeon General, 1996.

[a] Professional opinions vary regarding the most appropriate markers and thresholds for obesity, and therefore, allied health professionals should use clinical judgment when evaluating this risk factor.

[b] Accumulating 30 minutes or more of moderate physical activity on most days of the week.

[c] It is common to sum risk factors in making clinical judgments. If HDL is high, subtract one risk factor from the sum of positive risk factors, because high HDL decreases CAD risk.

she has begun to experience new or additional signs and symptoms that they have not yet communicated to others (i.e., healthcare providers).

Clients transitioning out of cardiopulmonary rehabilitation, physical therapy, or another medically supervised program will still need written medical clearance even if their physician referred them to a Personal Trainer or to a club or recommended that they continue their exercise The advantage for the Personal Trainer is that he or she will be able to access the client's exercise records and clinical documentation. This can be accomplished by asking the client to get a copy of his or her file from the healthcare provider or sign a waiver for you to obtain a copy directly from the healthcare provider.

Coronary Artery Disease Risk Factors

ACSM risk stratification is based, in part, on the presence or absence of the coronary artery disease (CAD) risk factors listed in Table 14.1 (7–16). The risk factors in Table 14.1 should not be viewed

HIGH RISK IF ONE OF THESE IS Present.

Table 14.2	MAJOR SIGNS OR SYMPTOMS SUGGESTIVE OF CARDIOVASCULAR, PULMONARY, OR METABOLIC DISEASE[a]

Sign or Symptom	Clarification/Significance

Pain, discomfort (or other anginal equivalent) in the chest, neck, jaw, arms, or other areas that may result from ischemia	One of the cardinal manifestations of cardiac disease, in particular coronary artery disease
	Key features *favoring an ischemic origin* include:
	    Character: Constricting, squeezing, burning, "heaviness" or "heavy feeling"
	    Location: Substernal, across midthorax, anteriorly; in both arms, shoulders; in neck, cheeks, teeth; in forearms, fingers in interscapular region
	    Provoking factors: Exercise or exertion, excitement, other forms of stress, cold weather, occurrence after meals
	Key features *against an ischemic origin* include:
	    Character: Dull ache; "knifelike," sharp, stabbing; "jabs" aggravated by respiration
	    Location: In left submammary area; in left hemithorax
	    Provoking factors: After completion of exercise, provoked by a specific body motion

Shortness of breath at rest or with mild exertion	Dyspnea (defined as an abnormally uncomfortable awareness of breathing) is one of the principal symptoms of cardiac and pulmonary disease. It commonly occurs during strenuous exertion in healthy, well-trained persons and during moderate exertion in healthy, untrained persons. However, it should be regarded as abnormal when it occurs at a level of exertion that is not expected to evoke this symptom in a given individual. Abnormal exertional dyspnea suggests the presence of cardiopulmonary disorders, in particular left ventricular dysfunction or chronic obstructive pulmonary disease.
Dizziness or syncope (loss of consciousness)	Syncope (defined as a loss of consciousness) is most commonly caused by a reduced perfusion of the brain. Dizziness and, in particular, syncope *during* exercise may result from cardiac disorders that prevent the normal rise (or an actual fall) in cardiac output. Such cardiac disorders are potentially life-threatening and include severe coronary artery disease, hypertrophic cardiomyopathy, aortic stenosis, and malignant ventricular dysrhythmias. Although dizziness or syncope shortly *after* cessation of exercise should not be ignored, these symptoms may occur even in healthy persons as a result of a reduction in venous return to the heart.
Orthopnea or paroxysmal nocturnal dyspnea	Orthopnea refers to dyspnea occurring at rest in the recumbent position that is relieved promptly by sitting upright or standing. Paroxysmal nocturnal dyspnea refers to dyspnea, beginning usually 2 to 5 hours after the onset of sleep, which may be relieved by sitting on the side of the bed or getting out of bed. Both are symptoms of left ventricular dysfunction. Although nocturnal dyspnea may occur in persons with chronic obstructive pulmonary disease, it differs in that it is usually relieved after the person relieves himself/herself of secretions rather than specifically by sitting up.
Ankle edema	Bilateral ankle edema that is most evident at night is a characteristic sign of heart failure or bilateral chronic venous insufficiency. Unilateral edema of a limb often results from venous thrombosis or lymphatic blockage in the limb. Generalized edema (known as anasarca) occurs in persons with the nephrotic syndrome, severe heart failure, or hepatic cirrhosis.

High Risk if one of these is present

Table 14.2	**MAJOR SIGNS OR SYMPTOMS SUGGESTIVE OF CARDIOVASCULAR, PULMONARY, OR METABOLIC DISEASE[a] (CONTINUED)**
Palpitations or tachycardia	Palpitations (defined as an unpleasant awareness of the forceful or rapid beating of the heart) may be induced by various disorders of cardiac rhythm. These include tachycardia, bradycardia of sudden onset, ectopic beats, compensatory pauses, and accentuated stroke volume resulting from valvular regurgitation. Palpitations also often result from anxiety states, such as anemia, fever, thyrotoxicosis, arteriovenous fistula, and the so-called idiopathic hyperkinetic heart syndrome.
Intermittent claudication	Intermittent claudication refers to the pain that occurs in a muscle with an inadequate blood supply (usually as a result of atherosclerosis) that is stressed by exercise. The pain does not occur with standing or sitting, is reproducible from day to day, is more severe when walking upstairs or up a hill, and is often described as a cramp, which disappears within 1 or 2 minutes after stopping exercise. Coronary artery disease is more prevalent in persons with intermittent claudication. Diabetics are at increased risk for this condition.
Known heart murmur	Although some may be innocent, heart murmurs may indicate valvular or other cardiovascular disease. From an exercise safety standpoint, it is especially important to exclude hypertrophic cardiomyopathy and aortic stenosis as underlying causes because these are among the more common causes of exertion-related sudden cardiac death.
Unusual fatigue or shortness of breath with usual activities	Although there may be benign origins for these symptoms, they also may signal the onset of, or change in the status of, cardiovascular, pulmonary, or metabolic disease.

Reprinted from Guidelines for Exercise Testing and Prescription, 7th ed. Baltimore: Lippincott Williams & Wilkins, 2006:23–24.

[a] These signs or symptoms must be interpreted within the clinical context in which they appear because they are not all specific for cardiovascular, pulmonary, or metabolic disease.

Table 14.3	**ACSM RISK STRATIFICATION CATEGORIES**
Low risk	Men <45 years of age and women <55 years of age who are asymptomatic and meet no more than one risk factor threshold from Table 14.1
Moderate risk	Men ≥45 years of age and women ≥55 years of age *or* those who meet the threshold for two or more risk factors from Table 14.1
High risk	Individuals with one or more signs and symptoms listed in Table 14.2 *or* known cardiovascular,[a] pulmonary,[b] or metabolic[c] disease

Reprinted from Guidelines for Exercise Testing and Prescription, 7th ed. Baltimore: Lippincott Williams & Wilkins, 2006:27.

[a] Cardiac, peripheral vascular, or cerebrovascular disease.

[b] Chronic obstructive pulmonary disease, asthma, interstitial lung disease, or cystic fibrosis (see American Association of Cardiovascular and Pulmonary Rehabilitation. Guidelines for pulmonary rehabilitation programs. 2nd ed. Champaign, IL: Human Kinetics, 1998:97–112.

[c] Diabetes mellitus (IDDM, NIDDM), thyroid disorders, renal or liver disease.

Table 14.4 ACSM PRE-PARTICIPATION SCREENING ALGORITHM

	Screening Recommended Prior to Self-Guided[a] Physical Activity	Screening Recommended Prior to Professionally Guided[b] Exercise Testing/Prescription
Level - 1 Risk Stratification & Medical Clearance (Chapter 2)	1. Complete ACSM/AHA Questionnaire or PAR-Q (Figures 14.1 and 14.2) 2. Determine need for medical clearance and obtain if recommended 3. Proceed to Level 2	1. Identify presence of major CAD risk factors (Table 14.1) and major signs/symptoms suggestive of cardiovascular, pulmonary or metabolic disease (Table 14.2). This process could include the use of the ACSM/AHA Questionnaire (Figure 14.2)(2). This process may also include a more elaborate, facility-specific medical/health history questionnaire. 2. Determine ACSM risk category from Table 14.3 for use in Levels 2 and 3. 3. Determine need for medical clearance prior to testing and/or participation and obtain if recommended. 4. Proceed to Level 2 and follow recommendations based on ACSM risk category.

		Low Risk	Moderate Risk	High Risk
Level - 2 Additional Pre-Participation Assessment (Chapter 3-4)	• Initiate general physical activity recommendations as outlined by the United States Surgeon General[6] • For a specific self-guided exercise assessment and examples of both aerobic and resistance training regimens, see Chapters 4-6 of the ACSM Fitness Book[10] • Individuals identified as needing medical clearance in Level 1 may benefit from participation in a professionally guided pre-exercise assessment and prescription	• Perform informed consent for testing and/or training[c] • Complete appropriate assessment procedures • Medical history, physical examination, laboratory tests, body composition, etc.	• Perform informed consent for testing and/or training[c] *Both the depth and breadth of pre-exercise test assessment should increase as a function of risk category.*	
Level - 3 Exercise Test Considerations (Chapter 4-5)		• Further medical examination and exercise testing not necessary[d] prior to initiation of exercise training • Medical supervision[e] for submaximal exercise testing not necessary	• Medical examination and exercise testing recommended prior to initiation of vigorous exercise training • Medical supervision[e] recommended for maximal exercise testing	• Medical examination and exercise testing recommended prior to initiation of moderate or vigorous exercise training • Medical supervision[e] recommended for maximal or submaximal exercise testing

Moderate exercise intensity = 40-59% V̇O₂R; Vigorous exercise intensity = > 60% V̇O₂R.

[a] Physical activity regimen that is initiated and guided by the individual with little or no input or supervision from an exercise program professional.

[b] Professionally guided implies that the fitness/clinical assessment is conducted by, and exercise program designed and supervised by, appropriately trained personnel that possess academic training and practical/clinical knowledge, skills and abilities commensurate with the credentials defined in the Appendix, or the ACSM Program Director or Health/Fitness Director.

[c] Published samples of appropriate consent forms for participation in preventive and rehabilitative exercise programs are found in references 3 & 9.

[d] The designation of not necessary reflects the notion that a medical examination, exercise test, and medical supervision of exercise training would not be essential in the pre-activity screening; however, they should not be viewed as inappropriate.

[e] When medical supervision of exercise testing is "recommended," the physical should be in proximity and readily available should there be an emergent need.

PAR-Q & YOU

(A Questionnaire for People Aged 15 to 69)

Regular physical activity is fun and healthy, and increasingly more people are starting to become more active every day. Being more active is very safe for most people. However, some people should check with their doctor before they start becoming much more physically active.

If you are planning to become much more physically active than you are now, start by answering the seven questions in the box below. If you are between the ages of 15 and 69, the PAR-Q will tell you if you should check with your doctor before you start. If you are over 69 years of age, and you are not used to being very active, check with your doctor.

Common sense is your best guide when you answer these questions. Please read the questions carefully and answer each one honestly: check YES or NO.

YES	NO		
☐	☐	1.	**Has your doctor ever said that you have a heart condition <u>and</u> that you should only do physical activity recommended by a doctor?**
☐	☐	2.	**Do you feel pain in your chest when you do physical activity?**
☐	☐	3.	**In the past month, have you had chest pain when you were not doing physical activity?**
☐	☐	4.	**Do you lose your balance because of dizziness or do you ever lose consciousness?**
☐	☐	5.	**Do you have a bone or joint problem (for example, back, knee or hip) that could be made worse by a change in your physical activity?**
☐	☐	6.	**Is your doctor currently prescribing drugs (for example, water pills) for your blood pressure or heart condition?**
☐	☐	7.	**Do you know of <u>any other reason</u> why you should not do physical activity?**

If you answered

YES to one or more questions

Talk with your doctor by phone or in person BEFORE you start becoming much more physically active or BEFORE you have a fitness appraisal. Tell your doctor about the PAR-Q and which questions you answered YES.

- You may be able to do any activity you want — as long as you start slowly and build up gradually. Or, you may need to restrict your activities to those which are safe for you. Talk with your doctor about the kinds of activities you wish to participate in and follow his/her advice.
- Find out which community programs are safe and helpful for you.

NO to all questions

If you answered NO honestly to **all** PAR-Q questions, you can be reasonably sure that you can:
- start becoming much more physically active — begin slowly and build up gradually. This is the safest and easiest way to go.
- take part in a fitness appraisal — this is an excellent way to determine your basic fitness so that you can plan the best way for you to live actively. It is also highly recommended that you have your blood pressure evaluated. If your reading is over 144/94, talk with your doctor before you start becoming much more physically active.

DELAY BECOMING MUCH MORE ACTIVE:
- if you are not feeling well because of a temporary illness such as a cold or a fever — wait until you feel better; or
- if you are or may be pregnant — talk to your doctor before you start becoming more active.

PLEASE NOTE: If your health changes so that you then answer YES to any of the above questions, tell your fitness or health professional. Ask whether you should change your physical activity plan.

<u>Informed Use of the PAR-Q</u>: The Canadian Society for Exercise Physiology, Health Canada, and their agents assume no liability for persons who undertake physical activity, and if in doubt after completing this questionnaire, consult your doctor prior to physical activity.

No changes permitted. You are encouraged to photocopy the PAR-Q but only if you use the entire form.

NOTE: If the PAR-Q is being given to a person before he or she participates in a physical activity program or a fitness appraisal, this section may be used for legal or administrative purposes.

"I have read, understood and completed this questionnaire. Any questions I had were answered to my full satisfaction."

NAME _____

SIGNATURE _____ DATE_____

SIGNATURE OF PARENT _____ WITNESS _____
or GUARDIAN (for participants under the age of majority)

Note: This physical activity clearance is valid for a maximum of 12 months from the date it is completed and becomes invalid if your condition changes so that you would answer YES to any of the seven questions.

 © Canadian Society for Exercise Physiology

 Health Canada Santé Canada

FIGURE 14.1. PAR-Q & You. (Reprinted with permission from the Canadian Society for Exercise Physiology. Physical Activity Readiness Questionnaire, 2002: http:///www.csep.forms.asp; Guidelines for Exercise Testing and Prescription, 7th ed. Baltimore: Lippincott Williams & Wilkins, 2006:26.)

AHA/ACSM Health/Fitness Facility Preparticipation Screening Questionnaire

Access your health status by marking all *true* statements

History

You have had:

- a heart attack
- heart surgery
- cardiac catheterization
- coronary angioplasty (PTCA)
- pacemaker-implantable cardiac
- defibrillatory/rhythm disturbance
- heart valve disease
- heart failure
- heart transplantation
- congenital heart disease

Symptoms

- You experience chest discomfort with exertion
- You experience unreasonable breathlessness
- You experience dizziness, fainting, or blackouts
- You take heart medications

> If you marked any of these statements in this section, consult your physician or other appropriate health care provider before engaging in exercise. You may need to use a facility with a **medically qualified staff.**

Other health issues

- You have diabetes
- You have asthma or other lung disease
- You have burning or cramping sensation in your lower legs when walking short distances
- You have musculoskeletal problems that limit your physical activity
- You have concerns about the safety of exercise
- You take prescription medications
- You are pregnant

Cardiovascular risk factors

- You are a man older than 45 years
- You are a woman older than 55 years, have had a hysterectomy, or are postmenopausal
- You smoke, or quit smoking within the previous 6 months
- Your blood pressure is > 140/90 mm Hg
- You do not know your blood pressure
- You take blood pressure medication
- Your blood cholesterol level is >200 mg/dL
- You do not know your cholesterol level
- You have a close blood relative who had a heart attack or heart surgery before age 55 (father or brother) or age 65 (mother or sister)
- You are physically inactive (ie, you get < 30 minutes of physical activity on at least 3 days/week)
- You are >20 pounds overweight.

> If you marked two or more of the statements in this section, you should consult your physician or other appropriate healthcare provider before engaging in exercise. You might benefit from using a facility with a **professionally qualified exercise staff†** to guide your exercise program.

† Professionally qualified exercise staff refers to appropriately trained individuals who posses academic training, practical and clinical knowledge, skills and abilities commensurate with the credentials defined in Appendix F.

- None of the above

> You should be able to exercise safely without consulting your physician or other appropriate health care provider in a self-guided program or almost any facility that meets your exercise program needs.

Modified from **American College of Sports Medicine and American Heart Association ACSM/AHA** joint position statement. Recommendations for cardiovascular screening, staffing and emergency policies at health fitness facilities. Med Sci Sports Exerc 1998:1018.

FIGURE 14.2. AHA/ACSM Health/Fitness Facility Preparticipation Screening Questionnaire (From American College of Sports Medicine and American Heart Association. ACSM/AHA Joint Position Statement: Recommendations for cardiovascular screening, staffing, and emergency policies at health/fitness facilities. Med Sci Sports Exerc 1998:1018; Guidelines for Exercise Testing and Prescription, 7th ed. Baltimore: Lippincott Williams & Wilkins, 2006:25.)

Sample medical clearance form

Dear Dr. White,

Your patient, Michelle Jean Smith, a 42-year-old female (DOB: June 1, 1963), has indicated that you are her primary physician. This individual is beginning a moderate to vigorous intensity exercise program under the supervision of a certified Personal Trainer. Please provide your recommendation regarding exercise participation for this individual and any restrictions and/or limitations you suggest for her program. Should you have any questions or concerns, please contact me at the number below. Thank you.

Physician recommendation:

☐ Patient may participate in unrestricted activity.

☐ Patient may participate in light to moderate activities only.

☐ Patient should not participate in activity at this time.

☐ Other: please specify: _____

_____

Please specify any restrictions or limitations you feel appropriate: _____

_____

Physician: _____ Telephone: _____

Signature: _____

Personal Trainer: _____ Telephone: _____

FIGURE 14.3. Sample medical clearance form.

Release of medical information form

Dear Dr._____,

I, (name of client), hereby authorize the immediate release of a copy of all my medical information to the following persons:

(Personal Trainer name and contact information)

Patient information:

Name: _____ Date of birth: _____

Signature: _____ Date: _____

FIGURE 14.4. Release of medical information form.

as an all-inclusive list, but rather as a group with *clinically relevant thresholds* that should be considered collectively when making decisions about the level of medical clearance, the need for exercise testing prior to initiating participation, and the level of supervision for both exercise testing and exercise program participation. The *scope* of the list and the *threshold* for each risk factor should not be viewed as inconsistent with other risk factor lists that are intended for use in predicting coronary events during long-term follow-up (8), because the intended use for the list in Table 14.1 is to aid in the prediction or identification of as yet undiagnosed coronary artery disease.

SIGNS OR SYMPTOMS OF CARDIOVASCULAR, PULMONARY, AND METABOLIC DISEASE

Table 14.2 presents a list of major signs or symptoms that suggest cardiovascular, pulmonary, and/or metabolic disease, along with additional information to aid in the clarification and significance of each sign or symptom (8). The presence of most of these risk factors can be detected using a questionnaire; however, a few (e.g., orthopnea, ankle swelling or edema, heart murmur) require a more thorough medical history and/or examination.

Informed consent for an exercise test

— Purpose and explanation of the test

You will perform an exercise test on a cycle ergometer or motor-driven treadmill. The exercise intensity will begin at a low level and will be advanced in stages depending on your fitness level. We may stop the test at any time because of signs of fatigue or changes in your heart rate, ECG, or blood pressure, or symptoms you may experience. It is important for you to realize that you may stop when you wish because of feelings of fatigue or any other discomfort.

— Attendant risks and discomforts

There exists the possibility of certain changes occurring during the test. These include abnormal blood pressure, fainting, irregular, fast or slow heart rhythm, and in rare instances, heart attack, stroke, or death. Every effort will be made to minimize these risks by evaluation of preliminary information relating to your health and fitness and by careful observation during the testing. Emergency equipment and trained personnel are available to deal with unusual situations that may arise.

— Responsibilities of the participant

Information you possess about your health status or previous experiences of heart-related symptoms (e.g., shortness of breath with low-level activity, pain, pressure, tightness, heaviness in the chest, neck, jaw, back, and/or arms) with physical effort may affect the safety of your exercise test. Your prompt reporting of these and any other unusual feelings with effort during the exercise test itself is very important. You are responsible for fully disclosing your medical history, as well as symptoms that may occur during the test. You are also expected to report all medications (including non-prescription) taken recently and, in particular, those taken today, to the testing staff.

— Benefits to be expected

The results obtained from the exercise test may assist in the diagnosis of your illness, in evaluating the effect of your medications or in evaluating what type of physical activities you might do with low risk.

— Inquiries

Any questions about the procedures used in the exercise test or the results of your test are encouraged. If you have any concerns or questions, please ask us for further explanations.

— Use of medical records

The information that is obtained during exercise testing will be treated as privileged and confidential as described in the Health Insurance Portability and Accountability Act of 1996. It is not to be released or revealed to any person except your referring physician without your written consent. However, the information obtained may be used for statistical analysis or scientific purposes with your right to privacy retained.

— Freedom of consent

I hereby consent to voluntarily engage in an exercise test to determine my exercise capacity and state of cardiovascular health. My permission to perform this exercise test is given voluntarily. I understand that I am free to stop the test at any point if I so desire.

I have read this form, and I understand the test procedures that I will perform and the attendant risks and discomforts. Knowing these risks and discomforts, and having had an opportunity to ask questions that have been answered to my satisfaction, I consent to participate in this test.

Signature of Patient _____   Date _____

Signature of Witness _____   Date _____

Signature of Physician or _____   Date _____
Authorized Delegate

The client or patient can prepare adequately the following points which should be considered for inclusion in such preliminary instructions: however, specific instructions vary with test type and purpose.

- Participants should refrain from ingesting food, alcohol or caffeine or using tobacco products within 3 hours of testing.
- Participants should be rested for the assessment, avoiding significant exertion or exercise on the day of the assessment.
- Clothing should permit freedom of movement and include walking or running shoes. Women should bring a loose-fitting, short-sleeved blouse that buttons down the front and should avoid restrictive undergarments.
- If the evaluation is on an outpatient basis, participants should be made aware that the evaluation may be fatiguing and that they may wish to have someone accompany them to the assessment to drive home afterwards.
- If the test is for diagnostic purposes, it may be helpful for patients to discontinue prescribed cardiovascular medications, but only with physician approval. Currently prescribed antianginal agents alter the hemodynamic response to exercise and significantly reduce the sensitivity of ECG changes for ischemia. Patients taking intermediate- or high-dose ß-blocking agents may be asked to taper their medication over a 2 to 4-day period to minimize hyperadrenergic withdrawal responses.
- If the test is for functional purposes, *patients should continue their medication regimen* on their usual schedule so that the exercise responses will be consistent with responses expected during exercise training.
- Participants should bring a list of their medications, including dosage and frequency of administration, to the assessment and should report the last actual dose taken. As an alternative, participants may wish to bring their medications with them for the exerise testing staff to record.
- Drink ample fluids over the 24-hour period preceding the test to ensure normal hydration testing.

FIGURE 14.5. Sample of informed consent form for a symptom-limited exercise test. (From Guidelines for Exercise Testing and Prescription, 7th ed. Baltimore: Lippincott Williams & Wilkins, 2006:52–54.)

ACSM RISK CATEGORIES

Once symptom and risk factor information is known, candidates for exercise testing or training can be stratified on the basis of the likelihood of events during exercise program participation. Risk stratification becomes progressively more important as disease prevalence increases in the population under consideration. Using age, health status, symptoms, and risk factor information, potential clients can be classified into one of three risk strata (see Table 14.3) for referral to other healthcare providers for further screening prior to participation.

Inherent within the concept of risk stratification is the impression that signs and symptoms (see Table 14.2) represent a higher level of concern for decision making than do risk factors (see Table 14.1). However, high blood pressure (hypertension) represents a unique risk factor in that it may be aggravated by short-term exercise such as weight training. Therefore, although it appears within Table 14.1, special consideration should be given to hypertensive clients when screening for exercise testing or training. The Seventh Report of the Joint National Committee on Prevention, Detection, Evaluation, and Treatment of High Blood Pressure (JNC7) (11) recommends a thorough medical history, physical examination, routine laboratory tests, and other diagnostic procedures in the evaluation of clients with documented hypertension. Because hypertension is commonly clustered with other risk factors associated with cardiovascular disease (e.g., dyslipidemia, obesity, diabetes), most hypertensive clients who want to start an exercise program fall into the *moderate-* or *high-*risk category as defined in Table 14.3. For such clients, the medical examination in Table 14.4 is consistent with the screening recommendations for hypertensive clients outlined in JNC7 (11). However, in cases of isolated hypertension (i.e., hypertension is the only risk factor from those conditions in listed in Table 14.1), prudent recommendations for pre-participation screening should be based on the severity of the hypertension and the desired intensity of exercise. For *low-*risk clients with isolated stage 1 hypertension (<160/100 mm Hg), exercise testing generally is not necessary for clearance to engage in up to moderate-intensity exercise. However, it is advisable for such clients to have physician clearance prior to participation. On the other hand, if the client has documented stage 2 hypertension or if a client with stage 1 hypertension desires to engage in more intense exercise training, an exercise assessment is recommended to quantify blood pressure responses during exercise to aid in establishing prudent guidelines for exercise training (8).

Exercise Testing and Testing Supervision Recommendations

No set of guidelines for exercise testing and participation can cover all situations. Circumstances, policies, and program procedures vary by location. To provide some general guidance on the need for a medical examination and exercise testing prior to participation in a moderate-to-vigorous exercise program, ACSM suggests the recommendations presented in Table 14.4 for determining when a medical examination and diagnostic exercise test are appropriate and when physician supervision is recommended. Although the testing guidelines are less rigorous for those clients considered to be at low risk, the information gathered from an exercise test may be useful in establishing a safe and effective exercise prescription for these clients. The exercise testing recommendations found in Table 14.1 reflect the notion that the risk of cardiovascular events increases as a function of increasing physical activity intensity. Personal Trainers should choose the most appropriate definition (i.e., relative or absolute) for their setting when making decisions about the level of screening to use prior to exercise training and whether or not it is necessary to have physician supervision during exercise testing.

Medical supervision of exercise tests varies appropriately from physician-supervised tests to situations in which there may be no physician present (15). The degree of physician supervision may differ, depending on local policies and circumstances, the client's health status, and the experience of the staff conducting the test. The appropriate protocol should be based on the age, health status, and physical activity level of the potential client to be tested. In all situations in which exercise testing is performed, site personnel should at least be certified at a level of basic life support (8, 15) (including operation of automated external defibrillators—AEDs); preferably, one or more staff members should be certified in advanced cardiac life support (2). Because of their knowledge, skills, and abilities, ACSM-certified professionals should, ideally, be the individuals performing exercise testing.

Health History Evaluation

Conducting a thorough health history will provide the Personal Trainer with valuable information for developing a client's program. Specifically, the purposes of a health history are to identify known disease and risk factors for disease (especially cardiovascular disease) and to identify conditions that warrant special consideration when developing an exercise program or require referral to a healthcare provider.

Although health history forms vary depending on the setting, a description of the kinds of information to include on a health history from is discussed below. A sample health history form is shown in Figure 14.2. While traditionally not viewed as health history information, assessments of physical activity level, dietary habits, and learning style are included on this form because they are part of the initial client consultation format that is recommended in this text.

Medical history—Current and previous medical conditions, injuries, surgical procedures, and therapies are all vital factors that influence the development of an exercise plan. The Personal Trainer should always include dates for each and discuss each one with the client so that there is a full understanding of the extent or severity of any medical condition.

Medications—Some medications, such as calcium channel blockers and beta-blockers, affect heart rate and/or blood pressure response to exercise, thus altering the exercise prescription. Because medications change frequently, clients need to be instructed to report any significant alterations in their prescriptions immediately to their Personal Trainer.

Exercise history—A client's experience with exercise is an important factor to consider when developing a program, as it could affect his or her ability to advance to more difficult movements, attitude toward exercise, and the kinds of exercise in which he or she is willing to engage.

Nutrition—Dietary intake affects many aspects of a client's life, such as weight and body composition, risk for disease, mood, and energy level. Nutrition analysis is discussed in more depth in Chapter 11.

Documentation

Documentation is an important aspect of risk management. Personal Trainers should maintain accurate records of client responses to testing and training, changes in reported health status, and how these are referred to appropriate healthcare providers. Client health information should be updated regularly to document any changes in medications and conditions. Although there is no set rule for how long records should be maintained, 3–5 years is a typical length of time.

MEDICAL CLEARANCE AND REFERRAL

Obtaining Medical Clearance

Initial clearance to exercise should be obtained from a physician when necessary, according to the ACSM risk stratification process. Clearance should also be obtained when clients have had any significant or recent change in health status that has not yet been evaluated by a physician. This can be accomplished by sending a Medical Clearance Form (see Fig. 14.3) to the physician's office.

It is common for clients to have multiple healthcare providers, such as a general practitioner, specialists (e.g., cardiologist, orthopedist, oncologist, obstetrician), and therapists. As all of these professionals work together as a team, they rely on one another to make decisions that are beyond their scope of practice and expertise. Many times the general practitioner will defer clearance to the specialist based on specific medical conditions. Although necessary, it can slow down the clearance process because the Personal Trainer may need to contact multiple providers.

The Personal Trainer should keep in mind, however, that there is a difference between obtaining medical clearance to exercise and obtaining expert opinion that will help create the best possible exercise program for the client. Obtaining medical clearance means that the Personal Trainer will not exercise the client until the physician provides approval to do so. When seeking an expert opinion, the Personal Trainer typically proceeds with training, even if modified, and incorporates the recommendations of the physician into the program. The Personal Trainer should make sure that communication with healthcare providers clearly explains the intent of the questions. More information on working with healthcare providers is discussed in subsequent sections in this chapter.

When to Refer?

By screening and assessing a new client, the Personal Trainer becomes a part of the healthcare team, which may include physicians, specialists, clinical exercise physiologists, physical therapists, physical therapy assistants, registered dietitians, athletic trainers, nurses, nurse practitioners, and physician assistants. Therefore, it is the responsibility of the Personal Trainer to refer clients to other members of the team when problems or potential problems arise or are identified that are beyond the Personal Trainer's expertise. Referring clients for medical clearance based on the ACSM risk stratification process or information obtained during the health history evaluation has already been briefly discussed, but referral may take place at any time, such as during the physical assessment process or once exercise training has begun.

REFERRAL DURING SCREENING

The physical assessments described in detail in Chapter 15 are designed to provide the Personal Trainer with more information regarding the client's abilities and potential limitations. Potential problems may be discovered during these assessments. When this occurs, the Personal Trainer must decide whether or not to refer the client to a healthcare provider for a more in-depth assessment. It is certainly advisable to err on the side of caution. If in doubt, the Personal Trainer should refer the client to an appropriate physician or specialist.

For example, a new client reports no joint problems on the health history evaluation but during an initial assessment the Personal Trainer discovers that the client's left arm can only abduct 45° while maintaining scapular retraction. Upon questioning, the Personal Trainer learns that the client injured his left shoulder when he was in grade school and has not had complete range of motion since that time. However, because it does not cause him pain and he has learned to live with the limitation, he did not feel that it was important enough to report on the health history form. Given the significant limitation of the shoulder joint and the risk of further damage during upper body strength movements, the Personal Trainer may decide to refer the client to a physician for further assessment. In the meantime, the Personal Trainer proceeds with cardiovascular, lower body, and core exercises so that the client can begin training without risking further injury to the shoulder joint.

REFERRAL DURING TRAINING

Once exercise training begins, it is the responsibility of Personal Trainers to continually re-evaluate the health status of their clients through either formal (direct questions or assessments) or informal (casual conversation, observation) means. The onset of new signs and symptoms, aggravation of existing medical conditions, or occurrences of injury may warrant stopping or modifying exercise training until after further consultation with the physician. Recognizing these situations and communicating effectively with the healthcare team will maximize the safety of clients, increase their probability of successfully reaching established health and fitness goals, and raise the stature of the Personal Trainer in the eyes of the medical community. Any incident of a client reporting new signs or symptoms as listed in Table 14.2 requires that the Personal Trainer stop exercise training and initiate an immediate examination by a medical professional. Likewise, significant change in the frequency, intensity, or nature of a client's existing signs and symptoms should also prompt immediate referral to a physician.

Serious joint injuries or those that do not resolve quickly should, at a minimum, prompt modification of training techniques to protect or minimize strain on the joint and a recommendation to follow up with a healthcare professional. In addition, clients reporting a muscle or joint problem (e.g., redness, swelling, pain, stiffness, burning sensation) that has either been brought on or aggravated by exercise should be referred to a healthcare professional. Sometimes this is a gray area that depends on the Personal Trainer's experience and interpretation of the information. It can be difficult to determine the difference between discomfort associated with exercise and signs of an injury or other orthopedic condition. When in doubt, the Personal Trainer should seek the advice of healthcare professionals.

When referring a client for consultation, it is helpful to send documentation directly to the physician. The Personal Trainer should be sure to include any measurements taken of the client, such as heart rate and blood pressure before, during, and after exercise, along with any observed signs and symptoms (e.g., sweating, pain). A clear and accurate description of the situation will allow the physician to make an informed decision as to the best course of action for the client.

Communicating with Healthcare Providers

Communicating with healthcare providers can be intimidating at first, but when done properly and consistently, it can lead to great benefits for both the Personal Trainer and client. The Personal Trainer can follow these simple guidelines to maximize the effectiveness of communications with healthcare providers:

➤ Always include information that clearly identifies the client, such as his or her full name, age, and date of birth
➤ Be clear and to the point as to the purpose of the communication (physicians, especially, have very little time to read long documents)
➤ Set a response date (if something needs to be turned around quickly, write "URGENT" in big letters at the top of the form)
➤ Provide options that can be checked off easily
➤ Allow room for additional comments
➤ Faxing is typically more effective and quicker than the mail system (for a quicker reply, call the office staff and notify them that a fax that needs attention is on the way)
➤ If requesting a release or personal medical information, then automatically include a Release of Medical Information Form (see Fig. 14.4) signed by your client

Not all communications need to request a response. Simply informing and educating the medical community about the Personal Trainer's training, experience, and services can be a valuable marketing tool. Some Personal Trainers find it useful to personally visit medical offices, provide in-service training over lunch hours for medical staff, send introductory packets or letters to physicians of new clients, and provide brief periodic updates on clients.

Informed Consent

Although some locations do not require informed consent for fitness assessments, it is widely accepted within the health/fitness industry to do so. The informed consent form is intended to ensure that the client:

➤ Has full knowledge of what tests are going to be performed
➤ Understands the relevant risks associated with those tests
➤ Knows about alternative procedures
➤ Understands the benefits associated with the assessments

Written consent is preferable to verbal or implied consent. A sample informed consent form is included in Figure 14.5; however, you should always obtain legal counsel when creating or adopting an informed consent document.

SUMMARY

The pre-participation health screening that takes place during the initial client consultation is an extremely important process yielding valuable information concerning a client's risk and health status. It is essential that the Personal Trainer obtain as much information as possible about a client's health status to maximize benefit and minimize risk. This information should serve as the Personal Trainer's foundation to developing a safe and effective exercise program.

REFERENCES

1. Fletcher GF, Balady GJ, Amsterdam EA, et al. Exercise standards for testing and training. A statement for health care professionals from the American Heart Association. Circulation 2001;104:1694–1740.
2. American College of Sports Medicine and American Heart Association. ACSM/AHA Joint position statement: recommendations for cardiovascular screening, staffing, and emergency policies at health/fitness facilities. Med Sci Sports Exerc 1998:1018.
3. American Association of Cardiovascular and Pulmonary Rehabilitation. Guidelines for Cardiac Rehabilitation and Secondary Prevention Programs. 4th ed. Champaign, IL: Human Kinetics, 2003.
4. Thompson PD, Funk EJ, Carleton RA, et al. Incidence of death during jogging in Rhode Island from 1975 through 1980. JAMA 1982;247:2535–2538.
5. Siscovick DS, Weiss NS, Fletcher RH, et al. The incidence of primary cardiac arrest during vigorous exercise. N Engl J Med 1984;311:874–877.
6. Mittleman MA, Maclure M, Tofler GH, et al. Triggering of acute myocardial infarction by heavy physical exertion. Protection against triggering by regular exertion. Determinants of Myocardial Infarction Onset Study Investigators. N Engl J Med 1993;329:1677–1683.
7. Giri S, Thompson PD, Kiernan FJ, et al. Clinical and angiographic characteristics of exertion-related acute myocardial infarction. JAMA 1999;282:1731–1736.
8. American College of Sports Medicine. ACSM's Guidelines for Exercise Testing and Prescription. 7th ed. Baltimore: Lippincott Williams & Wilkins, 2005.
9. Physical Activity and Health: A Report of the Surgeon General, Atlanta: U.S. Department of Health and Human Services, Centers for Disease Control and Prevention, National Center for Chronic Disease Prevention and Health Promotion, 1996.
10. Third Report of the National Cholesterol Education Program (NCEP) Expert Panel on Detection, Evaluation, and Treatment of High Blood Cholesterol in Adults (Adult Treatment Panel III) Final Report. National Cholesterol Education Program, National Heart, Lung and Blood Institute, National Institutes of Health. NIH Publ no. 02-5215, 2002.
11. Seventh Report of the Joint National Committee on Prevention, Detection, Evaluation, and Treatment of High Blood Pressure (JNC7). U.S. Department of Health and Human Services, National Institutes of Health, National Heart, Lung and Blood Institute, National High Blood Pressure Education Program. NIH Publ no. 03-5233, 2004.
12. Genuth S, Alberti KG, Bennett P, et al. Follow-up report on the diagnosis of diabetes mellitus. Diabetes Care 2003;26:3160–3167.
13. Expert Panel on Detection Evaluation and Treatment of Overweight and Obesity in Adults. National Institutes of Health. Clinical guidelines on the identification, evaluation, and treatment of overweight and obesity in adults—the evidence report. Arch Intern Med 1998;158:1855–1867.
14. Wilson PW, D'Agostino RB, Levy D, et al. Prediction of coronary heart disease using risk factor categories. Circulation 1998;97:1837–1847.
15. American College of Sports Medicine. ACSM's Resource Manual for Guidelines for Exercise Testing and Prescription. Baltimore: Lippincott Williams & Wilkins, 2005.
16. American College of Sports Medicine. Position stand: exercise and hypertension. Med Sci Sports Exerc 2004;36:533–553.

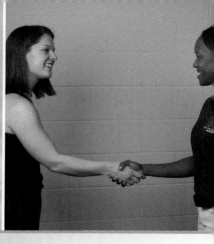

CHAPTER

15 Client Health-Related Physical Fitness Assessments

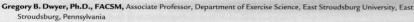

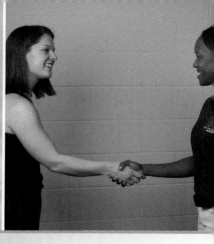

CHAPTER

15 Client Health-Related Physical Fitness Assessments

Gregory B. Dwyer, Ph.D., FACSM, Associate Professor, Department of Exercise Science, East Stroudsburg University, East Stroudsburg, Pennsylvania

Shala E. Davis, Ph.D., FACSM, Associate Professor/Graduate Coordinator, Department of Exercise Science, East Stroudsburg University, East Stroudsburg, Pennsylvania

Kenneth E. Baldwin, M.Ed., A.H. Ismail Center for Health, Exercise & Nutrition, Department of Health and Kinesiology, College of Liberal Arts, Purdue University, West Lafayette, Indiana

Chapter Outline

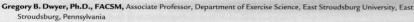

Assessments to Meet Client Needs

Selection and Sequence of Assessments

Heart Rate: Resting, Exercise, and Recovery
- Measurement of Heart Rate
  - Palpation of Pulse
  - Measurement of Exercise Heart Rate

Blood Pressure: Resting and Exercise
- Measurement of Blood Pressure
  - Korotkoff Sounds
  - Instruments Used for Blood Pressure Measurement
- Procedures for Resting Blood Pressure Measurement

Body Composition
- Height and Weight
- Body Mass Index
- Waist-to-Hip Ratio
- Waist Circumference Alone
- Skinfolds
  - Procedures for Skinfold Measurements
  - Jackson-Pollock 3-Site Skinfold Formula for Percentage Body Fat
  - Calculation of Ideal or Desired Body Weight

Cardiorespiratory Assessment
- Pretest Considerations
- Field Tests for Prediction of Cardiorespiratory Fitness
- Walk/Run Performance Tests
  - 1.5-Mile Run Test Procedures
  - Rockport 1-Mile Walk Test Procedures
- Step Tests
  - Queens College Step Test Procedures
- Norms for CRF ($\dot{V}O_{2max}$)

Flexibility Assessment

Postural Analysis and Body Alignment Assessments
- Postural Improvement Takes Time
- The Center of Gravity and Base of Support
- Line of Gravity
- Static and Dynamic Posture
- Posture-related Injuries and Health Concerns
- Equipment Needs for Posture Assessment
- The Posture Screening and Assessment Process
- Analysis of Posture
  - Analysis of Posture: Anterior/Posterior
  - Analysis of Posture: Lateral

Correction of Posture and Body Alignment

Exercise Program Design and New Skills Application

Goniometry and Joint Range-of-Motion Assessments
- Client Involvement in the Range-of-Motion Assessment
- The Goniometry/Range-of-Motion Assessment
- Range of Motion (ROM)
  - Active Range of Motion (AROM)
  - Passive Range of Motion (PROM)
  - Factors Affecting ROM
- The Goniometer
  - Assessment Process and Techniques
- ROM and Postural Alignment Assessments
  - Sample ROM Assessments: Neck, Spine, Shoulder, Hip
  - Specific ROM Assessments
- Goniometry and Its Usefulness as an Assessment Tool

Assessments as a Motivational Device

Objectives

- **Understand the concept of the selection of the proper sequence of fitness assessments**
- **Know how to take a resting and exercise blood pressure**
- **Know and understand the different techniques to determine body composition**
- **Present information on how to perform some basic health-related physical fitness assessments that are common to the field of personal training**
  - **Resting heart rate and blood pressure**
  - **Body composition: height, weight, body mass index, circumferences (waist and hip), skinfolds**
  - **Cardiovascular: field tests and step tests**
  - **Flexibility and posture assessments**

Individualizing an exercise program for a client, as discussed in other chapters in this book, is best achieved by having some preliminary assessment data. In addition, the collection of assessment results periodically during a client's program is important to assess progress toward established short-term and long-term goals. The Personal Trainer needs to consider the client's needs/desires in the selection of which assessment test to perform.

ASSESSMENTS TO MEET CLIENT NEEDS

The assessment process can be extremely intimidating to clients, especially those who are conscientious about their appearance and intimidated by the idea of joining a "gym." As their Personal Trainer, it is important that you make your clients feel as comfortable as possible in any situation. During the assessment process, share with your client what you will be doing. Clients may feel uncomfortable during certain parts of the assessment, such as weight assessment, waist circumference, and skinfold assessment. For example, if a client is overweight and a skinfold measurement at the abdomen site would be unsuccessful, do not attempt to take the abdomen site measurement. If the client is apprehensive about any part of the assessment process, explain the importance of accurately recording the measurements. If this explanation does not change the client's feelings, record any modifications to the measurement/assessment process for future reference. The success of the Personal Trainer–client relationship is built on a foundation of respect for the client. How can the Personal Trainer make the client feel comfortable during the assessment process?

SELECTION AND SEQUENCE OF ASSESSMENTS

A Personal Trainer has many alternatives available to assess a client's health-related physical fitness. Among the considerations are the client's needs/desires, the situation or setting, and the Personal Trainer's training and experience. The exact sequence of assessments is dictated most by the setting and equipment available; however, a few generalizations regarding sequencing can be made. Resting measures (i.e., resting heart rate, resting blood pressure, body composition, and goniometry measurements) typically should be taken prior to any exertional assessments, such as cardiorespiratory fitness and muscular fitness. The Personal Trainer should perform assessments after the client has completed the health and physical activity questionnaire. One recommended order for performing assessments is the following (1):

1. Heart rate: resting
2. Blood pressure: resting
3. Body composition: height and weight, body mass index, waist-to-hip ratio, and skinfolds

4. Postural analysis and body alignment assessments
5. Goniometry and joint range-of-motion assessments
6. Cardiovascular assessment: Rockport 1-mile walk test procedures, 1.5-mile run test procedures, and Queens College Step Test

HEART RATE: RESTING, EXERCISE, AND RECOVERY

Heart rate (HR) is the number of times that the heart contracts, usually reported in beats per minute (bpm). Although there are no known or accepted standards for resting HR, resting HR has often been thought of as an indicator of cardiorespiratory fitness because it tends to decrease as the client becomes more physically fit. There are also no standards for exercise HR, but the HR response to a standard amount of exercise is an important fitness variable and the foundation for many cardiorespiratory endurance tests. Recovery HR is often thought of as an excellent index of cardiorespiratory fitness and is used as a variable in some cardiorespiratory fitness tests (e.g., Queens College Step Test).

Measurement of Heart Rate

There are many ways to assess HR, including manual palpation at various anatomical sites, use of an HR watch, or an electrocardiogram.

PALPATION OF PULSE

There are three common anatomical sites for the measurement of HR (2):

➤ Radial: Lightly press the index and middle fingers against the radial artery in the groove on the anterior surface of the lateral wrist (bordered by the abductor pollicis longus and extensor pollicis longus muscles). The radial palpation site has been described earlier in this book and is shown in Figure 6.2.
➤ Brachial: Located in a groove between the triceps and biceps muscles on the medial side of the arm, anterior to the elbow, and palpated with the first two fingers in the medial part of this groove (see Fig. 6.3).
➤ Carotid: May be more visible or easily found than the radial pulse; press fingers lightly along the medial border of the sternocleidomastoid muscle in the lower neck region (on either side). Avoid the carotid sinus area (stay well below the thyroid cartilage) to avoid the reflexive slowing of HR or drop in blood pressure (BP) by the baroreceptor reflex. The carotid palpation site is shown in Figure 6.4 and should be used only if the client fails to feel the pulse in the radial or brachial sites.

When clients experience difficulty in palpating the pulse, the use of an HR monitor as a learning tool to check the accuracy of the palpated HR with the monitor's HR may be desirable.

All the above methods, when applied correctly, should yield similar results. The palpation of the pulse method for HR measurement can be mastered through practice and should to be taught to your clients. However, some clients, as a result of anatomical aberrations, are more difficult to palpate (2).

The measurement of HR by palpation of the carotid artery may lead to an underestimation of the true HR because the baroreceptors in the carotid sinus region often become stimulated when touched. This may reflexively reduce the client's HR as the baroreceptors sense a false increase in BP. This concept is discussed in more detail Chapter 6. Therefore, the radial or brachial arteries are the locations of choice for palpation.

The baroreceptor reflex becomes a more important issue with HR counts longer than 15 seconds. It is recommended that a full 60-second count be performed for accuracy in resting HR. However, a 30-second time period may be sufficient for the count. "Resting" conditions must be present, such as the client should be seated for at least 5 minutes with the back supported. Clients should be free of stimulants such as tobacco and caffeine for at least 30 minutes prior to taking the measurements (similar to resting BP). A resting HR may alternatively be assessed by having clients take their own pulse at home in bed upon waking in the morning. This resting heart rate may prove to be useful for the calculation of the exercise target heart rate.

MEASUREMENT OF EXERCISE HEART RATE

By either palpation method, measure the number of beats felt in a 15- or 30-second period and multiply by 4 (for 15 seconds) or 2 (for 30 seconds) to convert to a 1-minute value (bpm). Although the 30-second count may be more accurate and less prone to error than a 15-second count, the latter is typically used immediately postexercise because HR will decrease during recovery. When counting the exercise HR for a time count period less than 1 minute, you should start the count at zero (reference) at the first beat felt and start the time period at that beat (2).

The use of HR monitors has increased in popularity as these monitors have become more available and affordable. Some monitors are prone to error (i.e., not always consistent in measuring HR); however, newer technology has resolved the reliability problem previously associated with many of these monitors. HR monitors that rely on the opacity of blood at the earlobe or fingertip to measure/count flow are generally not as accurate as are the monitors that use a chest electrode strap.

BLOOD PRESSURE: RESTING AND EXERCISE

Blood pressure (BP) is the force of blood against the walls of the arteries and veins created by the heart as it pumps blood to every part of the body. BP is typically expressed in millimeters of mercury (mm Hg). BP is a dynamic variable with regard to location (i.e., artery versus vein and the level in an artery). Personal Trainers are most concerned with arterial BP at the level of the heart. This arterial, heart-level BP is the one typically measured at rest and during exercise (2). More discussion concerning the regulation of BP can be found in Chapter 6.

➤ Systolic blood pressure (SBP) is the maximum pressure in the arteries when the ventricles of the heart contract during a heartbeat. The term derives from systole, or contraction of the heart. The SBP occurs late in ventricular systole. SBP is thought to represent the overall functioning of the left ventricle and is thus an important indicator of cardiovascular function during exercise. SBP is typically measured from the brachial artery at the heart level and is expressed in units of mm Hg.

➤ Diastolic blood pressure (DBP) is the minimum pressure in the arteries when the ventricles relax. The term is derived from diastole, or relaxation of the heart. The DBP occurs late in ventricular diastole and reflects the peripheral resistance to blood flow in the arterial vessels. DBP is typically measured from the brachial artery at the heart level and is expressed in units of mm Hg.

"Hypertension," or high BP, is a condition in which the resting BP, either SBP and/or DBP, is chronically elevated above the optimal or desired level. The standards for classifying resting hypertension are presented later in this chapter. "Hypotension" is the term for low BP, and there are no excepted standards for a value that classifies an individual with hypotension. Hypotension exists medically if the individual has symptoms related to the low BP, such as lightheadedness, dizziness, or fainting (2). BP is typically assessed using the principle of indirect auscultation. Auscultation is discussed further in this chapter and involves the use of a BP cuff, a manometer, and a stethoscope. Measurement of BP is a fundamental skill and is covered in detail in this chapter (3).

Measurement of Blood Pressure

The measurement of BP is an integral component of a resting physical fitness assessment session. BP measurement is a relatively simple technique and may be used in risk stratification, as discussed in Chapter 14. Hypertension cannot be diagnosed from a single measurement; serial measurements must be used on separate days. The BP of a client should be based on the average of two or more resting BP recordings during each of two or more visits (2).

For accurate resting BP readings, it is important that the client be made as comfortable as possible. To accomplish this, take a few minutes to talk to the client after having him or her sit in a chair. Make sure the client does not have the legs crossed. Also, be sure to use the correct size BP cuff. As with many other physiological and psychological measures, there exists a "white coat syndrome" in the measurement of BP. This white coat syndrome with regard to resting BP refers to an elevation of BP because of the effect of being in a doctor's office or in a clinical setting (i.e., clinician wearing a white lab coat). Thus, having a client in a relaxed state is important when taking a resting BP measurement.

KOROTKOFF SOUNDS

To measure BP, the Personal Trainer must be able to hear and distinguish between the sounds of the blood as it makes its way past the pumped-up cuff. These sounds are known as Korotkoff sounds. The sounds can be divided into five phases (2):

➤ Phase 1 (SBP)
  • The first, initial sound or the onset of sound
  • Sounds like clear, repetitive tapping
  • Sound approximates the SBP, the maximum pressure that occurs near the end of systole of the left ventricle
➤ Phase 2
  • Sounds like a soft tapping or murmur; sounds are often longer than in the first phase; these sounds have also been described as having a swishing component
  • The phase 2 sounds are typically 10–15 mm Hg after the onset or just below the phase 1 sounds
➤ Phase 3
  • Sounds like loud tapping; high in both pitch and intensity
  • Sounds are crisper and louder than the phase 2 sounds
➤ Phase 4 (also known as the true DBP)
  • Sounds like muffling of the sound; sounds become less distinct and less audible; another way of describing this sound is as soft or blowing
  • This is often considered the true DBP and is typically recorded as the DBP
➤ Phase 5 (also known as the clinical DBP)
  • Sounds like the complete disappearance of sound

The true disappearance of sound usually occurs within 8 to 10 mm Hg of the muffling of sound, also known as phase 4. Phase 5 is considered by some to be the clinical DBP. Phase 5 is the reading most often used for resting DBP in adults, while phase 4 is considered the true DBP and should be recorded, if discerned.

INSTRUMENTS USED FOR BLOOD PRESSURE MEASUREMENT

A sphygmomanometer consists of a manometer and a BP cuff. The prefix *sphygmo-* refers to the occlusion of the artery by a cuff. A manometer is simply a device used to measure pressure. Two common types of manometers are available for BP measurement: mercury *(Fig. 15.1)* and aneroid *(Fig. 15.2)*. Mercury is the standard for accuracy; however, because of the toxic nature of mercury, aneroid sphygmomanometers are becoming more common in the workplace.

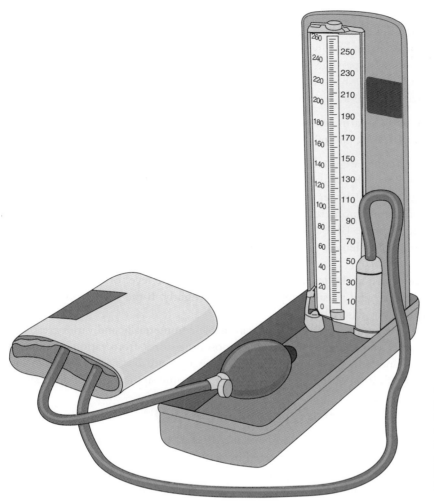

FIGURE 15.1. Sphygmomanometer, gravity mercury. Freestanding pressure manometer of the gravity mercury type, which uses the height of a mercury column in a glass tube to indicate cuff pressure. (Reprinted with permission from LifeART, Lippincott Williams & Wilkins. All rights reserved.)

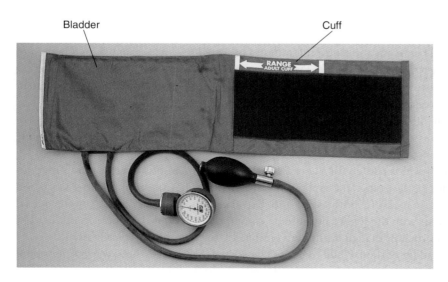

FIGURE 15.2. Aneroid sphygmomanometer, blood pressure cuff, and stethoscope. (Reprinted with permission from Bickley LS, Szilagyi P. Bates' Guide to Physical Examination and History Taking. 8th ed. Philadelphia: Lippincott Williams & Wilkins, 2003.)

Position the manometer at your eye level to eliminate the potential for any reflex errors when reading either the mercury level or the needle if using the aneroid manometer. This is very important. Aneroid manometers are usually of a dial type (round), while mercury manometers are usually of a straight tube/column type. The cuff typically consists of a rubber bladder and two tubes, one to the manometer and one to a hand bulb with a valve that is used for inflation. The bladder must be of appropriate size for accurate readings. The sizing of a BP cuff should be:

➤ Width of bladder = 40–50% of arm circumference
➤ Length of bladder = almost long enough (;80%) to circle arm

Three BP cuff sizes commonly are used in the health and fitness field, a pediatric or child cuff for small arm sizes (13–20 cm; 5–8 in); a normal adult cuff for arm size between 24 and 32 cm (9–11 in); and a large adult cuff for larger arm sizes (32–42 cm; 12–16 in). There are index lines on many of the newer sphygmomanometers cuffs to help "fit" the cuff for a client's arm circumference. In general, the appropriate BP bladder should encircle at least 80% of the arm's circumference. A cuff that is too small in length or width will generally result in a BP measurement that will be falsely high.

The cuff should be positioned at the level of the heart; if below the level of the heart, the BP reading will be falsely high. The cuff must be applied snugly or tightly. If the cuff is too loose, the BP measurement will typically be falsely high.

Equipment used in the measurement of BP is widely available commercially and varies greatly in quality. BP sphygmomanometer units can be purchased in most drug stores, from various health and fitness commercial catalogs, and at medical supply stores. Stethoscopes are also widely available and vary in quality. Electric amplification of the sounds is available on some stethoscope models (2).

Procedures for Resting Blood Pressure Measurement (2)

1. Position yourself to have the best opportunity to hear the BP and see the manometer scale. Take control of the client's arm while having it supported by some piece of furniture when listening for the sounds. Make sure your stethoscope is flat and placed completely over the brachial artery. The room noise should be at a minimum, and the temperature should be comfortable (21–23°C; 70–74 °F). If you have some form of sinus congestion, your ability to hear the BP sounds may be diminished. Clearing your throat prior to attempting a BP measurement may be helpful. Of course, practice in the skill of resting BP measurement is important for its mastery.

2. Your client should be sitting, with the feet flat, the legs uncrossed, the arm free of any clothing, and relaxed. The arm you are using for the BP measurement should be supported. Your client's back should be well supported.

3. Measurement should begin after at least 5 full minutes of seated rest. The client should be free of stimulants (nicotine products, caffeine products, recent alcohol, or other cardiovascular stimulants) for at least 30 minutes prior to the resting measurement. In addition, your client should not have exercised strenuously for at least the prior 60 minutes.

4. There is no practical difference between a seated and supine resting BP; however, statistically, BP tends to be higher by about 6 to 7 mm Hg for SBP and 1 mm Hg for DBP in the supine position.

5. It matters little which arm is chosen for the resting BP measurement; however, it is important to use the same arm for both resting and exercise measurements. The American Heart Association recommends that you measure both right and left arm BPs on your client on the initial evaluation and the arm with the higher pressure be chosen. However, if BP is normal in the right arm, it tends to be normal in the left arm. Conventionally, the left arm is typically used.

6. Center the rubber bladder of the BP cuff over the client's brachial artery; the lower border of the cuff should be 2.5 cm (1 in) above the antecubital fossa or crease of the elbow. Be sure to use the appropriate-size BP cuff, as discussed above. Make sure you palpate your client's brachial artery to determine its location.

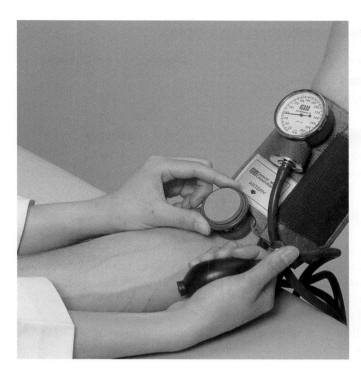

FIGURE 15.3. Position of the stethoscope head and blood pressure cuff. (Reprinted with permission from Bickley LS, Szilagyi P. Bates' Guide to Physical Examination and History Taking. 8th ed. Philadelphia: Lippincott Williams & Wilkins, 2003.)

7. Secure the BP cuff snugly around the arm. Again, be sure to use the appropriate-size cuff. The client should have no clothing on the upper arm to secure the cuff properly. (Clothing on the arm where you place the stethoscope will also muffle the intensity of the sound.)

8. Position the client's arm so it is slightly flexed at the elbow; support the arm or rest it on some piece of furniture. If the client supports his or her own arm, the constant isometric contraction by the client may elevate the DBP. By having the client support the arm on a table, you can reduce the "noise" heard during the procedure, which may increase measurement accuracy. Figure 15.3 depicts how the client's arm should be positioned with the BP cuff and stethoscope.

9. Position the BP cuff on the upper arm with the cuff at heart level. For every centimeter the cuff is below heart level, the BP tends to be higher by 1 mm Hg. The reverse is true for a BP cuff that is above heart level.

10. Find the client's brachial artery. This artery, and thus pulse, is just medial to the biceps tendon. Mark the artery with an appropriate marker (water color) to "locate" the artery for the stethoscope bell placement. To best find the client's brachial artery, have the client face the palm upward and rotate the arm outward on the thumb side with the arm hyperextended.

11. Firmly place the bell of the stethoscope over the artery located in the antecubital fossa. Do not place the bell of the stethoscope under the lip of the BP cuff. There should be no air space or clothing between the bell of the stethoscope and the arm. The stethoscope earpieces should be directed facing slightly forward, toward your nose and in the same direction as your ear canal. Do not press too hard with the stethoscope bell on the arm. The earpieces of a stethoscope should be cleaned with rubbing alcohol before use each time.

12. Be sure to position the manometer (either mercury or aneroid) so that the dial or tube is clearly visible and at eye level to avoid any parallax (distortion from looking up or down) error.

13. Choose between any one of the following three accepted methods for BP cuff inflation. Quickly inflate the BP cuff to about:
    - 20 mm Hg above the SBP, if known
    - Up to 150–180 mm Hg for a resting BP
    - Up to 30 mm Hg above disappearance of the radial pulse, if you palpate for radial pulse first. This is called the palpation method. Many educators favor the palpation method

Table 15.1	CLASSIFICATION OF RESTING BLOOD PRESSURE FOR ADULTS	
Classification	**Systolic (mm Hg)**	**Diastolic (mm Hg) (5th phase)**
Normal	<120	<80
Prehypertension	120–139	80–89
Hypertension		
Stage 1	140–159	90–99
Stage 2	>160	>100

Reprinted with permission from the National High Blood Pressure Education Program; The Seventh Report of the Joint National Committee on the Prevention, Detection and Treatment of High Blood Pressure; JNC7, 2003.

when the technician is first learning BP measurement, to "feel" for and then listen to the SBP.

14. Deflate the pressure slowly; 2–3 mm Hg per heart beat (or 2–5 mm Hg per second) by opening the air exhaust valve on the hand bulb. Rapid deflation leads to underestimation of SBP and overestimation of DBP. Slow the deflation rate to 2 mm Hg per pulse beat when in the anticipated range of the systolic to diastolic BP; this will compensate for slow HRs. A falsely low BP tends to result from too rapid deflation of the cuff.

15. Record measures of SBP and DBP in even numbers. Always round off upward to the nearest 2 mm Hg. Always continue to listen for any BP sounds for at least 10 mm Hg below the fifth phase (to be sure you have correctly identified the fifth phase).

16. Rapidly deflate the cuff to zero after the DBP is obtained.

Wait one full minute before repeating the BP measurement. Average at least two BP readings to get a "true sense" of an individual's BP. It is suggested that BP readings on clients be taken on at least two separate occasions to screen for hypertension. Also, the two readings on your client in any given session should be within 5 mm Hg of each other. If they are not, you should take another BP.

The norms (4) presented in Table 15.1 for resting BP are for adults older than 18 years of age. To use these norms, individuals should not be taking any antihypertensive medications and should not be acutely ill during the measurement. When SBP and DBP fall into two different classifications, the higher classification should be selected. This classification is based on two or more readings taken at each of two or more visits after an initial BP screening. Generally, these norms are revised periodically. It is generally recommended that all persons older than 30 years of age have their BP checked annually (5).

BODY COMPOSITION

Body composition is defined as the relative proportion of fat and fat-free tissue in the body. The assessment of body composition is necessary for numerous reasons. There is a strong correlation (6) between obesity and increased risk of an assortment of chronic diseases (e.g., coronary artery disease, diabetes, hypertension, certain cancers, hyperlipidemia). There is a frequent need to evaluate body weight and body composition in the health and fitness field. Most often this evaluation is done to establish a target, desirable, or optimal weight for an individual. There are several ways to evaluate the composition of the human body. Body composition can be estimated with both laboratory and field techniques that vary in terms of complexity, cost, and accuracy. For the purposes of this text, the following techniques are reviewed:

➤ Height and weight
➤ Body mass index
➤ Waist-to-hip ratio (waist circumference)
➤ Skinfolds

Height and Weight

Measure the client's height. With shoes removed, instruct the client to stand straight up, take a deep breath and hold, and look straight ahead. Record the height in centimeters or inches.

➤ 1 in = 2.54 cm
➤ 1 m = 100 cm
➤ For example: 6 feet = 72 inches = 183 cm = 1.83 m

Measure the client's weight with his or her shoes removed and as much other clothing removed as is practical and possible. Convert weight from pounds to kilograms when necessary.

➤ 1 kg = 2.2 lb
➤ For example: 187 lb = 85 kg

Compare the client's height and weight with the several height–weight tables that are still available. One such source for height and weight tables is the *American College of Sports Medicine Health-Related Physical Fitness Assessment Manual* (2). With the many criticisms of the validity of the height–weight tables (including using a select group of individuals for development and the imprecise concept of "frame size"), there has been a strong trend recently to discontinue their use. Thus, this chapter discusses more advanced methods of anthropometry and body composition analysis.

Body Mass Index

Body mass index (BMI), also called the Quetelet's Index, is used to assess weight relative to height. BMI has a similar association with body fat as the height–weight tables previously discussed. This technique compares an individual's weight (in kilograms) with their height (in meters, squared), much like a height–weight table would. The BMI gives a single number for comparison, as opposed to the weight-to-height ranges located in the tables.

$$\text{Body mass index (kg} \cdot \text{m}^{-2}) = \frac{\text{weight (kg)}}{\text{height (m}^2)}$$

For example: an individual who weighs 150 lb and is 5 feet, 8 inches tall has a BMI of:

$$5 \text{ ft } 8 \text{ in} = 173 \text{ cm} = 1.73 \text{ m} = 2.99 \text{ m}^2$$

$$\text{and } 150 \text{ lb} = 68.18 \text{ kg}$$

$$\text{BMI} = \frac{68}{2.99} = 22.8 \text{ kg} \cdot \text{m}^{-2}$$

The major shortcoming with using BMI for body composition is that it is difficult for a client to relate to or interpret needed weight loss or weight gain. Also, the BMI does not differentiate fat weight from fat-free weight and has only a modest correlation with percentage body fat predicted from hydrostatic weighing (2). Norms for BMI are presented in Table 15.2 and Figure 15.4.

Waist-to-Hip Ratio

The waist-to-hip ratio is a comparison between the circumference of the waist and the circumference of the hip. This ratio best represents the distribution of body weight, and perhaps body fat, in an individual. The pattern of body fat distribution is recognized as an important predictor of health risks of obesity. Individuals with more weight or circumference on the trunk are at higher risk of hypertension, type 2 diabetes, hyperlipidemia, and coronary artery disease

Table 15.2 **CLASSIFICATION OF DISEASE RISK BASED ON BODY MASS INDEX (BMI) AND WAIST CIRCUMFERENCE**

| | BMI (kg · m⁻²) | Disease Risk[a] Relative to Normal Weight and Waist Circumference | |
		Men ≤102 cm Women ≤88 cm	Men >102 cm Women >88 cm
Underweight	<18.5	—	—
Normal	18.5–24.9	—	—
Overweight	25.0–29.9	Increased	High
I	30.0–34.9	High	Very high
II	35.0–39.9	Very high	Very high
III	≥40	Extremely high	Extremely high

Modified from Expert Panel. Executive Summary of the clinical guidelines on the identification, evaluation, and treatment of overweight and obesity in adults. Arch Intern Med 1998;158:1855–1867. Reprinted from American College of Sports Medicine. ACSM's Guidelines for Exercise Testing and Prescription. 7th ed. Baltimore: Lippincott Williams & Wilkins, 2006:58.

[a] Disease risk for type 2 diabetes, hypertension, and cardiovascular disease. Dashes (—) indicate that no additional risk at these levels of BMI was assigned. Increased waist circumference can also be a marker for increased risk, even in persons of normal weight.

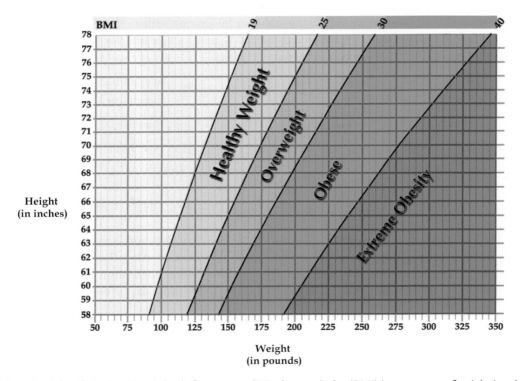

FIGURE 15.4. The risks of obesity. How is body fat measured? Body mass index (BMI) is a measure of weight in relation to a person's height. For most people, BMI has a strong relationship to weight. For adults, BMI can also be found by using this table. To use the BMI table, first find your weight at the bottom of the graph. Go straight up from that point until you reach the line that matches your height. Then look to see what weight group you fall in. (Reprinted with permission from Anatomical Chart Co.)

than individuals who are of equal weight but have more of their weight distributed on the extremities. Some experts suggest that the waist circumference alone may be used as an indicator of health risk (1):

➤ Waist: The waist circumference has been frequently defined as the smallest waist circumference, typically measured 1 inch (2.54 cm) above the umbilicus or navel and below the xiphoid process.
➤ Hip: The hip circumference has been defined as the largest circumference around the buttocks, above the gluteal fold (posterior extension).
➤ WHR is a ratio (thus, there are no units).
➤ $\text{WHR} = \dfrac{\text{Waist circumference}}{\text{Hip circumference}}$

Measure the waist and hip circumferences in either inches or centimeters (1 in = 2.54 cm). Take multiple measurements until each is within 1/4 inch of each other. Health risk is very high for young men when the WHR is more than 0.95 and for young women when the WHR is more than 0.86. For example: A male client has a waist circumference of 32 in (81.3 cm) and a hip circumference of 35 in (88.9 cm). The WHR is 32/35 = 0.91.

Waist Circumference Alone

Some experts suggest that the waist circumference alone may be used as an indicator of health risk. For example, the health risk is very high when the waist circumference is greater than or equal to 43 in (110 cm) for women and 47 in (120 cm) for men. A very low risk is associated with a waist circumference less than 27.5 in (70 cm) for women and 31.5 in (80 cm) for men.

Skinfolds

Skinfold determination of percentage body fat can be quite accurate if the technician is properly trained in the use of skinfold calipers. It should be remembered, however, that skinfold determination of percentage body fat is still an estimate or prediction of percentage body fat, not an absolute measurement. This estimate is based on the principle that the amount of subcutaneous fat is proportional to the total amount of body fat; however, the proportion of subcutaneous to total fat varies with gender, age, and ethnicity. Regression equations considering these factors have been developed to predict body density or percentage fat from skinfold measurements (7).

Standardized descriptions as well as pictorial descriptions of skinfold sites are provided in Box 15.1 and Figure 15.5.

PROCEDURES FOR SKINFOLD MEASUREMENTS

The following procedures help to standardize the measure (2):

1. Firmly grasp a double fold of skin (a skinfold) and the subcutaneous fat between the thumb and index finger of your left hand and lift up and away from the body. Be certain that you have not grasped any muscle in this procedure and that you have taken up all the fat. You can also have the subject first flex the muscle below the site to help distinguish muscle from fat before you measure. Be sure, however, to have the subject relax the area prior to measurement.
2. You should grasp the skinfold site with your two fingers about 8 cm (3 inches) apart on a line that is perpendicular to the long axis of the skinfold site. You should be able to form a fold that has roughly parallel sides. Larger skinfolds (obese individuals) will require separating your fingers farther than 8 cm.
3. Hold the calipers in your right hand with the scale facing up to ease your viewing. Place the contact surfaces of the calipers 1 cm (0.5 in) below your fingers. The calipers should be placed on

---

BOX 15.1   **Standardized Description of Skinfold Sites and Procedures**

SKINFOLD SITE

Abdominal	Vertical fold; 2 cm to the right side of the umbilicus
Triceps	Vertical fold; on the posterior midline of the upper arm, halfway between the acromion and olecranon processes, with the arm held freely to the side of the body
Biceps	Vertical fold; on the anterior aspect of the arm over the belly of the biceps muscle, 1 cm above the level used to mark the triceps site
Chest/pectoral	Diagonal fold; one-half the distance between the anterior axillary line and the nipple (men), or one-third of the distance between the anterior axillary line and the nipple (women)
Medial calf	Vertical fold; at the maximum circumference of the calf on the midline of its medial border
Midaxillary	Vertical fold; on the midaxillary line at the level of the xiphoid process of the sternum. An alternate method is a horizontal fold taken at the level of the xiphoid/sternal border in the midaxillary line
Subscapular	Diagonal fold (at a 45° angle); 1 to 2 cm below the inferior angle of the scapula
Suprailiac	Diagonal fold; in line with the natural angle of the iliac crest taken in the anterior axillary line immediately superior to the iliac crest
Thigh	Vertical fold; on the anterior midline of the thigh, midway between the proximal border of the patella and the inguinal crease (hip)

PROCEDURES

- All measurements should be made on the right side of the body with the subject standing upright
- Calipers should be placed directly on the skin surface, 1 cm away from the thumb and finger, perpendicular to the skinfold, and halfway between the crest and the base of the fold
- Pinch should be maintained while reading the calipers
- Wait 1 to 2 seconds (no longer) before reading calipers
- Take duplicate measures at each site and retest if duplicate measurements are not within 1 to 2 mm
- Rotate through measurement sites or allow time for skin to regain normal texture and thickness

Reprinted with permission from ACSM's Guidelines for Exercise Testing and Prescription. 7th ed. Baltimore: Lippincott Williams & Wilkins, 2006:62.

---

the exact skinfold site, while your fingers should be above the site by 1 cm. Place the tips of the calipers on the doublefold of skin and fat.

4. Release the scissor grip of the calipers claws with your hand and continue to support the weight of the calipers with that hand.

5. Record the reading on the calipers scale 1 to 2 seconds (no longer) after releasing the scissor grip lever to allow the jaws of the calipers to measure the skinfold site. Measure the skinfold to the nearest 0.5 mm (using the Lange calipers). Be careful to avoid jaw slippage of the calipers.

6. Measure each skinfold site at least twice. Rotate through the measurement sites or allow time for the skin to regain its normal texture and thickness. If duplicate measurements are not within 1 or 2 mm, retest this site.

7. Sum the mean, or average, of each skinfold site to determine percentage body fat by consulting tables found in other sources (1, 7).

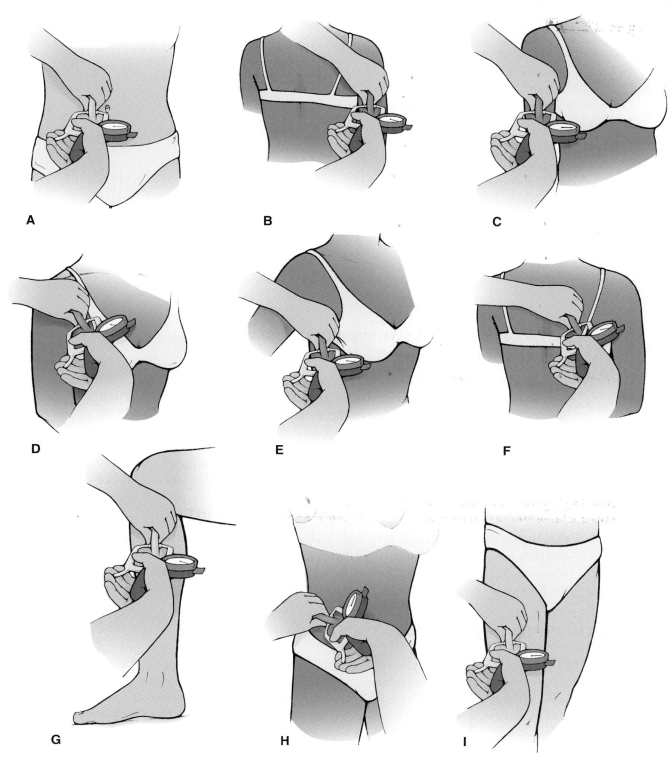

FIGURE 15.5. Anatomical sites for skinfold measurement. (Reprinted with permission from ACSM's Health-related Physical Fitness Assessment Manual. Baltimore: Lippincott Williams & Wilkins, 2005:63.)

Table 15.3 IDEAL BODY WEIGHT CALCULATIONS

Ideal Body Weight (IBW) Calculations

- IBW = $\dfrac{\text{LBM (Lean Body Mass)}}{1.00 \text{ (Desired \% Body Fat/100)}}$

- For example, if a man weighs 190 lb (86.4 kg) and is determined to have 22.3% body fat then

- Fat Weight = Body Weight × (% Body Fat/100)

    = 190 × (22.3/100)

    = 42.37 lb (19.25 kg)

- Lean Body Mass (LBM) = Body Weight − Fat Weight

    = 190 − 42.37

    = 147.63 lb

- Ideal Body Weight (IBW) = $\dfrac{147.63 \ (67.1 \text{ kg})}{1.00 - (15/100)}$ (15% used for a man; as a guideline)

    = 173.68 (78.9 kg)

In this example, 190 − 173.7 = 16.3 lb (7.4 kg) to lose to achieve ideal body weight.

JACKSON-POLLOCK 3-SITE SKINFOLD FORMULA FOR PERCENTAGE BODY FAT

Jackson and Pollock (9) have developed several skinfold formulas for the prediction of percentage body fat or body composition (often referred to as the Jackson-Pollock formulas) (6, 9). The 3-site formula, published in 1985, has been used successfully by many practitioners. Jackson and Pollock developed another 3-site skinfold formula in 1980, as well as a 7-site skinfold formula (10). The 1985 formula provides percentage body fat averages for the skinfold measurement for the triceps, chest, and subscapula (for men) and triceps, suprailiac, and abdomen (for women). Sum the means of the three skinfold site measures and use tables for percentage body fat estimation published in other resources (7).

CALCULATION OF IDEAL OR DESIRED BODY WEIGHT

Along with the determination of percentage body fat, it is often desirable to determine an ideal or desired body weight based on a desired percentage of fat for the individual (Table 15.3). Obviously, this process can be problematic in that a desirable percentage body fat for an individual must be determined. The determination of a desirable body weight is useful in weight loss or weight maintenance (8).

CARDIORESPIRATORY ASSESSMENT

Cardiorespiratory fitness (CRF) is related to the ability to perform large muscle, dynamic, moderate-to high–intensity exercise for prolonged periods of time and reflects the functional capabilities of the heart, blood vessels, blood, lungs, and relevant muscles during various types of exercise demands. CRF is a synonym for many terms that may be used for the same thing (2). The following is a list of the terms that all mean essentially the same thing:

➤ Maximal aerobic capacity
➤ Functional capacity
➤ Physical work capacity (PWC)
➤ Maximal oxygen uptake ($\dot{V}O_{2max}$)
➤ Cardiovascular endurance, fitness, or capacity
➤ Cardiopulmonary endurance, fitness, or capacity

CRF can be measured or predicted by many methods. This chapter discusses the prediction of CRF by the use of field tests such as the 1.5-mile run test and step tests, as well as laboratory tests. The Personal Trainer needs to decide which test may be the most appropriate for CRF determination for a client. The measurement of CRF can be used in:

➤ Exercise prescription and programming: in helping to set up an exercise program
➤ Progress in, and motivation of, an individual in an exercise program (providing both feedback and motivation to keep a client interested in exercise)
➤ Prediction of medical conditions such as coronary artery disease (to further identify or diagnose health problems)

A laboratory prediction of CRF, using a cycle ergometer, is popular, but this procedure is likely beyond the scope of practice of many Personal Trainers. The true measurement of CRF involves maximal exertion or exercise along with the collection of expired gases. The measurement of expired gases is not always applicable, nor desirable, in many settings such as corporate fitness and wellness programs that wish to measure or quantify CRF. Thus, there are many approaches to the assessment of CRF that do not involve the use of maximal exercise and/or the use of sophisticated gas analyzers (2, 10).

Pretest Considerations

It is important to standardize pretesting conditions for all clients who undergo these various tests for CRF. Standardization can also increase the accuracy of prediction of CRF as well as aid in client safety. Instructions to clients prior to the test can increase their comfort as well. These general instructions are (1):

➤ Abstain from prior eating (>4 hours)
➤ Abstain from prior strenuous exercise (>24 hours)
➤ Abstain from prior caffeine ingestion (>12–24 hours)
➤ Abstain from prior nicotine use (>3 hours)
➤ Abstain from prior alcohol use (>24 hours)
➤ Medication considerations (if the client's medications affect resting or exercise HR, it will invalidate the test)

Field Tests for Prediction of Cardiorespiratory Fitness

A field test generally requires the client to perform a task in a non-laboratory or field setting, such as running 1.5 miles at near maximal exertion. Thus, field tests, perhaps considered by some to be submaximal, may be inappropriate for safety reasons for sedentary individuals at moderate to high risk for cardiovascular or musculoskeletal complications.

Two types of field tests are commonly used for the prediction of aerobic capacity: a timed completion of a set distance (e.g., 1.5-mile run) or a maximal distance for a set time (e.g., 12-minute walk/run). Field tests are relatively easy and inexpensive to administer and thus are ideal for testing large groups of subjects (2, 8). Although the CRF assessment test to select can be difficult to choose, there are some criteria you may use to help you select the best one for your client:

➤ What the data will be used for (e.g., exercise programming)
➤ Need for data accuracy
➤ Client's age and health status
➤ Available resources

In general, both walk/run performance tests and step tests are applicable to a wide range of clients, as long as the appropriate health risk screening has occurred first. One note of importance here: in the performance of a step test, the client can approach a level of near-maximal exertion, and this clearly may not be desirable.

Walk/Run Performance Tests

There are two common field test protocols that use a walk or run performance test to predict aerobic capacity. These walk or run tests tend to be more accurate (i.e., less error in prediction) than the step tests discussed on page 331. The performance tests can be classified into two groups: walk/run tests or pure walk tests. In the walk/run test, the subject can walk, run, or use a combination of both to complete the test. In the pure walking test, the subjects are strictly limited to walking (always having one foot on the ground at any given time) the entire test. Another classification for these tests is whether the test is performed over a set distance (e.g., 1 mile or 1.6 km) or over a set time period (e.g., 12 minutes). The first test discussed uses a 1.5-mile distance and requires the subject to complete the distance in the shortest time possible, either by running the whole distance, if possible, or by combining periods of running and walking to offset the fatigue of continuous running in an untrained individual. The second test uses a set 1-mile course and requires the subject to walk the entire distance.

1.5-MILE RUN TEST PROCEDURES (2)

1. This test is contraindicated for unconditioned beginners, individuals with symptoms of heart disease, and those with known heart disease or risk factors for heart disease. Clients should be able to jog for 15 minutes continuously to complete this test and obtain a reasonable prediction of their aerobic capacity.
2. Ensure that the area for performing the test measures 1.5 miles in distance. A standard 1/4 mile (400 m) track would be ideal (6 laps = 1.5 miles).
3. Inform clients of the purposes of the test and the need to pace themselves over the 1.5-mile distance. Effective pacing and the subject's motivation are key variables in the outcome of the test.
4. Have clients start the test and start a stopwatch to coincide with the start. Give your clients feedback on time to help them with pacing.
5. Record the total time to complete the test, and use the formula below to predict CRF as measured by $\dot{V}O_{2max}$ and recorded in $mL \cdot kg^{-1} \cdot min^{-1}$:

   - For men and women
   - $\dot{V}O_{2max}\ (mL \cdot kg^{-1} \cdot min^{-1}) = 3.5 + 483/time$

where time = time to complete 1.5 miles in nearest hundredth of a minute (for example, 15:20 = 15.33 minutes).

ROCKPORT 1-MILE WALK TEST PROCEDURES

This test may be useful for those who are unable to run because of a low fitness level and/or injury. The client should be able to walk briskly (get the exercise heart rate above 120 bpm) for 1 mile to complete this test.

The 1-mile walk test requires that subjects walk as fast as they can around a measured 1-mile course. The client must not break into a run! Walking can be defined as having one foot in contact with the ground at all times, whereas running involves an airborne phase. The time it takes to walk this 1 mile is measured and recorded (10, 12).

Immediately at the end of the 1-mile walk, the client counts the recovery heart rate (or pulse) for 15 seconds and multiplies by 4 to determine a 1-minute recovery heart rate (bpm). In another version of the test, heart rate is measured in the final minute of the 1-mile walk (during the last quarter mile).

The formula for $\dot{V}O_2max$ ($mL \cdot kg^{-1} \cdot min^{-1}$) is gender specific (the constant 6.315 is added to the formula for men only). This formula was derived on apparently healthy individuals ranging in age from 30 to 69 years (12).

$$\dot{V}O_{2max} (mL \cdot kg^{-1} \cdot min^{-1}) = 132.853 - (0.1692 \cdot WT) - (0.3877 \cdot AGE) + (6.315, \text{ for men}) - (3.2649 \cdot TIME) - (0.1565 \cdot HR)$$

where WT = weight in kilograms, AGE = age in years, TIME = time for 1 mile in nearest hundredth of a minute (e.g., 15:42 = 15.7 [42/60 = 0.7], and HR = recovery HR in bpm.

Step Tests

Step tests have been around for more than 50 years in fitness testing. We will discuss the use of the Queens College Step Test (2) for the prediction of CRF (there are several popular step test protocols). This test relies on having the subject step up and down on a standardized step or bench (standardized for step height) for a set period of time at a set stepping cadence. After the test time period is complete, a recovery HR is obtained and used in the prediction of aerobic capacity. The lower the recovery HR, the more fit the individual. Most step tests use the client's HR response to a standard amount of exertion (2).

In general, step tests require little equipment to conduct (a watch, a metronome, and a standardized height step bench). Special precautions for safety are needed for those clients who may have balance problems or difficulty with stepping. It should also be remembered that while step tests may be considered submaximal for many clients, they might be at or near maximal exertion for other clients.

QUEENS COLLEGE STEP TEST PROCEDURES (2)

1. The Queens College Step Test requires that the individual step up and down on a standardized step height of 16.25 inches (41.25 cm) for 3 minutes. Many gymnasium bleachers have a riser height of 16.25 inches.
2. The men step at a rate (cadence) of 24 per minute, while women step at a rate of 22 per minute. This cadence should be closely monitored and set with the use of an electronic metronome. A 24-steps-per-minute cadence means that the complete cycle of step up with one leg, step up with the other, step down with the first leg, and finally step down with the last leg is performed 24 times in a minute (up one leg—up the other leg—down the first leg—down the second leg). Set the metronome at a cadence of four times the step rate, in this case 96 beats per minute for men, to coordinate each leg's movement with a beat of the metronome. The women's step rate would be 88 beats per minute. Thus, while it may be possible to test more than one client at a time, depending on equipment, it is problematic to test men and women together.
3. After the 3 minutes are up, the client stops and has his or her pulse taken (preferably at the radial site) while standing and within the first 5 seconds. A 15-second pulse count is then taken. Multiply this pulse count by 4 to determine heart rate in beats per minute. The recovery heart rate should occur between 5 and 20 seconds of immediate recovery from the end of the step test.
4. The subject's $\dot{V}O_{2max}$ (in $mL \cdot kg^{-1} \cdot min^{-1}$) is determined from the recovery heart rate (Table 15.4).

Table 15.4	**CALCULATION OF MAXIMAL OXYGEN CONSUMPTION AS DETERMINED FROM THE RECOVERY HEART RATE**
For Men:	**For Women:**
$\dot{V}O_{2max} (mL \cdot kg^{-1} \cdot min^{-1}) = 111.33 - (0.42 \cdot HR)$	$\dot{V}O_{2max} (mL \cdot kg^{-1} \cdot min^{-1}) = 65.81 - (0.1847 \cdot HR)$

HR, recovery heart rate (bpm).

Table 15.5 PERCENTILE VALUES FOR MAXIMAL AEROBIC POWER

Percentile Values for Maximal Aerobic Power ($mL \cdot kg^{-1} \cdot min^{-1}$) in Men

	Age				
Percentile	20–29 (N = 2,234)	30–39 (N = 11,158)	40–49 (N = 13,109)	50–59 (N = 5,641)	60+ (N = 1,244)
90	55.1	52.1	50.6	49.0	44.2
80	52.1	50.6	49.0	44.2	41.0
70	49.0	47.4	45.8	41.0	37.8
60	47.4	44.2	44.2	39.4	36.2
50	44.2	42.6	41.0	37.8	34.6
40	42.6	41.0	39.4	36.2	33.0
30	41.0	39.4	36.2	34.6	31.4
20	37.8	36.2	34.6	31.4	28.3
10	34.6	33.0	31.4	29.9	26.7

Percentile Values for Maximal Aerobic Power ($mL \cdot kg^{-1} \cdot min^{-1}$) in Women

Percentile	20–29 (N = 1,223)	30–39 (N = 3,895)	40–49 (N = 4,001)	50–59 (N = 2,032)	60+ (N = 465)
90	49.0	45.8	42.6	37.8	34.6
80	44.2	41.0	39.4	34.6	33.0
70	41.0	39.4	36.2	33.0	31.4
60	39.4	36.2	34.6	31.4	28.3
50	37.8	34.6	33.0	29.9	26.7
40	36.2	33.0	31.4	28.3	25.1
30	33.0	31.4	29.9	26.7	23.5
20	31.4	29.9	28.3	25.1	21.9
10	28.3	26.7	25.1	21.9	20.3

Data were obtained from the initial examination of apparently healthy men and women enrolled in the Aerobics Center Longitudinal Study (ACLS), 1970 to 2002. The study population for the data set was predominantly white and college educated. Maximal treadmill exercise tests were administered using a modified Balke protocol. Maximal oxygen uptake was estimated from the final treadmill speed and grade using the current ACSM equations found in this edition of the *Guidelines* (1). The data are provided courtesy of the ACSL investigators, The Cooper Institute, Dallas, TX. The ACLS is supported in part by a grant from the National Institute on Aging (AG06945), SN Blair, Principal Investigator. The following may be used as descriptors for the percentile rankings: well above average (90), above average (70), average (50), below average (30), and well below average (10). (Originally sourced from the Aerobics Center Longitudinal Study, 1970–2002). Reprinted with permission from American College of Sports Medicine. ACSM's Guidelines for Exercise Testing and Prescription. 7th ed. Baltimore: Lippincott Williams & Wilkins, 2006:79.

Norms for CRF ($\dot{V}O_{2max}$)

Cardiorespiratory fitness is commonly expressed as maximal oxygen uptake ($\dot{V}O_{2max}$). $\dot{V}O_{2max}$ is expressed as milliliters of oxygen consumed per kilogram of body weight per minute ($mL \cdot kg^{-1} \cdot min^{-1}$). Table 15.5 shows the norms for $\dot{V}O_{2max}$ for men and women.

FLEXIBILITY ASSESSMENT

The most common flexibility assessment is the sit-and-reach test. While there exists no single best test of overall flexibility, the sit-and-reach test is the most common and most practical in use. Preceded by a proper warm-up, the sit-and-reach test can be easy to administer and interpreted. The

Table 15.6 TRUNK FLEXION (SIT-AND-REACH) TEST PROCEDURES

Pretest: Participant should perform a short warm-up prior to this test and include some stretches (e.g., modified hurdler's stretch). It is also recommended that the participant refrain from fast, jerky movements, which may increase the possibility of an injury. The participant's shoes should be removed.

1. For the YMCA sit-and-reach test, a yardstick is placed on the floor and tape is placed across it at a right angle to the 15-inch mark. The participant sits with the yardstick between the legs, with legs extended at right angles to the taped line on the floor. Heels of the feet should touch the edge of the taped line and be about 10 to 12 inches apart.

2. The participant should slowly reach forward with both hands as far as possible, holding this position momentarily. Be sure that the participant keeps the hands parallel and does not lead with one hand. Fingertips can be overlapped and should be in contact with the yardstick or measuring portion of the sit-and-reach box.

3. The score is the most distant point (in inches or centimeters) reached with the fingertips. The best of three trials should be recorded. To assist with the best attempt, the participant should exhale and drop the head between the arms when reaching. Testers should ensure that the knees of the participant stay extended; however, the participant's knees should not be pressed down. The participant should breathe normally during the test and should not hold his or her breath at any time. Norms for the YMCA test are presented in Table 15.7.

4. The sit-and-reach test is also done using a sit-and-reach box. The participant sits with the legs fully extended with the soles of the feet against the box. The other directions are as described above. Note that these norms use a sit-and-reach box in which the "zero" point is set at the 26 cm mark. If you are using a box in which the zero point is set at 23 cm (e.g., Fitnessgram), subtract 3 cm from each value in this table.

Reprinted with permission from American College of Sports Medicine. ACSM's Health-Related Physical Fitness Assessment Manual. Baltimore: Lippincott Williams & Wilkins, 2005:81.

[a] Diagrams of these procedures are available elsewhere.

Personal Trainer should be made aware that this test only measures flexibility of the hamstrings, hip, and lower back. It is a specific measure of those regions. Its practical significance and the reason for it being a very good measure of flexibility is the significant number of people who complain of low back pain. It is likely that this pain is caused by decreased flexibility primarily of the hamstrings (which have their anatomical origin in the posterior hip region). For a detailed description of the procedure, see Table 15.6. Percentile rankings for men and for women can be found in Table 15.7.

Table 15.7 PERCENTILES BY AGE GROUPS AND GENDER FOR YMCA SIT-AND-REACH TEST (INCHES)

Percentile	Age											
	18–25		26–35		36–45		46–55		56–65		> 65	
Gender	M	F	M	F	M	F	M	F	M	F	M	F
90	22	24	21	23	21	22	19	21	17	20	17	20
80	20	22	19	21	19	21	17	20	15	19	15	18
70	19	21	17	20	17	19	15	18	13	17	13	17
60	18	20	17	20	16	18	14	17	13	16	12	17
50	17	19	15	19	15	17	13	16	11	15	10	15
40	15	18	14	17	13	16	11	14	9	14	9	14
30	14	17	13	17	13	15	10	14	9	13	8	13
20	13	16	11	15	11	14	9	12	7	11	7	11
10	11	14	9	13	7	12	6	10	5	9	4	9

Based on data from YMCA of the USA (reprinted from YMCA Fitness Testing and Assessment Manual. 4th ed. 2000 with permission of YMCA of the USA, 101 N. Wacker Drive, Chicago, IL 60606). The following may be used as descriptors for the percentile rankings: well above average (90), above average (70), average (50), below average (30), and well below average (10).

POSTURAL ANALYSIS AND BODY ALIGNMENT ASSESSMENTS

Improved posture is often a central goal on a Personal Trainer's agenda. A successful exercise program, presented in an education-based way, can help the client achieve the goal of better posture. Posture is the position or "attitude" of the body or bodily parts that requires a minimum amount of muscular energy to maintain a mechanically efficient function of the joints and muscular systems. Unfortunately, incorrect positions and attitudes of the body often lead to chronic muscle and skeletal problems that require the Personal Trainer's skill and guidance to correct. Correct posture is more than "standing up straight and tall." Physical well-being depends on correct postures while sitting, standing, walking, and exercising. In an optimal postural alignment, the line of gravity (LOG) falls through the center of most joint axes, evenly distributing the body weight throughout the body's joint structures. This correct weight distribution allows the correct balance of ligament and muscle tension surrounding a given joint (13).

By implementing a posture program for your clients, based on the fundamentals of observation, evaluation, and feedback, clients and Personal Trainers can achieve their goals and objectives of improved structural alignment. Discuss and educate clients on the following benefits of good posture:

➤ Proper alignment for the vertebral column
➤ Improved balance within joint structures
➤ Better overall muscular balance
➤ A safer body alignment while moving throughout the day
➤ Improved daily and activity performance
➤ Increased self-confidence

Postural Improvement Takes Time

The information provided in this section will help the Personal Trainer develop a thoughtful program for his or her clients that will educate and train them for improved posture and health. Remind your clients that improving one's posture can be initiated at any age, whether you are young or old (14). However, if a client is 60 years old, it will likely take more than a few sessions of training in most cases to break the 60-year habit of poor posture. Personal Trainers are there to educate and provide guidance and feedback to help clients achieve their goals. The time factor involved in postural realignment must be emphasized. This process takes time, and the Personal Trainer will need to observe and evaluate the client over weeks and sometimes months to successfully achieve postural changes.

The Center of Gravity and Base of Support

The center of gravity (COG) is located at about the second sacral segment and is the point in the body where all forces acting upon it are in equilibrium or balance. The COG may move outside of equilibrium when playing a sport and/or performing a dynamic movement such as walking or running. The proprioceptors send impulses from the muscles, tendons, joints, and other structures to the central nervous system, telling the body when movement is occurring and also whether or not the appropriate response necessary to maintain equilibrium is functioning (15).

Line of Gravity

The line of gravity (LOG) is the imaginary vertical line passing through the body's center of gravity. The effect of forces acting on joint structures is related to the location of the LOG. The LOG in "optimal" posture comes close to, but does not fall evenly through, each joint structure (16). Performing posture assessments requires that the Personal Trainer understand the location of the client's current LOG and the required or ideal LOG to obtain a client's optimal posture. The client's current LOG can be changed toward a more ideal posture and body alignment based on the exercise program designed by the Personal Trainer.

Static and Dynamic Posture

Posture and body alignment can assume a multitude of positions that may be either static or dynamic (17). Static posture means alignment that is commonly viewed as not moving or limited in motion. Sitting, standing, and lying would be considered static postures. The Personal Trainer must consider this when designing a client's exercise program (18). In contrast to static posture, dynamic posture refers to posture with moving body segments such as when walking, running, exercising, or performing an activity such as tennis. By understanding the characteristics that develop from the client's postural habits, the Personal Trainer can accurately build an exercise process to balance and correct unhealthy postural positions and movements.

Posture-Related Injuries and Health Concerns

Many people do not realize that common injuries to muscles and joints can develop through prolonged incorrect posture and poor body alignment. Problems and injuries that occur from habitually poor posture include the following (19):

➤ Joint problems
➤ Muscle imbalances
➤ Low back pain (20)

When clients learn of the potential injuries that can occur with poor posture, they will have an increased incentive to be more conscious about maintaining better postural alignment throughout the day. In this way, the Personal Trainer can play an important role in creating an awareness of unhealthy current or potential postural conditions and in educating clients on the potential injuries they can cause. Most importantly, however, the Personal Trainer can teach the client how to end bad postural habits and start new patterns of movement.

Equipment Needs for Posture Assessment

A competent practitioner of posture and body alignment can identify structural landmarks relative to a client's LOG (21). Through observation and evaluation, Personal Trainers can determine whether a body segment or joint structure deviates from the ideal or normal alignment. Sophisticated electronic equipment may be used to assess a client, such as radiography or electromyography. However, a successful and professional posture and body alignment assessment can be done inexpensively with a digital camera and posture grid. The camera technique also provides another way to actively involve the client in the training process if the Personal Trainer explains what is being photographed and why as he or she takes the pictures. Communication is the key to involving clients and motivating them to do their best in their training sessions. Most clients like this process and think it is fun when they are approached by someone with good communication skills (see Chapters 4 and 5).

The equipment listed below can provide a detailed and thorough postural analysis with visual feedback via printed handouts for your clients:

➤ A digital camera
➤ Posture and body alignment grid or matrix (22)
➤ Computer, printer, and software provided by the camera manufacturer to immediately print posture photos
➤ Optional: Extra batteries and memory card(s) are recommended if performing multiple posture assessments within your facility or organization

The Posture Screening and Assessment Process

Posture screening and assessment is a tool that Personal Trainers may use to evaluate the standing posture for signs of deviations and misalignments. The client's standing posture can be evaluated in relation to his or her body segments compared with the LOG. To determine if a client has postural deviations, a posture screening is appropriate (23). At some point in a client's training program, analysis and evaluation of the client's sitting positions may also be helpful in improving postural positions.

First, hang the posture and body alignment grid against the wall. Then, stand the client in front of the grid and take photos of the client's standing position. It is recommended that you take pictures of the client standing with the back, front, and both sides facing the grid, to get all of the viewing angles. It is recommended that additional photos and reassessments be taken as often as every week to every 4 weeks, depending on the client's degree of misalignment. When taking the photos, follow these steps:

➤ Subject should wear minimal clothing to better observe body alignment
➤ No shoes
➤ Clients should stand in their normal posture
➤ Stand far enough away from the client to enable pictures of the full view of the body from the feet to the top of the head
➤ A total of four photos are needed: anterior, posterior, and lateral positions (right/left sides) *(Fig. 15.6)*
➤ Print the photos
➤ Evaluate the photos with the client

Show the posture pictures to the client and ask what he or she sees there. Give clients a chance to point out their own weaknesses before you start identifying them. Listen well and pay attention to what the client sees in the pictures. When the client is finished responding, comment on the points the client discussed and then add your own observations. The client's curiosity about how you will go about solving his or her posture problems will be peaked at this point, so reassure the client that you will prepare a personally tailored program by the next session.

Analysis of Posture

The Personal Trainer's analysis of posture and body alignment should be made from three different positions: anterior, posterior, and laterally from both sides. The trainer should be looking at the whole person, from the head (superiorly) all the way down to the client's feet (inferiorly). When observing the client's posture, begin to consider and visualize the sequence of exercise movements and the training process. Each primary joint structure in the body, including the glenohumeral, spine, elbow, wrist, hip, knee, and ankle, should be evaluated individually and also as an integrated or whole system that is working together with all the other structures to perform a movement (24). Identified in the following sections are some (not all) of the anatomical structures and a description of terms with relevant information for the cause of various postural deviations.

ANALYSIS OF POSTURE: ANTERIOR/POSTERIOR

In an anterior/posterior view, the LOG bisects the middle of the body into right and left halves. The LOG divides the vertebral bodies of the spine and is equidistant from the glenohumeral, elbow, wrist, hip, knee, and ankle joints. Again, in an optimal posture, the body has little to no muscular activity to maintain balance and equilibrium. Unfortunately, most individuals do not have perfectly symmetrical bodies and have joint, muscle, and ligamentous structures that are unbalanced (25). The following structures are important to anterior/posterior observation and analysis (26):

➤ Head and neck area: upper trapezius and sternocleidomastoid (SCM) muscles
➤ Vertebral column for scoliosis
➤ Glenohumeral joint for balance
➤ Scapula for balance

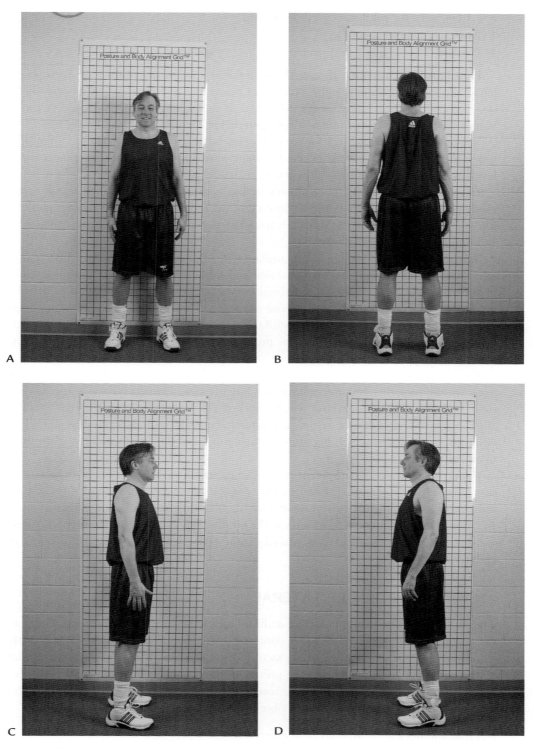

FIGURE 15.6. Anterior, posterior, and lateral positions (right/left sides).

➤ Elbow/wrist for palm forward or backward
➤ Knee for valgus/varus stress
➤ Flat feet

Head and Neck Area. Observe the head for an upward, downward, or sideways (either to the left or right) tilt. Also check the muscles of the upper trapezius and SCM area for balance and symmetry. Often these muscles are not balanced and are either too shortened or too lengthened. Note whether the client's shoulders look rounded in the upper back and neck area.

Vertebral Column. Check for scoliosis or lateral deviations in the vertebral column of the spine. Often these conditions may be detected through observing or palpating the spinous process, scapula level, or differences in arm-to-body space.

Glenohumeral Joint. The muscles of the glenohumeral joint that compose the anterior, middle, and posterior deltoid often assume a position of imbalance. One shoulder is often lower than the other. Check whether the shoulders round forward, thus improperly lengthening the posterior, and middle deltoid and rotator cuff.

Scapula. The scapula often is in a constant state of protraction due to lengthened muscles caused by forward shoulder rounding and weakness within the middle trapezius and rhomboid muscles.

Elbow/Wrist. Forward-rounded shoulders can cause an internal rotation of the glenohumeral joint. Thus, the elbow and wrist positions need to be checked, as these will rotate the palms of the hands to face posteriorly instead of toward the sides of the body. This internal rotation derives from several misaligned areas, including the protraction of the scapula and shortened muscles in the anterior shoulder area.

Knees. Knees in the genu valgum ("knock knees") or genu varum ("bow legs") positions create stress within the joint structures and surrounding muscles. Trainers must take special care in the design of personal training programs when these conditions are present, as they are usually irreversible and can significantly limit the client's comfortable range of motion. Significant damage can be done when the cardiovascular training and/or other programs do not adequately adapt their design to these conditions.

Feet. A common foot problem is pes planus, or flat foot. Flat feet are characterized by feet that have no noticeable arch. Flat feet may result in knee and hip problems because of rotational imbalances caused by turned-in ankles that then disturb the LOG of the knee and hip joints. Again, Personal Trainers need to look at the whole body as a kinetic chain of reactions and watch for the ways in which the stresses placed on the body in one area may be affecting the stress in another location.

ANALYSIS OF POSTURE: LATERAL

The LOG passes through the external auditory meatus posterior to the coronal suture and through the odontoid process (27). The LOG continues through the midline of the trunk of the vertebral column to pass slightly anterior to the sacroiliac joint. From there, the LOG moves slightly posterior to the hip joint axis, through the greater trochanter, anterior to the midline of the knee (but posterior to the patella) through to the anterior of the lateral malleolus of the ankle. The following list of structures is important to lateral observation and analysis:

➤ Head and neck area: forward head protrusion
➤ Vertebral column: exaggerated kyphosis and lordosis
➤ Glenohumeral joint: centered or off-center
➤ Elbow/wrist position: in front of or behind the LOG
➤ Hip and pelvis

Head and Neck Area. Individuals often show forward head protrusion or cervical flexion. This deviation is common among office workers who sit in front of the computer all day.

Kyphosis and Lordosis. Kyphosis is an exaggerated curve primarily in the thoracic region. Two improperly stressed muscle groups cause this deviation: lengthening of the middle trapezius and rhomboids in the posterior, and shortening of the pectoralis major and anterior deltoid in the anterior. Lordosis is an exaggerated curve in the lumbar region of the lower back. Typically, shortening of the erector spinae muscles in the posterior and weakening of the rectus abdominis in the anterior create the curve known as lordosis.

Glenohumeral Joint. A combination of an imbalanced scapula and exaggerated internal rotation of the glenohumeral joint limit the shoulder muscle structures, including the anterior, middle, and posterior deltoid to an anterior movement. This creates shoulders that are rounded forward. With such rounding, the shoulders typically will not be level.

Elbow/Wrist. Because of the internal rotation of the glenohumeral joint when shoulders are rounded forward, the elbow and wrist often shift in front of the LOG. Often the elbows and wrists will be in front of, or parallel to, the rib cage instead of the palms hanging evenly with the sides of the legs.

Hip and Pelvis. Various muscle imbalances can develop either an anterior or posterior pelvic tilt. In an anterior pelvic tilt, the pelvis tilts forward, increasing the lumbar curve, which exaggerates lordosis in combination with hip flexion. A posterior pelvic tilt creates a flattening of the lumbar curve as a result of increased lumbar flexion and hip extension.

CORRECTION OF POSTURE AND BODY ALIGNMENT

Postural alignment of body segments can be strengthened with well-designed and effective exercise programs. The best results are obtained when the implementation of the well-designed program is monitored with assessments and the client is actively involved through a communicative Personal Trainer–client relationship. A regular program of exercise can change body deviations created by poor posture, but this change can be difficult for the Personal Trainer and the client. Therefore, the creative combination of a variety of tools can help to overcome this challenging task. A combination of education, training, and cueing a client on exercise techniques (28) can help the client move toward a life with better posture and overall well-being (29).

EXERCISE PROGRAM DESIGN AND NEW SKILLS APPLICATION

The topics in Chapters 16–19 include the process of exercise program design integrating resistance, flexibility, and cardiovascular training as applied to client alignment, posture, and positioning while performing specific exercise modalities. Clients need to apply the new skills they learn in their posture training sessions to their daily lives when at home and at work, as well as during recreation time, to fully integrate the posture lessons learned in the personal training sessions into their permanent movement habits.

GONIOMETRY AND JOINT RANGE-OF-MOTION ASSESSMENTS

Many of the joints of the body can perform several different movements. Joints can perform movements in different planes and angles depending on the type of joint structure and its designed function (30). The specific joint range of motion (JROM or joint ROM) is measurable using an instrument known as a goniometer. Goniometry consists of assessment techniques that measure and compare the change in joint angles in degrees of motion (31).

Client Involvement in the Range-of-Motion Assessment

Clients need to understand that it is important for the Personal Trainer to assess the client's joints and their range of motion so that the Personal Trainer knows whether the client can safely perform a given exercise. The Personal Trainer can again involve clients in their training by showing them the goniometer and explaining the assessment. Go over the assessment vocabulary—goniometry, joint, ranges of motion, and dysfunction—with clients so that they understand how the goniometric assessment will support the Personal Trainer in designing the exercise sessions. Above all, remember to remind clients that any pain they feel in moving a joint is extremely important to the Personal Trainer, and they must not "grin and bear it" but instead tell the Personal Trainer if any movement hurts or causes pain in any way.

The Goniometry/Range-of-Motion Assessment

Information obtained through goniometry assessments, in cooperation with the posture and body alignment assessment and client's health and medical history, provides the Personal Trainer with the information he or she needs to design a successful client-oriented exercise program. As discussed in Chapter 14, if the goniometry assessments are performed on a client who is unable to move pain free through a normal range of motion for a particular joint, this is a strong indicator that the client should not perform that exercise/movement with that joint structure and in that plane until he or she has been seen by a medical professional and cleared to begin the exercise program.

Goniometry assessment serves the Personal Trainer in five critically important ways:

1. Provides immediate range of motion feedback. The Personal Trainer and the client know immediately whether the client is able to perform the given movement with the given body segment weight against gravity and pain free. It provides a "pre-resistance training" assessment without the risk of injuring the client. The client can be injured if not assessed using a goniometer before attempting the resistance-training phase of an exercise program.

2. Identifies muscle imbalances. When assessing joint range of motion for a bilateral comparison, the goniometer may indicate differences in range of motion between the left and right structures being evaluated. Range of motion deviations may lead to muscle imbalances and cause adjacent joint and muscle structures to overcompensate within the kinetic chain of movement. This can result in dysfunction within the related joint structures and cause potential injuries, trauma, and movement pattern complications.

3. Identifies the client's current ranges of motion before the exercise program starts. This assessment in turn provides a base of departure for the progress of the exercise program, specifically when implementing the flexibility and resistance components. Reassessments can be performed every 4 to 12 weeks to determine if the client and Personal Trainer are achieving their goals and objectives.

4. Provides insight into the client's learning preferences. The trainer can observe the client's ways of responding, and his or her preferences in responding to verbal instructions (see Chapter 5).

5. Provides a base measurement from which plans can be made for future exercise goals. The first range of motion test of primary joints necessary to future exercise movements tells trainers what can be achieved within the client's time and schedule limitations. Personal Trainers will be able to design safer resistance, flexibility, cardiovascular, and other training programs based on the client's original assessment.

Range of Motion (ROM)

The range of motion (ROM) is defined as the amount of available motion, or arc of motion, that occurs at a specific joint (32). All ROM assessments start with the client in the anatomical start position, except motions in rotation. In the anatomical start position, the body is set at 0° (0 degrees) of flexion, extension, abduction, and adduction. ROM can be assessed in two ways using the goniometer: active range of motion (AROM) or passive range of motion (PROM).

ACTIVE RANGE OF MOTION (AROM)

The client performs AROM without assistance from the Personal Trainer. For purposes of this book, the trainer will test AROM only. The Personal Trainer observes the client's AROM performance for *(a)* the ability to move pain free, *(b)* neuromuscular control, *(c)* muscle strength, and *(d)* joint ROM. The AROM test provides the Personal Trainer with an excellent screening process to determine if a client can move pain free. It also measures the client's available range of motion and flexibility. If the client is in pain while performing a specific AROM assessment, testing of that joint should be stopped immediately. Refer to Chapter 14 for appropriate screening and medical referral procedures.

PASSIVE RANGE OF MOTION (PROM)

Although not applied in this book to personal training, PROM is performed by allied medical professionals such as orthopedic surgeons, sports medicine physicians, and physical therapists without assistance from the patient. It is used when the patients themselves are not independently active and are unable to move the body segment being tested as a result of severe injury or because the medical professional wants to assess the ROM manually to a joint's end-feel. PROM is tested by bringing the joint structure to the physiological end-feel of the movement. Physiological end-feel occurs when the joint reaches an end-point in its possible ROM. Since this book is written for the personal training setting, the clients will be independently active, and the PROM assessment process would not be needed and should only be performed by an experienced medical professional.

FACTORS AFFECTING ROM

Five factors are significant to a joint structure's ROM. Personal Trainers need to be aware of the following:

➤ The shape of the articular or bony surfaces between body segments
➤ The structure of the joint, including ligaments, cartilage, bursae, fascia, and joint capsule
➤ Structure of muscles and tendons
➤ Joint diseases such as chondromalacia, osteoarthritis, and bursitis
➤ Neurological conditions such as cerebral palsy, stroke, multiple sclerosis

The Goniometer

The goniometer comes in many different shapes, sizes, and materials (metal or plastic). The design of the goniometer includes a body, axis or center point, a stabilization arm, and a movement arm *(Fig. 15.7)*. The body of a goniometer is similar to a protractor and consists of the arc of a circle.

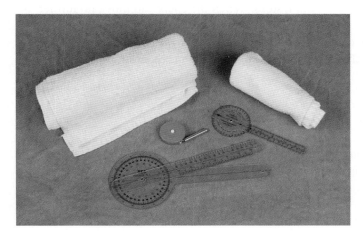

FIGURE 15.7. A goniometer including the body, axis (or center point), a stabilization arm, and a movement arm.

Around the circle are degree measurements that will range from 0° to 180° or a circle from 0° to 360°. The axis is the centering point of the goniometer. The axis point is centered to the identified anatomical landmark required for a given ROM assessment. The stabilization arm is the body segment of the goniometer that will remain fixed and stable during the test. The stabilization arm establishes the starting position of the measurement. The movement arm is the body segment of the goniometer that will move in relation to the client's movement during the test. The movement arm establishes the ending position.

ASSESSMENT PROCESS AND TECHNIQUES

As explained earlier, before the assessment begins, the client needs to understand what the goniometry test is and what it involves. The Personal Trainer can do this by providing the client with an overview of the goniometry process and the purpose of the assessment. The Personal Trainer should provide a demonstration of a sample ROM test on a joint to explain how the assessment works. As each joint's ROM is assessed, the Personal Trainer can demonstrate the proper starting position, performance of the ROM test, and the ending position before actually doing it. The Personal Trainer needs to remind the client to speak up when any joint is painful during the test.

Starting Position. The client's and the goniometer's position before assessing the joint's range of motion is important to attaining an accurate measurement. The following process needs to be completed first to attain the client's starting measurement:

➤ Client is stable and the body is balanced and level in all planes.
➤ Client needs to assume optimal posture in most goniometry assessments.
➤ Client's joint structure is in 0° starting position.
➤ Special starting position considerations are identified under specific joint range of motion tests, explained later in this chapter.
➤ The goniometer starts at the joint axis or hinge point where the axis of rotation occurs for the two body segments.
➤ The goniometer's stabilization and movement arms are centered along each body segment by the trainer.

Client ROM Assessment. The client needs to move his or her body segment slowly through the ROM as instructed by the Personal Trainer. The Personal Trainer can remind the client that the assessment is not a competition, and as soon as the client feels that the body segment cannot move further without compensating the body through shifting or pushing beyond the ROM, the client can stop the movement. Again, stress to clients that they move the given body segment SLOWLY through its ROM. One arm of the goniometer needs to be stabilized by the trainer, while the other arm moves with the second body segment until it stops. When the client can move no further, the joint angle is measured and recorded.

Recording Measurements. Accurate recording of goniometry measurements is perhaps one if the most important parts of the assessment. The following recording procedures are recommended:

➤ Client information: name
➤ Personal Trainer: name
➤ Date of assessment
➤ The joint and type of motion being measured: right or left side of the body, joint, and motion being measured (example: right hip extension)
➤ The starting ROM in degrees
➤ The ending ROM in degrees
➤ Any discomfort or pain felt by the client

➤ Client's performance as observed by the trainer

➤ Notes on the client's apparent learning preferences

➤ Any adaptations or changes to normal assessment procedures made by the Personal Trainer

Obtaining Accurate Measurements. The use of goniometry can be an accurate measure of a joint's ROM when the following procedures are properly performed (33):

➤ All anatomical landmarks are identified by the trainer.

➤ The joint axis point has been clearly defined.

➤ The Personal Trainer is able to stabilize the client in proper body alignment from the start to ending positions.

➤ The Personal Trainer is able to instruct the client to move slowly through the proper range of motion and can keep the goniometer aligned to each body segment.

➤ The Personal Trainer reads and records measurements correctly.

➤ The Personal Trainer is familiar with the normal ROM for each joint structure.

➤ The Personal Trainer observes whether the client is performing each joint's ROM assessment pain free.

➤ Each Personal Trainer on the staff is using the same procedures and techniques to obtain reliable and valid recordings.

ROM and Postural Alignment Assessments

The ROM assessment, when combined with the posture and body alignment assessment, works well as a guide for the Personal Trainer's choices of resistance and flexibility exercises appropriate and helpful to a client's specific needs.

SAMPLE ROM ASSESSMENTS: NECK, SPINE, SHOULDER, HIP

Joint ROM assessments require that Personal Trainers instruct their clients on accurate procedures and confidently demonstrate the movements for the client. The ROM assessments provided below focus on primary joint and muscle structures essential to the exercise program design. These goniometry assessments are by no means a complete list of all the possible joint movements that could be measured on a client. These particular goniometry assessments have been chosen because they show the Personal Trainer the client's weaknesses and deficiencies in the ROM in certain joints, so that the Personal Trainer can accurately design the client's exercise program (Box 15.2).

Box 15.2   **Range of Motion Assessment Sequence**

STRUCTURE
- Movement
- The plane of motion
- The axis of motion
- Average range
- Goniometer position

1. Axis point
2. Stabilization arm
3. Movement arm
   - Stabilization
   - Starting/ending body position

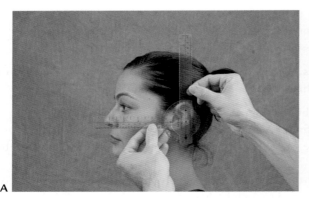
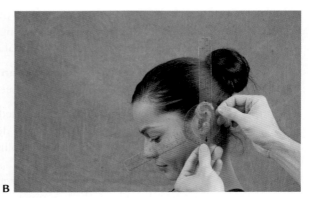

A

B

FIGURE 15.8. Cervical flexion.

SPECIFIC ROM ASSESSMENTS

Structure: The Neck

Movement: Cervical flexion (*Fig. 15.8*)
The plane of motion: Sagittal
The axis of motion: Coronal
Average range: 0–45°
Goniometer position
1. Axis point: External auditory meatus
2. Stabilization arm: Perpendicular to the floor
3. Movement arm: Parallel to the floor, with midline of goniometer level with the inferior bottom of the nose
Stabilization: Client is in good posture with a stabilized scapula and thoracic and lumber spine.
Starting/ending body position: Client is seated with cervical spine in 0° of flexion, extension, rotation, or lateral flexion. Head is in neutral position. Client performs cervical flexion until the first sign of resistance.

Movement: Cervical extension (*Fig. 15.9*)
The plane of motion: Sagittal
The axis of motion: Coronal
Average range: 0–45°

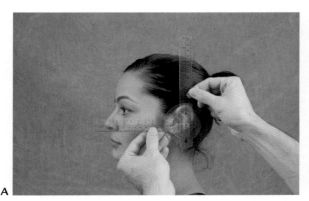
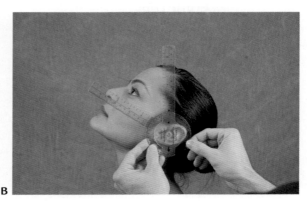

A

B

FIGURE 15.9. Cervical extension.

Goniometer position

1. Axis point: External auditory meatus
2. Stabilization arm: Perpendicular to the floor
3. Movement arm: Parallel to the floor, with midline of goniometer level with the inferior bottom of the nose

Stabilization: Client is in good posture with a stabilized scapula and thoracic and lumber spine.

Starting/ending body position: Client is seated with cervical spine in 0° of flexion, extension, rotation, or lateral flexion. Head is in neutral position. Client performs cervical extension until the first sign of resistance.

Movement: Lateral flexion (*Fig. 15.10*)

The plane of motion: Frontal

The axis of motion: Anterior–posterior

Average range: 0–45°

Goniometer position

1. Axis point: Cervical 7
2. Stabilization arm: Perpendicular to the floor
3. Movement arm: Midline of the head; occipital protuberance for reference

Stabilization: Client is in good posture with a stabilized scapula and thoracic and lumber spine.

Starting/ending body position: Client is seated with cervical spine in 0° of flexion, extension, rotation, or lateral flexion. Head is in neutral position. Client performs lateral flexion until the first sign of resistance.

Structure: The Spine

Movement: Lumbar flexion (*Fig. 15.11*)

The plane of motion: Sagittal

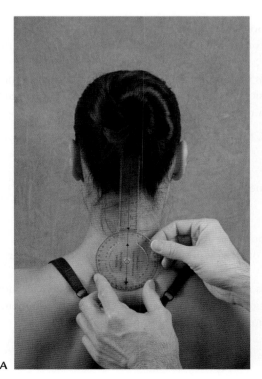 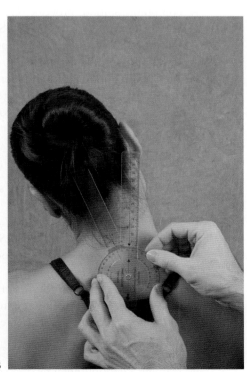

A   B

FIGURE 15.10. Client performing lateral flexion.

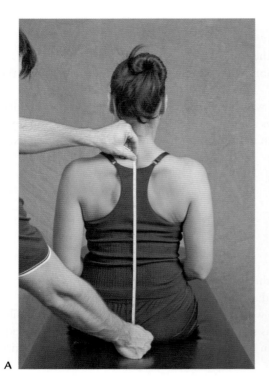 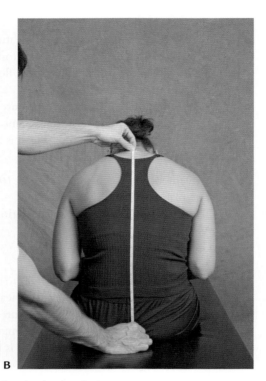

A B

FIGURE 15.11. Client performing lumbar flexion.

The axis of motion: Coronal
Average range: 4-inch increase
Tape measure position
1. Top point: Spinous processes C7
2. Bottom point: S1 or level to PSIS (posterior superior iliac spine)
Stabilization: Subject is seated on floor or table with pelvis stabilized to prevent anterior/posterior tilting with legs extended.
Starting/ending body position: Client is in good posture with a stabilized cervical, thoracic, and lumbar spine in 0° of flexion, extension, rotation, or lateral flexion. Head is in neutral position. Client performs lumbar flexion until the first sign of resistance.

Movement: Lumbar extension (*Fig. 15.12*)
The plane of motion: Sagittal
The axis of motion: Coronal
Average range: 2-inch difference as spine extends
Tape measure position
1. Top point: Spinous processes C7
2. Bottom point: S1 or level to PSIS (posterior superior iliac spine)
Stabilization: Subject is seated on floor or table with pelvis stabilized to prevent anterior/posterior tilting with legs extended.
Starting/ending body position: Client is in good posture with a stabilized cervical, thoracic, and lumbar spine in 0° of flexion, extension, rotation, or lateral flexion. Head is in neutral position. Client performs lumbar extension until the first sign of resistance.

Structure: The Shoulder

Movement: Glenohumeral flexion (*Fig. 15.13*)
The plane of motion: Sagittal

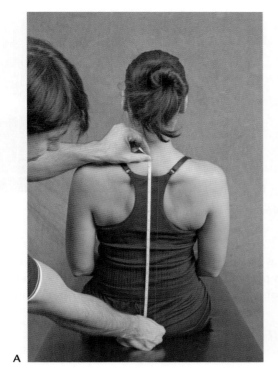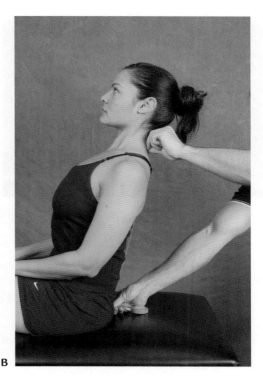

A   B

FIGURE 15.12. Client performing lumbar extension.

The axis of motion: Coronal
Average range: 0–90°
Goniometer position
1. Axis point: Lateral aspect of greater tubercle
2. Stabilization arm: Perpendicular to the floor
3. Movement arm: Align with midline of humerus and reference the lateral epicondyle.
Stabilization: Client is in good posture with a stabilized scapula (retracted) and thoracic and
    lumber spine. Stabilize scapula to prevent tilting, rotation, or elevation.

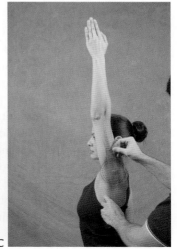

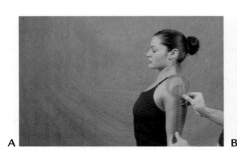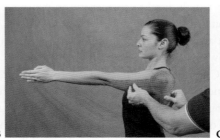

A   B   C

FIGURE 15.13. Client performing glenohumeral flexion.

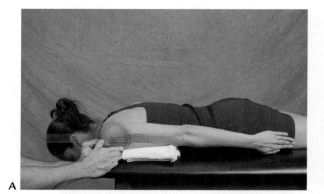
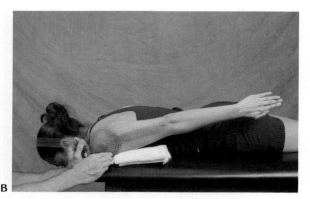

FIGURE 15.14. Client performing glenohumeral extension.

Starting/ending body position: Client is seated with glenohumerus in 0° of flexion, extension, abduction, or adduction. Head is in neutral position. Palm of hand should be facing the body. Elbow should be extended completely. Client performs glenohumeral flexion until the first sign of resistance.

Movement: Glenohumeral extension (*Fig. 15.14*)
The plane of motion: Sagittal
The axis of motion: Coronal
Average range: 0–60°
Goniometer position
1. Axis point: Lateral aspect of greater tubercle
2. Stabilization arm: Perpendicular to the floor
3. Movement arm: Align with midline of the lateral humerus and reference the lateral epicondyle.
Stabilization: Client is in good posture with a stabilized scapula (retracted) and thoracic and lumber spine. Stabilize scapula to prevent tilting, rotation, or elevation. Place towel under humerus to stabilize and align with acromion process.
Starting/ending body position: Client is prone on the table with glenohumerus in 0° of flexion, extension, abduction, or adduction. Head is in neutral position. Palm of hand should be facing the body. Elbow should be extended completely. Client performs glenohumeral extension until the first sign of resistance.

Movement: Glenohumeral abduction (palm facing body)
The plane of motion: Frontal
The axis of motion: Anterior–posterior
Average range: 0–90°
Goniometer position
1. Axis point: 1 inch distal to the acromion process at the posterior shoulder
2. Stabilization arm: Perpendicular to the floor
3. Movement arm: Align with midline of posterior humerus and reference the olecranon process of the elbow.
Stabilization: Client is in good posture with a stabilized scapula (retracted) and thoracic and lumber spine. Stabilize scapula to prevent tilting, rotation, or elevation.
Starting/ending body position: Client is seated with glenohumerus in 0° of flexion, extension, abduction, or adduction. Head is in neutral position. Palm of hand should be facing the body. Arm should be extended completely. Client performs glenohumeral abduction until the first sign of resistance.

Movement: Glenohumeral abduction (palm facing away from body)

The plane of motion: Frontal

The axis of motion: Anterior–posterior

Average range: 0–180°

Goniometer position

1. Axis point: 1 inch distal to the acromion process at the posterior shoulder
2. Stabilization arm: Perpendicular to the floor
3. Movement arm: Align with midline of posterior humerus and reference the olecranon process of the elbow.

Stabilization: Client is in good posture with a stabilized scapula (retracted) and thoracic and lumber spine. Stabilize scapula to prevent tilting, rotation, or elevation.

Starting/ending body position: Client is seated with glenohumerus in 0° of flexion, extension, abduction, or adduction. Head is in neutral position. Palm of hand should be facing away from the body. Arm should be extended completely. Client performs glenohumeral abduction until the first sign of resistance.

Movement: Glenohumeral internal rotation (*Fig. 15.15*)

The plane of motion: Transverse

The axis of motion: Longitudinal

Average range: 0–70°

Goniometer position

1. Axis point: Olecranon process of the elbow
2. Stabilization arm: Perpendicular to the floor
3. Movement arm: Align with lateral midline of ulna and reference the ulnar styloid.

Stabilization: Client is in good posture with a stabilized scapula (retracted) and thoracic and lumber spine. Stabilize scapula to prevent tilting, rotation, or elevation. Place towel under humerus to stabilize and align with acromion process.

Starting/ending body position: Client is supine on table with humerus abducted at 90° and elbow is flexed at 90°. Elbow is at 0° of supination and pronation. Client performs glenohumeral internal rotation until the first sign of resistance.

Movement: Glenohumeral external rotation (see Fig. 15.15)

The plane of motion: Transverse

The axis of motion: Longitudinal

Average range: 0–90°

Goniometer position

1. Axis point: Olecranon process of the elbow
2. Stabilization arm: Perpendicular to the floor
3. Movement arm: Align with lateral midline of ulna and reference the ulnar styloid.

Stabilization: Client is in good posture with a stabilized scapula (retracted) and thoracic and lumber spine. Stabilize scapula to prevent tilting, rotation, or elevation. Place towel under humerus to stabilize and align with acromion process.

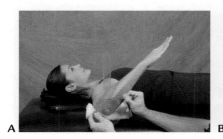
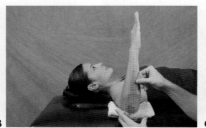
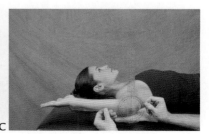

FIGURE 15.15. Client performing glenohumeral internal and external rotation

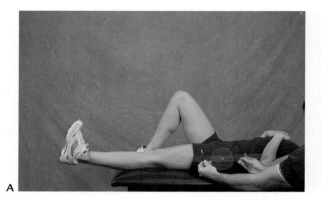
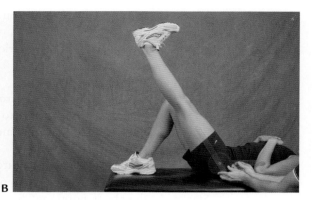

FIGURE 15.16. Client performing hip flexion

Starting/ending body position: Client is supine on table with humerus abducted at 90° and elbow flexed at 90°. Elbow is at 0° of supination and pronation. Client performs glenohumeral external rotation until the first sign of resistance.

Structure: The Hip

Movement: Hip flexion (testing leg fully extended) (*Fig. 15.16*)
The plane of motion: Sagittal
The axis of motion: Coronal
Average range: 0–90°
Goniometer position
1. Axis point: Greater trochanter of the lateral thigh
2. Stabilization arm: Lateral midline of the pelvis
3. Movement arm: Lateral midline of the femur, using the lateral epicondyle as a reference
Stabilization: Client is in good posture with a stabilized scapula, thoracic and lumber spine, and pelvic area. Pelvis should not rise off table. Opposite leg not being assessed should have knee flexed and foot flat on table for added stability and protection for the back.
Starting/ending body position: Client is supine on table with hip in 0° of flexion, extension, abduction, adduction, and rotation. Testing leg has knee fully extended. Client performs hip flexion until the first sign of resistance or until the pelvis rotates or knee breaks extension.

Movement: Hip flexion (testing knee flexed 90° and hip flexed 90°) (*Fig. 15.17*)
The plane of motion: Sagittal
The axis of motion: Coronal

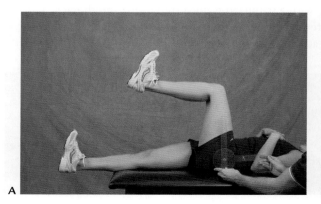
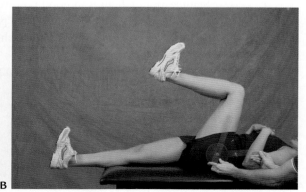

FIGURE 15.17. Client performing hip flexion.

Average range: 0–120°

Goniometer position

1. Axis point: Greater trochanter of the lateral thigh

2. Stabilization arm: Lateral midline of the pelvis

3. Movement arm: Lateral midline of the femur, using the lateral epicondyle as a reference

Stabilization: Client is in good posture with a stabilized scapula, thoracic and lumber spine, and pelvic area. Pelvis should not rise off table. Opposite leg not being assessed should have knee extended on table for added stability and protection for the back.

Starting/ending body position: Client is supine on table with knee flexed at 90° and hip flexed at 90°; hip is in 0° of abduction, adduction, and rotation. Knee is flexed to reduce contraction of hamstrings. Client performs hip flexion until the first sign of resistance or until the pelvis rotates.

Movement: Hip extension (testing leg fully extended) (*Fig. 15.18*)

The plane of motion: Sagittal

The axis of motion: Coronal

Average range: 0–30°

Goniometer position

1. Axis point: Greater trochanter of the lateral thigh

2. Stabilization arm: Lateral midline of the pelvis

3. Movement arm: Lateral midline of the femur, using the lateral epicondyle as a reference

Stabilization: Client is in good posture with a stabilized scapula, thoracic and lumber spine, and pelvic area. Pelvis should not rise off table. Opposite leg not being assessed should have leg fully extended on table for added stability.

Starting/ending body position: Client is prone on table with hip in 0° of flexion, extension, abduction, adduction, and rotation. Testing leg has knee fully extended. Client performs hip extension until the first sign of resistance or until the pelvis rotates.

Movement: Hip abduction (*Fig. 15.19*)

The plane of motion: Frontal

The axis of motion: Anterior–posterior

Average range: 0–45°

Goniometer position

1. Axis point: Locate at the ASIS (anterior superior iliac spine)

2. Stabilization arm: Imaginary horizontal line connecting axis point ASIS to the other ASIS

3. Movement arm: Anterior midline of the femur, using the midline of the patella as a reference

Stabilization: Client is in good posture with a stabilized scapula, thoracic and lumbar spine, and pelvic area. Stabilize for lateral trunk flexion on both sides.

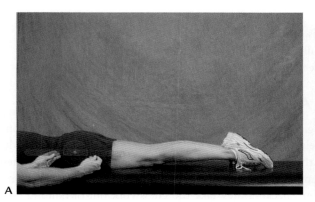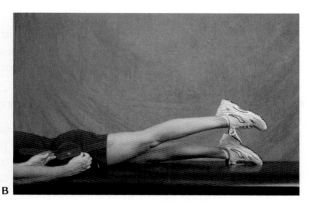

FIGURE 15.18. Client performing hip extension.

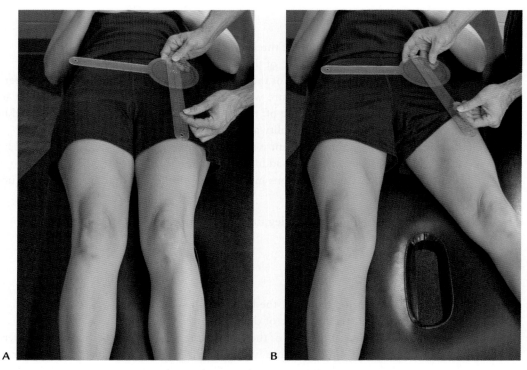

FIGURE 15.19. Client performing hip abduction.

Starting/ending body position: Client is supine on table with hip in 0° of flexion, extension, and rotation. Testing leg has knee fully extended. Client performs hip abduction until the first sign of resistance or lateral trunk flexion occurs on either side.

Movement: Hip adduction

The plane of motion: Frontal

The axis of motion: Anterior–posterior

Average range: 0–30°

Goniometer position

1. Axis point: Locate at the ASIS (anterior superior iliac spine)

2. Stabilization arm: Imaginary horizontal line connecting axis point ASIS to the other ASIS

3. Movement arm: Anterior midline of the femur, using the midline of the patella as a reference

Stabilization: Client is in good posture with a stabilized scapula, thoracic and lumbar spine, and pelvic area. Opposite leg not being tested should be abducted fully to allow for testing hip to be assessed.

Starting/ending body position: Client is supine on table with hip in 0° of flexion, extension, and rotation. Testing leg has knee fully extended. Client performs hip adduction until the first sign of resistance or lateral trunk flexion or pelvic rotation occurs.

Goniometry and Its Usefulness as an Assessment Tool

Both clients and Personal Trainers benefit greatly from the information provided by goniometry and its ROM assessments. Clients learn how their bodies move and understand more clearly how and why a given exercise is beneficial or harmful to their physiology. This increases their participation in their own training process and increases the potential for their success as self-motivated exercisers. Personal Trainers benefit from goniometry assessments because they take the guesswork out of training program design, and it provides them with a reliable point of departure in the measurement of the clients' progress in their personal training program. Moreover, goniometry is not complicated technically and can be performed in the most simple of exercise settings. In combination with postural alignment assessments, the goniometry assessment gives a solid basis for a satisfying and successful training experience for both the client and the Personal Trainer.

ASSESSMENTS AS A MOTIVATIONAL DEVICE

Health-related physical fitness assessments can serve not only for exercise programming, but also for motivational purposes when the results of the various assessments are explained and used in the goal-setting approach. It is important to note that a particular physical fitness assessment that is not used in programming decisions and not used to instill motivation should be questioned as to its use. In other words, simply testing all clients for all available assessments should be avoided.

Physical fitness assessment should likely be performed on a regular basis to determine if established goals have been met. As goals are set, often a time frame for the attainment of those goals is included (e.g., lose 5% body fat in 3 months). For instance, if the individual has a goal to improve his or her overall flexibility in 3 months, then the goniometry measurements (and possibly other assessments) should be performed every 4 to 6 weeks to measure progress toward that goal. A word of caution about follow-up assessments is that frequent assessments may fail to demonstrate desired changes as some components of physical fitness may take time and effort to change (for instance, significant and lasting body composition changes are not likely to occur in short time intervals). A standard for follow-up may be 4 weeks to 3 months, depending on what is being assessed.

SUMMARY

Just as the spring season represents a time of change, so should the results of a physical fitness assessment. If a client has failed to demonstrate progress in certain areas (such as muscular strength with 1RM strength testing), then answers should be sought as to why the changes were not evident and how the exercise program should be adjusted to produce the desired changes in the future. Once again, the results of the physical fitness assessments should be used with some kind of an outcome in mind. As Personal Trainers, we need to realize that not all individuals are going to adapt to our programming suggestions in the same way. Thus, each round of physical fitness assessments calls for a re-examination of the client's goals and objectives. Perhaps new measurable goals may be identified for that individual at some distant time interval.

REFERENCES

1. American College of Sports Medicine. ACSM's Guidelines for Exercise Testing and Prescription. 7th ed. Baltimore: Lippincott Williams & Wilkins, 2006.
2. American College of Sports Medicine. ACSM Health-Related Physical Fitness Assessment Manual. Baltimore: Lippincott Williams & Wilkins, 2005.
3. Prisant LM, Alpert BS, Robbins CB, et al. American national standard for nonautomated sphygmomanometry. Am J Hypertens 1995;8:210–213.
4. Seventh Report of the Joint Committee on Prevention, Detection, Evaluation, and Treatment of High Blood Pressure (JNC7), Public Health Service, National Institutes of Health, National Heart, Lung and Blood Institute, NIH Publ no. 03-5233, 2003.
5. Perloff D, Grimm C, Flack J, et al. Human blood pressure determination by sphygmomanometry. Circulation 1993;88:5(pt 1):2460–2470.
6. Heyward V. Advanced Fitness Assessment and Exercise Prescription. 3rd ed. Champaign, IL: Human Kinetics, 1998.
7. Howley E, Franks B. Health Fitness Instructor's Handbook. 4th ed. Champaign, IL: Human Kinetics, 2003.
8. Golding LA, Myers CR, Sinning WE, eds. Y's Way to Physical Fitness. 3rd ed. Champaign, IL: Human Kinetics, 1989.
9. Jackson AS, Pollock ML. Practical Assessment of Body Composition. Physician Sports Med 1985;13(5):85.
10. Nieman D. Fitness and Sports Medicine: A Health-related Approach. 4th ed. Mountain View, CA: Mayfield, 1999.
11. Powers S, Howley E. Exercise Physiology: Theory and Application to Fitness and Performance. 4th ed. New York: McGraw-Hill, 2001.
12. Kline GM, Porcari JP, Hintermeister R, et al. Estimation of VO_2max from a one-mile track walk, gender, age, and body weight. Med Sci Sports Exerc 1987;19:253–259.

13. Norkin C, Levangie P. Standing Posture. Joint Structure and Function. Philadelphia: FA Davis, 1992.

14. Luttgens K, Hamilton N. Standing posture. In: Dorwick T, Malinee V, Turenne M, eds. Kinesiology. 10th ed. New York: McGraw-Hill, 2002.

15. Lehmkuhl LD, Smith LK, Weiss EL. Standing and Walking. In: McNichol CS, ed. Brunnstrom's Clinical Kinesiology. 5th ed. Philadelphia: FA Davis, 1996.

16. Adrian M, Cooper J. Static and Dynamic posture. In: Spoolman S, Klein J, eds. Biomechanics of Human Movement. 2nd ed. Dubuque, IA: McGraw-Hill, 1997.

17. Howley ET, Franks BD. Flexibility and low back pain. In: Bahrke M, Crist R, Washington S, eds. Health Fitness Instructors Handbook. 4th ed. Champaign: Human Kinetics, 2003.

18. Nieman DC. Prevention and treatment of low back pain. In: Malinee V, Seely C, eds. Exercise Testing and Prescription. New York: McGraw-Hill, 2003.

19. Magill RA. Mental practice. In: Malinee V, Seely C, eds. Motor Learning and Control. New York: McGraw-Hill, 2001.

20. Floyd RT, Thompson C. Muscular analysis of the upper extremity. In: Malinee V, Martin M, eds. Manual of Structural Kinesiology. 14th ed. New York: McGraw-Hill, 2001.

21. Norkin CC White DJ. Basic concepts. In: Biblis M, Seitz A, eds. Measurement of joint motion. Philadelphia: FA Davis, 2003.

22. Griffin JC. Client-centered musculoskeletal assessments. In: Wilgren S, Mustain E, Graham M, eds. Client-Centered Exercise Prescription. Champaign, IL: Human Kinetics, 1998.

Developing Your Client's Exercise Program

PART

V

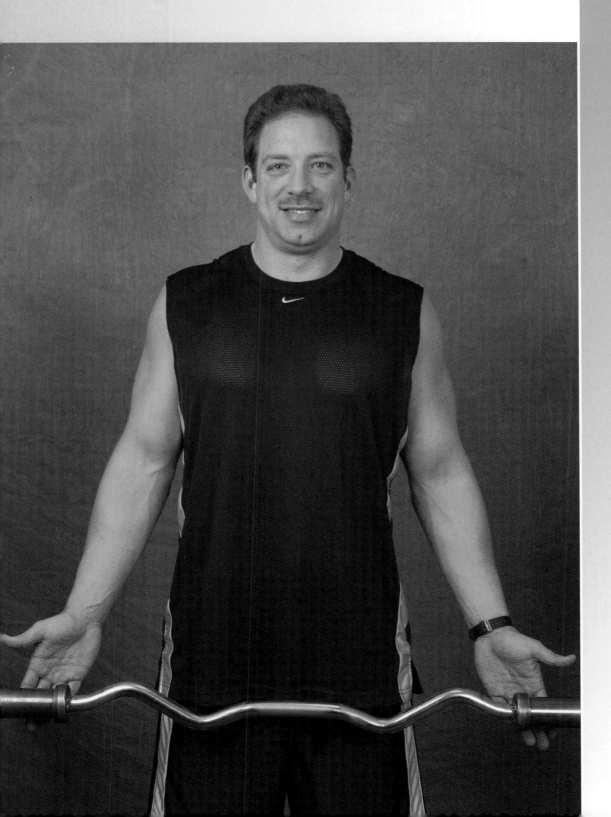

Client Exercise Program Design

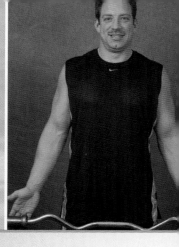

Nikki Carosone, M.S., General Manager, Personal Training Director, Plus One Health Management,
New York, New York

Chapter Outline

Objectives

- Provide the Personal Trainer with the fundamentals needed to safely and effectively design a client exercise program
- Review the basic physiological systems of the body to better facilitate the client's needs
- Identify the different modes of resistance, cardiovascular, and flexibility training
- Educate the certified Personal Trainer on communication skills and client–trainer relationships
- Prepare the certified Personal Trainer for the first training session, as well as subsequent sessions and program variables

This chapter provides the Personal Trainer with the key elements needed to design a safe and effective client exercise program. It provides the Personal Trainer with the tools needed to structure the client exercise program by incorporating a review of basic anatomy, applied physiology, exercise protocol, and program design. This process begins with the initial consultation and the fitness assessment—which are fully explained in Chapter 12. This chapter applies the fundamentals of exercise programming, through to the actual personal training session. This chapter specifically focuses on program design, client objectives, and assessment results, the various phases of an exercise program, and methods of strength, resistance, balance, flexibility, and functional training. Other chapters in this book explain, in detail, the physiological responses to the specific types of training programs detailed in this chapter. This chapter briefly addresses the musculoskeletal system, cardiovascular system, and respiratory system, as well as posture and body alignment.

OVERVIEW OF ANATOMY AND PHYSIOLOGY

Musculoskeletal System

This is a brief overview of the structural anatomy of the musculoskeletal system. It is not intended to replace the valuable information in other chapters of this book. In particular, please refer to Chapter 7 for a more detailed explanation of the etymology and function of each of these components.

Muscles cause movement by pulling on the skeleton. The muscular system supplies the forces that enable the body to perform physical activity. When a muscle acts (shortens), it moves a bone by pulling on the tendon that attaches the muscle to the bone. Beyond being the support system for soft tissue, providing protection for internal organs, and acting as an important source of nutrients and blood constituents, the bones are the rigid levers for locomotion. The axial skeleton consists of the skull, the vertebral column, sternum, and ribs. The appendicular skeleton is made up of the bones of the upper and lower extremities. The major bones of the body are illustrated in Chapter 7.

An outer layer of fibrous connective tissue attaches the bone to muscles, deep fascia, and joint capsules. Just beneath this fibrous outer layer is a highly vascular inner layer that contains cells that provide the creation of new bone. These outer and inner layers that cover the bones make up the periosteum. The periosteum, along with adjacent articulated structures, anchors the muscles to bone. Tendons are continuous with the epimysium (outer layer of connective tissue that covers muscle). Muscles consist of individual cells, or fibers, connected in bundles. A single muscle is made up of many bundles of muscle fibers, called "fasciculi." Connective tissue runs from end to end of muscle (from the tendon origin to the tendon insertion) and exists within the muscle tissue surrounding the fibers and giving rise to muscle bundles.

On the basis of structure and function, muscle tissue is categorized into three types: *smooth, skeletal* (sometimes referred to as striated), and *cardiac*. Refer to Chapter 6 for a full explanation of the muscle fibers and types. Although skeletal muscles are grouped together, they function either separately or along with others (1). Which, and how many, skeletal muscles become involved in a workout depends on which exercises are selected and the techniques used during their execution. For example, the width of stance or grip, or the angle and path that a bar is pushed or pulled all have an effect on which muscles are recruited and to what extent (2).

Power and muscle force are created by the action of skeletal muscles. However, there are different types of muscle actions; *concentric muscle actions* occur when the muscle fibers shorten. In this case, the muscle force exceeds the resistance, causing the muscle insertion point and point of origin to move closer together. Concentric actions are what are typically thought of as muscle contractions. In contrast, *eccentric muscle actions* are muscle actions in which active muscle fibers lengthen. That is, the muscle is generating force, but the resistance exceeds the muscle force, and the muscle point of origin and insertion point move farther apart. Note that eccentric muscle actions occur constantly, in normal regular body movements. Examples include the action of the quadriceps muscles when walking down steps or sitting down into a chair and the action of the forearm flexors when throwing a baseball. Indeed, everyday tasks such as walking or running cause simultaneous actions both concentrically and eccentrically. Finally, *isometric* or static muscle actions refer to a type of muscular activity in which there is tension in the muscle but it does not shorten. The bony attachments are fixed, or the forces functioning to lengthen the muscle are countered by forces that are equal to or greater than those generated by the muscles to shorten. In this case, muscle force and resistance are equal.

ANATOMICAL LOCATIONS AND DEFINITIONS

The following are terms that the Personal Trainer will have to become familiar with to explain anatomical locations to the client (3):

➤ **Anterior:** refers to the front of the body
➤ **Anatomical position:** the body is standing erect with feet together and the upper limbs hanging at the sides, with palms of the hands facing forward, thumbs facing away from the body, and fingers extended
➤ **Distal:** farther away from any reference point
➤ **Inferior:** away from the head
➤ **Lateral:** away from the midline of the body
➤ **Medial:** toward the midline of the body
➤ **Posterior:** refers to the back of the body
➤ **Proximal:** closer to any point of reference
➤ **Superior:** toward the head

COMMON MOVEMENT TERMS AND DEFINITIONS

The following are terms that the Personal Trainer should be familiar with when explaining and demonstrating common movement actions to the client (4) (*Fig. 16.1* and Tables 16.1–16.4):

➤ **Abduction:** a movement away from the axis or midline of the body when in the anatomical position
➤ **Adduction:** a movement toward the axis or midline of the body when in the anatomical position
➤ **Agonist:** the prime mover—the muscle directly engaged in muscle action as distinguished from muscles that are relaxing at the same time
➤ **Antagonist:** a muscle that has an action opposite that of the agonist and yields to the movement of the agonist
➤ **Circumduction:** a movement in which the distal end of a bone inscribes a circle within the shaft rotating
➤ **Extension:** a movement that increases the joint angle between two articulating bones (e.g., extending the knee joint)

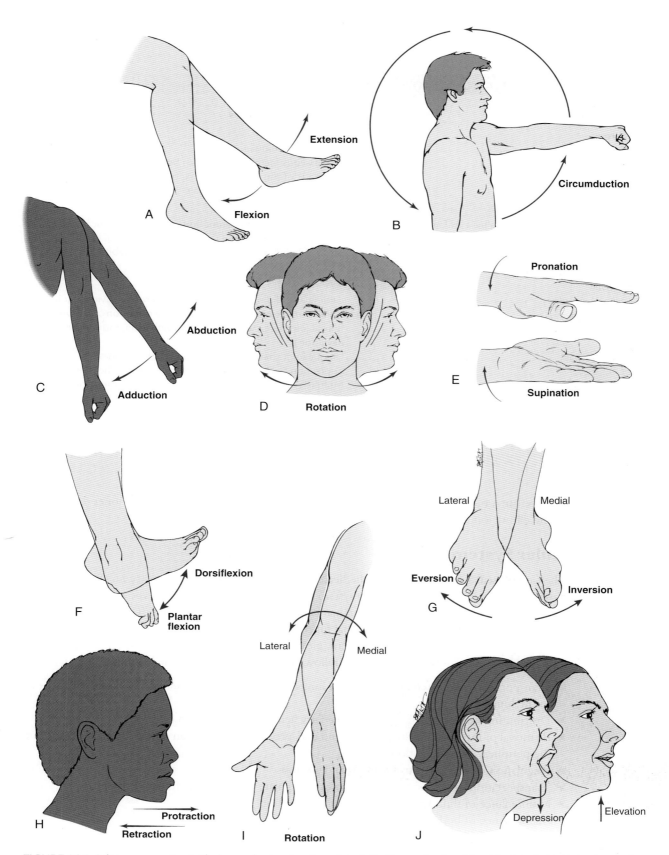

FIGURE 16.1. Joint movements. **A.** Flexion and extension (knee joint). **B.** Circumduction (shoulder joint). **C.** Abduction and adduction (shoulder joint). **D.** Rotation (atlantoaxial joint). **E.** Pronation and supination (elbow joint). **F.** Dorsiflexion and plantar flexion (ankle joint). **G.** Inversion and eversion (ankle joint). **H.** Protraction and retraction (temporomandibular joint). **I.** Medial and lateral rotation (shoulder joint). **J.** Depression and elevation (temporomandibular joint). (Reprinted with permission from Smeltzer SCO, Bare BG. Brunner and Suddarth's Textbook of Medical-Surgical Nursing, 9th ed. Philadelphia: Lippincott Williams & Wilkins, 2002.)

Table 16.1	CLASSIFICATION OF JOINTS IN THE HUMAN BODY
Joint Classification	**Features and Examples**
Fibrous	
Suture	Tight union unique to the skull
Syndesmosis	Interosseous membrane between bone (e.g., the union along the shafts of the radius and ulna, tibia and fibula)
Gomphosis	Unique joint at the tooth socket
Cartilaginous	
Primary (synchondroses; hyaline cartilaginous)	Usually temporary to permit bone growth and typically fuse; some do not (e.g., at the sternum and rib [costal cartilage])
Secondary (symphyses; fibrocartilaginous)	Strong, slightly movable joints (e.g., intervertebral disks, pubic symphysis)
Synovial	
Plane (arthrodial)	Gliding and sliding movements (e.g., acromioclavicular joint)
Hinge (ginglymus)	Uniaxial movements (e.g., elbow, knee extension and flexion)
Ellipsoidal (condyloid)	Biaxial joint (e.g., wrist flexion and extension, radioulnar deviation)
Saddle (sellar)	Unique joint that permits movements in all planes, including opposition (e.g., the carpometacarpal joint of the thumb)
Ball and socket (enarthrodial)	Multiaxial joints that permit movements in all directions (e.g., hip and shoulder joints)
Pivot (trochoidal)	Uniaxial joints that permit rotation (e.g., humeroradial joint)

Reprinted with permission from ACSM's Resource Manual for Guidelines for Exercise Testing and Prescription. 5th ed. Baltimore: Lippincott Williams & Wilkins, 2006:20.

> **Flexion:** a movement that decreases the joint angle between two articulating bones (e.g., flexing the elbow joint)

Cardiovascular System

The cardiovascular system consists of the heart and the blood vessels. The primary function of the cardiovascular system is to act as a transport system that delivers nutrients and removes waste products. The cardiovascular system plays a major role in maintaining homeostasis in the body. The cardiovascular system also assists with maintenance of normal function at rest and during exercise. For a full explanation of the functions of the cardiovascular system, please refer to Chapter 6. As discussed in Chapter 6, the cardiovascular system is responsible for the following specific functions in the body (10–12):

> Transporting oxygenated blood from the lungs to tissues and deoxygenated blood from the tissues to the lungs
> Distributing nutrients (e.g., glucose, free fatty acids, amino acids) to cells
> Removal of metabolic waste products and end-products (e.g., carbon dioxide, urea, lactate) from the periphery for elimination or reuse
> Regulation of pH to control acidosis and alkalosis
> Transportation of hormones and enzymes to regulate physiological function
> Maintenance of fluid volume to prevent dehydration
> Maintenance of body temperature by absorbing and redistributing heat

Respiratory System

The primary function of the respiratory system is the basic exchange of oxygen and carbon dioxide. This will help the certified Personal Trainer to better understand the role of this system in exercise selection and programming. Please read Chapter 6 for a full explanation of this system and its components.

Table 16.2	**MAJOR JOINT MOTIONS AND PLANES OF MOTION**		
Major Joints	**Type of Joints**	**Joint Movements**	**Planes**
Scapulothoracic	Not a true joint	Elevation–depression	Frontal
		Upward–downward rotation	Frontal
		Protraction–retraction	Transverse
Glenohumeral	Synovial: ball and socket	Flexion–extension	Sagittal
		Abduction–adduction	Frontal
		Internal–external rotation	Transverse
		Horizontal abduction–adduction	Transverse
		Circumduction	
Elbow	Synovial: hinge	Flexion–extension	Sagittal
Proximal radioulnar	Synovial: pivot	Pronation–supination	Transverse
Wrist	Synovial: ellipsoidal	Flexion–extension	Sagittal
		Ulnar–radial deviation	Frontal
Metacarpophalangeal	Synovial: ellipsoidal	Flexion–extension	Sagittal
		Abduction–adduction	Frontal
Proximal interphalangeal	Synovial: hinge	Flexion–extension	Sagittal
Distal interphalangeal	Synovial: hinge	Flexion–extension	Sagittal
Intervertebral	Cartilaginous	Flexion–extension	Sagittal
		Lateral flexion	Frontal
		Rotation	Transverse
Hip	Synovial: ball and socket	Flexion–extension	Sagittal
		Abduction–adduction	Frontal
		Internal–external rotation	Transverse
		Horizontal abduction–adduction	Transverse
		Circumduction	
Knee	Synovial: hinge	Flexion–extension	Sagittal
Ankle: talocrural	Synovial: hinge	Dorsiflexion–plantar flexion	Sagittal
Ankle: subtalar	Synovial: gliding	Inversion–eversion	Frontal

Reprinted with permission from ACSM's Resource Manual for Guidelines for Exercise Testing and Prescription. 5th ed. Baltimore: Lippincott Williams & Wilkins, 2006:21.

TYPES OF TRAINING

Resistance Training

GENERAL TRAINING PRINCIPLES

Resistance training has become an integral part of physical activity programs designed to promote health and wellness. Resistance training has been shown to have a positive impact on many health measures, and the collective impact may significantly improve functionality, well-being, and quality of life. When mapping out a plan for an effective resistance training program, the Personal Trainer must follow these three general training principles: specificity, overload, and progression.

SPECIFICITY

The specificity principle dictates that training a client in a specific way will produce a specific result and that to reach a specific goal the client has to follow a specific type of training program (1). For example, a client who wants to strengthen the muscles of the chest must perform exercises such as the bench press or dumbbell flys, to target that area, not a dumbbell row, which will work the mus-

| Table 16.3 | MAJOR MOVEMENTS OF THE UPPER EXTREMITY |

Joint	Movement	Major Agonist Muscles	Examples of Resistance Exercises
Scapulothoracic	Fixation	Serratus anterior	Push-ups
		Pectoralis minor	Parallel bar dips
		Trapezius	Upright rows
		Levator scapulae	Shoulder shrugs
		Rhomboids	Seated rows
Glenohumeral	Flexion	Anterior deltoid	Front raises
		Pectoralis major (clavicular head)	Incline bench press
	Extension	Latissimus dorsi	Dumbbell pullovers
		Teres major	Chin-ups
		Pectoralis major (sternocostal head)	Bench press
	Abduction	Middle deltoid	Lateral raises, dumbbell press
		Supraspinatus	Low pulley lateral raises
	Adduction	Latissimus dorsi	Lats pulldown
		Teres major	Seated row
		Pectoralis major	Cable crossover fly
	Medial (internal) rotation	Latissimus dorsi	Back latissimus pulldowns, bent rows
		Teres major	
		Subscapularis	One-arm dumbbell rows
		Pectoralis major	
		Anterior deltoid	Rotator cuff exercises
			Dumbbell press, parallel bar dips
			Front raises
	Lateral (external) rotation	Infraspinatus	External rotation exercises
		Teres minor	
		Posterior deltoid	Back press, bent-over lateral raises
Elbow	Flexion	Biceps brachii	Curls
		Brachialis	Preacher curls
		Brachioradialis	Hammer curls
	Extension	Triceps brachii	Triceps dips, triceps extensions
		Anconeus	Pushdowns, triceps kickback
Radioulnar	Supination	Supinator	Dumbbell supination
		Biceps brachii	
	Pronation	Pronator teres, pronator quadratus	Dumbbell pronation
Wrist	Flexion	Flexor carpi radialis and ulnaris	Wrist curls
		Palmaris longus	
		Flexor digitorum superficialis	
	Extension	Extensor carpi radialis longus, brevis, ulnaris	Reverse wrist curls
		Extensor digitorum	
	Adduction (ulnar deviation)	Flexor and extensor carpi ulnaris	Wrist curls, reverse wrist curls
	Abduction (radial deviation)	Extensor carpi radialis longus and brevis	Wrist curls, reverse wrist curls
		Flexor carpi radialis	

Reprinted with permission from ACSM's Resource Manual for Guidelines for Exercise Testing and Prescription. 5th ed. Baltimore: Lippincott Williams & Wilkins, 2006:23.

Table 16.4 MAJOR MOVEMENTS OF THE LOWER EXTREMITY

Joint	Movement	Major Agonist Muscles	Examples of Resistance Exercises
Intervertebral	Trunk flexion	Rectus abdominis	Sit-ups, crunches, leg raises
		External obliques	Machine crunches
		Internal obliques	High pulley crunches
	Trunk extension	Erector spinae	Back extensions, dead lifts
	Lateral flexion	Rectus abdominis	Roman chair side bends
		External obliques	Dumbbell side bends
		Internal obliques	Hanging leg raises
	Rotation	External obliques	Broomstick twist
		Internal obliques	Machine trunk Rotations
Hip	Flexion	Iliacus	Leg raises
		Psoas major	Incline leg raises
		Rectus femoris	Machine crunches
		Sartorius	Leg raises
		Pectineus	Cable adductions
	Extension	Gluteus maximus	Squats, leg presses, lunges
		Hamstrings (semitendinosus, semimembranosus, long head of biceps femoris)	Leg curls (standing, seated, lying) Good mornings
	Abduction	Tensor fasciae latae	Cable hip abductions
		Sartorius	Standing machine abductions
		Gluteus medius	Floor hip abductions
		Gluteus minimus	Seated machine abductions
	Adduction	Adductor longus, brevis, and magnus	Power squats
		Gracilis	Cable adductions
		Pectineus	Machine adductions
	Medial rotation	Semitendinosus	Leg curls (standing, seated, lying)
		Semimembranosus	Floor hip adduction
		Gluteus medius	Machine abductions
		Tensor fascia latae	
		Gracilis	
	Lateral rotation	Biceps femoris	
		Adductor longus, brevis, magnus	
		Gluteus maximus	
Knee	Flexion	Hamstrings	Leg curls (standing, seated, lying)
		Gracilis	
		Sartorius	
	Extension	Quadriceps femoris (rectus femoris, vastus lateralis, medialis, and intermedius)	Lunges, squats, leg extensions
Ankle: talocrural	Dorsiflexion	Tibialis anterior	Ankle dorsiflexion against resistance
		Extensor digitorum longus	
		Extensor hallucis longus	
	Plantar flexion	Gastrocnemius, soleus, tibialis posterior	Standing calf raises, donkey calf raises
		Flexor digitorum longus	
Ankle: subtalar	Eversion	Peroneus longus and brevis	Exercises against resistance
	Inversion	Tibialis anterior and posterior	Exercises against resistance

Reprinted with permission from ACSM's Resource Manual for Guidelines for Exercise Testing and Prescription. 5th ed. Baltimore: Lippincott Williams & Wilkins, 2006:24.

cles of the back. The term "specificity" is also important when the Personal Trainer is trying to train a client for a specific sport or activity. The actions of the exercises selected should be very similar to those of the activity. For example, a golf-specific training program should focus on exercises that will strengthen the core and trunk muscles, such as swing drills and trunk twists, because they carry over to the specified activity.

OVERLOAD

The overload principle states that each workout should place a demand on the muscle or muscles that is greater than that in the previous workout session. Even the most specifically based training programs will only produce limited results if the client does not experience overload regularly. The degree of overload depends on the load, number of repetitions (refers to the number of times a load is administered), rest between sets, and frequency (number of training sessions per week). To produce strength and endurance gains, resistance training programs should progressively overload the muscular system. This can be done by:

➤ Increasing the resistance or weight
➤ Increasing repetitions
➤ Increasing sets
➤ Decreasing the rest period between sets or exercises

Training that incorporates this principle challenges the body to meet and adapt to greater-than-normal physiological stress. As it does, a new threshold is established that requires an even greater stress to produce an overload (2). The amount of overload clients need to attain their goal is based on their level of muscular fitness. For example, a hockey player requires a different level of overload than a sedentary person. To best determine the load at which your client should be working (either starting from or progressing to), please refer to Chapter 15.

PROGRESSION

Progression is defined as an increase in workload to maintain overload. The concept of progression may also include the practice of using very modest weights during the initial sessions of an exercise program. Guidelines for the progression of exercise become a factor in the success of individuals who are beginning exercise programs or who are engaging in specific types of exercise programs. An example of exercise progression for beginning exercisers (9) is provided in Table 16.5.

GOAL SETTING

When developing a resistance training program, the most valuable tool that a certified Personal Trainer can have is knowing the client's primary goal. Goal setting is an essential preliminary step when designing an effective training program. Goals should be realistic and attainable and should focus on attempting to meet the client's medical, emotional, and functional needs, within the limitations of time, interest, and actual physical ability.

The three primary resistance training goals are hypertrophy, muscular strength, and muscular endurance. Explaining the specifics of each of these three primary resistance training goals to the client will not only educate them but also help to establish strong client–trainer rapport.

Hypertrophy. Hypertrophy refers to an increase in muscle size or mass. For example, a client who states that he wants to look more "sculpted" or "wants bigger biceps" is referring to the aesthetic look of the enlarged muscle groups. Physiologically, hypertrophy occurs when there is an increase in size of the existing muscle fibers. Chapter 6 in this text explores the physiology of hypertrophy of the muscle fibers.

Table 16.5	TRAINING PROGRESSION FOR SEDENTARY LOW-RISK[a] PARTICIPANTS			
Program Stage	Week	Exercise Frequency (sessions/week)	Exercise Intensity (%HRR)	Exercise Duration (min)
Initial stage	1	3	40–50	15–20
	2	3–4	40–50	20–25
	3	3–4	50–60	20–25
	4	3–4	50–60	25–30
Improvement stage	5–7	3–4	60–70	25–30
	8–10	3–4	60–70	30–35
	11–13	3–4	65–75	30–35
	14–16	3–5	65–75	30–35
	17–20	3–5	70–85	35–40
	21–24	3–5	70–85	35–40
Maintenance stage[b]	24+	3–5	70–85	20–60

Reprinted with permission from ACSM's Guidelines for Exercise Testing and Prescription. 7th ed. Baltimore: Lippincott Williams & Wilkins, 2006:149.

[a] Defined as low-risk category in Table 14-3.

[b] Depending on long-term goals of program, the intensity, frequency, and duration may vary.

HRR, heart rate reserve; it is recommended that low-risk cardiac patients train at the lower end of these ranges.

Muscular Endurance. A client who states that she "wants more stamina" or wants to feel "less winded" after a workout is typically is looking for a resistance program that will increase her muscular endurance. The outcome of training for greater endurance is an enhanced ability of the targeted muscles to perform at a submaximal level for many repetitions or for an extended period of time. A common example is what the muscles do during an aerobic workout: the lower body muscles contract and relax thousands of times during a 20-minute run (1).

Muscular Strength. Many clients will state that they "want to be stronger." These types of clients generally want to exercise at heavier workloads to enhance their strength and power. Typically, these are athletes who are looking to improve their performance and are already familiar with resistance-based training programs. However, a client who is just starting out should start with a program that emphasizes hypertrophy or a muscle endurance training program first to acclimate his or her body to this type of training.

Cardiovascular Training

Cardiovascular training is often referred to as aerobic endurance training or cardiovascular exercise, or even more commonly as "cardio" or "aerobics." These terms are synonymous because they all encompass exercise that recruits cardiovascular and respiratory systems (heart, blood vessels, and lungs). This mode of training is an integral part of any exercise session. To effectively and safely design a client's cardiovascular training program, the Personal Trainer must be familiar with the client's current level of fitness, previous fitness history, and, of course, established goals. Most commonly, the goal of most people who begin or continue a cardiovascular program is fat loss.

As with a resistance training program, the same principal of specificity applies to designing a cardiovascular exercise program. Therefore, the results of a cardiovascular-based program will be more specific to aerobic-based training. In other words, resistance training will not significantly improve maximal aerobic power (5, 6). In addition, training that involves one mode of aerobic exercise will not necessarily improve a different mode. For example, a client who has a high level of aerobic endurance as a runner may not be able to achieve that same level of endurance as a cyclist. The muscle activation patterns and oxygen requirement varies greatly among different modes of exercise. Therefore, the responses and adaptations will not be equal (7).

As with all types of training programs, cardiovascular training programs are composed of different components. These components are meant to be manipulated in a variety of ways to ultimately produce the desired outcome. These components include the mode of exercise, intensity of exercise, frequency of exercise sessions, and duration of each session. The first logical step is to decide on the mode of exercise. Exercise selection plays a major role in all types of training programs. Cardiovascular exercise modes consist of machine- and non-machine–based exercises. There are several factors that need to be considered when choosing the mode of cardiovascular exercise for the client. Some of those factors include, but are not limited to:

➤ Availability
➤ Client's ability to perform the specified exercise
➤ Client's preference
➤ Client's goals

It is also important to note that when training athletes, the athletes should choose modes of cardiovascular exercise that most closely mimic their sport or activity. Some of the more popular modes of machine-based cardiovascular exercises include StairMaster, treadmills, rowers, cycle ergometers, and elliptical trainers. If the Personal Trainer is in a facility that does not have access to equipment, activities such as walking, jogging, running, and swimming all encompass non-machine–based cardiovascular exercise modes. As with resistance training, the mode of exercise should also be based on the client's goals. For example, a client who is preparing to run his or her first 10K will spend the bulk of the session focusing on running, whether on the treadmill or on the track. If you have a client whose goal is to lose body fat, you should implement a cardiovascular program in which that individual uses a variety of exercise modes (e.g., 15 minutes on the treadmill, 15 minutes of boxing drills, and 10 minutes of cycling). This type of training is referred to as "cross training" and is very effective in fat loss and caloric expenditure.

EXERCISE INTENSITY

Before the Personal Trainer can establish frequency and duration of the exercise sessions, he or she must determine the appropriate intensity level to attain the client's goals. To design the best aerobic training program for a client, the Personal Trainer must be able to monitor and regulate the exercise intensity. As explained in Chapter 6, a certain threshold of oxygen consumption or heart rate reserve, which is the difference between a client's resting heart rate and their maximal heart rate, must be attained during an aerobic exercise session before improvements in the cardiorespiratory system are seen (8). Ultimately, the necessary aerobic exercise threshold depends on the client's initial fitness level. In apparently healthy adults, that threshold is generally between 50 and 80% of heart rate reserve (9).

Understanding the Body's Response to Cardiorespiratory Exercise

➤ **Heart Rate (HR).** Heart rate is the number of times the heart beats per minute. Heart rate increases as the work rate and oxygen uptake during dynamic exercise increase. The actual magnitude of the HR increase is related to age, fitness level, medications, body position, blood volume, presence of heart disease, and environmental factors such as temperature and humidity. Maximum attainable HR decreases with age (10).

➤ **Stroke Volume (SV).** Stroke volume is the amount of blood ejected per heart beat. As explained in Chapter 6, during exercise, SV increases in a curvilinear pattern with the work rate until it reaches near-maximal level equivalent to approximately 50–70% of aerobic capacity, increasing only slightly thereafter (11).

➤ **Cardiac Output.** The product of SV and HR determines cardiac output. In apparently healthy adults, the cardiac output increases as the work rate increases. However, like HR, the maximal level of cardiac output is dependent on factors such as age, posture, body size, level of physical conditioning, and presence of cardiovascular disease (11).

Table 16.6	**THE BENEFITS OF INCREASED FLEXIBILITY**

Reduced muscle tension and increased relaxation

Ease of movement

Improved coordination through greater ease of movement

Increased range of motion

Injury prevention

Improvement and development of body awareness

Improved circulation and air exchange

Decreased muscle viscosity, causing contractions to be easier and smoother

Decreased soreness associated with other exercise

Reprinted with permission from ACSM's Resources for the Personal Trainer. 1st ed. Baltimore: Lippincott Williams & Wilkins, 2005:44.

➤ **Blood Pressure.** With increasing levels of exercise comes an increase in systolic blood pressure (SBP). Maximal values typically reach 190–220 mm Hg and should not exceed 260 mm Hg. Diastolic blood pressure (DBP) should decrease slightly or remain unchanged.

Flexibility Training

Proper flexibility and stretching techniques are essential when designing a program to fit a client's needs. Everyone can learn to stretch, regardless of age, level of fitness, or initial flexibility. The way that the body responds to stretching depends on how the sensory organs respond to the stretch stimulus. When educating the client on the importance of proper stretching techniques, refer to Table 16.6 to discuss the many benefits that are associated with increased levels of flexibility.

It is important that the Personal Trainer learn proper stretching techniques when assisting with or assigning stretching exercises to a client. There is no right or wrong answer as to when is the best time to stretch; it is based on individual preference. Stretching may be performed just before or after exercise. When designing an exercise program, the Personal Trainer should allow for stretching exercise to be part of both the warm-up and cool-down phases of the session. As with all exercise programs, there are contraindications and precautions to flexibility training (Tables 16.7 and 16.8).

HOW TO STRETCH

Table 16.9 outlines the guidelines Personal Trainers should follow for proper stretching techniques.

Table 16.7	**CONTRAINDICATIONS TO FLEXIBILITY TESTING**

Motion limited by bony block at a joint interface

Recent unhealed fracture

Infection and acute inflammation affecting the joint or surrounding tissues

Sharp pain associated with stretch or uncontrolled muscle cramping when attempting to stretch

Local hematoma as a result of an overstretch injury

Contracture (desired functional shortening) requiring stability to a joint capsule or ligament contracture that is intentional to improve function, particularly in clients with paralysis or severe muscle weakness (e.g., tenodesis of finger flexors to allow grasp in an individual with quadriplegia)

Reprinted with permission from ACSM's Resources for the Personal Trainer. 1st ed. Baltimore: Lippincott Williams & Wilkins, 2005:45.

Table 16.8   **PRECAUTIONS FOR FLEXIBILITY TRAINING**
Stretch a joint through limits of normal ROM only.
Do not stretch at healed fracture sites for about 8–12 weeks postfracture, after which gentle stretching may be initiated.
In individuals with known or suspected osteoporosis, stretch with particular caution (e.g., men older than 80 years and women older than 65 years, older persons with spinal cord injury).
Avoid aggressive stretching of tissues that have been immobilized (e.g., cast or splinted). Tissues become dehydrated and lose tensile strength during immobilization.
Mild soreness should take no longer than 24 hours to resolve after stretching. If more recovery time is necessary, the stretching force was excessive.
Use active comfortable ROM to stretch edematous joints or soft tissue.
Do not overstretch weak muscles. Shortening in these muscles may contribute to joint support that muscles can no longer actively provide. Combine strength and stretching exercise so that gains in mobility coincide with gains in strength and stability.
Be aware that physical performance may vary from day to day.
Set individual goals.

Reprinted with permission from ACSM's Resources for the Personal Trainer. 1st ed. Baltimore: Lippincott Williams & Wilkins, 2005:45.

TYPES OF STRETCHES

There are various ways to gain flexibility through proper stretching programs. The following techniques focus on a different stimulus to elicit a response.

Static Stretching. This type of stretching is slow and sustained to increase movement at a particular joint when one segment is manipulated relative to another. Passive, active, active assistive, and proprioceptive neuromuscular facilitation (PNF) stretches are all examples of static stretches. The benefits of this type of stretching include:

➤ Decreased possibility of exceeding normal ROM
➤ Lower energy requirements
➤ Lower instance of muscle soreness

Passive Stretching. Passive stretching requires assistance from another person. This form of stretching is widely used by Personal Trainers during the client exercise session. To obtain optimal results when performing a passive stretch, the person being stretched must remain relaxed and refrain from any reflexive movements.

Table 16.9   **GUIDELINES FOR PROPER STRETCHING**
Determine posture or position to be used. Ensure proper position and alignment prior to the stretch.
Emphasize proper breathing. Inhale through the nose and exhale through pursed lips during the stretch. One may stretch with the eyes closed to increase concentration and awareness.
Hold end points progressively for 30–90 seconds and take another deep breath.
Exhale and feel the muscle being stretched, relaxed, and softened so that further ROM is achieved.
Discomfort may increase slightly, but continue to focus on breathing.
Repeat the inhale–exhale–stretch cycle until the end of the available range for the day.
Do not bounce or spring while stretching.
Do not force a stretch while holding the breath.
Increased stretching range during exhalation encourages full body relaxation.
Slowly reposition from the stretch posture and allow muscles to recover at natural resting length.

Reprinted with permission from ACSM's Resources for the Personal Trainer. 1st ed. Baltimore: Lippincott Williams & Wilkins, 2005:45.

Active Stretching. During an active stretch, the muscle being stretched is actively moved through its ROM. This particular technique requires greater energy than passive or static stretching.

Active Assistive Stretching. In this type of stretch, the muscle being stretched may require some assistance to go through its ROM, because of muscular weakness. This is what is considered a "partner stretch."

Proprioceptive Neuromuscular Facilitation. There are different types of PNF stretching that can be performed to elicit the best response to the stretch stimulus. These types include the contract–relax (hold–relax), and the contract–relax–contract (hold–relax–hold). When performing the contract–relax stretch, the muscle is contracted then relaxed, then further stretched into its available ROM during the brief relax phase. Contract–relax–contract follows the same procedure; however, a subsequent contraction of the antagonist muscle gains slightly more ROM.

Dynamic, Phasic, or Ballistic Stretching. These terms, when associated with stretching, refer to quick jerking and often bounce-like movements such as bouncing when trying to touch the toes. Generally it is thought that the disadvantages of this type of stretching far outweigh the benefits. Performing these jerking movements can predispose the muscles to injury. When educating the client on the different types of stretches, the Personal Trainer should provide some flexibility exercises that will help the client gain more flexibility

Plyometrics and Sports Performance

Plyometric exercise programming is very similar to resistance and cardiovascular training. For the Personal Trainer to safely design a plyometric-based training program that will enhance the client's sports performance, the client's goals, needs, and preferences must be established. Plyometric training is not for everyone. This method of training is sport-specific and requires the client to be well conditioned. For athletes to achieve optimal performance in their chosen sport, they must train for speed, strength, and power, endurance and flexibility, and coordination. Plyometrics was first introduced as jumping exercises for the lower extremities. Now, however, there are a variety of upper-body plyometric exercises that athletes and trainers are using to improve skills in almost every sporting platform. These upper-body exercises are performed using weighted balls, bands, and bars. Plyometrics has been described (12) as beginning with rapid stretching (eccentric muscle actions), followed by a shortening of the same muscle (concentric muscle action). This is known as the stretch–shortening cycle. Plyometric training is based on the principle of using the elastic properties of the muscle. These conditions will create a greater force.

Balance and Stability

Another, less obvious form of sports performance training is balance or stability training. Balance is defined as the ability to maintain a position for a given period of time without moving. There are many sports performance drills that require the athlete to jump, slide, or step in non-traditional movement patterns (i.e., single leg hop or squat hops). These drills rely on the client's proprioception and balance to safely and successfully complete the exercise. Working on clients' core muscles will enhance their ability to maintain the balance and stability needed for their sport. There are several balance drills that can be performed, at various fitness levels, to help develop core strength. Some of these drills include standing on one leg at the beginner level or single leg half squat at the advanced level.

FUNCTIONAL TRAINING

Functional training is another variation of sports performance training. This technique allows the client to perform movements that imitate those used in their everyday lives. For example, if the client has a career in which lifting heavy boxes is part of everyday activity, a training program that works the muscles of the lower extremities and strengthens the core muscles would be beneficial, as well as doing exercises that will enhance proper-posture lifting techniques. When training an athlete, functional training plays a key role in training the body the way it will be used in competition, making it a very effective training tool for the Personal Trainer.

PROGRAM DESIGN

The process of **exercise programming** can be divided into three steps. The first step is assessing health and fitness information. The second step is interpreting that information. The third step is combining the information with the interpreted results as well as the client's goals, to formulate an exercise program. When designing the actual client program, there are certain variables that the Personal Trainer must take into consideration, such as what exercises to include in the program, the sequence of the selected exercises, how often the client wants to train, the load, repetition, and set assignment, as well as rest periods.

Each individual potential client has specific goals related to health and fitness. Being able to understand and identify this range of goals is an essential step in program design and exercise selection. To most efficiently and effectively design a client exercise program, the Personal Trainer must fully assess the needs of the client based not only on goals but also on the results of the fitness assessment. The measurement or assessment of health-related physical fitness is a common practice by most fitness professionals. The Personal Trainer should be able to identify and understand the different components of fitness assessment results to do the following (13):

➤ Educate individuals about their current health-related physical fitness
➤ Use data from the assessments to individualize exercise programs
➤ Provide baseline and follow-up data to evaluate exercise programs
➤ Motivate individuals toward more specific exercises
➤ Assist with client's risk stratification

Before the initial exercise selection process begins, the Personal Trainer must take into consideration the client's physiological capacity for beginning and maintaining an exercise program. Exercise training is defined as planned, structured, and repetitive bodily movement done to improve or maintain one or more components of physical fitness. In Chapter 6, the body's response to exercise and the principles of adaptation are fully explained. Each of these principles guides the design of an exercise program. In exercise training, the mode of exercise, as well as the frequency, duration, and intensity of training, are critical in achieving fitness, athletic, or health outcomes (2). When designing a client exercise program, the mode must be specific to the targeted component of fitness, and the frequency, duration, and intensity must be combined in a systematic overload that will result in physiological adaptations.

Anatomy of an Exercise Session

The three basic components to any personal training session are the warm-up, the conditioning stimulus, and the cool-down. Workouts should always begin with some warm-up exercises so the body is better prepared to meet the challenges that will be presented by the succeeding conditioning stimulus phase.

Warm-up and cool-down phases are the periods of metabolic and cardiorespiratory adjustment from rest to exercise and exercise to rest, respectively. Therefore, the most appropriate types of warm-up and cool-down are activities similar to the conditioning stimulus activities, performed at approximately 50% of the stimulus intensity (14).

An appropriate warm-up can improve performance and decrease the risk of cardiac disease events (14). Cool-down has these benefits as well as helping to clear metabolic waste from skeletal muscle. Older individuals and those at risk of cardiac disease events benefit from longer periods of warm-up and cool-down. The conditioning stimulus may contain a period of aerobic conditioning, muscle conditioning, or both. Depending on the allotted session time, this may be as short as 20 minutes or as long as 60 minutes (9).

Exercise Selection

The exercises selected, as well as the order in which they are selected, will determine the intensity of the client's workout. An advanced training program with a client who is an experienced athlete may include as many as 20 exercises, focusing on sports-specific exercises as well as total-body conditioning. However, a beginning or basic exercise program may only include one exercise for each large muscle group of the body. As previously stated, the order of the exercises affects the intensity of the training session and is therefore a very important consideration. For instance, alternating upper and lower body exercises does not produce as high an intensity level as performing all lower body exercises first. Exercises that involve multiple joints and muscles (referred to as multi-joint exercises) are more intense than those that involve only one joint (referred to as single-joint exercises) (1). Two of the most common arrangements for exercise arrangement are:

➤ Exercise large muscle groups (i.e., bench press, leg press squats) before smaller muscle groups (i.e., wrist curls, calf raises). This method of exercise arrangement is the most widely used.
➤ Alternate push and pull exercises (extension = push, flexion = pull). An example of this would be a triceps extension (push) followed by a biceps curl (pull).

The next step to designing a client exercise program, after determining exercise selection and arrangement, is determining workload. Load refers to the weight used or intensity of the exercise. To best determine the load at which the client should be working, please refer to Chapter 17.

SUMMARY

This chapter is designed to provide the Personal Trainer with a solid base of knowledge in all of the variables that create a client exercise program. This chapter serves as a review for previous chapters in the book that discuss anatomy, physiology, exercise science, exercise physiology, and human behavior. This chapter applies the fundamentals of the previously mentioned topics and applies them within the scope of the Personal Trainer.

REFERENCES

1. Fleck SJ, Kraemer WJ. Designing Resistance Training Programs. 2nd ed. Champaign, IL: Human Kinetics, 1997.
2. Baechle TR, Groves BR. Weight Training Instruction: Steps to Success. Champaign, IL: Human Kinetics, 1994.
3. Spence AP. Reading: Basic Human Anatomy. 3rd ed. Redwood, CA: Benjamin/Cummings, 1991.
4. Cooper JM, Adrian M, Glassow RB. Kinesiology. St. Louis: Mosby, 1982
5. Luthi, JM, Howald H Claasen H, et al. Structural changes in skeletal muscle tissue with heavy-resistance exercise. Int J Sports Med 1986;7:123–127.
6. McGee D, Jessee TC, Stone MH, Blessing D. Leg and hip endurance adaptations to three weight training programs. J Appl Sports Sci Res 1992;6:92–95.
7. Bressel E, Heise GD, Bachman G. A neuromuscular and metabolic comparison of forward and reverse pedaling. J Appl Biomech 1998;14(4):401–411.
8. Hickson RC, Foster C, Pollock ML, et al. Reduced training intensities and loss of aerobic power, endurance, and cardiac growth. J Appl Physiol 1985;58(2):492–499.
9. American College of Sports Medicine. Guidelines for Exercise Testing and Prescription. 7th ed. Philadelphia: Lippincott Williams & Wilkins, 2006.
10. Dehn MM, Mullins CB. Physiologic effects and importance of exercise in patients with coronary artery disease. J Cardiovasc Med 1977;2:365–367.
11. Mitchell JH, Blomqvist G. Maximal oxygen uptake. N Engl J Med 1971;284:1018–1022.
12. Chu D. Plyometrics. Livermore, CA: Bittersweet, 1989:8–15, 78–79.
13. American College of Sports Medicine. Health-related Physical Fitness Assessment Manual. Philadelphia: Lippincott Williams & Wilkins, 2005.
14. McArdle WD, Katch FL, Katch VL. Exercise Physiology. Baltimore: Williams & Wilkins, 1996.

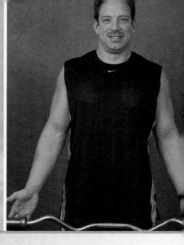

CHAPTER

17 Resistance Training Programs

William J. Kraemer, Ph.D., FACSM, Jakob L. Vingren, M.S., Disa L. Hatfield, M.A., Barry A. Spiering, M.S., Maren S. Fragala, M.S.,
Human Performance Laboratory, Department of Kinesiology, University of Connecticut, Storrs, Connecticut

Chapter Outline

- **Define resistance training principles**
- **Review how and why resistance training should be performed**
- **Provide direction to the Personal Trainer on how to design, evaluate, and implement resistance training programs**
- **Provide the fundamental tools to evaluate clients' resistance training needs and progress**

Resistance training, also known as strength training or weight training, is now a standard part of a comprehensive personal training program. The benefits of resistance training are numerous and include increases in strength, muscle mass, and bone density, to mention a few. All of these aspects are important to maintain good health in both men and women, and almost every population, from adolescents to senior citizens, can benefit from resistance training.

THE SCIENCE BEHIND RESISTANCE TRAINING

At the end of the second World War, Captain Thomas Delorme, M.D., experimented with the use of progressive resistance exercise as a rehabilitation tool for injured soldiers (1). A few years later, he and A. L. Watkins published the first paper in a scientific journal on the topic of long-term resistance training (2). After the initial work by DeLorme and Watkins, the science of resistance training lay somewhat dormant until the 1980s. Two notable former lifters, Dr. Patrick O'Shea from Oregon State University and Dr. Richard Berger from Temple University, became scientists, and their pioneering work in the 1960s and 1970s fueled the eventual explosion in scientific work on this topic (3, 4). Prior to that, the most influential personalities in resistance training during the last century were Mr. Bob Hoffman of York Barbell, who pioneered the interest in weightlifting and weight training with free weights through his publications and sales of barbells and dumbbells, and then Mr. Joe Weider and his brother Ben, who promoted bodybuilding. Since the 1980s, published research on resistance training has grown exponentially in both scientific manuscripts and books on the topic. A resistance training program can affect almost every system in the body, and add is used in a wide variety of scenarios, from helping young children prepare for sport to offsetting the effects of aging. With an explosion of information from books, magazines, and the Internet, a demanding challenge has been placed on the Personal Trainer to study and be able to evaluate information and its veracity as the resistance training mythology and marketing ploys still remain very dominant in the field today. Once information has passed a critical evaluation, it is of even greater importance to understand how it can be used in the implementation of a resistance training program that ultimately affects the health, fitness, and performance of a client.

In the later 1980s, the focus of much of the research changed from enhancement of athletic performance, especially in men, to improvement of health and fitness for both men and women in the general population (5). Research on resistance training now appears in a wide range of specialized medical and physiological scientific journals such as the American College of Sports Medicine's *Medicine and Science in Sports and Exercise* and the National Strength and Conditioning Association's *Journal of Strength and Conditioning Research*. There are literally thousands of scientific articles examining different aspects of resistance training, which have led to a large and still growing knowledge base of physiological adaptations and mechanisms, gender differences, biomechanical influences, and specificity considerations needed to understand resistance training exercise prescription. As a result, resistance training programs and exercise protocols can be guided by scientific facts and not by purely anecdotal evidence or, worse yet, marketing "mythology" as was the case for much of the last century.

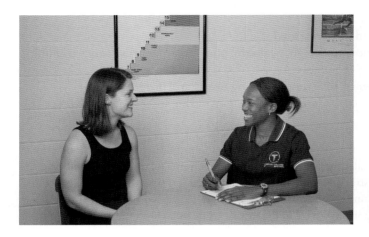

FIGURE 17.1. Exercise prescription in resistance training is an individualized process that requires a series of steps, from a needs analysis and goal setting to evaluations and making changes in the workouts over time.

GENERAL RESISTANCE TRAINING PRINCIPLES

The terms "resistance exercise" and "resistance training" are often used interchangeably; however, there is an important distinction between the two terms. *Resistance exercise* refers to a single exercise session; whereas, *resistance training* refers to the combination of many consecutive resistance exercise sessions over time. Thus, a resistance exercise protocol is an exercise prescription for a single session (also called a "workout") and a resistance training program is an overall program guiding the specific exercise parameters chosen for each exercise protocol.

Designing a resistance training program is a very individualized process, and the needs and goals of the client are paramount to the selection of program characteristics (*Fig 17.1*). Even though an individual may be training to maximize muscle hypertrophy, the client will also develop some muscular strength and endurance. The general principles of any effective resistance training program are:

1. *Specificity of Training:* Only the muscles that are trained will adapt and change in response to a resistance training program. For this reason, resistance programs must target all muscles for which a training effect is desired.

2. *SAID Principle:* Specific adaptations to imposed demands relate to the fact that the adaptation will be specific to the demands that the characteristics of the workout places upon the individual. If a high number of repetitions are used, the muscles will increase their ability to perform a high number of repetitions (muscular endurance).

3. *Progressive Overload:* As the body adapts to a given stimulus, an increase in the stimulus is required for further adaptations and improvements. Thus, if the load or volume is not increased over time, progress will be limited.

4. *Variation in Training:* No one program should be used without changing the exercise stimulus over time. Periodized training is the major concept related to the optimal training and recovery programming.

5. *Prioritization of Training:* It is difficult to train for all aspects of muscular fitness. Thus, within a periodized training program, one needs to focus or prioritize the training goals for each training cycle.

PROGRAM DESIGN PROCESS

The key to improved program design is the identification of specific variables, which need to be controlled to better predict the training outcomes. The most challenging aspect of resistance training exercise prescription is making decisions related to the development and changes of an individual's training goals and program design. One is faced with making appropriate changes in the resistance training program over time. This means that sound "clinical decisions" must be made based on factual understanding of resistance training, the needs of the sport or activity, individual training responses, and testing data. Therefore, planning and changing the exercise prescription is vital for the success of any resistance training program.

An understanding of resistance training exercise prescription allows better quantification of the exercise stimulus. Planning ranges from the development of a single exercise session to the variation of the training program over time. The ability to quantify the workout and evaluate the progress made toward a specific training goal is the basic hallmark of the Personal Trainer who is capable of designing solid programs that lead to optimal physical development.

Training Potential

The gains made in any variable related to muscular performance will ultimately be linked to an individual's genetic potential. If an individual starts to train in a relatively deconditioned state, the initial gains are great because of the large adaptational potential that is available. As training proceeds, gains decrease as an individual approaches his or her genetic potential. At this point, some goals are maintained; whereas other target goals for the resistance training program must be adjusted to prevent the client from losing interest and quitting because of a lack of progress or boredom. Appreciation of this concept is important in understanding the adaptations and changes that occur over time. Furthermore, one can see how almost any program might work for an untrained individual in the early phases of training.

Initial Assessments

When working with a new client, the Personal Trainer should always devote adequate time to learn about the client's prior resistance exercise experience before beginning any exercise sessions. The initial assessment should include a needs analysis focusing on learning about the client's goals and needs, the intended time frame for achieving these goals, targeted areas or muscle groups, health issues (e.g., hypertension, asthma, diabetes), musculoskeletal limitations, recent surgeries, chronic injuries, sites of pain, etc. Furthermore, Personal Trainers should try to understand why reaching these goals is important and the level of support the clients feel they are receiving from their loved ones (see Chapter 10 for additional discussion of social support). Also, Personal Trainers should try to elucidate past experiences with resistance training to uncover challenges, barriers, and strategies for motivation that their clients may face. The needs analysis will help the Personal Trainer determine which muscle groups, energy systems, and muscle actions are to be trained and how these and the other acute program variables should be manipulated to meet the specific needs of the training program. Furthermore, the Personal Trainer will be able to develop strategies to help the client overcome potential barriers to resistance training.

Prior to developing a resistance training program, Personal Trainers should take the time to conduct a baseline fitness assessment, consisting of anthropometric measurements (height, weight, circumferences, etc.), body composition, and tests of muscular strength and endurance. Initial determination of the level of the different fitness variables can help in the development of an effective training program. Examples of tests of muscular strength include 1 repetition maximum (1RM) testing on a variety of exercises, especially those exercises that involve the major muscle groups such as bench press and squat, but only if tolerable to the client (6). Muscular endurance testing might include 1-minute timed tests of curl-ups or push-ups or maximal amount of repetitions that can be performed at a given percentage of the 1RM load.

Follow-Up Assessments

It is exciting and motivating for clients to see improvements toward reaching their goals. To see these improvements, it is important that Personal Trainers keep records of their clients' progression. Individualized training logs are a useful tool for monitoring progress. These logs should record specific exercises, resistance or load, number of sets, and number of repetitions. Kept over time, these logs provide the Personal Trainer with a means to examine and evaluate progress and the effectiveness of the program. Another very important benefit of the training log is that it allows the Personal Trainer to assign the appropriate resistance to be used during an exercise on the basis of the resistance and performance of previous exercise sessions.

Reassessments of a client's progress should occur periodically for encouragement, but not so often that there has not been adequate time for noticeable changes to develop. These follow-up assessments should include measures similar to those of the baseline assessment, including anthropometric measurements and tests of muscular strength, power, and endurance.

Based on these assessments, the concepts of progression, variation, and overload can be applied to the resistance training program to achieve physiological performance and to accommodate changing fitness levels and goals of clients. These assessments will give the Personal Trainer a basis for modifying the acute program variables, including choice of exercise, order of exercises, intensity, number of sets, set structure, rest periods, load or resistance, and repetition speed. Variation can be incorporated by altering joint angles and positioning, primary exercises versus assistance exercises, or multi-joint versus single-joint exercises to stress the muscles and joints specified by the client's needs analysis. Progressive overload can be accomplished by increasing the intensity and/or volume by increasing the resistance, number of sets, number of repetitions, or number of exercises or by decreasing or increasing the rest intervals.

Individualization

Clients are not cookie cutter replicas of each other. Therefore, the better Personal Trainers do not give standard programs to multiple clients. Similar training programs provided to different clients will result in varied training responses. Therefore, the exercises that are given to one client may need to be modified to better suit the anatomical characteristics, needs, and abilities of another client. Additionally, the Personal Trainer must make modifications in response to the training adaptations of the specific client. Adjustments to programs should focus on optimizing the individual's physiological adaptations.

Client Feedback

When designing a resistance training program that meets and/or surpasses the needs and expectations of the client, it is critical that the Personal Trainer pay special attention to feedback from the client. This feedback can be openly expressed, a client may request a favorite exercise or muscle group they hope to focus on during the training session, or they may complain of pain or fatigue. It is important for the Personal Trainer to pick up on this feedback and encourage further feedback, to ensure that the program and strategy meet the expectations of the client. This can be accomplished by asking the client for feedback, for example, "How do you think the workout went?" "Did you feel that you worked out hard enough?" "Was the exercise protocol too hard? Just right?" Furthermore, Personal Trainers must learn to recognize physical signs of dizziness and lightheadedness as well as complexion changes, profuse sweating, facial expressions, and muscle exhaustion. Working a client to the point of vomiting or passing out will not leave a good impression with clients or any spectators who are present when medical attention arrives.

Personal Trainers should always explain the muscle groups the exercise is intended to target, and clients should be taught how to differentiate between muscle fatigue and unintentional pain. That way, if any pain is felt in any joint or non-synergistic or stabilizer muscle, the exercise may not be a good match for the client, but it should be kept in mind that new exercises often feel uncomfortable or awkward. Exercises should be stopped immediately if clients complain of pain or the Personal Trainer suspects the client is in pain. The last thing a Personal Trainer wants to do is induce or aggravate an injury.

Feedback from the client can also come from paying close attention to the technique of the client during an exercise. Reduction in technique often results from fatigue or insufficient flexibility in the range of motion involved in the exercise. Proper technique should always be a priority. When the technique breaks down during an exercise, the exercise should be either stopped or modified to re-establish correct technique to avoid injury.

Setting and Evaluating Goals

Personal Trainers encounter an assortment of clients with a plethora of goals including weight loss, weight gain, building strength, building muscle, shaping/toning, improving overall health, improving speed, agility, power, balance, coordination, decreasing blood pressure or cholesterol, managing diabetes, or sport-specific training. Often the desired goals of clients are unrealistic. When improvements do not meet expectations, motivation can be lost, frustration may set in, and non-adherence to the program can occur. Therefore, it is crucial that the Personal Trainer help the client understand what obtainable goals may be, considering the individual's beginning status, fitness level, and genetic potential. Also, the expectations of the client must be realistic considering the physiological time course of neural and muscle protein adaptations as well as weight loss. Goal setting and time frame should also be taken into consideration, as well as the individual's age, physical maturity, training history, and psychological and physical tolerance. It is important to set testable goals (such as increase in 1RM or fat mass loss), and progression toward the goals must be gradual to decrease the risk of injury. Resistance training program design and modifications should consider these individualized goals.

Common program goals in resistance training are related to improvements in function, such as increased muscular strength, power, and local muscular endurance or decreased body fat (*Fig. 17.2*). Other functional gains such as increased coordination, agility, balance, and speed are also common goals of a program. It is becoming clear that such factors as balance may have implications for injury prevention by limiting falls in older individuals. Physiological changes related to increased body mass through muscle hypertrophy and improvement of other physiological functions such as improved blood pressure, decreased body fat, and increased metabolic rate to help burn calories are also goals that can be reached with resistance training.

For the most part, training goals or objectives should be testable variables (e.g., 1RM strength, vertical jump height) so that one can objectively judge whether or not gains were made or goals achieved. Examination and evaluation of a workout log is invaluable in assessing the effects of various resistance training programs. Formal strength tests to determine functional changes in strength can be done on a variety of equipment, including isokinetic dynamometers, free weights, and machines. Using the results of these objective tests can help in modifying the exercise program to reach previous training goals or to develop new goals.

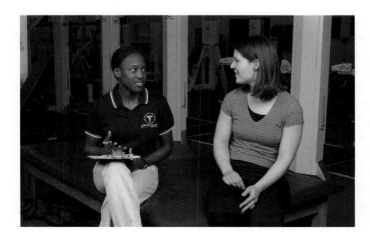

FIGURE 17.2. Setting goals and evaluating progress in a resistance training program is vital to see realistic progress and gains.

It should be noted here that athletic performance and health are not always the same thing. Many elite athletes do things in their training program that far exceed what is needed for good health because of the need for performance gains (e.g., lifting 7 days a week or running 140 miles in a week or training 4–6 hours a day). Thus, goals in resistance training have to be put in the context of the needed outcome for the individual. Factors such as age, physical maturity, training history, and psychological and physical toleration need to be considered in any goal development process and individual program design. Decisions on the use of the available training time must be made to affect the training goals, which directly influence performance in the sport or activity. This is what makes an optimal program design.

Maintenance of Training Goals

A concept called "capping" may need to be applied to various training situations in which small gains will require very large amounts of time to achieve, and yet in the long run, these small gains are not necessary for success. This may be related to a performance (e.g., bench press 1RM strength) or some form of physical development (e.g., calf size). This is a tough decision that comes only after an adequate period of training time and observation of what the realistic potential for further change is for a particular variable. At some point, one must make a value judgment on how to best spend training time. By not adding any further training time to develop a particular muscle characteristic (e.g., strength, size, power), one decides to go into a maintenance training program. Thus, more training time is available to address other training goals. Ultimately, this decision may result in greater total development of the individual.

Decisions such as capping are part of the many types of clinical decisions that must be made when monitoring the progress of resistance training programs. Are the training goals realistic in relation to the sport or health enhancement for which the client is being trained? Is the attainment of a particular training goal vital to the program's success? These are difficult questions that need to be continually asked in the goal development phase of each training cycle for any program.

Unrealistic Goals

Careful attention must be paid to the magnitude of the performance goal and the amount of training time needed to achieve it. While scientific studies may last up to 6 months, most real-life training programs are developed as a part of a lifestyle for an individual's sports career or whole life. Goals change, and resistance training programs must change to reflect these changing needs.

Too often, goals are open-ended and unrealistic. For most men, the 23-inch biceps, the 36-inch thighs, the 20-inch neck, the 400-pound bench press, or the 50-inch chest are unrealistic goals. This is because of genetic limitations most men have for such extreme muscle size and performance. Women too can develop unrealistic goals. Usually this is in an opposite direction from men, in that goals many times include desire for drastic decreases in limb size and body shape. Again, based on genetics, such changes may not be possible in many women because of a naturally larger anatomical structure. Many women mistakenly believe large gains in strength, muscle definition, and body fat loss can be achieved through the use of very light resistance training programs (e.g., 2- to 5-lb hand-held weights) that attempt to "spot build" a particular body part or muscle. Although one may be able to "spot hypertrophy" on a particular body part, it is not done with resistances that are this light. In addition, the "fear of getting big" has produced unrealistic fears about lifting heavy weights, and thus many women do not gain the full benefits of resistance training. Ultimately, for both men and women, it is a question of whether the resistance training program used can stimulate the desired changes in their body. The desired changes must be carefully and honestly examined.

Unrealistic expectations of equipment and programs also exist when they are not evaluated on the basis of sound scientific principles. In today's "high tech" and "big hype" in marketing products, Internet information, programs, and equipment, unrealistic training expectations can be developed for the average person. In addition, movie actors, models, and elite athletes can also project a desired body image and/or performance level, but for most people such upper levels of physical development and performance are unrealistic. Proper goal development is accomplished by starting out small and making progress and then evaluating where the individual is and what is now possible. Most people make mistakes in goal development by wanting too much too soon, with too little effort expended. Making progress in a resistance training program is related to a long-term commitment to a total training program.

In addition to resistance exercise, appropriate cardiovascular conditioning and proper nutrition and lifestyle behaviors can help support training objectives and physical development. Careful evaluation of training goals, objectives, and the equipment needed to achieve these goals and objectives can eliminate wasted time, money, and effort.

RESISTANCE TRAINING MODALITIES

There are many different training tools (e.g., free weights, machines, medicine balls) that can be used in a resistance training programs. All of these tools can be placed into specific categories of training. From the following, it is clear that each category has certain inherent strengths and weaknesses, and therefore, the modality chosen should depend on the needs, goals, experiences, and limitations of the client.

Variable-Resistance Devices

Variable resistance equipment operates through a lever arm, cam, or pulley arrangement. Its purpose is to alter the resistance throughout the exercise's range of motion in an attempt to match the increases and decreases in strength (strength curve) throughout the exercise. Proponents of variable-resistance machines believe that by increasing and decreasing the resistance to match the exercise's strength curve, the muscle is forced to contract maximally throughout the range of motion, resulting in maximal gains in strength.

There are three major types of strength curves: ascending, descending, and bell shaped (*Fig. 17.3*). In an exercise with an ascending strength curve, it is possible to lift more weight if only the top 1/2 or 1/4 of a repetition is performed than if the complete range of motion of a repetition is performed. For example, an exercise with an ascending strength curve is the squat exercise. If an exercise has a descending strength curve, it is possible to lift more weight if only the bottom half of a repetition is performed. Such an exercise is upright rowing. A bell-shaped curve is an exercise in which it is possible to lift more resistance, if only the middle portion of the range of motion is performed and not the beginning or end portions of the range of the motion. Elbow curls have a bell-shaped strength

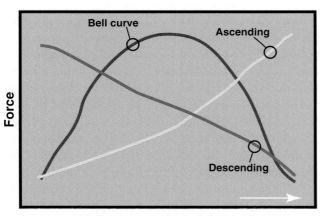

FIGURE 17.3. Three basic strength curves exist for every exercise, with hybrids of them for certain movements.

curve. Since there are three major types of strength curves, variable-resistance machines have to be able to vary the resistance in three major patterns to match the strength curves of all exercises. To date, this has not been accomplished. Additionally, because of variations in limb length, point of attachment of a muscle's tendon to the bones, and body size, it is hard to conceive of one mechanical arrangement that would match the strength curve of all individuals for a particular exercise.

Biomechanical research indicates that one cam type of variable-resistance equipment does not match the strength curves of the elbow curl, fly, knee extension, knee flexion and pullover exercises (7, 8). A second type of cam type equipment has been reported to match the strength curves of females fairly well (9). However, for females, the cam resulted in too much resistance near the end of the knee extension exercise. The cam also provided too much resistance during the first half and too little during the second half of the elbow flexion and extension exercises. The knee flexion machine matched the female's strength curve well throughout the range of motion.

Elastic bands have become popular within the fitness world because they are relatively easy to work with and less frightening to clients. Although very effective as a training modality if the resistance can be heavy enough (10), care must be taken when using elastic bands with certain types of exercises that do not match the ascending strength curve. A possible major drawback to elastic bands is that the resistance increases constantly as the band is stretched, a resistance pattern that only matches an ascending strength curve; thus at the beginning of a muscle flexion, the resistance is low, and at the end of the flexion the resistance is very high. This means that only the part of the muscle involved in the later part of the flexion may be optimally stimulated if the setup is not correct. Thus, proper starting fit and stretch is essential for the training outcome. Also because of the physics of elastic bands, the resistance during the extension phase will be lower than that during the flexion phase, again reducing the training stimulus. In addition, elastic bands give minimal feedback that may be important to some clients, especially men who like to see the weight stacks or plates move with each repetition.

Dynamic Constant External Resistance Devices

Isotonic is traditionally defined as a muscular contraction in which the muscle exerts a constant tension. The execution of free-weight exercises and exercises on various weight training machines, though usually considered isotonic, is not by nature isotonic. The force exerted by a muscle in the performance of such exercises is not constant, but varies with the mechanical advantage of the joint involved in the movement and the length of the muscle at a particular point in the movement. A more workable definition of isotonic is a resistance training exercise in which the external resistance or weight does not change and both a lifting (concentric) and lowering (eccentric) phase occurs during each repetition. Thus, free-weight exercises and exercise machines that do not vary the resistance are isotonic in nature. Because there is confusion concerning the term "isotonic," the term "dynamic constant external resistance (DCER) training" has been adopted.

The types of devices used for DCER include dumbbells, barbells, and medicine balls; these are generally devices that do not use pulleys or levers. The major disadvantage to this type of device is that it does not stimulate the neuromuscular systems involved maximally throughout the entire range of motion. The changes in the musculoskeletal leverage occurring during a movement also change the force requirement and thus the exercise stimulus. However, these types of devices require that muscles other than the primary movers of an exercise are recruited to act as stabilizers, and this increases the total amount of physiological work the body must do to perform the exercise, as well as produce exercise stimuli to the stabilizing muscles that are very important in a real-world setting or for athletic performance. We also call these types of modalities "free form" exercises, as they operate in multiple dimensions of space. Other benefits to most constant external resistance devices include little or no limitation in the range of motion allowed and easy adaptation of the exercise to accommodate individual differences such as the clients' body size or physical capabilities. Equipment fit is also not a limiting factor for large and small body sizes and limb lengths.

Static Resistance Devices

Specialized static contraction devices, in which a person pulls or pushes against an immovable apparatus for isometric exercise, are rarely used. Pushing an overloaded barbell against the safety racks, or using a wall or partner for an isometric contraction, are occasionally used for an individual to overcome a sticking point, and this is called "functional isometrics." Isometrics or static resistance training refers to a muscular action in which no change in the length of the muscle takes place. This type of resistance training is normally performed against an immovable object such as a wall, a barbell, or a weight machine loaded beyond the maximal concentric strength of an individual.

Isometrics can also be performed by having a weak muscle group contract against a strong muscle group. For example, trying to bend the left elbow by contracting the left elbow flexors maximally while resisting the movement by pushing down on the left hand with the right hand with just enough force to prevent any movement at the left elbow. If the left elbow flexors are weaker than the right elbow extensors, the left elbow flexors would be performing an isometric action at 100% of a maximal voluntary contraction.

Review of subsequent studies demonstrated that isometric training leads to static strength gains but that the gains are substantially less than 5% per week (11). Increases in strength resulting from isometric training are related to the number of muscle actions performed, the duration of the muscle actions, whether the muscle action is maximal or submaximal, and the frequency of training. Most studies involving isometric training manipulate several of these factors simultaneously. It is difficult, therefore, to evaluate the importance of any one factor. Enough research has been conducted, however, to allow some recommendations concerning isometric training.

Other Resistance Devices

Isokinetic devices allow one to maintain a maximum resistance throughout the whole range of motion by controlling the speed of the movement. These devices use either friction, compressed air, or pneumatics, which allow for both the concentric and the eccentric component of a repetition, or hydraulics for the concentric component of a repetition. Isokinetic exercises, although popular in the rehabilitation setting, have never caught on as a typical modality used in a weight room. The initial excitement for this training modality was related to the ability to train at fast velocities similar to the high-speed movements seen in sport and real life. Isokinetic refers to a muscular action performed at constant angular limb velocity. Unlike other types of resistance training, there is no set resistance to meet; rather, the velocity of movement is controlled. The resistance offered by the isokinetic machine cannot be accelerated; any force applied against the equipment results in an equal reaction force. The reaction force mirrors the force applied to the equipment by the user throughout the range of movement of an exercise, making it theoretically possible for the muscle(s) to exert a continual, maximal force through the movement's full range of motion.

Pneumatic resistance (compressed air) exercise has caught on to the greatest extent as it has both the concentric and eccentric portion of a repetition and can be adjusted during a repetition or set of exercises with hand-held buttons. This type of device has been popular for working with older populations. In addition, with no deceleration, it can be used effectively to train power with joint exercises not possible with conventional machines. Power is important for older adults to maintain function as well as for athletes. Because of the fixed nature of the configuration for most pneumatic machines, they are unable to address key factors such as balance and control in a multi-dimensional environment.

Hydraulics has also caught on, with many fitness clubs selling it as a safe and non-intimidating form of resistance exercise. Although this modality has no deceleration in its repetition range and has been used as a type of power training modality, it also has no eccentric component, which limits its efficiency as twice the number of repetitions may be required to get the same effect as a typical concentric/eccentric repetition (12). The eccentric phase is important to protect the body from injury and also enhance the ability to recover from injury. Further, concentric-only training appears to be less resistant to detraining.

MACHINES VERSUS FREE-WEIGHT EXERCISES

A topic of great debate, especially in the health and fitness world, is the use of free weights versus machine resistance exercises. The two different exercise modalities were covered during the sections on constant external resistance and variable-resistance devices, respectively. Below is a comparison of the two modalities:

1. Machines are not always designed to fit the proportions of all individuals. Clients who are obese, have special physical considerations or disabilities, and those shorter, taller, or wider than the norm may not be able to fit comfortably in the machines and use them with ease. Free-weight exercises can easily be adapted to fit most clients' physical size or special requirements.

2. Machines use a fixed range of motion, thus the individual must conform to the movement limitations of the machine. Often, these movements do not mimic functional or athletic movements. Free weights allow full range of motion, and the transfer to the real-world movements is greater than for machines.

3. Most machines isolate a muscle or muscle group, thus negating the need for other muscles to act as assistant movers and stabilizers. Free-weight exercises almost always involve assisting and stabilizing muscles. On the other hand, if the goal is to isolate a specific muscle or muscle group, as in some rehabilitation settings or because of physical disabilities, machine exercises can be used.

4. Although it is never advisable to perform resistance exercise alone, machines do allow greater independence, as the need for a spotter or helper is usually diminished once the client has learned the technique of the exercise. However, there is a misconception of extra safety that may lead to a lack of attention being paid to the exercise. It is still possible to be injured when using machines.

5. Machine exercises may be more useful than free-weight exercises in some special populations. One reason for this is that machines are often perceived to be less intimidating to a beginner. As the resistance training skill and experience level increases, free-weight exercise can gradually be introduced if desired. However, it is important to inform clients of the benefits that free weights have compared with machines (e.g., increased musculoskeletal loading that reduces the risk of developing osteoporosis, improved balance).

6. Certain free-weight exercises (e.g., Olympic-style lifts) and hydraulic and pneumatic machines allow training of power, as no joint deceleration occurs.

7. Rotational resistance accommodates certain body movements (e.g., shoulder adduction) that would be difficult to work through a full range of motion with free weights.

From the comparison above, it should be clear that variable resistive devices (machines) in general are at a comparative disadvantage to constant resistance devices (free weights), but machine exercises can still be useful in resistance training when used appropriately. Actually, a solid resistance training program has a combination of both free-weight and machine exercises, taking into consideration many aspects of the client's needs and the advantages of the different modalities. They can also be used differently to add variation to the training program and it as effective tools in your fitness "tool box" of instruments. This being said, machines and other variable-resistance devices should only be used as an adjunct to training of mid-level and advanced clients and athletes.

THE NEEDS ANALYSIS

Before designing a training program, a needs analysis (see Chapter 13) of the client should be performed to design the most effective program (5). Once the needs and goals of the client have been established, the following areas should also be carefully considered so the resistance training program can address questions that will come up when designing the workout using the acute program variables. It is important to keep in mind the general principles of resistance training covered in the beginning of this chapter as one continues with the development of the exercise.

A needs analysis for strength training consists of answering some initial questions that affect the program design components (13). It is important to take time to examine such questions. The major questions asked in a needs analysis are:

1. What muscle groups need to be trained?
2. What are the basic energy sources (e.g., anaerobic, aerobic) that need to be trained?
3. What type of muscle action (e.g., isometric, eccentric actions) should be used?
4. What are the primary sites of injury for the particular sport or prior injury history of the individual?

Biomechanical Analysis to Determine What Muscles Need to Be Trained

The first question requires an examination of the muscles and the specific joint angles designated to be trained. For any activity, including a sport, this involves a basic analysis of the movements performed and the most common sites of injury. With the proper equipment and a background in basic biomechanics, a more definitive approach to this question is possible. With the use of a slow-motion videotape, the coach can better evaluate specific aspects of movements and can conduct a qualitative analysis of the muscles, angles, velocities, and forces involved. The decisions made at this stage help define one of the acute program variables—choice of exercise.

Specificity is a major tenet of resistance training and is based in the concept that the exercises and resistances used result in training adaptations that will transfer to better performance in sport or daily activity. Resistance training is used because it is often difficult if not impossible to overload sports movements without risk of injury or dramatically altering sport skill technique. Specificity assumes that muscles must be trained similarly to the sport or activity in terms of:

➤ The joint around which movement occurs
➤ The joint range of motion
➤ The pattern of resistance throughout the range of motion
➤ The pattern of limb velocity throughout the range of motion
➤ Types of limb movement (e.g., concentric, eccentric, or isometric)

Resistance training for any sport or activity should include full range of motion exercises around all the major body joints. However, training designed for specific sports or activity movements should also be included in the workout to maximize the contribution of strength training to performance. The best way to select such exercises is to biomechanically analyze, in quantitative terms, the sport or physical activity and match it to exercises according to the above variables. Few such analyses of sports or activities have been done to date. Yet biomechanical principles can be used in a qualitative manner to intelligently select exercises. Ideally, this analysis is followed up with appropriate resistance exercises in the weight room that train the specific muscles and joint angles involved. For general fitness and muscular development, the major muscle groups of the shoulders, chest, back, and legs are usually trained.

Each exercise and resistance used in a program will have various amounts of transfer to another activity or sport. When training for improved health and well-being, such a concept of transfer is more related to its effects on medical variables (e.g., bone mineral density) rather than to physical performance. The concept of "transfer specificity" is unclear to many Personal Trainers and health/fitness professionals. Every training activity has a percentage of carryover to other activities. Except for practicing the specific task (e.g., lifting groceries or shoveling snow) or sport (e.g., running, basketball) itself, no conditioning activity has 100% carryover. However, some activities have a higher percentage of carryover than others because of similarities in neuromuscular recruitment patterns, energy systems, and biomechanical characteristics. Most of the time, one cannot use the sport or activity to gain the needed "overload" on the neuromuscular system, and this is why resistance training is used in the conditioning process. The optimal training program maximizes carryover to the sport or activity.

Determining the Energy Sources Used in the Activity

Performance of every sport or activity uses a percentage of all three energy sources. The energy sources (see Chapter 6) to be trained have a major impact on the program design. Resistance training usually stresses the anaerobic energy sources (ATP–CP energy source and glycolytic energy source) more than aerobic metabolism (14). It is very difficult for individuals who have gained initial cardiovascular fitness to improve maximal oxygen consumption values using conventional resistance training alone (15). However, resistance training can be used to improve performance by improving running efficiency and economy (16).

Selecting a Resistance Modality

Decisions regarding the use of isometric, dynamic concentric, dynamic eccentric, and isokinetic modalities of exercise are important in the preliminary stages of planning a resistance training program for sport, fitness, or rehabilitation. The basic biomechanical analysis is used to decide what muscles to train and to identify the type of muscle action involved in the activity. Most resistance training programs use several types of muscle actions. It is important to understand that not all equipment uses concentric and eccentric muscle actions and that this can reduce the training effectiveness (e.g., hydraulics) (12).

Injury Prevention Exercises

It is also important to determine the primary sites of injury in the sport or recreational activity performed along with the prior injury profile of the individual. The prescription of resistance training exercises will be directed at enhancing the strength and function of tissue so that it better resists injury, recovers faster when injured, and reduces the extent of damage related to an injury. The term "prehabilitation" (the opposite of rehabilitation) has become popular. This term refers to preventing initial injury by training the joints and muscles that are most susceptible to injury in an activity. The prevention of reinjury is also an important goal of a resistance training program. Thus, understanding the sport's or activity's typical injury profile (e.g., knees in downhill skiing or elbows for baseball pitchers) and the individual's prior history of injury can help in properly designing a resistance training program.

THE ACUTE PROGRAM VARIABLES

Developed more than 20 years ago, the paradigm of acute program variables allows one to define every workout (17). Every resistance exercise protocol or workout is derived from the five acute program variables. In turn, the choices made for each of these variables defines the exercise stimuli and ultimately, with repeated exposure, the training adaptations. Essentially, the choices made for the specific combination of acute program variables creates an exercise stimulus "fingerprint" that is specific and unique to that workout protocol. Thus, by making specific choices for the acute program variables that are related to the needs and goals of the client, the Personal Trainer is able to create many different types of workouts (5). The classical acute program variables are choice of exercises, order of exercises, resistance and repetitions used, number of sets for each exercise, and duration of rest period between sets and exercises.

Choice of Exercises

The choice of exercise will be related to the biomechanical characteristics of the goals targeted for improvement. The number of possible joint angles and exercises are almost as limitless as the body's functional movements. As muscle tissue that is not activated will not benefit from resistance training, the exercises should be selected so they stress the muscles, joints, and joint angles specified by the client's needs analysis. To aid the Personal Trainer in making these correct choices of exercise, exercises can be divided into several different categories based on their function and/or muscle involvement.

Exercises can be designated as primary exercises or assistance exercises. Primary exercises train the prime movers in a particular movement and are typically major muscle group exercises (e.g., leg press, bench press, hang pulls). Assistance exercises are exercises that train predominantly a single muscle group (e.g., triceps press, biceps curls) that aids (synergists) in the movement produced by the prime movers.

Exercises can also be classified as multi-joint or single-joint exercises. Multi-joint exercises require the coordinated action of several muscle groups and joints. Power cleans, power snatches, dead lifts, and squats are good examples of whole-body multi-joint exercises. The bench press, which involves movement of both the elbow and shoulder joints, is also a multi-joint, multi-muscle group exercise, although it only involves movement in the upper body. Some examples of other multiple-joint exercises are the lat pull-down, military press, and squat.

Exercises that attempt to isolate a particular muscle group's movement of a single joint are known as single-joint and/or single-muscle group exercises. Biceps curls, knee extensions, and knee curls are examples of isolated single-joint, single-muscle group exercises. Many assistance exercises may be classified as single-muscle group or single-joint exercises.

Multi-joint exercises require neural coordination among muscles and thus promote coordinated multi-joint and multi-muscle group movements. It has recently been shown that multi-joint exercises require a longer initial learning or neural phase than single-joint exercises (18); however, it is important to include multiple-joint exercises in a resistance training program, especially when whole-body strength movements are required for a particular activity. Most sports and functional activities in everyday life (e.g., climbing stairs) depend on structural multi-joint movements, and for most sports, whole-body strength/power movements are the basis for success. Running and jumping, as well as activities such as tackling in American football, a take down in wrestling, or hitting a baseball, all depend on whole-body strength/power movements. Thus, incorporating multi-joint exercises in a resistance training program is important for both athletes and non-athletes.

In addition, it is important to consider the inclusion of both bilateral (both limbs) and unilateral (single limb) exercises in a program to make sure that proper balance is seen in the development of the body. Unilateral exercises (e.g., dumbbell biceps curl) play an important role in helping to maintain equal strength in both limbs. Bilateral differences in muscle force production can be developed with one limb working harder on every repetition than the other, leading to an obvious force production deficit and imbalances between limbs.

Many multi-joint exercises, especially those with an explosive component, involve the need for advanced lifting techniques (e.g., power cleans, power snatches). These exercises require additional technique coaching beyond just the simple movement patterns. An important advantage to multi-joint exercises is that they are time efficient, since several different muscle groups are activated at the same time. Therefore they can be especially useful for an individual or team with a limited amount of time for each training session. In addition, the other benefits of multi-joint exercises, in terms of muscle tissue activated, hormonal response, and metabolic demands, also far outweigh single-joint exercises, and most workouts should revolve around these exercises.

Order of Exercises

The order in which the chosen exercises are performed is an important variable that affects the quality and focus of the workout. It has been theorized that by exercising the larger muscle groups first, a superior training stimulus is presented to all of the muscles involved. This is believed to be mediated by stimulating a greater neural, metabolic, endocrine, and circulatory response, which potentially may augment the training with subsequent muscles or exercises trained later in the workout. This concept also applies to the sequencing of multi- and single-joint exercises. The more complex multi-joint exercises (e.g., squats) should be performed initially followed by the less complex single-joint exercises (e.g., biceps curls).

The sequencing rationale for this exercise order is that the exercises performed in the beginning of the workout require the greatest amount of muscle mass and energy for optimal performance. This has been observed by Simao et al. (19), who found that performing exercises of both the large and the small muscle groups at the end of an exercise sequence resulted in significantly fewer repetitions in the three sets of an exercise. This decrease in the number of repetitions performed was especially apparent in the third set, when an exercise was performed last in an exercise sequence (19). These sequencing strategies focus on attaining a greater training effect for the large muscle group exercises. If multi-joint exercises are performed early in the workout, more resistance can be used due to a limited amount of fatigue in the smaller muscle groups that assist the prime movers during the multi-joint exercises. Also, alternating upper and lower body exercises and/or pushing and pulling exercises allows more time for the assisting muscle to recover between exercises.

As the order of exercise affects the outcome of a training program, it is important to have the exercise order correspond to the specific training goals. In general, the sequence of exercises for both multiple and single muscle group exercise sessions should be as follows:

1. Large muscle group before small muscle group exercises
2. Multi-joint before single-joint exercises
3. Alternating push/pull exercises for total body sessions
4. Alternating upper/lower body exercises for total body sessions
5. Explosive/power type lifts (e.g., Olympic lifts) before basic strength and single-joint exercises
6. Exercises for weak areas (priority) performed before exercises for strong areas of the client
7. Most intense to least intense (particularly when performing several exercises consecutively for the same muscle group)

Resistance and Repetitions Used

The amount of resistance used for a specific exercise is one of the key variables in any resistance training program. It is the major stimulus related to changes observed in measures of strength and local muscular endurance. When designing a resistance training program, the resistance for each exercise must be chosen carefully. The use of either repetition maximums (RM, the maximal load that can be lifted the specified number of repetitions) or the absolute resistance, which only allows a specific number of repetitions to be performed, is probably the easiest method for determining a resistance. Typically, a single training RM target (e.g., 10RM) or a RM target range (e.g., 3–5RM) is used. Throughout the training program, the absolute resistance is then adjusted to match the changes in strength so a true RM target or RM target range resistance continues to be used. Performing every set until failure occurs can be stressful on the joints, but it is important to ensure that the resistance used corresponds to the targeted number of repetitions. This is because performing 3 to 5 repetitions with a resistance that allows for only 3–5 repetitions or using a resistance that would allow 13 or 15 repetitions produces quite different training results.

Another method of determining resistances for an exercise involves using a percentage of the 1RM (e.g., 70 or 85% of the 1RM). If the client's 1RM for an exercise is 200 lb (90.9 kg), a 70% resistance would be 140 lb (63.6 kg). This method requires that the maximal strength in all exercises used in the training program must be evaluated regularly. In some exercises, %1RM needs to be used, as going to failure or near-failure is not optimal (e.g., power cleans, Olympic-style lifts). Without regular 1RM testing (e.g., each week), the percentage of 1RM actually used during training, especially at the beginning of a program, will decrease, and the training intensity will be reduced. From a practical perspective, use of percentages of 1RM as the resistance for many exercises may not be administratively effective because of the amount of testing time required. In addition, for beginners, the reliability of a 1RM test can be poor. It is therefore recommended that the RM target or RM target range be used, as it gives the Personal Trainer the ability to alter the resistance in response to changes in the number of repetitions that can be performed at a given absolute resistance.

As is the case for the acute program variables, the loading intensity should depend on the goal and training status of the client. The intensity of the loading (as a percentage of 1RM) has an effect on the number of repetitions that can be performed, and vice versa. It is ultimately the number of repetitions that can be performed at a given intensity that will determine the effects of training on strength development (20, 21). If a given absolute resistance allows a specific number of repetitions (defined as the repetition maximum), then any reductions in the number of repetitions without an increase in the resistance will cause a change in the training stimulus. In this case, the change in the stimulus will lead to a change in the motor units recruited to perform the exercise and thus the neuromuscular adaptations. It is also important to understand that differences exist between free weights and machines for percentage of RM used. For example, in a squat exercise one may only be able to perform 8 to 10 repetitions, while in the leg press, 15 to 20 repetitions are possible. Differences exist owing to the amount of balance and control that is needed in the exercise, with free weight exercises requiring more neural control and activation of assistance muscle. In addition, the size of the muscle groups used influences this effect as well. With 80% (of 1RM) in an arm curl, a client may only be able to do 6 to 8 repetitions, so as the muscle group gets smaller, the response to a given percentage of the 1RM gets smaller.

Specific neuromuscular adaptations to resistance training depend in large part on the resistance used. These adaptations follow the SAID principle presented earlier in this chapter. Heavier resistances will produce lower numbers of repetitions (1–6) but will lead to greater improvements in maximal strength (22, 23). Thus, if maximal strength is desired, heavier loads should be used. Alternately, if muscular endurance is the goal, a lower load should be used, which will in turn allow a greater number of repetitions (12–15) to be returned (22, 23).

Number of Sets for Each Exercise

First, the number of sets does not have to be the same for all exercises in a workout program. In reality, apart from training mythologies, the number of sets performed for each exercise is one variable in what is referred to as the *volume* of exercise equation (e.g., sets × reps × resistance) calculation. As such, one of the major roles of the number of sets performed is to regulate the volume performed during a particular exercise protocol or training program. In studies examining resistance-trained individuals, multiple-set programs have been found to be superior for strength, power, hypertrophy, and high-intensity endurance improvements (24, 25). These findings have prompted the recommendation from the American College of Sports Medicine (22) for periodized multiple-set programs when long-term progression (not maintenance) is the goal. No study has shown single-set training to be superior to multiple-set training in either trained or untrained individuals. Thus, it appears that both single- and multi-set programs can be effective in increasing strength in untrained clients during short-term training periods (i.e., 6–12 weeks). However, some short-term (22, 23) and all long-term studies (22, 23) support the contention that the greater training stimulus associated with the higher volume from multiple sets is needed to create further improvement and progression in physical adaptation and performance. Yet variation in training stimuli, as is discussed in detail later, is also critical for continued improvement. This variation often includes a reduction in training volume during certain phases of the overall training program. The determining factor here is in the "periodization" of training volume rather than in the number of sets, which is only one of the components in the volume equation. Once initial fitness has been achieved, a multiple presentation of the exercise stimulus (three to six sets), with specific rest periods between sets to allow use of the desired resistance, is superior to a single presentation of the training stimulus. Some advocates of single-set programs believe that a muscle or muscle group can only perform maximal exercise for a single set; however, this has not been demonstrated. On the contrary, studies have found that with sufficient rest between sets, trained individuals can produce the same maximal effort during multiple sets (22).

Exercise volume is a vital concept in resistance training progression, especially for those who have already achieved a basic level of training or strength fitness. As mentioned earlier, the principle of variation in training or more specifically "periodized training" involves the number of sets performed. As the use of a constant-volume program can lead to staleness and lack of adherence to training, variations in training volume (i.e., both low- and high-volume exercise protocols) is important during a long-term training program to provide adequate rest and recovery periods. This concept is addressed later in this chapter under "Periodization of Exercise." Multiple-set programs are superior for long-term progression, but one-set programs are effective for developing and maintaining a certain level of muscular strength and endurance. For some fitness enthusiasts, this given level of muscular fitness may be adequate. Also, one-set programs sometimes result in greater compliance by those who are limited in their time for exercise and also need to perform cardiovascular exercise, flexibility exercise, etc. It is better for the client to do one set than no sets at all.

Duration of Rest Period between Sets and Exercises

The rest periods play an important role in dictating the metabolic stress of the workout and influence the amount of resistance that can be used during each set or exercise. A major reason for this is that the primary energy system used during resistance exercise, the ATP–creatine phosphate system, needs to be replenished, and this process takes time (see Chapter 6). Therefore, the duration of the rest period significantly influences the metabolic, hormonal, and cardiovascular responses to a short-term bout of resistance exercise, as well as the performance of subsequent sets (26, 27). For advanced training emphasizing absolute strength or power (few repetitions and maximal or near-maximal resistance), rest periods of at least 3–5 minutes are recommended for large muscle mass multi-joint exercises (such as squat, power clean, or dead lift); whereas shorter rest may be sufficient for smaller muscle mass exercises or single-joint movements (22). For a novice-to-intermediate resistance exercise protocol, rest periods of 2–3 minutes may suffice for large muscle mass multi-joint exercises, since the lower absolute resistance used at this training level seems to be less stressful to the neuromuscular system. Performance of maximal resistance exercises requires maximal energy substrate availability at the onset of the exercise and a minimum fatigue level and thus requires relatively long rest periods between sets and exercises.

Resistance training that stresses both the glycolytic and ATP–creatine phosphate energy systems appears to be superior in enhancing muscle hypertrophy (e.g., bodybuilding), thus less rest between sets appears to be more effective in high levels of muscular definition. If the goal is to optimize both strength and muscle mass, both long rest with heavy loading and short rest with moderate loading types of workout protocols should be used. However, it should be kept in mind that the short-rest resistance training programs can potentially cause greater psychological anxiety and fatigue because of the greater discomfort, muscle fatigue, and high metabolic demands of the program (28). Therefore, psychological ramifications of using short-rest workouts must be carefully considered and discussed with the client before the training program is designed. The increase in anxiety appears to be associated with the high metabolic demands found with short-rest exercise protocols (i.e., 1 minute or less). Despite the high psychological demands, the changes in mood states do not constitute abnormal psychological changes and may be a part of the normal arousal process before a demanding workout.

The key to rest-period lengths is the observation of symptoms of loss of force production in the beginning of the workout and clinical symptoms of nausea, dizziness, and fainting, which are direct signs of the inability to tolerate the workout. When such symptoms occur, the workout should be stopped and longer rest periods used in subsequent workouts. With aging, decreased ability to tolerate decreases in muscle and blood pH underscores the need for gradual progression when cutting rest period lengths between sets and exercises (26). Rest periods may be thought of as:

➤ Very short rest periods—1 minute or shorter
➤ Short rest periods—1 to 2 minutes
➤ Moderate rest periods—2 to 3 minutes
➤ Long rest periods—3 to 4 minutes
➤ Very long rest periods—5 minutes or longer

The more rest that is allowed between sets and exercises, the heavier the resistance and the greater the number of repetitions that can be performed at a specific RM load (26, 29). Improvements take place for a given rest period when the body's bicarbonate and phosphate, blood and muscle buffering systems, respectively, are improved by the gradual use of shorter rest period lengths (26, 29).

VARIATION OF THE ACUTE PROGRAM VARIABLES

The acute program variables can be manipulated to develop different workouts for the single-exercise sessions used over time. Also, the number of sets, number of repetitions, relative resistance used, and rest periods do not have to be the same for each exercise in a session. They can all be varied either within an exercise or, more frequently, between different exercises in an exercise protocol. Variation must seek to address the needed change in the demands placed on the neuromuscular system over time, with planned rest a vital part of this principle. It is also important to understand that one can use light exercise to rest higher threshold motor units (i.e., motor neuron and associated muscle fibers). Understanding the "size principle" in this regard is important, as not all motor units are recruited with each resistance loading experience of a muscle, and therefore, different loadings can result in different amounts of muscle tissue being used. Heavier loads with adequate volume recruit more muscle tissue and are one reason why women need to have heavy loading cycles in their resistance training programs (5). The use of the size principle is vital for understanding variation in resistance training and ultimately periodized training.

Muscle Actions

Muscles can produce force while performing one of three different actions:

1. When sufficient force is produced to overcome the external load and shorten the muscle, the actions is termed *concentric* muscle action or contraction.
2. If the muscle produces force but there is no change in length of the muscle, the action is termed *isometric*.
3. Production of force while the muscle is lengthening (i.e., resisting the movement) is termed *eccentric* muscle action.

In the past, the term *contraction* was used for each of the three muscle actions; however, this use is inappropriate, since only the concentric muscle actions actually involve a muscle contraction. An exercise can include one, all, or any combination of the three muscle actions; however, most exercises are performed using either isometric muscle action or both concentric and eccentric muscle actions. The force–velocity curve runs from high- to low-speed eccentric muscle actions to maximal isometric muscle action to slow- to high-velocity concentric muscle contractions, creating a descending hierarchy of force productions. However, the most effective training programs appear to use concentric/eccentric repetitions (12).

True Repetition and Range of Movement

Muscle actions involving movement of a joint are termed *dynamic,* and thus exercises involving joint movements are called dynamic exercises. A full-range dynamic exercise repetition usually contains both a concentric and an eccentric phase. The order of the phases depends on the choice of exercise. A squat, for example, starts with the eccentric phase; a pull-up normally starts with the concentric phase. It is important to perform the exercise so that the joints involved move through a large range of motion. For single-joint exercises especially, it is important to move the joint through the full range of motion. For example, in the arm curl, a full repetition should start with the elbow almost completely extended, progress until the elbow is maximally flexed, and finish with the elbow almost completely extended again. By using the whole range of motion, the whole length of the muscle is stimulated, leading to adaptations throughout the whole muscle and not just in parts of it.

PERIODIZATION OF EXERCISE

Periodization is a concept, and the exact design or workouts used are the program and its application (30). Understanding some of the basic concepts about periodization is important to create workouts and the actual periodized program using the acute program variables. Periodization refers to systematic changes in the prescribed volume and intensity during different phases of a resistance training program. A traditional periodization program contains four phases:

1. Hypertrophy, consisting of high volume and short rest period
2. Strength/power, consisting of reduced volume but increased load and rest periods
3. Peaking, consisting of low volume but high load and longer rest periods
4. Recovery, consisting of low volume and load

There is no set formula for how a program should be periodized, as it depends on the specific goals and needs of the clients (31). Table 17.1 presents an example of a traditional four-phase periodized training program aimed at producing maximal power and strength.

The reason for incorporating periodization into the training program is that by changing some of the acute program variables, the muscles are exposed to different stimuli to which they must adapt differently, leading to greater increases in performance. In addition, rest is encouraged at different points in the training program, which allows for recovery and the prevention of both short- and long-term overtraining. Another important benefit to periodization is that it can reduce the potential boredom found with repeating the same resistance exercise program over and over again. This may well affect adherence to a fitness program. Many different models for periodization have been

Table 17.1	TRADITIONAL AMERICAN STYLE PERIODIZATION SCHEDULE			
Goal	**Hypertrophy**	**Maximal Strength/Power**	**Peak**	**Recovery**
Reps	High	Moderate-low	Low	Moderate
Sets	High	Moderate	Low	Moderate
Rest	Short	Moderate	Long	Moderate
Load	Low	Moderate	Very high	Low
Volume	High-moderate	Moderate	Low	Low

developed, thus the model to be used should be selected on the basis of the needs and desires of the client.

The popular terms "micro-, meso-, and macrocycle" refer to different phases of periodization. The largest time frame for a training cycle is the *macrocycle*. In the example used in this chapter, a macrocycle refers to a year, and all phases are included in this cycle. A *mesocycle* refers to the next smaller group of training cycles that make up the macrocycle, usually four to six in a year. Finally, the *microcycle* is a the smallest component, which usually ranges in time from 1 to 4 weeks dedicated to one type of workout variable in that phase (e.g., high volume, low intensity, power). Anecdotally it has been found that more mesocycles are more beneficial to the overall training effect, and this leads to the concept that higher degrees of variation in the training stimulus are more effective in producing overall adaptations in the body. In part, this leads to many different variations in the classic periodization model, including non-linear periodization.

The use of periodized resistance training has been shown to be superior to constant training methods. Periodized training involves the planned variation in the intensity of exercises and in the volume of a workout. Typically, one periodizes large muscle group exercises. However, variation schemes can be created for smaller muscle groups. One must consider the type of periodized program to use. In general, there are two basic types that have developed, linear and non-linear periodized protocols for maximal strength development.

Linear Periodization

Classic periodization methods use a progressive increase in the intensity with small variations in each 1- to 4-week microcycle. An example of a classic four-cycle linear periodized program (4 weeks for each cycle) is presented in Table 17-2.

One can see that there is some variation within each microcycle due to the repetition range of each cycle. Still, the general trend for the 16-week program is a steady linear increase in the intensity of the training program. Microcycle 5 is a 2-week active rest period in which no lifting is done or at best very light, low-volume training is used prior to the next mesocycle. Because of the straight-line increase in the intensity of the program, it has been termed "linear" periodized training. Since most training programs from which periodization evolved were of the single-peaking nature (e.g., track and field, weightlifting), consecutive build-up to the peak was used in this so-called classic method. Now many more models exist that are hybrids of this classical model.

The volume of the training program will also vary with the classic program, starting with a higher initial volume, and as the intensity of the program increases, the volume gradually decreases. The drop-off between the intensity and volume of exercise can decrease as the training status of the individual advances. In other words, advanced athletes can tolerate higher volumes of exercise during the heavy and very heavy microcycles.

It is important to point out here that one must be very careful not to progress too quickly to train with high volumes and heavy weights. Pushing too hard has the potential for a serious overtraining

Table 17.2	**AN EXAMPLE OF A CLASSIC LINEAR PERIODIZED PROGRAM USING 4-WEEK MICROCYCLES**
Microcycle 1 3–5 sets of 12–15RM	**Microcycle 4** 3–5 sets of 1–3RM
Microcycle 2 4–5 sets of 8–10RM	**Microcycle 5 (2 weeks)** Active rest/recovery
Microcycle 3 3–4 sets of 4–6RM	

syndrome. Overtraining can compromise progress for weeks or even months. While it takes a great deal of excessive work to produce such a long-term overtraining effect, highly motivated individuals can easily make mistakes out of sheer desire to make gains and see rapid progress in their training. So it is important to monitor the stress of the workouts and the total conditioning program. Exercises within a program can interact to compromise each other.

The purpose of the high-volume exercise in the early microcycles is that it has been thought to promote the muscle hypertrophy needed to eventually enhance strength in the later phases of training. Thus, the late cycles of training are linked to the early cycles of training, and they enhance each other as strength gains are related to size changes in the muscle. Programs that attempt to gain strength without the needed muscle tissue are limited in their potential.

The increases in the intensity of the periodized program then start to develop the needed nervous system adaptations for enhanced motor unit recruitment. This happens as the program progresses and heavier resistances are used. Heavier weights demand higher threshold motor units to become involved in the force production process. The subsequent increase in muscle protein from the early cycle training enhances force production from the motor units. Here again one sees integration of the different parts of the 16-week training program.

The completion of all of the cycles in this 16-week program would be one mesocycle, and a year training program (macrocycle) is made up of several mesocycles. Again, shorter mesocycles have been used to better delineate the different trainable features of muscle. Each mesocycle attempts to progress the body's musculature upward toward one's theoretical genetic maximum for a given variable. Thus, the theoretical basis for a linear method of periodization consists of developing the body with a sequential loading from light to heavy and from high volume to low volume, thereby addressing the goals of the program for that training cycle while providing active rest at the completion of the mesocycle. This is repeated again and again with each mesocycle, and progress is made in the training program over an entire macrocycle.

Non-Linear Periodized Programs

More recently, the concept of non-linear periodized training programs has been developed to maintain variation in the training stimulus. However, non-linear periodized training makes implementation of the program possible because of schedule, business, or competitive demands placed on the individual. The non-linear program allows variation in the intensity and volume within each week over the course of the training program (e.g., 12 weeks). Active rest is then taken after the 12-week mesocycle. The change in the intensity and volume of training will vary within the cycle, which could be 7–14 days. An example of a non-linear periodized training program over a 12-week mesocycle is shown in Table 17.3.

Table 17.3 **EXAMPLE OF A NON-LINEAR PERIODIZED TRAINING PROTOCOL**
This protocol uses a 4-day rotation with 1-day rest between workouts.
Monday 1 set 12–15RM
Wednesday 3 sets of 8–10RM
Friday 4 sets of 4–6RM
Monday Power day, 6 sets of 3 at 30–45% of 1RM in using power exercises (e.g., hang pulls etc) /*Plyometrics*

The variation in training is much greater within the 7-day period. One can easily see that intensity spans a wide range. This is but just one set of workout options for intensity and volume, and many others can be created. This span in training variation appears to be as effective as linear programs. One can also add a "power" training day in which loads may be from 30 to 45% of 1RM and exercises must not have a high deceleration component, so the choice of exercise and/or equipment used is vital (e.g., Olympic lifts or pneumatic resistance) so that no deceleration exists with the movement of the joint(s), or one can have a plyometric training day of different exercises and intensities (e.g., jumps, bounds, medicine ball exercises).

Unlike the linear programs, one trains the different components of muscle size, strength, and power within the same week. Unlike the linear methods, non-linear programs attempt to train different features of muscle within the same week (e.g., hypertrophy and power and strength). Thus, one is working at two different physiological adaptations together within the same 7- to 10-day period of the 12-week mesocycle. Such a periodization model may be more conducive to many individual's schedules, especially when travel, school, competitions, or other schedule conflicts can make adherence to the traditional linear method difficult.

In this program, one just rotates through the different protocols. The workout rotates different workouts with the different training sessions. If one misses the Monday workout, the rotation order is just pushed forward, meaning one just performs the rotated workout scheduled. For example, if the light 12–15 workout was scheduled for Monday and you miss it, you just perform it on Wednesday and continue with the rotation sequence. In this way, no workout stimulus is missed in the training program. One can also say that a mesocycle will be completed when a certain number of workouts are completed (e.g., 48) and not use training weeks to set the program length.

One of the new advances in periodization is called "unplanned non-linear periodization." The name is somewhat of a misnomer, as an overall plan is developed for a 12-week mesocycle, but the actual day that a given workout will be performed is based on the readiness to train. In other words, in unplanned non-linear periodization, a workout plan is set for the mesocycle but deciding what workout is to be done on what day is left to the Personal Trainer, who will base it on the client's fatigue level, psychological state, or fitness, to use only the most optimal workout that can be performed on a given day. In this model, the training session category (e.g., light, moderate, power, or heavy) is prescribed based on the physiological ability or state of the client at the time of the session. Thus, if the client is very fatigued before a particular exercise session, some workouts would not be prescribed (e.g., a power training or plyometrics training day or a high-volume, low-rest training day would not be a good choice because prior fatigue would dramatically reduce the workout quality). After a workout is done, it is checked off in the major planning matrix for the 12-week mesocycle.

In any periodization model, it is the primary exercises that are typically periodized, but one can also use a two-cycle periodization program to vary the small muscle group exercises. For example in the "triceps pushdown" one could rotate between the moderate (8–10RM) and the heavy (4–6RM) cycle intensities. This would provide the hypertrophy needed for such isolated muscles of a joint but also provide the strength needed to support heavier workouts of the large muscle groups.

In summary, two different approaches can be used to periodize a resistance training program, specifically, linear and non-linear program workout schedules. The programs appear to accomplish the same effect and appear superior to constant-intensity training programs. This seems to be accomplished by training either the hypertrophy component first and then the neural strength component second in the linear method and both components within a 7- to 14-day time period, depending on the number of workout types one uses in the non-linear method. The key to workout success is variation, and different approaches can be used over the year to accomplish this training need.

PROGRESSION FROM BEGINNER TO ADVANCED

The level of fitness and resistance training experience of the client is maybe the most important factor to be considered when designing a resistance training program. Resistance exercise can place a large stress on the body, and certain exercises require a high level of technique to avoid injury.

The most important aspect for beginners is resistance exercise techniques. At the beginning of the training program, correct technique of the exercises involved should be stressed, and the resistance and volume should be kept low. From a strictly short-term performance-enhancement point of view, a single set per exercise may be enough for beginners to achieve the stimulus needed from an exercise.

Although multiple sets may not lead to greater improvements in performance for beginners in the short term, there may still be benefits to using multiple sets from the onset of the training program (25, 32). One reason for this is that more repetitions can lead to faster improvements in the technique of the exercises involved in the training program, especially for multi-joint exercises. The squat exercise is an example of an exercise that requires a great deal of technique to be performed correctly. In addition, some studies have found that multiple sets even for beginners create larger improvements than single sets; whereas no study has found that single sets are superior (32).

As the client progresses past the initial few months of training, multi-sets should be used for each exercise session. As the skill level and experience of the client improves, more technical exercises can be taught. Advanced resistance training can include highly technical exercises such as the clean or the snatch, as well as advanced modalities such as plyometric exercises. The progression will differ among individuals, and the Personal Trainer must evaluate each client extensively and continuously before including more advanced exercises, to ensure that the exercises match the client's skill and experience level.

CLIENTS

Client Interactions

As a Personal Trainer working with clients, it is important to encourage and motivate them as well as to provide innovative, optimal, individualized resistance training programs. Many clients hire a Personal Trainer because they feel they need constant guidance. In addition, it provides them with a support system. Most importantly, they are hiring a professional with training and knowledge in conditioning science. They are also hiring a professional to help them perform exercises properly and who understands exercise prescription to allow them to achieve their personal goals and objectives. For some clients, it is an important part of their sports conditioning program. Ultimately, the Personal Trainer must form a special relationship with each and every client that is based on professionalism, trust, and openness (*Fig. 17.4*).

Clients should feel that their Personal Trainer genuinely cares about them and is personally vested in helping them achieve their goals. Clients expect their Personal Trainer to be a source of knowledge and an educator. Clients expect their Personal Trainer to be able to explain things or answer the question "Why?" Thus, clients appreciate having their Personal Trainer explain why they are doing this exercise or this combination of sets and reps in their program. Personal training has been found to be superior to unsupervised training, even for people who understand resistance training (33).

Additionally, Personal Trainers should convey the specific benefits of resistance training, including increases in strength, muscle mass, and bone mass, particularly to clients who may be skeptical about why resistance training is important. Many uneducated clients may have false impressions of the outcome from resistance training. In particular, some women often perform programs that are not optimal, excluding a heavy loading workout or cycles because of the "fear of

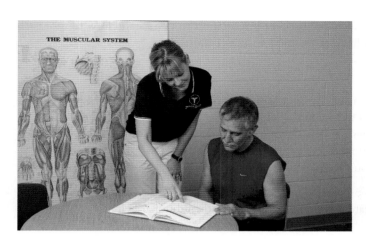

FIGURE 17.4. Education and being a credible source of knowledge as a fitness expert is part of what Personal Trainers must provide to their clients. This takes continual study and preparation to stay current and up to date on basic topics and hot topics of the day.

getting big muscles." This misunderstanding of resistance training effects has held many women back in achieving optimal gains in muscle tissue mass and bone mineral density, which are challenged to a greater extent in women as they age.

Clients consider Personal Trainers experts and will often want to hear their opinion on fads facing the fitness industry. Often clients' knowledge of resistance training comes from infomercials and magazine marketing products, which often mislead clients by encouraging the sales of the various products. It is important for Personal Trainers to stay educated and ideally current with the scientific literature and know how to do research on topics of interest to their clients. Clients will also ask questions the Personal Trainer cannot answer (nobody knows everything). In these cases, it is best for the Personal Trainer to admit that he or she does not know the answer but will find it from experts in the field, thus showing a broader network of people who can act as resources. This is always a better strategy than conveying potentially incorrect information. Furthermore, Personal Trainers are often required to obtain continuing education credits to maintain their certifications; therefore, staying current is critical to success.

SPOTTING IN RESISTANCE EXERCISE

In comparison with other components of a complete fitness program (such as cardiovascular conditioning), resistance training often requires more physical interaction between the client and Personal Trainer to ensure proper positioning, fit and set-up of a machine, and techniques in both machine and free-weight exercises. It is important for the Personal Trainer to explain to clients the spotting procedures in resistance training and the level of physical interaction required between the client and the Personal Trainer. Always ask your client before physically touching them, to ensure that they are comfortable with it. For example, when performing elbow extension exercises, it is sometimes helpful for the Personal Trainer to place his or her hands on the client's elbows as a reminder to keep the elbow from pointing outward. In these cases, explain to the client, "I am going to put my hands on your elbows to remind you to keep them from pointing outward. Is this okay with you?" In most cases, clients will have no problem with this physical contact, but it is always better to ask than to assume.

Know Proper Spotting Technique

Good spotting technique is vital for a safe resistance training program. It is important for the Personal Trainer to understand proper technique for every exercise and how to position clients for the exercise, whether it is in a machine that may not fit all people or with free weights to get the proper anatomical positioning throughout the exercises. Most important is to understand how to spot each and every exercise in a program. A checklist for the Personal Trainer is:

1. Know proper exercise technique
2. Know proper spotting technique
3. Be sure you are strong enough to assist the lifter with the resistance being used or get help
4. Know how many repetitions the lifter intends to do
5. Be attentive to the lifter at all times
6. Stop lifters if exercise technique is incorrect or they break form
7. Know the plan of action if a serious injury occurs

The goal of correct spotting is to prevent injury. A lifter should always have an exercise spotted, and the Personal Trainer must mediate this process, alone or with additional help.

RESISTANCE EXERCISES

A large number of resistance exercises can be used in a program. It is beyond the scope of this chapter to go through each and every exercise. The reader is referred to a comprehensive list of over 125 exercise descriptions of both machine and free-weight exercises along with spotting techniques, by Kraemer and Fleck (34). Each program should be designed on the basis of the principles outlined in this chapter. Free weights and machines can be used for each exercise as well as bilateral and unilateral exercises. See Figure 17.5, A–O, for examples.

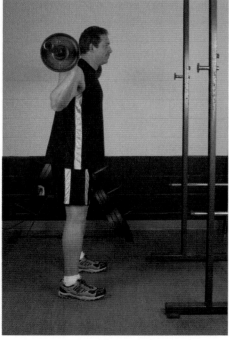
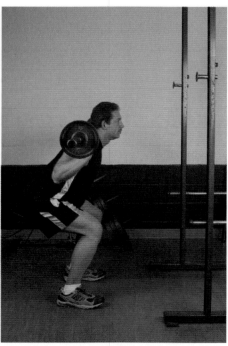

A Start Finish

FIGURE 17.5. A. Back squat (thighs). Place the barbell on the back of the shoulders and grasp the barbell at the sides, with feet shoulder-width apart, toes slightly out. Dismount bar from rack. Descend until thighs are just past parallel to the floor and then extend the knees and hips until legs are straight, returning you to the starting position. Repeat for the appropriate number of repetitions. Keep the head forward with the chin level, back straight, and feet flat on the floor; keep equal distribution of weight throughout forefoot and heel and either squat within the power rack or have spotter(s).

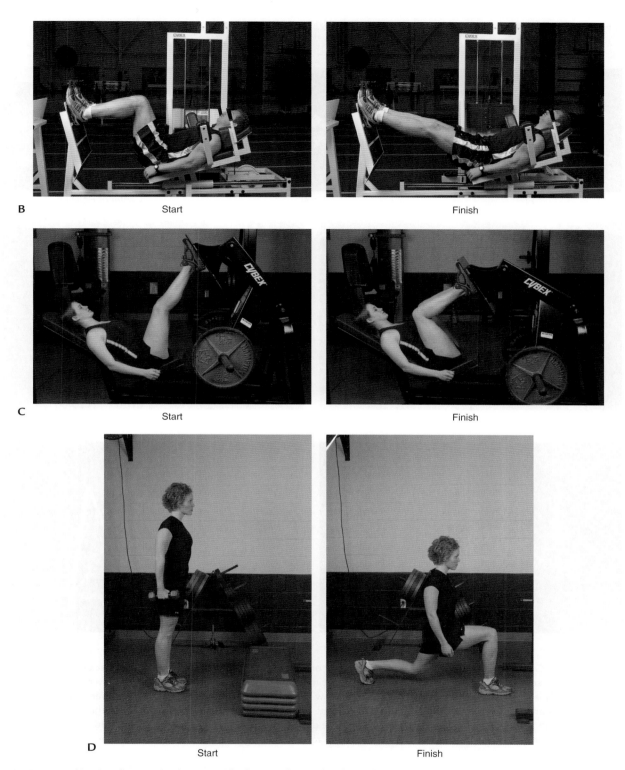

FIGURE 17.5. *(Continued)* **B.** Supine leg press (thighs). Lie flat on the sled with shoulders against the pad. Place the feet on the platform, making sure they are securely on the base plate. Extend the hips and knees. Flex the hips and knees until the knees are just short of complete flexion and return to the starting position to complete the repetition. Keep the feet flat on the platform and do not lock the knees. A full range of motion should be used; keep the knees in the same direction as the feet. **C.** 45° leg press (thighs). Lie down on the machine with the back on the padded supports. Place the feet on the platform. Grasp the handles on the side and release the weight. Lower the weight by flexing the hips and knees until the hips are completely flexed and then extend the knees to complete the repetition. Make sure the feet are flat on the platform and the knees track over the feet. **D.** Lunge (thighs, unilateral). Standing straight up with feet shoulder-width apart, stand holding the dumbbells at the sides. Lunge forward with one leg at a time, keeping the hips in the middle of the two legs, with the trailing knee just above the ground. Return to the standing position to complete the repetition and then repeat with the opposite leg. Keep the back straight and chin level with the ground.

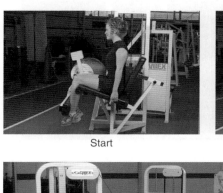
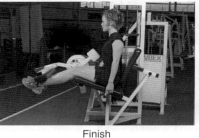
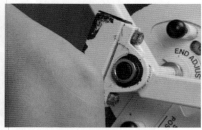

E   Start   Finish   Center of Rotation

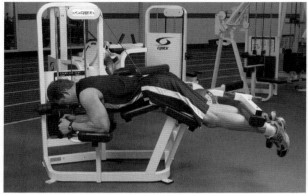
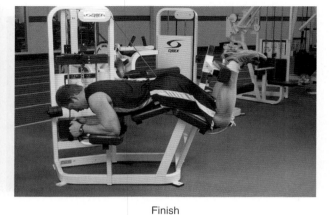

F   Start   Finish

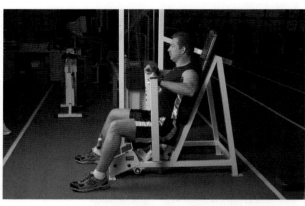
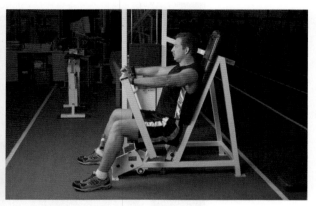

G   Start   Finish

FIGURE 17.5. *(Continued)* **E.** Leg extensions (thighs, bilateral or unilateral). Sit on the machine with the back straight against the back pad or seat and grasp the handles on the side of the machine. Place the legs under the padded lever, making sure they are positioned just above the ankles. Most machines will allow adjusting the length of the lever. Lift the lever until the legs are almost straight and return to the starting position to complete the repetition. It is important not to "rip" the plates off the stack, as this can add stress to the knees. This exercise can be done with a single leg (unilateral) or with both legs (bilateral). Make sure the knees are aligned with the machine's center of rotation. **F.** Leg curls (hamstrings, bilateral or unilateral). Lying face down, grab the support handles in the front of the machine with the heels just beyond the edge of the lever pads. Lift the lever arm by flexing the knees until they are straight. Return to the starting position to complete the repetition. Keep the body on the bench and focus on moving only the legs. Many machines are angled so that the user is in a better position for the exercise movement, to reduce stress on the lower back. Other forms of leg curls are standing and seated forms. This exercise can be done with a single leg (unilateral) or with both legs (bilateral). **G.** Vertical machine bench press (chest–triceps, bilateral). Sit on the seat, making sure that the line of the grips are just below the chest. The bar line should be an inch above the chest. Grasp the handles with an overhand grip and make sure the feet are flat on the ground. Push the lever arm straight out until the elbows are straight. Return to the starting position to complete one repetition.

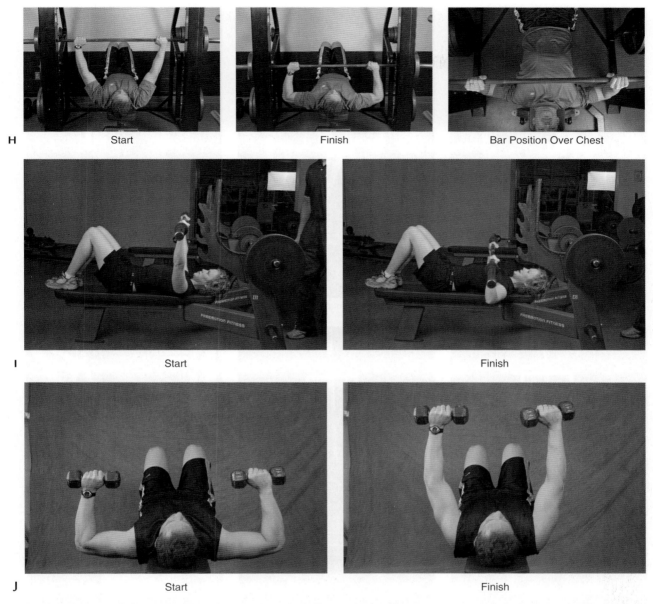

H   Start   Finish   Bar Position Over Chest

I   Start   Finish

J   Start   Finish

FIGURE 17.5. *(Continued)* **H.** Smith supine bench press (chest–triceps, bilateral). Lie flat on the bench with the upper chest under the bar, as shown in the bar position figure above. Place the feet flat on the floor unless the bench is too high, in which case put them flat on the bench. Keep the shoulders and hips on the bench at all times during the lift. Grasp the bar with elbows at 45° angles. Disengage the bar hooks from the Smith machine. Lower the weight to the chest and then press the bar up until arms are extended to complete the repetition. When completed, re-hook the bar to the machine. **I.** Free weight supine bench press (chest–triceps, bilateral). Lie flat on the bench with the upper chest under the bar, as shown in the bar position figure above. Place the feet flat on the floor unless the bench is too high, in which case put them flat on the bench. Keep the shoulders and hips on the bench at all times during the lift. Grasp the bar with elbows at 45° angles. Lower the weight to the chest and then press the bar up until the arms are extended to complete the repetition. When completed, re-rack the bar with a spotter's help. **J.** Dumbbell bench press (chest–upper arms–triceps, unilateral). Start in a seated position on the bench with a dumbbell in each hand resting on the lower thigh. Lift the weights to the shoulder and lie back on the bench or have the spotter give you the dumbbells once you are in position. Position the dumbbells to the side of the upper chest. Press the dumbbells up until the arms are extended and then return to complete a repetition. When completed, return to the seated position with the dumbbells on your thighs or have the spotter take the dumbbells. If heavy weights are used, two spotters may be necessary.

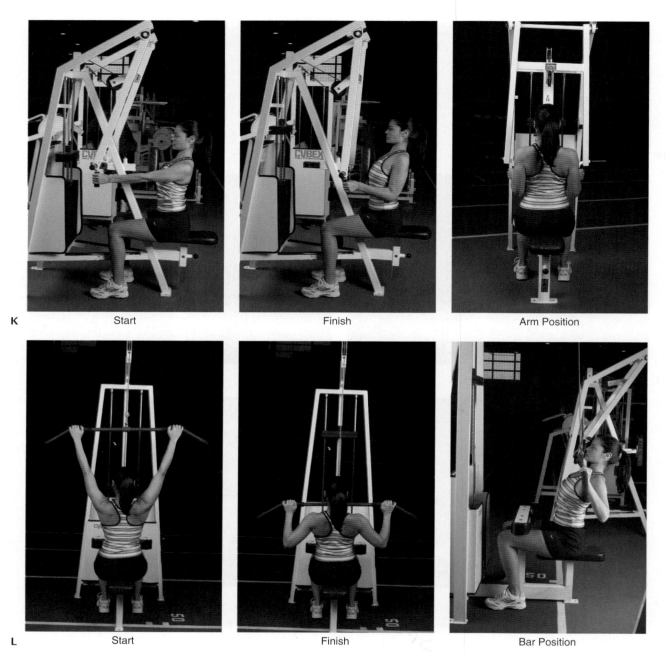

K   Start   Finish   Arm Position

L   Start   Finish   Bar Position

FIGURE 17.5. *(Continued)* **K.** Machine seated rows (upper back, bilateral). Take a seated position with the chest against the pad. Grasp the lever vertical handles with a vertical or horizontal overhand grip. Pull the lever back until the elbows are in line with the upper body and return to complete the repetition. Check the seat height so that the chest is directly in front of the lever handles and check that the client is pulling in a straight line parallel to the ground. The client can use an overhand grip as a variation to the movement using the other horizontal handles. **L.** Front lat pull down (upper back, bilateral). Use a locked grip (thumb around the bar) and grasp the cable bar with a wide grip. Sit with thighs under machine support. Proceed to pull down the bar to the upper chest. Return to the starting position to complete the repetition.

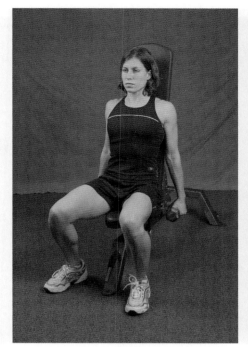
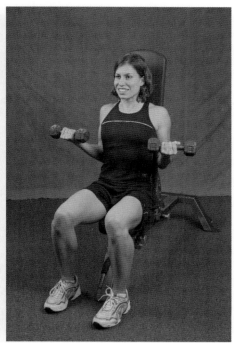

M   Start   Finish

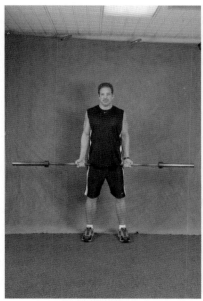
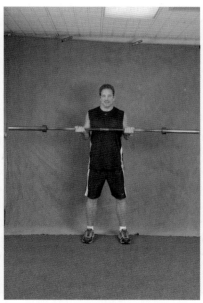
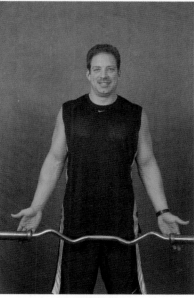

N   Start   Finish   E-Z Bar

FIGURE 17.5. *(Continued)* **M.** Dumbbell arm curls (upper arm–biceps, unilateral). Take a seated position with two dumbbells held at the sides, with the palms facing in and the arms hanging straight down. Raise the dumbbells and rotate the forearm so that the palms face the shoulder. Lower to the original position to complete one repetition. One can also alternate one arm at a time. **N.** Barbell arm curls (upper arm–biceps, bilateral). In the standing position with the feet shoulder-width apart, grasp the straight barbell with an underhand grip and palms facing up. Raise the bar until the forearms are vertical and then lower the bar to the starting position to complete a repetition. One can also perform this exercise with an E-Z bar with the palms facing inward.

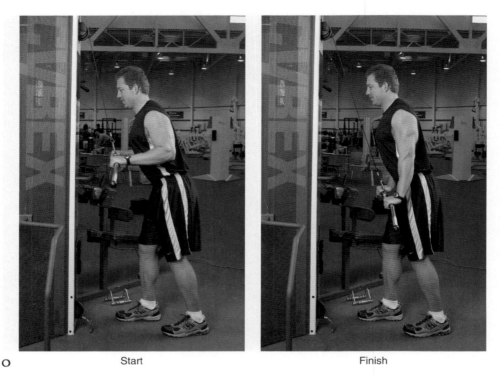

O   Start   Finish

FIGURE 17.5 *(Continued)* **O.** Triceps push down (upper arm–triceps, bilateral). Stand in front of the lat pull station or high pulley station and take an overhand grasp on the bar with your elbows at the sides. Start at chest level and extend the arms down until straight and return to the starting position to complete the repetition. Position the hands above the bar prior to the push-down phase of the repetition.

SUMMARY

Development of a resistance training program is a systematic process in which science and art come together to allow the Personal Trainer to specifically address a client's needs for neuromuscular fitness. A sequence of events in the exercise prescription process consists of getting a client's medical clearance, personal training history, goal generation, a needs analysis, and a general preparation phase of initial training and testing prior to putting together workouts based on the acute program variables that will be used in a resistance training program. This program is then updated and revised with the same process over time. Education, client interactions, and a motivation are vital components of successful resistance training programs that meet each client's goals and objectives.

REFERENCES

1. Delorme TL. Restoration of muscle power by heavy resistance exercises. J Bone Joint Surg 1945;27:645.
2. Delorme TL, Watkins AL. Techniques of progressive resistance exercise. Arch Phys Med 1948;29:263–273.
3. Todd T, Todd J. Pioneers of strength research: the legacy of Dr. Richard A. Berger. J Strength Cond Res 2001;15(3):275–278.
4. Todd T, Todd J. Dr. Patrick O'Shea: a man for all seasons. J Strength Cond Res 2001;15(4):401–404.
5. Fleck SJ, Kraemer WJ. Designing Resistance Training Programs. 3rd ed. Champaign, IL: Human Kinetics, 2004.
6. Kraemer WJ, Fry AC. Strength testing: development and evaluation of methodology. In: Maud P, Foster C, eds. Physiological Assessment of Human Fitness. Champaign IL: Human Kinetics, 1995:115–138.
7. Harman E. Resistive torque analysis of 5 Nautilus exercise machines. Med Sci Sports Exerc 1983;15:113.
8. Pizzimenti MA. Mechanical analysis of the Nautilus leg curl machine. Can J Sport Sci 1992;17:41–48.
9. Johnson JH, Colodny S, Jackson D. Human torque capability versus machine resistive torque for four Eagle resistance machines. J Appl Sport Sci Res 1990;4:83–87.
10. Kraemer WJ, Keuning M, Ratamess NA, et al. Resistance training combined with bench-step aerobics enhances women's health profile. Med Sci Sports Exerc 2001;33(2):259–269.
11. Fleck SJ, Schutt RC. Types of strength training. Clin Sports Med 1985;4:159–169.

12. Dudley GA, Tesch PA, Miller BJ, Buchanan P. Importance of eccentric actions in performance adaptations to resistance training. Aviat Space Environ Med 1991;62(6):543–550.

13. Kraemer WJ. Exercise prescription in weight training: a needs analysis. Natl Strength Cond Assoc J 1983;5(1):64–65.

14. Hickson JF, Bruno MJ, Wilmore JH, Constable SH. Energy cost of weight training exercise. Natl Strength Cond Assoc J 1984;6:522–523.

15. Kraemer WJ, Patton JF, Gordon SE, et al. Compatibility of high-intensity strength and endurance training on hormonal and skeletal muscle adaptations. J Appl Physiol 1995;78(3):976–989.

16. Johnson RE, Quinn TJ, Kertzer R, Vroman NB. Strength training in female distance runners: impact on running economy. J Strength Cond Res 1997;11(4):224–229.

17. Kraemer WJ. Exercise prescription in weight training: manipulating program variables. Natl Strength Cond Assoc J 1983;5:58–59.

18. Chilibeck PD, Calder AW, Sale DG, Webber CE. A comparison of strength and muscle mass increases during resistance training in young women. Eur J Appl Physiol Occup Physiol 1998;77(1–2):170–175.

19. Simao R, Farinatti T, Polito MD, et al. Influence of exercise order on the number of repetitions performed and perceived exertion during resistance exercises. J Strength Cond Res 2005;19(1):152–156.

20. Hoeger WWK, Barette SL, Hale DF, Hopkins DR. Relationship between repetitions and selected percentages of one repetition maximum. J Applied Sport Sci Res 1990;4(2); 47–54.

21. Hoeger WWK, Hopkins DR, Barette SL, Hale DF. Relationship between repetitions and selected percentages of one repetition maximum: a comparison between untrained and trained males and females. J Appl Sport Sci Res 1987;1(1):1–13.

22. American College of Sports Medicine Position Stand. Progression models in resistance training for healthy adults. Med Sci Sports Exerc 2002;34:364–380.

23. Tan B. Manipulating resistance training program variables to optimize maximum strength in men: a review. J Strength Cond Res 1999;13(3):289–304.

24. Kraemer WJ, Ratamess N, Fry AC, et al. Influence of resistance training volume and periodization on physiological and performance adaptations in collegiate women tennis players. Am J Sports Med 2000;28(5):626–633.

25. Marx JO, Ratamess NA, Nindl BC, et al. Low-volume circuit versus high-volume periodized resistance training in women. Med Sci Sports Exerc 2001;33(4):635–643.

26. Kraemer WJ, Noble BJ, Culver BW, Clark MJ. Physiologic responses to heavy-resistance exercise with very short rest periods. Intl J Sports Med 1987;8:247–252.

27. Kraemer WJ, Marchitelli L, McCurry D, et al. Hormonal and growth factor responses to heavy resistance exercise. J Appl Physiol 1990;69(4):1442–1450.

28. Tharion WJ, Rausch TM, Harman EA, Kraemer WJ. Effects of different resistance exercise protocols on mood states. J Appl Sport Sci Res 1991;5(2):60–65.

29. Kraemer WJ. A series of studies: the physiological basis for strength training in American football: fact over philosophy. J Strength Cond Res 1997;11(3):131–142.

30. Matveyev L. Fundamentals of sports training. Moscow: Progress, 1981.

31. Plisk SS, Stone MH. Periodization strategies. Strength Cond J 2003;25(6):19–37.

32. Rhea MR, Ball SD, Phillips WT, Burkett LN. A comparison of linear and daily undulating periodized programs with equated volume and intensity for strength. J Strength Cond Res 2002;16(2):250–255.

33. Mazzetti SA, Kraemer WJ, Volek JS, et al. The influence of direct supervision of resistance training on strength performance. Med Sci Sports Exerc 2000;32(6):1175–1184.

34. Kraemer WJ, Fleck SJ. Strength Training for Young Athletes. 2nd ed. Champaign, IL: Human Kinetics, 2005.

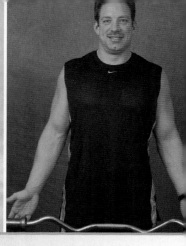

CHAPTER

18 Cardiorespiratory Training Programs

Barbara Bushman, Ph.D., FACSM, Associate Dean, Graduate College, Professor, Department of Health, Physical Education, and Recreation, Missouri State University, Springfield, Missouri

Kenneth E. Baldwin, M.Ed., A.H. Ismail Center for Health, Exercise & Nutrition, Department of Health and Kinesiology, College of Liberal Arts, Purdue University, West Lafayette, Indiana

Chapter Outline

- Identify the components of a cardiovascular training program
- Learn to identify and instruct clients on proper posture and alignment while performing different forms of cardiovascular exercise
- Assess the interaction of frequency, duration, and intensity
- Describe the recommended range of training based on current research

Personal Trainers interact directly with clients as they design and integrate the three primary components of the exercise program, including resistance, cardiorespiratory, and flexibility training. Determination of the "best" exercise program must be made with regards to the client's health and fitness status, risk factors, and goals as described in Chapters 12 through 15. This chapter outlines the basic training principles as well as the specific variables that are manipulated when designing a cardiorespiratory training program.

Cardiorespiratory training is one of the primary components of a balanced exercise program. The other two major components, resistance and flexibility training, are described in Chapters 17 and 19. The ACSM Position Stand (1) on "The Recommended Quantity and Quality of Exercise for Developing and Maintaining Cardiorespiratory and Muscular Fitness, and Flexibility in Health Adults" emphasizes the importance of these three components:

> As a result of specificity of training and the need for maintaining muscular strength and endurance, and flexibility of the major muscle groups, a well-rounded training program including aerobic and resistance training and flexibility exercise is recommended.

GENERAL TRAINING PRINCIPLES

Cardiorespiratory endurance or training refers to the ability of a client to perform large muscle, repetitive, moderate- to high-intensity exercise for an extended period of time. The goal is to increase heart rate and respiration to place an appropriate physiological stress on the cardiorespiratory system. This required stress is often referred to as "overload." The term overload is most commonly used when referring to resistance or strength training (i.e., lifting a weight heavier than typically done in daily activity, to stress the muscle, resulting in increased strength and potential hypertrophy). In a similar manner, overload of the cardiovascular and respiratory systems is required to have beneficial adaptations in cardiorespiratory endurance. Cardiorespiratory fitness is improved by enhanced heart function (i.e., oxygen delivery to the working muscles) and the ability of the working muscles to use the oxygen in metabolic processes, allowing for increased energy production (2). Typical measurements used to determine improvements include increases in maximal oxygen consumption and decreases in heart rate or oxygen consumption in response to a given submaximal workload. The benefits of cardiorespiratory endurance include the following (2):

➤ Decreased risk of premature death from all causes, and specifically from heart disease
➤ Reduction in death from all causes
➤ Increased likelihood of increased habitual activity levels, which is also associated with health benefits

More specific benefits are found in Box 18.1 (2). Inclusion of cardiorespiratory endurance provides many benefits and thus is an important element of a balanced exercise program.

The training methods used to bring about these adaptations are quite varied. There is no single exercise program to apply universally. A Personal Trainer must have the knowledge, skills, and abilities to individualize programs based on the client's current health status, risk factors for heart disease, and individual goals. Various options for exercise modes are presented below in this chapter.

BOX 18.1	**Benefits of Regular Physical Activity and/or Exercise**

Improvement in cardiovascular and respiratory function
- Increased maximal oxygen uptake resulting from both central and peripheral adaptations (*improving the body's ability to take in and use oxygen is a result of adaptations within both the cardiorespiratory system and the muscular system*)
- Decreased minute ventilation at a given absolute submaximal intensity (*at any given submaximal workload, fewer liters of air will be breathed with training*)
- Decreased myocardial oxygen cost for a given absolute submaximal intensity (*at any given submaximal workload, less oxygen will be required because of improved efficiency*)
- Decreased heart rate and blood pressure at a given submaximal intensity (*at any given submaximal workload, the heart rate and blood pressure will be lower following training*)
- Increased capillary density in skeletal muscle (*the number of capillaries [small blood vessels around the muscle cells] is increased around muscles, allowing better oxygen delivery*)
- Increased exercise threshold for the accumulation of lactate in the blood (*exercise workload will be higher before lactate begins to build up in the blood and thus limits performance*)
- Increased exercise threshold for the onset of disease signs or symptoms (e.g., angina pectoris, ischemic ST-segment depression, claudication) (*exercise workload will be higher before signs/symptoms of disease, such as chest pain or abnormal EKG changes, are displayed*)

Reduction in coronary artery disease risk factors
- Reduced resting systolic/diastolic pressures (*blood pressure decreases*)
- Increased serum high-density lipoprotein cholesterol and decreased serum triglycerides (*HDL or "good" cholesterol increases and blood levels of fats decrease*)
- Reduced total body fat, reduced intra-abdominal fat (*both total fat stores and fat within the abdominal region are decreased*)
- Reduced insulin needs, improved glucose tolerance (*the body's ability to deal with sugars/carbohydrates is improved*)
- Reduced blood platelet adhesiveness and aggregation (*blood "stickiness" and clotting [which could lead to a heart attack or stroke] are decreased*)

Decreased morbidity and mortality
- Primary prevention (i.e., interventions to prevent the initial occurrence)
  - Higher activity and/or fitness levels are associated with lower death rates from coronary artery disease
  - Higher activity and/or fitness levels are associated with lower incidence rates for combined cardiovascular diseases, coronary artery disease, stroke, type 2 diabetes, osteoporotic fractures, cancer of the colon and breast, gallbladder disease
- Secondary prevention (i.e., interventions after a cardiac event [to prevent another])
  - Based on meta-analysis (pooled data across studies), cardiovascular and all-cause mortality are reduced in post-myocardial infarction patients who participate in cardiac rehabilitation exercise training, especially as a component of multifactorial risk factor reduction
  - Randomized controlled trials of cardiac rehabilitation exercise training involving postmyocardial infarction patients do not support a reduction in the rate of nonfatal reinfarction

Other postulated benefits
- Decreased anxiety and depression
- Enhanced physical function and independent living in older patients
- Enhanced feelings of well-being
- Enhanced performance of work, recreational, and sport activities

Adapted from American College of Sports Medicine. ACSM's Guidelines for Exercise Testing and Prescription. 7th ed. Baltimore: Lippincott Williams & Wilkins, 2006:8–9.

Different modes, or types, of exercise will bring about specific adaptations as well as more generalized cardiorespiratory fitness gains. The principle of adaptation states that if endurance training at a certain level for a certain period of time challenges the cardiorespiratory system, function (translated as fitness or performance) will improve. Determining how to tax the system for a given individual is one of the roles of a Personal Trainer. This determination is not a one-size-fits-all option. Rather, each client comes with specific health and fitness levels (and risk factors) that should be considered when preparing an exercise program. See Table 14.1 for a list of the risk factors, which must be considered prior to engaging a client in a fitness program. These risk factors place individuals into general risk classifications, which can be used to determine the need for physician oversight of testing as well as the level of exercise to be prescribed.

To challenge the cardiorespiratory system, an overload must be applied. To overload, activities that increase heart rate and respiration are prescribed. The minimal amount of overload needed to bring about the desired adaptation is referred to as the "threshold." If the training level exceeds the threshold, then physiological adaptations occur because of the prescribed overload. A properly constructed exercise program includes frequency (number of days per week), duration (minutes per workout), and intensity (how hard the workout is for the client). According to the ACSM Position Stand (1), cardiorespiratory training for less than 2 days per week, for less than 40–50% of oxygen uptake reserve (described later in this chapter), and for less than 10 minutes will not provide sufficient overload to develop and maintain fitness in apparently healthy adults.

Although exceeding the threshold is required for physiological adaptations to occur, excessive overload can result, paradoxically, in diminished performance. When either a single bout or long-term period of excessive stress is placed on the cardiorespiratory system (resulting in decreased physiological capacities), the term "retrogression" is used (3). The Personal Trainer must carefully balance the frequency, intensity, and duration of the workouts to avoid over-challenging the client beyond an appropriate amount of overload.

The principle of specificity states that the particular exercise(s) involved also influences adaptation. Training of the upper (arms) or lower (legs) extremities is one example. When training only lower extremities, researchers found favorable heart rate adaptations (i.e., lowering of the heart rate at a given workload) only occurred with similar exercise, not with upper extremity exercise (4). The same situation occurred when training upper extremities. Adaptations occurred when doing arm exercises and not for leg exercises. Similarly, an arm-only training program was not sufficient to maintain fitness gains achieved with leg-only training (5). Therefore, at least some of the training adaptations are occurring because of positive alterations within the muscles (peripheral adaptations) not because of general adaptations in the cardiorespiratory system (central adaptations).

Other physiological changes have been identified in studies between trained and untrained limbs, suggesting a central adaptation (i.e., central circulatory adaptations). For example, maximal oxygen consumption has been found to be increased even when using untrained limbs (6). The balance between peripheral and central contributions to changes in fitness is not consistent and is difficult to determine. Differences have also been identified within various populations. The general viewpoint is that approximately half of the positive changes can be attributed to central and the other half to peripheral adaptations (2).

Although the desire is for all clients to continue to improve through appropriate levels of overload, there are times when clients stop exercising or decrease the overload below their threshold level. The result will be a loss of physiological adaptations as the person regresses toward pre-overload status. This process of losing fitness gains is referred to as regression or de-adaptation (3). Anticipating periods of decreased physical activity (e.g., travel, excessive work obligations) can allow a planned "re-entry" into the exercise program. Chapter 10 includes information on how to keep clients motivated and promote positive behavior changes.

DESIGN OF A CARDIORESPIRATORY TRAINING SESSION

A cardiorespiratory exercise session includes a warm-up, the endurance phase, and a cool-down. The warm-up prepares the person for the focal point of the workout (the endurance phase) when a target intensity is achieved, allowing appropriate overload. The cool-down allows the person to transition back toward resting levels following the endurance phase. Personal Trainers may want to have clients perform the primary cardiorespiratory portion of the workout before, during, or after the scheduled personal training session. Developing the structure of the entire exercise program is presented in Chapter 16.

Warm-Up

A properly constructed exercise program will include a transition period from rest to the target exercise intensity. This transition period is called the "warm-up." During the warm-up, the client should gradually increase body temperature by incorporating low-level activity similar to what will be done during the endurance phase. For example, an appropriate warm-up for a brisk walking exercise program would include slow walking. The muscle groups used are similar in the two activities—slow walking being a low-intensity activity that leads naturally to the brisk walking of the exercise program. The warm-up may also include stretching activities, although stretching should only be done following some activity to warm the muscles. The activities included in a warm-up will vary depending on the target activity to be included in the endurance phase. General recommendations for a warm-up include (2):

➤ 5–10 minutes of low-intensity large muscle activity (Personal Trainers may consider a warm-up timeline that is longer when a client is entering from an externally cooler environment)
➤ Intensity progression to the lower end of the target exercise range for the endurance phase

The intent of a warm-up is to prepare the muscles and cardiorespiratory system for the upcoming workout. It is a time of transition and should provide a gradual (rather than an abrupt) increase in heart rate, respiration, and body temperature. Taking sufficient time to prepare the body for physical activity increases the safety and enjoyment of the target exercise during the endurance phase. The benefits of completing a warm-up include the following (2):

➤ May reduce the susceptibility of injury to muscles or joints by increasing the extensibility of connective tissue
➤ Improve joint range of motion and function
➤ Improve muscle performance
➤ Potentially help to prevent ischemia (lack of oxygen) of the heart muscle, which may occur in clients with sudden strenuous exertion

Endurance Phase

The endurance phase is the target of the workout. The warm-up has provided the client with a transition from rest to a higher level of intensity. During the endurance phase, the proper overload promotes beneficial cardiorespiratory adaptations. The Personal Trainer should consider the appropriate mode (i.e., type) of exercise as well as how to balance exercise intensity, duration, and frequency.

EXERCISE MODE

The selection of exercise mode is made with consideration for the client's fitness, health, and interests. Cardiorespiratory exercises involve the use of large muscle groups in a repetitive, or rhythmic, fashion for an extended period of time. Some activities are weight-dependent, meaning that body weight is moved during the exercise (e.g., walking, running). In other activities, body weight is not a factor

Table 18.1	GROUPING OF CARDIORESPIRATORY EXERCISE AND ACTIVITIES		
	Group 1	**Group 2**	**Group 3**
Definition	• Ease of maintaining constant intensity • Low interindividual variation in energy expenditure	• Ease of maintaining constant intensity • Energy expenditure is related to skill	• Skill highly variable • Energy expenditure highly variable
Use	Desirable for more precise control of exercise intensity: • Beginning an exercise program • Rehabilitation	Not contraindicated for the early stages of conditioning, but skill must be considered	Good for group inter-actions, but caution must be taken for: • High risk-low fit • Symptomatic patients
Examples	• Treadmill walking • Cycle ergometry	• Swimming • Cross-country skiing	• Racquet sports • Basketball • Soccer

Reprinted with permission from American College of Sports Medicine. ACSM's Resource Manual for Guidelines for Exercise Testing and Prescription. 5th ed. Baltimore: Lippincott Williams & Wilkins, 2006:338.

because the body is supported (e.g., cycling, swimming). These activities are referred to as weight-bearing and non–weight-bearing exercises, respectively (3). Non–weight-bearing exercises may be useful in avoiding injuries of the lower limbs as a result of overuse (3). Table 18.1 lists a number of cardiorespiratory endurance activities (3). ACSM has classified these activities into three groups. The groups do not necessarily represent an optimal progression, but rather present the Personal Trainer with information on important characteristics of the exercise modes when selecting activities.

Treadmill walking and stationary cycling are two examples of group 1 activities (3). The classification is based on the ability to maintain a consistent intensity and a relatively constant energy expenditure (2). As a result of the consistency of the activities, a Personal Trainer may find them effective to use when initiating an exercise program with a client. Individuals unfamiliar with exercise may have difficulty maintaining the prescribed intensity. The use of group 1 activities provides new exercisers with more precise control of the exercise intensity.

Swimming and cross–country skiing are examples of group 2 exercises (3). This classification reflects the relationship between skill level and individual energy expenditure. For example, an experienced swimmer may be able to maintain a constant intensity while swimming, while a person with poor skills would struggle to swim at an appropriate, constant intensity to receive cardiorespiratory benefits.

Sports like basketball, soccer, tennis and other racquet sports are classified as group 3 activities because both skill and intensity can vary greatly among individuals (3). Maintaining a constant, controlled intensity is difficult because of the nature of the activities and becomes even more challenging when competition is involved (2). As a result, group 3 activities should be used with caution for clients with low fitness or who are high risk or symptomatic of disease.

The groupings outlined provide the Personal Trainer with guidance on selection of an appropriate exercise mode. Group 1 activities are appropriate to use with clients beginning an exercise program when precisely controlling the exercise intensity can be challenging. Group 2 activities may be appropriate but will require discussion with the client regarding skill levels for the activities in question. Group 3 activities may best be included after a baseline level of fitness is in place because of the variations in intensity and the concerns about monitoring intensity in competitive environments. The Personal Trainer and client must maintain open lines of communication regarding the selection of exercise modes. In some situations, individuals will be satisfied with continuing with various group 1 activities. Other clients may have skills or desire to learn new skills to include group 2 activities, or may enjoy the variety and challenge of group 3 activities.

Posture and Body Alignment. Detailed instruction by the Personal Trainer includes a discussion about proper posture and body alignment while conducting cardiorespiratory training and group 1 exercises. Having a client perform these exercises in a proper biomechanical position is just as important as when clients are performing resistance training exercises, as discussed in Chapter 17. Often overlooked by many Personal Trainers, repetitive stress injuries can occur if clients are not taught the required body alignment.

Common alignment observations while clients perform group 1 cardiovascular-type exercises include forward head protrusion, exaggerated kyphosis or lordosis, and overextension of the knee joint, causing a lock-out position for the joint structure. Awareness and instruction to clients when deviating from the optimal line of gravity should be presented by the Personal Trainer. The following examples are provided to compare the "common" and "required" performance necessary to conduct cardiovascular exercise and training safely:

➤ Stationary bikes (*Figs. 18.1–18.4*)
➤ Treadmills-walking (*Figs. 18.5* and *18.6*)
➤ Treadmills-running (*Figs. 18.7* and *18.8*)
➤ Stair steppers and cross trainers (*Figs. 18.9* and *18.10*)
➤ Recumbent bikes (*Figs. 18.11* and *18.12*)

EXERCISE INTENSITY

Intensity can be determined using various methods. For a quick overview of the intensity classifications for cardiorespiratory endurance, refer to Table 18.2 (3). Details on these various methods are outlined in this section. Some methods require knowledge of maximal oxygen consumption, or maximal and/or resting heart rate. Others rely on estimations of maximal heart rate based on age. Personal Trainers must use the information available to determine the more appropriate exercise prescription, realizing the shortcomings of the various methods. When using maximal oxygen consumption (as described within this section), a range of values will be determined. These values

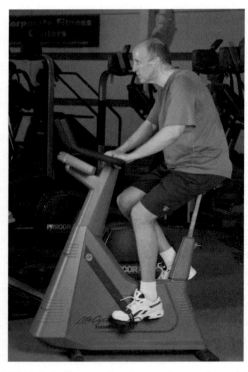

FIGURE 18.1. A client performing cardiovascular training on a stationary bike (group 1 exercise) in poor posture.

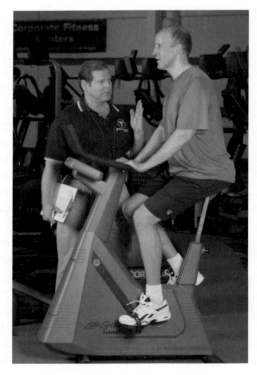

FIGURE 18.2. A client is being educated by his trainer on how to sit properly and maintain proper alignment while on the bike.

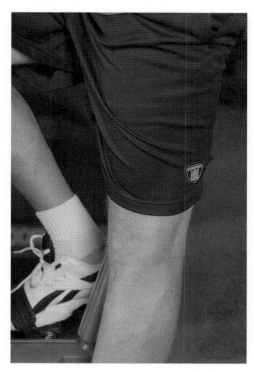

FIGURE 18.3. Full extension of the knee while pedaling on the stationary bike is not recommended to reduce compression on the joint structure.

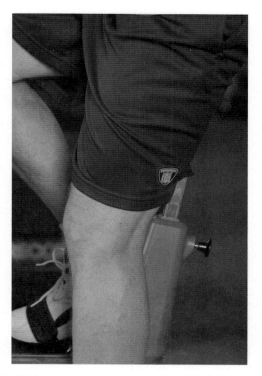

FIGURE 18.4. Personal trainers may instruct clients to adjust seat heights to maintain a 5–10° bend in the knee before reaching full extension.

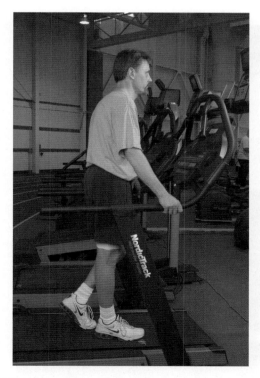

FIGURE 18.5. Individuals tend to lean forward in improper posture and body alignment while walking on treadmills (group 1 exercise).

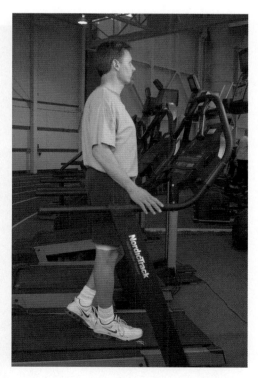

FIGURE 18.6. Personal trainers should teach clients to maintain proper alignment while using a treadmill.

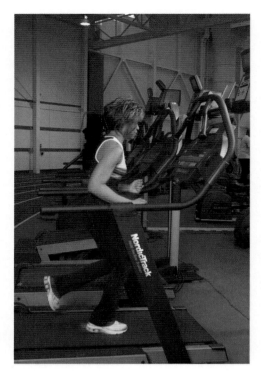

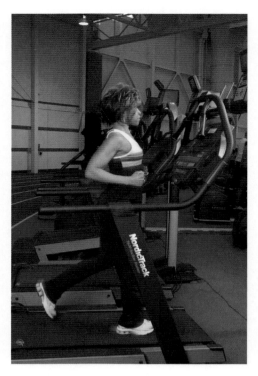

FIGURE 18.7. Individuals tend to lean forward in improper posture and body alignment while running on treadmills (group 1 exercise).

FIGURE 18.8. Proper alignment while running on a treadmill.

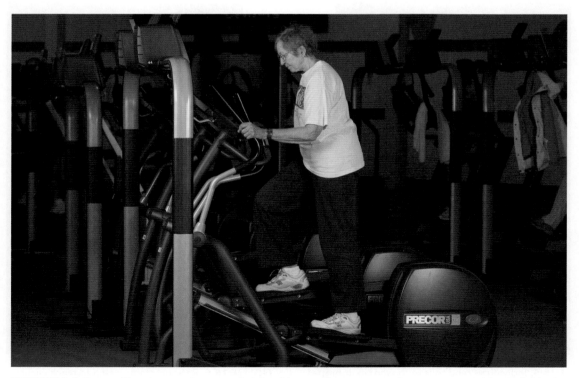

FIGURE 18.9. Forward head protrusion, rounded shoulders, and poor posture is a common position individuals assume while using stair steppers and cross training machines (group 1 exercise).

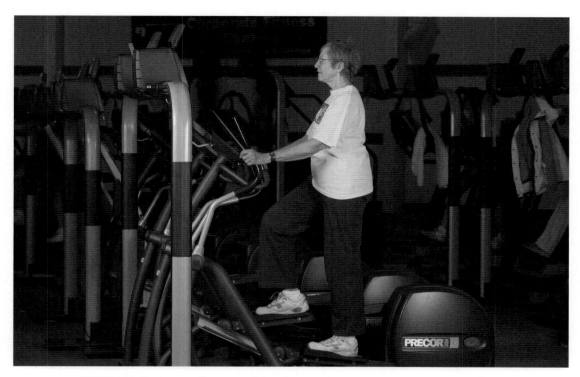

FIGURE 18.10. Proper alignment while using a stair stepper or cross training machine.

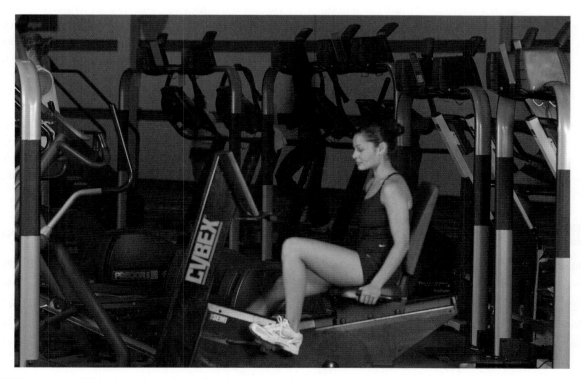

FIGURE 18.11. Individuals tend to relax and maintain poor alignment while training on recumbent bikes (group 1 exercise).

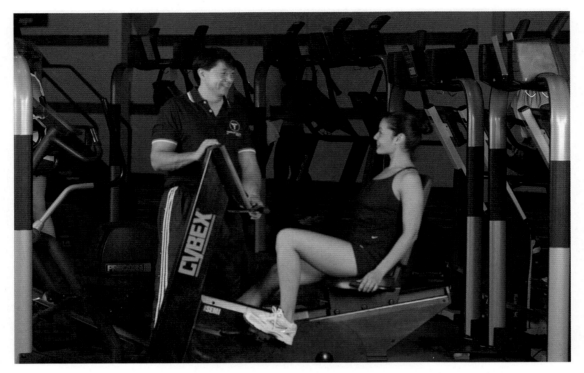

FIGURE 18.12. A trainer teaching his client proper alignment when using a recumbent bike.

can be used to determine the workload for various activities using charts or metabolic calculations. A shortcoming of this technique is the outcome, which is a determination of workload, not the individual's response. For example, determining an outdoor running pace based on oxygen consumption alone might pose the problem of inaccuracy when faced with a hot, humid environment. Factors such as environmental conditions may make the relative intensity higher than prescribed. Blindly using workloads can be a concern if physiological responses (such as heart rate) are not monitored during exercise.

Use of heart rate can be helpful because it represents a client's response, but it too has shortcomings. Accuracy can be compromised when estimations of maximal heart rate are used or when medications are taken that may influence heart rate (e.g., beta-blockers, drugs that suppress heart rate at rest and during exercise). When a measured maximal heart rate taken during a graded exercise test

Table 18.2 **CLASSIFICATION OF EXERCISE INTENSITY FOR CARDIORESPIRATORY ENDURANCE**

Intensity	Percentage of HRR or $\dot{V}O_2R$	Percentage of HR_{max}	RPE
Very light	<20	<35	<10
Light	20–39	35–54	10–11
Moderate	40–59	55–69	12–13
Hard	60–84	70–89	14–16
Very hard	>85	>90	17–19
Maximal	100	100	20

Reprinted with permission from American College of Sports Medicine. ACSM's Resource Manual for Guidelines for Exercise Testing and Prescription. 5th ed. Baltimore: Lippincott Williams & Wilkins, 2006:340.
HRR, heart rate reserve; $\dot{V}O_2R$, oxygen uptake reserve; HR_{max}, maximum heart rate; RPE, rating of perceived exertion.

is unavailable, the Personal Trainer commonly uses an age-predicted estimate (220 − age). The concern with this method (2) is the variability for a given single age (1 standard deviation equals ±10–12 beats per minute). The role of the Personal Trainer is to use the information available, realizing the shortcomings of the various techniques, to determine an appropriate exercise prescription. A willingness and ability to modify the exercise program to provide an appropriate overload is the sign of a good Personal Trainer.

The ACSM recommends intensity levels for exercise between 64 and 70% (64/70%) and 94% of maximal heart rate (2). The following calculation would be used to determine the target heart rate (HR):

$$\text{Target HR (lower end of range)} = [\text{maximal HR}] \times 0.64$$

$$\text{Target HR (upper end of range)} = [\text{maximal HR}] \times 0.94$$

For example, for a 20-year-old client with an estimated maximal heart rate of 200 (220 − 20 = 200), the range would be 128–188 beats per minute. The resulting target heart rate range may be so wide that it is not helpful for guiding the client's exercise session. Personal Trainers must therefore consider the client's health history as well as his or her goals to narrow the range. For apparently healthy individuals, the range is often narrowed to 70 to 85% of maximal heart rate (2). Therefore, for the 20-year-old, moderately active client, the target heart rate range would be 140–170 beats per minute. If the client were very deconditioned or very unfit, then a lower percentage would be used (e.g., 55–70%). Selection of the intensity range must be made with the client's health status and fitness goals in mind.

Exercise intensity can also be determined from oxygen uptake reserve or heart rate reserve. ACSM recommends a range of between 40 and 50% up to 85% of oxygen uptake reserve or heart rate reserve (2). The oxygen uptake reserve (commonly designated $\dot{V}O_2R$) is the difference between maximal oxygen consumption ($\dot{V}O_{2max}$) and resting oxygen consumption ($\dot{V}O_{2rest}$). In the $\dot{V}O_2R$ method to determine intensity, the following equations would be used:

$$\text{Target } \dot{V}O_2 \text{ (lower end of range)} = ([0.40] \times [\dot{V}O_{2max} - \dot{V}O_{2rest}]) + \dot{V}O_{2rest}$$

$$\text{Target } \dot{V}O_2 \text{ (upper end of range)} = ([0.85] \times [\dot{V}O_{2max} - \dot{V}O_{2rest}]) + \dot{V}O_{2rest}$$

$\dot{V}O_{2rest}$ has been estimated to be $3.5 \text{ mL} \cdot \text{kg}^{-1} \cdot \text{min}^{-1}$ (also referred to as one metabolic equivalent, or 1 MET) and is used for all individuals. If a Personal Trainer has access to $\dot{V}O_{2max}$ information, then these equations can be used. The percentages used to determine the appropriate range must be made with the client's fitness level and goals in mind. Low-fit clients will need to start on the lower end of the range, while more active clients will require intensities toward the upper end of the range to receive the appropriate overload. Normative values for $\dot{V}O_{2max}$ are found in Table 18.3, which allows the Personal Trainer to see the percentile rank for males and females of various ages.

To determine an appropriate workload, various metabolic equations are available (2). These equations are found in Box 18.2. These equations can estimate the oxygen consumption required by the body during constant, submaximal activity (including walking, jogging/running, stationary cycling, arm cranking, and stepping). Box 18.3 presents an extended example showing the application of the various equations to a client's exercise prescription. Underestimating the workload may leave a person below the appropriate target intensity (and the accompanying health benefits). Overestimating commonly results in frustration with exercise and poor adherence. These equations will give initial starting points. Intensity levels may still need to be adjusted based on individual heart rate responses and perceived levels of exertion.

A simpler method, not requiring extensive calculations, is to take the oxygen consumption values (for the upper and lower end of the target range) and convert them to MET values. This is accomplished by taking the oxygen consumption values and dividing by 3.5 (as 1 MET = $3.5 \text{ mL} \cdot \text{kg}^{-1} \cdot \text{min}^{-1}$). Tables are available that will help the Personal Trainer determine

Table 18.3 **PERCENTILE VALUES FOR MAXIMAL AEROBIC POWER (mL · kg^{-1} · min^{-1})^a**

Percentile Values for Maximal Oxygen Uptake (mL · kg^{-1} · min^{-1}) in Men

| Percentile | Age (years) | | | | |
	20–29 (N = 2,234)	30–39 (N = 11,158)	40–49 (N = 13,109)	50–59 (N = 5,641)	60+ (N = 1,244)
90	55.1	52.1	50.6	49.0	44.2
80	52.1	50.6	49.0	44.2	41.0
70	49.0	47.4	45.8	41.0	37.8
60	47.4	44.2	44.2	39.4	36.2
50	44.2	42.6	41.0	37.8	34.6
40	42.6	41.0	39.4	36.2	33.0
30	41.0	39.4	36.2	34.6	31.4
20	37.8	36.2	34.6	31.4	28.3
10	34.6	33.0	31.4	29.9	26.7

^{a}Data were obtained from the initial examination of apparently healthy men enrolled in the Aerobics Center Longitudinal Study (ACLS), 1970 to 2002. The study population for the data set was predominantly white and college educated. Maximal treadmill exercise tests were administered using a modified Balke protocol. Maximal oxygen uptake was estimated from the final treadmill speed and grade using the current ACSM equations (2). The data are provided courtesy of the ACLS investigators, The Cooper Institute, Dallas, TX. The ACLS is supported in part by a grant from the National Institute on Aging (AG06945), SN Blair, Principal Investigator. The following may be used as descriptors for the percentile rankings: well above average (90), above average (70), average (50), below average (30), and well below average (10).

Percentile Values for Maximal Oxygen Uptake (mL · kg^{-1} · min^{-1}) in Women

| Percentile | Age (years) | | | | |
	20–29 (N = 1,223)	30–39 (N = 3,895)	40–49 (N = 4,001)	50–59 (N = 2,032)	60+ (N = 465)
90	49.0	45.8	42.6	37.8	34.6
80	44.2	41.0	39.4	34.6	33.0
70	41.0	39.4	36.2	33.0	31.4
60	39.4	36.2	34.6	31.4	28.3
50	37.8	34.6	33.0	29.9	26.7
40	36.2	33.0	31.4	28.3	25.1
30	33.0	31.4	29.9	26.7	23.5
20	31.4	29.9	28.3	25.1	21.9
10	28.3	26.7	25.1	21.9	20.3

^{a}Data were obtained from the initial examination of apparently healthy women enrolled in the Aerobics Center Longitudinal Study (ACLS), 1970 to 2002. The study population for the data set was predominantly white and college educated. Maximal treadmill exercise tests were administered using a modified Balke protocol. Maximal oxygen uptake was estimated from the final treadmill speed and grade using the current ACSM equations (2). The data are provided courtesy of the ACLS investigators, The Cooper Institute, Dallas, TX. The ACLS is supported in part by a grant from the National Institute on Aging (AG06945), SN Blair, Principal Investigator. The following may be used as descriptors for the percentile rankings: well above average (90), above average (70), average (50), below average (30), and well below average (10).

Reprinted with permission from American College of Sports Medicine. ACSM's Guidelines for Exercise Testing and Prescription. 7th ed. Baltimore: Lippincott Williams & Wilkins, 2006:79.

Box 18.2	**Metabolic Equations for Gross $\dot{V}O_2$ in Metric Units***

Walking

$\dot{V}O_2 \; (mL \cdot kg^{-1} \cdot min^{-1}) = (0.1 \cdot S) + (1.8 \cdot S \cdot G) + 3.5 \; mL \cdot kg^{-1} \cdot min^{-1}$

$\dot{V}O_2 \; (mL \cdot kg^{-1} \cdot min^{-1}) = [0.1 \; mL \cdot kg^{-1} \cdot meter^{-1} \cdot S \; (m \cdot min^{-1})]$
$+ \; [1.8 \; mL \cdot kg^{-1} \cdot meter^{-1} \cdot S \; (m \cdot min^{-1}) \cdot G] + 3.5 \; mL \cdot kg^{-1} \cdot min^{-1}$

Running

$\dot{V}O_2 \; (mL \cdot kg^{-1} \cdot min^{-1}) = (0.2 \cdot S) + (0.9 \cdot S \cdot G) + 3.5 \; mL \cdot kg^{-1} \cdot min^{-1}$

$\dot{V}O_2 \; (mL \cdot kg^{-1} \cdot min^{-1}) = [0.2 \; mL \cdot kg^{-1} \cdot meter^{-1} \cdot S \; (m \cdot min^{-1})]$
$+ \; [0.9 \; mL \cdot kg^{-1} \cdot meter^{-1} \cdot S \; (m \cdot min^{-1}) \cdot G] + 3.5 \; mL \cdot kg^{-1} \cdot min^{-1}$

Leg Cycling

$\dot{V}O_2 \; (mL \cdot kg^{-1} \cdot min^{-1}) = 1.8 \; (work \; rate)/(BM) + 3.5 \; mL \cdot kg^{-1} \cdot min^{-1}$
$+ \; 3.5 \; mL \cdot kg^{-1} \cdot min^{-1}$

$\dot{V}O_2 \; (mL \cdot kg^{-1} \cdot min^{-1}) = (1.8 \; mL \cdot kg^{-1} \cdot min^{-1})$
$\times \; (work \; rate \; in \; kg \cdot m \cdot min^{-1}) \; (body \; mass \; in \; kg)$
$+ \; 3.5 \; mL \cdot kg^{-1} \cdot min^{-1} + 3.5 \; mL \cdot kg^{-1} \cdot min^{-1}$

Arm Cycling

$\dot{V}O_2 \; (mL \cdot kg^{-1} \cdot min^{-1}) = 3 \; (work \; rate)/(BM) + 3.5 \; mL \cdot kg^{-1} \cdot min^{-1}$

$\dot{V}O_2 \; (mL \cdot kg^{-1} \cdot min^{-1}) = (3 \; mL \cdot kg^{-1} \cdot meter^{-1})$
$\times \; (work \; rate \; in \; kg \cdot m \cdot min^{-1}) \; (body \; mass \; in \; kg) + 3.5 \; mL \cdot kg^{-1} \cdot min^{-1}$

Stepping

$\dot{V}O_2 \; (mL \cdot kg^{-1} \cdot min^{-1}) = (0.2 \cdot f) + (1.33 \cdot 1.8 \cdot H \cdot f) + 3.5 \; mL \cdot kg^{-1} \cdot min^{-1}$

$\dot{V}O_2 \; (mL \cdot kg^{-1} \cdot min^{-1}) = 0.2 \; (steps \cdot min^{-1})$
$+ \; (1.33 \; mL \cdot kg^{-1} \cdot meter^{-1}) \; (1.8 \; mL \cdot kg^{-1} \cdot meter^{-1})$
$\times \; (step \; height \; in \; meters) \; (steps \cdot min^{-1}) + 3.5 \; mL \cdot kg^{-1} \cdot min^{-1}$

$\dot{V}O_2$ is gross oxygen consumption in $mL \cdot kg^{-1} \cdot min^{-1}$; S is speed in $m \cdot min^{-1}$; BM is body mass (kg); G is the percent grade expressed as a fraction; work rate ($kg \cdot m \cdot min^{-1}$); f is stepping frequency in minutes; H is step height in meters.

From American College of Sports Medicine. ACSM's Guidelines for Exercise Testing and Prescription. 7th ed. Baltimore: Lippincott Williams & Wilkins, 2006:289.

appropriate workloads. See Tables 18.4 through 18.8 for walking, jogging/running, leg cycle ergometry, arm ergometry, and stair stepping (2). Although simpler than the calculations found in Box 18.2, the limitation of using the tables is more restricted to specific workout options. For example, for the walking table, only certain grade and speed options are presented. In Box 18.4, an example is included regarding use of these tables to determine exercise workload ranges. Other tables (3) are available with more diverse activities (ranging from cleaning the house to hunting to sports and fitness activities).

Anytime a workload is determined using oxygen consumption, the Personal Trainer must recognize individual differences in skill and efficiency doing the particular exercise. In addition to using the metabolic calculations or MET tables, a Personal Trainer should monitor the client's

BOX 18.3	Example of Metabolic Calculations

Client (Anne) characteristics:

Age = 29 years
Weight = 150 lb (68.2 kg)
Height = 69 inches (1.75 meters)
$\dot{V}O_{2max}$ = 45 mL · kg^{-1} · min^{-1} (12.9 METs)

To calculate $\dot{V}O_2R$ use the following formula:

$$\text{Target } \dot{V}O_2 = [(\text{percentage}) \times (\dot{V}O_{2max} - \dot{V}O_{2rest})] + \dot{V}O_{2rest}$$

Since Anne's $\dot{V}O_{2max}$ puts her just above the 80th percentile (see Table 18.3), she is considered to be above average. As a result, her Personal Trainer decides to prescribe a range of 60–80% $\dot{V}O_2R$. To determine the target $\dot{V}O_2$ range, the calculations are as follows for Anne:

$$\text{Target } \dot{V}O_2 \text{ (lower end)} = [(0.60) \times (45 - 3.5)] + 3.5 = 28.4 \text{ mL} \cdot \text{kg}^{-1} \cdot \text{min}^{-1} \text{ (8.1 METs)}$$
$$\text{Target } \dot{V}O_2 \text{ (upper end)} = [(0.80) \times (45 - 3.5)] + 3.5 = 36.7 \text{ mL} \cdot \text{kg}^{-1} \cdot \text{min}^{-1} \text{ (10.5 (METs)}$$

Thus, the workouts will range between 28.4 and 36.7 mL · kg^{-1} · min^{-1} (8.1 − 10.5 METs). Anne indicates that using her club membership, she enjoys brisk walking and jogging on the treadmill as well as some stationary cycling and bench stepping. She has had trouble determining the right speed and grade, resulting in either an insufficient stress or working too hard, exhausting her in a short period of time.

WALKING

Taking the equation for walking from Box 18.2, the Personal Trainer uses walking on the treadmill as the lower end of the intensity range. The Personal Trainer must determine the grade necessary to reach 28.4 mL · kg^{-1} · min^{-1}, as Anne has indicated that she feels comfortable walking at about 4.0 mph (6.4 km per hour).
   The walking equation is as follows:

$$\dot{V}O_2 \text{ (mL} \cdot \text{kg}^{-1} \cdot \text{min}^{-1}) = (0.1 \times \text{speed}) + (1.8 \times \text{speed} \times \text{grade}) + 3.5 \text{ mL} \cdot \text{kg}^{-1} \cdot \text{min}^{-1}$$

Therefore, if Anne enjoys walking at 4.0 mph (6.4 km per hour), the first thing the Personal Trainer must calculate is the speed in m · min^{-1} (as required in the formula). This can be accomplished by multiplying speed in mph by 26.8 (26.8 m · min^{-1} = 1 mph). Therefore, 4.0 mph (6.4 km per hour) is 107.2 m · min^{-1}.

$$28.4 \text{ mL} \cdot \text{kg}^{-1} \cdot \text{min}^{-1} = (0.1 \times 107.2) + (1.8 \times 107.2 \times \text{grade}) + 3.5 \text{ mL} \cdot \text{kg}^{-1} \cdot \text{min}^{-1}$$
$$\text{Grade} = 0.07 = 7\%$$

For the lower end of the intensity range, Anne will walk on the treadmill at 4.0 mph (6.4 km per hour) with a 7% grade.

RUNNING

When working toward the upper end of the intensity range, Anne will be running on the treadmill. She prefers to have little grade, and thus, the formula for running will be used to determine the speed. The running equation (see Box 18.2) is as follows:

$$\dot{V}O_2 \text{ (mL} \cdot \text{kg}^{-1} \cdot \text{min}^{-1}) = (0.2 \times \text{speed}) + (0.9 \times \text{speed} \times \text{grade}) + 3.5 \text{ mL} \cdot \text{kg}^{-1} \cdot \text{min}^{-1}$$

Therefore, if Anne wants to run with a 1% grade (*Note:* 1% = 0.01) on the treadmill, the running formula will be used to determine the speed.

$$36.7 \text{ m mL} \cdot \text{kg}^{-1} \cdot \text{min}^{-1} = (0.2 \times \text{speed}) + (0.9 \times \text{speed} \times 0.01) + 3.5 \text{ mL} \cdot \text{kg}^{-1} \cdot \text{min}^{-1}$$
$$\text{Speed} = 158.9 \text{ m} \cdot \text{min}^{-1} = 5.9 \text{ mph (9.4 km per hour)}$$

continued >

Box 18.3. Example of Metabolic Calculations, cont.

CYCLING

Anne will be cycling on a Monark cycle ergometer. As with treadmill exercise, her Personal Trainer will determine the workload at the lower and upper end of her target range (corresponding to 28.4 and 36.7 mL · kg^{-1} · min^{-1}). The formula for cycling from Box 18.2 is as follows:

$$\dot{V}O_2 \, (\text{mL} \cdot \text{kg}^{-1} \cdot \text{min}^{-1}) = \frac{1.8 \times \text{work rate in kg} \cdot \text{m} \cdot \text{min}^{-1}}{\text{Body mass}} + 3.5$$

The Personal Trainer discussed a preferred cycling cadence with Anne and found that she is most comfortable at 70 revolutions per minute. This will be used to determine the resistance level. First the overall work rate is calculated as follows:

$$28.4 \, \text{mL} \cdot \text{kg}^{-1} \cdot \text{min}^{-1} = \frac{1.8 \times \text{work rate in kg} \cdot \text{m} \cdot \text{min}^{-1}}{68.2} + 3.5$$

Thus for the lower end of the range, the work rate is 943 kg · m · min^{-1}. To determine the resistance (weight) to place on the flywheel, the following calculation is used:

Work rate (kg · m · min^{-1}) = revolutions per minute × length of flywheel in meters × resistance in kg

Since Anne desires to pedal at a rate of 70 revolutions per minute on a Monark bike (whose distance per revolution is a constant of 6 meters), the calculation of resistance:

$$943 \, \text{kg} \cdot \text{m} \cdot \text{min}^{-1} = 70 \, \text{rpm} \times 6 \, \text{meters} \times \text{resistance}$$
$$\text{Resistance} = 2.2 \, \text{kg}$$

For the upper end of the target intensity, the work rate is determined using the following formula:

$$36.7 \, \text{mL} \cdot \text{kg}^{-1} \cdot \text{min}^{-1} = \frac{1.8 \times \text{work rate in kg} \cdot \text{m} \cdot \text{min}^{-1}}{68.2} + 3.5$$

Thus the work rate is 1258 kg · m · min^{-1} and then, assuming 70 rpm, the resistance at this level would be 3.0 kg.

$$1258 \, \text{kg} \cdot \text{m} \cdot \text{min}^{-1} = 70 \, \text{rpm} \times 6 \, \text{meters} \times \text{resistance}$$
$$\text{resistance} = 3.0 \, \text{kg}$$

STEPPING

Anne owns a 12-inch step (12 in = 30.48 cm = 0.3048 m) and is interested in knowing how quickly she would need to step to be within her target intensity range. A step is defined as a four-part movement (2): "lifting one leg onto a box, fixed bench or step; pushing with this leg to raise the body; placing the other leg on the box; and stepping down with the first and then second leg in a repetitive fashion." Once again, her Personal Trainer references the formulas in Box 18.2. For stepping, the formula is as follows:

$$\dot{V}O_2 \, (\text{mL} \cdot \text{kg}^{-1} \cdot \text{min}^{-1}) = (0.2 \times \text{frequency}) + (1.33 \times 1.8 \times \text{height} \times \text{frequency}) + 3.5$$

For the lower end of Anne's target range, the frequency would be 26 steps per minute:

$$28.4 \, \text{mL} \cdot \text{kg}^{-1} \cdot \text{min}^{-1} = (0.2 \times \text{frequency}) + (1.33 \times 1.8 \times 0.3048 \times \text{frequency}) + 3.5$$

For the upper end of Anne's target range, the frequency would be 36 steps per minute:

$$36.7 \, \text{mL} \cdot \text{kg}^{-1} \cdot \text{min}^{-1} = (0.2 \times \text{frequency}) + (1.33 \times 1.8 \times 0.3048 \times \text{frequency}) + 3.5$$

Anne now has some starting points for her exercise. Initially she can begin toward the lower end of the range. Over time, she will progress toward the higher end of her intensity range. Heart rate and ratings of perceived exertion will be monitored to fine-tune this prescription.

For Personal Trainers interested in more details on the metabolic equations, please see Appendix D in the ACSM's Guidelines for Exercise Testing and Prescription. 7th ed. (2).

Table 18.4	**APPROXIMATE ENERGY REQUIREMENTS IN METs FOR HORIZONTAL AND GRADE WALKING**					
	mph	**1.7**	**2.0**	**2.5**	**3.0**	**3.4**	**3.75**
% Grade	**m · min⁻¹**	**45.6**	**53.6**	**67.0**	**80.4**	**91.2**	**100.5**
0		2.3	2.5	2.9	3.3	3.6	3.9
2.5		2.9	3.2	3.8	4.3	4.8	5.2
5.0		3.5	3.9	4.6	5.4	5.9	6.5
7.5		4.1	4.6	5.5	6.4	7.1	7.8
10.0		4.6	5.3	6.3	7.4	8.3	9.1
12.5		5.2	6.0	7.2	8.5	9.5	10.4
15.0		5.8	6.6	8.1	9.5	10.6	11.7
17.5		6.4	7.3	8.9	10.5	11.8	12.9
20.0		7.0	8.0	9.8	11.6	13.0	14.2
22.5		7.6	8.7	10.6	12.6	14.2	15.5
25.0		8.2	9.4	11.5	13.6	15.3	16.8

Reprinted with permission from American College of Sports Medicine. ACSM's Guidelines for Exercise Testing and Prescription. 7th ed. Baltimore: Lippincott Williams & Wilkins, 2006:292.

Table 18.5	**APPROXIMATE ENERGY REQUIREMENTS IN METs FOR HORIZONTAL AND GRADE JOGGING/RUNNING**						
	mph	**5**	**6**	**7**	**7.5**	**8**	**9**	**10**
% Grade	**m · min⁻¹**	**134**	**161**	**188**	**201**	**214**	**241**	**268**
0		8.6	10.2	11.7	12.5	13.3	14.8	16.3
2.5		9.5	11.2	12.9	13.8	14.7	16.3	18.0
5.0		10.3	12.3	14.1	15.1	16.1	17.9	19.7
7.5		11.2	13.3	15.3	16.4	17.4	19.4	
10.0		12.0	14.3	16.5	17.4	18.8		
12.5		12.9	15.4	17.7	18.8			
15.0		13.8	16.4	18.9				

Reprinted with permission from American College of Sports Medicine. ACSM's Guidelines for Exercise Testing and Prescription. 7th ed. Baltimore: Lippincott Williams & Wilkins, 2006:292.

Table 18.6	**APPROXIMATE ENERGY REQUIREMENTS IN METs DURING LEG AND CYCLE ERGOMETRY**						
Body Weight		**Power Output (kg · m · min⁻¹ and W)**						
kg	**lb**	**300**	**450**	**600**	**750**	**900**	**1,050**	**1,200 (kg · m · min⁻¹)**
		50	**75**	**100**	**125**	**150**	**175**	**200 (W)**
50	110	5.1	6.6	8.2	9.7	11.3	12.8	14.3
60	132	4.6	5.9	7.1	8.4	9.7	11.0	12.3
70	154	4.2	5.3	6.4	7.5	8.6	9.7	10.8
80	176	3.9	4.9	5.9	6.8	7.8	8.8	9.7
90	198	3.7	4.6	5.4	6.3	7.1	8.0	8.9
100	220	3.5	4.3	5.1	5.9	6.6	7.4	8.2

Reprinted with permission from American College of Sports Medicine. ACSM's Guidelines for Exercise Testing and Prescription. 7th ed. Baltimore: Lippincott Williams & Wilkins, 2006:292.

| Table 18.7 | APPROXIMATE ENERGY REQUIREMENTS IN METS DURING ARM ERGOMETRY |

Body Weight		Power Output (kg · m · min⁻¹ and W)					
		150	300	450	600	750	900 (kg · m · min⁻¹)
kg	Lb	25	50	75	100	125	150 (W)
50	110	5.1	6.6	8.2	9.7	11.3	12.8
60	132	4.6	5.9	7.1	8.4	9.7	11.0
70	154	4.2	5.3	6.4	7.5	8.6	9.7
80	176	3.9	4.9	5.9	6.8	7.8	8.8
90	198	3.7	4.6	5.4	6.3	7.1	8.0
100	220	3.5	4.3	5.1	5.9	6.6	7.4

Reprinted with permission from American College of Sports Medicine. ACSM's Guidelines for Exercise Testing and Prescription. 7th ed. Baltimore: Lippincott Williams & Wilkins, 2006:293.

response to the exercise (including HR, rating of perceived exertion, and any other signs or symptoms of overexertion). The Personal Trainer should assist the client with making adjustments to workload based on the individual's response to the exercise load (2).

Often, a Personal Trainer will not have access to oxygen consumption information. Heart rate and oxygen consumption have a linear relationship, or in other words, when one increases, the other increases as well. Therefore, in the absence of oxygen consumption information, heart rate can be used. Heart rate reserve is the difference between maximal heart rate and resting heart rate. This method is often referred to as the Karvonen method (2). The formulas used resemble those used with the $\dot{V}O_2R$ method:

$$\text{Target HR (lower end of range)} = ([0.40] \times [\text{HR}_{max} - \text{HR}_{rest}]) + \text{HR}_{rest}$$

$$\text{Target HR (upper end of range)} = ([0.85] \times [\text{HR}_{max} - \text{HR}_{rest}]) + \text{HR}_{rest}$$

Thus, when using this method for a 20-year-old client who has a resting HR of 75, the range would be 125–181 beats per minute. This range is too wide to be useful, and thus, the client's fitness must be considered. If the client is moderately active, using a range of 60–80% may be more appropriate. The heart rate range program is therefore 150–175 beats per minute. If the client was deconditioned, then a range of 40–50% may be more appropriate.

| Table 18.8 | APPROXIMATE ENERGY REQUIREMENTS IN METS DURING STAIR STEPPING |

Step Height		Stepping Rate per Minute					
in	m	20	22	24	26	28	30
4	0.102	3.5	3.8	4.0	4.3	4.5	4.8
6	0.152	4.2	4.6	4.9	5.2	5.5	5.8
8	0.203	4.9	5.3	5.7	6.1	6.5	6.9
10	0.254	5.6	6.1	6.5	7.0	7.5	7.9
12	0.305	6.3	6.8	7.4	7.9	8.4	9.0
14	0.356	7.0	7.6	8.2	8.8	9.4	10.0
16	0.406	7.7	8.4	9.0	9.7	10.4	11.1
18	0.457	8.4	9.1	9.9	10.6	11.4	12.1

Reprinted with permission from American College of Sports Medicine. ACSM's Guidelines for Exercise Testing and Prescription. 7th ed. Baltimore: Lippincott Williams & Wilkins, 2006:293.

BOX 18.4   **Example of Use of MET Tables**

Client (Joe) characteristics:
    Age = 40 years
    Weight = 175 lb (80 kg)
    Height = 70 inches (1.78 meters)
    $\dot{V}O_{2max}$ = 45 mL · kg^{-1} · min^{-1}

To calculate $\dot{V}O_2$R use the following formula:

$$\text{Target } \dot{V}O_2 = [(\text{percentage}) \times (\dot{V}O_{2max} - \dot{V}O_{2rest})] + \dot{V}O_{2rest}$$

Since Joe's $\dot{V}O_{2max}$ puts him at approximately the 65th percentile (see Table 18-3), he is considered to be slightly above average. As a result, his Personal Trainer decides to prescribe a range of 60−75% $\dot{V}O_2$R. To determine the target $\dot{V}O_2$ range, the calculations are as follows for Joe:

$$\text{Target } \dot{V}O_2 \text{ (lower end)} = [(0.60) \times (45 - 3.5)] + 3.5 = 28.4 \text{ mL · kg}^{-1} \cdot \text{min}^{-1} \text{ (8.1 METs)}$$
$$\text{Target } \dot{V}O_2 \text{ (upper end)} = [(0.75) \times (45 - 3.5)] + 3.5 = 34.6 \text{ mL · kg}^{-1} \cdot \text{min}^{-1} \text{ (9.9 (METs)}$$

Thus, the workouts will range between 28.4 and 34.6 mL · kg^{-1} · min^{-1} (8.1–9.9 METs). Joe indicates that he wants to use the treadmill as well as a stationary bike.

Joe's Personal Trainer will use Tables 18.4, 18.5, and 18.6. To use these tables, the Personal Trainer must convert the oxygen consumption from units of mL · kg^{-1} · min^{-1} to METs. This is accomplished by dividing the lower and upper ends of the target zone by 3.5 as shown below.

$$28.4 \text{ mL · kg}^{-1} \cdot \text{min}^{-1}/3.5 = 8.1 \text{ METs}$$
$$34.6 \text{ mL · kg}^{-1} \cdot \text{min}^{-1}/3.5 = 9.9 \text{ METs}$$

Determination of a walking intensity on the lower end of the range (~8.1 METs) is possible by using Table 18.4. Note that many options are available close to the 8.1-MET target including walking at 1.7 mph (2.7 km per hour) with 25% grade (8.2 MET level) and walking at 2.5 mph (4 km per hour) with a 15% grade (8.1 METs). This would be a rather awkward workload due to the very steep grade. Therefore, the Personal Trainer would discuss various options with Joe. Joe indicated that he likes walking on incline when exercising on the treadmill, and thus the Personal Trainer suggests 3.4 mph with a 10% grade.

For the upper end of the workload range (9.9 METs), Joe would rather jog. He prefers to jog on a level treadmill. Using Table 18.5, the Personal Trainer sees that 6 mph (9.6 km per hour) with no grade will be 10.2 METs. Joe will be instructed to monitor his heart rate and rating of perceived exertion as well to make adjustments to these workloads as he becomes accustomed to the exercise.

Joe also requested guidance on determining appropriate settings on a stationary bike. To use Table 18.6 (leg cycle ergometry), the Personal Trainer must know Joe's body weight. Body weight is 175 lb (80 kg). Going across the row for 80 kg in Table 18.6, the workloads approximating 8.1 METs and 9.9 METs are slightly over 900 kg · m · min^{-1}kg (150 watts) and 1200 kg · m · min^{-1} (200 watts). These settings will provide Joe with guidance on what workloads to use to begin his exercise.

Rating of perceived exertion (RPE) is a guideline to use when setting exercise intensity. RPE is commonly used to monitor exercise tolerance (7). Two scales are typically used. Table 18.9 lists the 6 to 20 RPE scale as well as the category-ratio scale, which rates exercise intensity on a 0 to 10 scale (2). RPE can be used to subjectively rate overall feelings of exertion and so can be helpful in guiding exercise intensity (2). The threshold level for cardiorespiratory benefits appears to be between 12 and 16 on the original scale and 4 to 5 on the ratio scale (7). The verbal descriptors for this range include "somewhat hard" to "hard." When using RPE, the Personal Trainer should keep in mind the variability between individuals (e.g., the RPE value will not necessarily correspond directly with

Table 18.9	CATEGORY AND CATEGORY-RATIO SCALES FOR RATINGS OF PERCEIVED EXERTION[a]	

Category Scale	Category-Ratio Scale[b]	
6	0 Nothing at all	"No I"
7 Very, very light	0.3	
8	0.5 Extremely weak	Just noticeable
9 Very light	0.7	
10	1 Very weak	
11 Fairly light	1.5	
12	2 Weak	Light
13 Somewhat hard	2.5	
14	3 Moderate	
15 Hard	4	
16	5 Strong	Heavy
17 Very hard	6	
18	7 Very strong	
19 Very, very hard	8	
20	9	
	10 Extremely strong	"Strongest I"
	11	
	• Absolute maximum	Highest possible

[a] Copyright Gunnar Borg. Reproduced with permission. For correct usage of the Borg scales, it is necessary to follow the administration and instructions given in Borg G. Perceived Exertion and Pain Scales. Champaign, IL: Human Kinetics, 1998.
[b] *Note:* On the Category-Ratio Scale, "I" represents intensity.

a particular percentage of maximal heart rate or percentage of heart rate reserve) and must then make adjustments as needed (2). RPE is helpful for individuals having difficulty determining exercise heart rate or who are taking medications that influence heart rate.

Another very simple way to consider intensity is the "talk test" (8). This simply means that as clients exercise, they should be able to respond to someone. When comfortable speech is not possible (e.g., gasping for breath after every word or two), it may indicate that the intensity is moving above the level typically prescribed. Thus, the goal is to exercise close to the point at which speech first become difficult. Although very simple, it appears that use of the talk test does allow consistent training intensities.

EXERCISE SESSION DURATION

Duration and intensity are inversely related. As one increases, the other decreases. ACSM recommends 20 to 60 minutes of aerobic activity (2). This can be in one exercise session or could be accomplished intermittently (minimum number of minutes per session is 10 if done intermittently). Sedentary individuals should start exercising gradually. Short bouts (e.g., 5 minutes) of low-intensity exercise may be used until more extended periods of time can be completed without excessive fatigue. The rate of progression will vary depending on the health status and age of the individual.

Intensity of the exercise is a consideration when determining the duration. The intensity level may necessarily be higher for more fit individuals than that used for a sedentary individual because the threshold for cardiorespiratory benefits will be higher. Risk (2) does increase with higher intensity exercise (both cardiovascular and orthopedic). Also, exercise compliance (i.e., sticking with the exercise program) decreases as intensity increases. Therefore, for most individuals engaging in exercise to improve health and fitness, a prescription targeting 77–90% of maximal heart rate or 60–80% of heart rate reserve for 20 to 30 minutes is sufficient. This time frame does not include warm-up and cooldown, both of which would be done in addition to the time spent at the target exercise program (2).

EXERCISE FREQUENCY

Exercise frequency is the final component in a complete exercise program. For sedentary individuals, incorporating even a couple of days per week can initiate improvements in cardiorespiratory fitness (7). The optimal frequency appears to be 3 to 5 days per week (1, 2). As with intensity, although additional benefits may be achieved above the upper end of the target range, the risk of injuries also increases. Admittedly, individuals focused on competition or performance will likely train 6 or more days per week. Different goals will require different exercise programs and thus involve different associated risks. ACSM suggests that 3 days per week is sufficient to improve maximal oxygen consumption when exercising at 77–90% of maximal heart rate or 60–80% of heart rate reserve (2). If weight loss is a goal, then exercise may need to be more frequent (9). Similarly, if the exercise intensity is held at the lower end of the target range, then the frequency could be increased (2). In some situations, for deconditioned individuals, multiple short daily exercise sessions may be more appropriate (2).

CALORIES EXPENDED: A SUMMARY OF THE ENDURANCE PHASE

Selection of mode, intensity, duration, and frequency determines the calories expended during the activity. This caloric expenditure can be used to provide an overall summary of the workout. ACSM recommends expending 150 to 400 calories in physical activity each day (2). Previously sedentary individuals will begin on the lower end of the range and progress upward. Expenditures of approximately 1000 calories per week are associated with decreases in the risk of all-cause mortality (2). For weight loss, overweight and obese adults should strive toward expending 2000 calories per week or more (9).

Some shortcomings of caloric expenditure estimates include coordination and skill influences. An experienced swimmer, for example, will expend less energy to swim the same pace as someone with inefficient stroke patterns. Even though at a similar pace, the inexperienced swimmer will have a much higher caloric expenditure than the experienced athlete. Thus, inter-individual differences limit the precision of this estimation. Realizing the limitations, the Personal Trainer may use the following equation to approximate the number of calories expended per minute of a given activity (2):

$$(\text{METs} \times \mathbf{3.5} \times \text{body weight in kilograms})/\mathbf{200} = \text{calories per minute}$$

The attractive aspect of using this approach is the inclusion of both time and the intensity of the prescribed exercise mode. For example, if a client runs on the treadmill at 0% grade (level) and 7 mph (11.2 km/hour) for 45 minutes, the Personal Trainer can "summarize" the workout by using the formula for calories per minutes. Using Table 18.5, the MET level for 7 mph (11.2 km/hour) and 0% grade is 11.7 METs. If the client weighs 150 lb (68.2 kg), then the number of calories expended for the total workout can be determined as follows:

$$(11.7 \times 3.5 \times 68.2)/200 = 14 \text{ calories per minute}$$

$$14 \text{ calories per minute} \times 45 \text{ minutes} = 630 \text{ calories for the workout}$$

Tracking the calories expended can be helpful, since the time, intensity, and mode of exercise are all factors in the outcome. Also, for clients focusing on weight loss, it is very helpful to be able to calculate the number of calories expended in a given activity.

Finally, observation of the client performing higher intensity cardiovascular training requires close evaluation by the Personal Trainer. As cardiovascular intensity increases, signs of fatigue may be observed. Those signs may include more labored breathing and muscular fatigue resulting in possible faltered movement patterns and improper posture. Personal Trainers need to be cognizant of the results of client's fatigue and be prepared to offer suggestions and recommendations on maintaining proper alignment and movement patterns while reaching higher cardiovascular exercise stress levels.

Cool-Down

The cool-down is a transition from the higher intensity of the endurance phase back toward resting levels. The cool-down allows heart rate, blood pressure, and respiration rate to shift downward and back toward resting levels. By allowing a gradual progression toward resting rather than abruptly stopping exercise, the client will also avoid post-exercise hypotension (low blood pressure) and resulting dizziness (from lack of blood flow back to the heart and brain as a result of blood pooling in the legs). A gradual decrease in intensity also helps to dissipate body heat, promotes lactate removal (metabolic by-product that the body can actually break down for fuel during low levels of activity rather than being inactive), and attenuates the rise in catecholamines (hormones released that increase heart rate and blood pressure), which often follows exercise (2).

The cool-down period is one of gradual recovery from the endurance phase of the workout. As with the warm-up, approximately 10 minutes of activities of diminished intensities is appropriate (2). For higher intensity exercise, a longer cool-down may be warranted. For example, to return to the client who uses brisk walking as an exercise mode for the endurance phase, an appropriate cool-down would include slow walking for 5 minutes followed by 5 minutes of total body stretches.

SAMPLE CARDIOVASCULAR TRAINING PROGRAMS

In the following pages, examples of various cardiorespiratory endurance programs are presented. In Table 18.10, an overall scheme of training progression is shown for an apparently healthy client (2). The use of the terms to describe the program state—"initial," "improvement," and "maintenance"—is somewhat subjective. For some individuals, the initial stage may present too much of a challenge. If so, starting out with 5- to 10-minute bouts of exercise as tolerated may be more appropriate. The focus is not on starting aggressively or achieving target goals quickly, but rather on gradually increasing the overall workload to promote adherence. Progression should be individualized based on health status, age, individual goals, and current functional capacity (2).

For each of the stages, a range rather than a single number is included for frequency, intensity, and duration. The role of a Personal Trainer is to assist the client with the appropriate balance based on individual responses. Frequency of exercise progresses gradually over the 6-month period outlined, from 3 days per week up to a target of 3 to 5 days per week. Intensity increases from

Table 18.10 TRAINING PROGRESSION FOR SEDENTARY LOW-RISK PARTICIPANTS[a]

Program Stage	Week	Exercise Frequency (sessions/week)	Exercise Intensity (%HRR)	Exercise Duration (min)
Initial stage	1	3	40–50	15–20
	2	3–4	40–50	20–25
	3	3–4	50–60	20–25
	4	3–4	50–60	25–30
Improvement stage	5–7	3–4	60–70	25–30
	8–10	3–4	60–70	30–35
	11–13	3–4	65–75	30–35
	14–16	3–5	65–75	30–35
	17–20	3–5	70–85	35–40
	21–24	3–5	70–85	35–40
Maintenance stage[b]	24+	3–5	70–85	20–60

Reprinted with permission from American College of Sports Medicine. ACSM's Guidelines for Exercise Testing and Prescription. 7th ed. Baltimore: Lippincott Williams & Wilkins, 2006:149.

[a] Defined as the lowest risk categories in Table 14-3.

[b] Depending on long-term goals of program, the intensity, frequency, and duration may vary.

HRR, heart rate reserve; it is recommended that low-risk cardiac patients train at the lower end of these ranges.

relatively low to a target of 70–85% heart rate reserve. By slowly increasing the intensity, the client is able to adapt to the higher levels of exercise without becoming discouraged or experiencing retrogression (i.e., a reversal of gains as a result of excessive overload). The duration of the exercise session also increases in small steps to allow appropriate adaptations.

Fitness Progression for Beginners

Tables 18.11 through 18.13 include examples of training programs for various types of activities for a person who has not been previously active. Table 18.11 is a sample workout schedule for a walking program. Recall that walking (especially treadmill walking) is a group 1 activity because of the relative ease in maintaining a constant intensity. Table 18.12 is a sample workout schedule for a swimming program. Swimming is an example of a group 2 activity because of the skill level required to maintain a constant intensity for a sufficient period of time. Table 18.13 is a mixture of activities, which may be available at a health club. Note the sequence in time, intensity, and frequency as well as a progression in the different types of activities. New modes of exercise can provide much appreciated variety but should be introduced gradually so that appropriate adjustments can be made (i.e., appropriate overload).

Fitness Gains and Weight Loss

Clients who have not been active and are striving to achieve a healthier body weight often consult Personal Trainers. The ACSM Position Stand, "Appropriate Intervention Strategies for Weight Loss and Prevention of Weight Regain for Adults" (9) indicates that to assist in weight loss, increasing activity levels to 45 minutes per day may be required for overweight adults. In Box 18.5, an example is given for a male who is sedentary and overweight.

Table 18.11	**SAMPLE WALKING PROGRAM**			
Fitness Level	**Time Point**	**Warm-up**	**Workout**	**Cool-down**
Beginner	First week	Slow easy walking pace and gentle body stretches for 5 min	Walk at a pace that gives a fairly light level of exertion (RPE 11–12) for 10–15 min (3 days per week)	Slow easy walking pace for 5 min
	Later weeks	Slow easy walking pace and gentle body stretches for 10 min	Walk at a pace that gives a moderate level of exertion (RPE 12–13) for 20–25 min (3–4 days per week)	Slow easy walking pace for 10 min
Intermediate	Initial weeks	Slow easy walking pace and gentle body stretches for 10 min	Walk at a pace that feels somewhat hard (RPE 13–14) for 20–25 min (3–4 days per week)	Easy walking pace for 10 min
	Middle weeks	Slow easy walking pace and gentle body stretches for 10 min	Walk at a pace that feels somewhat hard to hard (RPE 13–15) for 25–30 min (3–5 days per week)	Easy walking pace for 10 min
	Later weeks	Slow easy walking pace and gentle body stretches for 10 min	Walk at a pace that feels hard (RPE 15–16) for 30–35 min (3–5 days per week)	Easy walking pace for 10 min
Established	Continue	Slow easy walking pace and gentle body stretches for 10 min	Walk at a pace that feels hard (15–16) for 30–40 min (3–5 days per week)	Easy walking pace for 10 min

Reprinted with permission from Bushman B, Young JC. Action Plan for Menopause. Champaign, IL: Human Kinetics 2005:142.

Table 18.12 SAMPLE SWIMMING PROGRAM

Fitness Level	Time Point	Warm-up	Workout	Cool-down
Beginner	First week	Gentle shoulder and arm stretches, easy swimming pace for 5 min (change strokes as needed)	Use kickboard and swim laps (alternating strokes and type of kicking) at a fairly light level of exertion (RPE 11–12) for 10–15 min (3 days per week)	Easy swim pace (use favorite stroke) for 5 min, stretch calf and shoulder muscles
	Later weeks	Shoulder and arm stretches, easy pace swim and kick (change strokes and kicks as needed) for 10 min	Use kickboard, pull buoy, and swim laps (alternating strokes and type of kicking) at a moderate level of exertion (RPE 12–13) for 20–25 min (3–4 days per week)	Easy swim pace (use 2 favorite strokes) for 10 min, stretch calf and shoulder muscles
				Total distance: approximately 500 yd (depends on skill level)
Intermediate	Initial weeks	Shoulder and arm stretches, easy pace swim and kick (change strokes and kicks as needed) for 10 min	Use kickboard, pull buoy, and swim laps (alternating strokes and type of kicking) at a pace that feels somewhat hard (RPE 13–14) for 20–25 min (3–4 days per week)	Easy swim and pull for 10 min, stretch calf and shoulder muscles
	Middle weeks	Shoulder and arm stretches, easy pace swim and kick (change strokes and kicks as needed) for 10 min	Use kickboard, pull buoy, and swim laps (alternating strokes and type of kicking), keeping RI at :15–:20, at a pace that feels somewhat hard to hard (RPE 13–15) for 25–30 min (3–5 days per week)	Easy swim and pull for 10 min, stretch calf and shoulder muscles
	Later weeks	Shoulder and arm stretches, easy pace swim and kick (change strokes and kicks as needed) for 10 min	Use kickboard, pull buoy, and swim laps (alternating strokes and type of kicking), keeping RI at :10–:15, at a pace that feels hard (RPE 15–16) for 30–35 min (3–5 days per week)	Easy swim and pull for 10 min, stretch calf and shoulder muscles
				Total distance: 900–1,350 yd (depends on skill level)
Established	Continue	Shoulder and arm stretches, easy pace swim and kick (change strokes and kicks as needed) for 10 min	Swim, kick, pull, keeping RI at :10–:15, at a pace that feels hard (RPE 15–16) for 30–40 min; use repeated sets, ascending, descending, or Fartlek swims (3–5 days per week)	Easy swim and pull for 10 min, stretch calf and shoulder muscles
				Total distance: 1,500–2,000 yd (depends on skill level)

Note: For the workout, those with more advanced swimming skill can alternate strokes (freestyle, backstroke, breaststroke) and add repeated sets of swims, pulls, and kicks. For example: intermediate-skill swimmers: swim 2 \X\ 50, 2 \X\ 100 with RI of :15–:20; established swimmers: swim 4 \X\ 100 with :10–:15 RI, kick 4 \X\ 75 with :10–:15 RI, pull 6 \X\ 50 with :10–:15 RI.

Reprinted with permission from Bushman B, Young JC. Action Plan for Menopause. Champaign, IL: Human Kinetics, 2005:144.

Table 18-13 SAMPLE CROSS TRAINING PROGRAM AT A HEALTH CLUB

Fitness Level	Time Point	Warm-up	Workout	Cool-down
Beginner	Early weeks	Slow easy walking pace and gentle body stretches for 5 min	Pick one activity each day at RPE 11–12 (fairly light level of exertion) for 10–15 min (3–4 days per week): • Walking on the treadmill • Stationary bike	Slow easy walking pace for 5 min
	Later weeks	Slow easy walking pace and gentle body stretches for 10 min	Pick one activity each day at RPE 12–13 (moderate level of exertion) for 20–25 min (3–4 days per week): • Brisk walking on the treadmill • Stationary bike • Stair stepper	Slow easy walking pace for 10 min
Intermediate	Early weeks	Slow easy walking pace and gentle body stretches for 10 min	Pick one activity each day at RPE 13–14 (somewhat hard level of exertion) for 20–25 min (3–4 days per week): • Brisk walking or jogging on the treadmill • Stationary bike • Stair stepper • Elliptical trainer • Nordic ski machine	Easy walking pace for 10 min
	Middle weeks	Slow easy walking pace and gentle body stretches for 10 min	Pick one activity each day at RPE 13–15 (somewhat hard to hard level of exertion) for 25–30 min (3–5 days per week): • Brisk walking or jogging on the treadmill • Stationary bike • Stair stepper • Elliptical trainer • Nordic ski machine • Floor or step aerobics class	Easy walking pace for 10 min
	Later weeks	Slow easy walking pace and gentle body stretches for 10 min	Pick one activity each day at RPE 15–16 (hard level of exertion) for 30–35 min (3–5 days per week): • Brisk walking or jogging on the treadmill • Stationary bike • Elliptical trainer • Stair stepper • Nordic ski machine • Floor or step aerobics class • Spinning class	Easy walking pace for 10 min
Established	Continue	Slow easy walking pace and gentle body stretches for 10 min	Pick an exercise that provides you with an intensity that feels hard (15–16) for 30–40 min (3–5 days per week)	Easy walking pace for 10 min

Reprinted with permission from Bushman B, Young JC. Action Plan for Menopause. Champaign, IL: Human Kinetics, 2005:145–146.

BOX 18.5

Example for Obese Client

Client (Bob) characteristics:
Age = 35 years
Weight = 210 lb (95.5 kg)
Height = 71 inches (1.80 meters)

Bob has led an inactive lifestyle with a desk/office job and desires to start an exercise program to assist him with his weight loss goals. He is consulting a dietitian regarding better food choices and realizes the importance of exercise in helping him lose the weight and maintaining the weight loss. Bob's Personal Trainer will develop a comprehensive program, including cardiorespiratory endurance training, resistance training, and flexibility. Listed below is the starting point for Bob's cardiorespiratory training program.

The Personal Trainer has reviewed Bob's health history and finds that other than his weight (which for his height results in a body mass index of 29.5), which places him in the overweight classification, and his sedentary lifestyle, he has no other risk factors for coronary artery disease. With this in mind, his ACSM risk stratification is "moderate risk" (see Table 14.3), so beginning a moderate intensity program is appropriate.

Using a cardiorespiratory fitness assessment (see examples in Chapter 15), the Personal Trainer estimates Bob's $\dot{V}O_{2max}$ to be 39 mL $\cdot$ kg^{-1} $\cdot$ min^{-1} ("below average" category according to Table 18.3). Bob's target range ($\dot{V}O_2$R method) will be lower than those in previous examples in this chapter because of his lower fitness level. The Personal Trainer decides to start with 45 to 60% $\dot{V}O_2$R. This is calculated as follows:

$$\text{Target } \dot{V}O_2 \text{ (lower end)} = [(0.45) \times (39 - 3.5)] + 3.5 = 19.5 \text{ mL} \cdot \text{kg}^{-1} \cdot \text{min}^{-1} \text{ (5.6 METs)}$$
$$\text{Target } \dot{V}O_2 \text{ (upper end)} = [(0.60) \times (39 - 3.5)] + 3.5 = 24.8 \text{ mL} \cdot \text{kg}^{-1} \cdot \text{min}^{-1} \text{ (7.1 METs)}$$

Getting an idea of a starting speed for treadmill walking can be done by consulting Table 18.4. To use this table, oxygen consumption values in mL $\cdot$ kg^{-1} $\cdot$ min^{-1} must be converted to METs (divide each by 3.5). This results in a range of 5.6 to 7.1 METs. Going to Table 18.4, the Personal Trainer selects 3.0 mph (4.8 km per hour) with a 5% grade as a starting point for the endurance of the exercise session.

To adjust the workout based on Bob's responses, the Personal Trainer has determined a heart rate range (using the HRR method). HR_{max} will be estimated from Bob's age (220 − age = 220 − 35 = 185). Bob's HR_{rest} is 70. To determine the lower end of the heart rate range, the following was calculated:

$$\text{Target HR (lower end of range)} = [(0.45) \times (HR_{max} - HR_{rest})] + HR_{rest}$$
$$\text{Target HR (lower end of range)} = [(0.45) \times (185 - 70)] + 70 = 122$$

To determine the upper end of the heart rate range, the following was calculated:

$$\text{Target HR (upper end of range)} = [(0.60) \times (HR_{max} - HR_{rest})] + HR_{rest}$$
$$\text{Target HR (upper end of range)} = [(0.60 \times (185 - 70)] + 70 = 139$$

Bob's Personal Trainer will use this information to make adjustments to Bob's exercise prescription.

After an initial warm-up, Bob begins walking on the treadmill at 3 mph (4.8 km per hour) with a 5% grade. Using a heart rate monitor to help track intensity, the Personal Trainer notes that Bob's heart rate is stabilizing at around 132 beats per minute. Noting that this is toward the upper end of the target heart rate range (122–139 beats per minute), the Personal Trainer lowers the grade to 3% and finds that Bob's heart rate responds by lowering to 126 beats per minute. The use of heart rate along with the pre-determined workload allows a well-controlled exercise prescription. Subjectively, Bob can also use the rating of perceived exertion and the talk test.

Initially Bob will walk for only 10 minutes. Establishing a baseline level of fitness and a pattern of activity is the goal for new exercisers. Bob's Personal Trainer will make small weekly adjustments to continue to provide an appropriate overload. Using Table 18.10 can be very helpful in providing appropriate exercise program progression.

A long-term goal for Bob to promote sustained weight loss will be to incorporate 200–300 minutes of physical activity each week (9) into his lifestyle. A regular exercise program, in addition to positive nutritional changes, is key to Bob's weight-loss goals as well as his ability to keep the weight off.

IMPLEMENTATION OF CARDIOVASCULAR TRAINING PROGRAMS

Implementation of effective cardiovascular endurance training programs requires the Personal Trainer to have knowledge of the current scientific basis of exercise. This chapter reviews in detail the ACSM guidelines regarding intensity, frequency, and duration. These guidelines provide a framework rather than a rigid checklist. The Personal Trainer must evaluate each client individually. This includes an understanding of health status and cardiovascular risks (see Chapters 14 and 15). Individual fitness assessments provide baseline information that is used to determine an appropriate initial level of exercise. Creating the exercise program is like being a master chef. Unlike a novice, who would be tied to a recipe, the master chef is able to take knowledge of various ingredients to create individualized dishes. In a similar manner, a qualified Personal Trainer does not try to fit all clients into a single mode (i.e., recipe approach) but rather has a solid understanding of the ingredients (i.e., mode, frequency, intensity, and duration) and is able to customize the combination of those ingredients for the benefit of the client.

SUMMARY

When considering the balance of intensity, duration, and frequency, the Personal Trainer must take into account the goals of the client (e.g., general fitness, weight loss, competition), life situations (e.g., work schedule, availability of exercise time), and client preferences (7). Cardiorespiratory endurance training is a pivotal piece within a client's exercise program. The other components of resistance and flexibility training are detailed in Chapters 17 and 19. A cardiorespiratory endurance training session includes three basic components: warm-up, endurance phase, and cool-down. A cardiorespiratory endurance program includes consideration of intensity, duration, and frequency. The Personal Trainer must determine the appropriate balance of these three factors on the basis of the client's current health status and fitness goals.

REFERENCES

1. American College of Sports Medicine. Position Stand: The recommended quantity and quality of exercise for developing and maintaining cardiorespiratory and muscular fitness, and flexibility in health adults. Med Sci Sports Exerc 1998;30:975–991.
2. ACSM's Guidelines for Exercise Testing and Prescription. 7th ed. Philadelphia: Lippincott Williams & Wilkins, 2006.
3. ACSM's Resource Manual for Guidelines for Exercise Testing and Prescription. 5th ed. Philadelphia: Lippincott Williams & Wilkins, 2006.
4. Clausen JP, Trap-Jensen J, Lassen NA. The effects of training on the heart rate during arm and leg exercise. Scand J Clin Lab Invest 1970;26:295–301.
5. Pate RR, Hughes RD, Chandler JV. Effects of arm training on retention of training effects derived from leg training. Med Sci Sports 1978;10:71–74.
6. McKenzie DC, Fox EL, Cohen K. Specificity of metabolic and circulatory responses to arm or leg interval training. Eur J Appl Physiol Occup Physiol 1978;39:241–248.
7. ACSM's Guidelines for Exercise Testing and Prescription. 6th ed. Philadelphia: Lippincott Williams & Wilkins, 2000.
8. Persinger R, Foster C, Gibson M, et al. Consistency of the talk test for exercise prescription. Med Sci Sports Exerc 2004;36:1632–1636.
9. American College of Sports Medicine. Position Stand: Appropriate intervention strategies for weight loss and prevention of weight regain for adults. Med Sci Sports Exerc 2001;33:2145–2156.

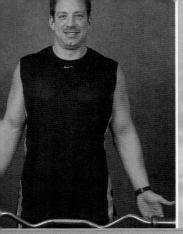

Guidelines for Designing Flexibility Programs

19

Christopher Berger, M.S., Department of Kinesiology & Health Promotion, University of Kentucky, Lexington, Kentucky
Jan Schroeder, Ph.D., Associate Professor, Department of Kinesiology, California State University, Long Beach, Long Beach, California

Chapter Outline

Determinants of Flexibility
- Age
- Gender
- Physical Activity History

Benefits and Risks of Flexibility Training
- Benefits
  - Improved ROM in Selected Joints
  - Improved Performance for Activities of Daily Living
- Risks
  - Joint Hypermobility
  - Decreased Strength
  - Ineffectiveness

Evaluating Flexibility

Three Types of Stretching
- Static
- Dynamic
- Proprioceptive Neuromuscular Facilitation

Rationale for Flexibility Training

General Guidelines to Consider When Designing a Flexibility Training Program
- Warm-Up
- Breathing
- Posture

Precautions for Individuals with Health Concerns
- Arthritis
- Muscular Imbalance
- Osteoporosis
- Hip Fracture/Replacement

Flexibility Program Development
- Frequency
- Intensity
- Duration
- Mode

Objectives

- Introduce flexibility as a health-related dimension of fitness
- Present three basic types of stretching (static, dynamic, proprioceptive neuromuscular facilitation)
- Discuss concepts and current controversy surrounding stretching
- Outline factors that influence flexibility and the response to training
- Suggest safe and effective stretches to perform
- Provide sample flexibility programs

Flexibility refers to the degree to which a joint moves throughout a normal, pain-free range of motion (ROM). As most physical activities and sports consist of numerous multi-joint movements, it is essential that musculoskeletal function not be compromised by inadequate flexibility. Stretching is the method used most commonly to increase joint ROM. In its current Position Stand on exercises to develop and maintain fitness and flexibility in adults, the American College of Sports Medicine recommends the inclusion of general stretching exercises that emphasize the major skeletal muscle groups at least 2 to 3 days a week (1).

Like body composition, cardiorespiratory fitness, or muscular strength, flexibility is classified as a health-related dimension of fitness (2). This means that flexibility not only has important performance implications for certain sports and day-to-day physical activities, but it also contributes to an overall improved quality of life in athletes and the general public alike.

The purpose of this chapter is to present flexibility as an essential ingredient of health-related fitness and to provide Personal Trainers with a basic understanding of how to properly incorporate flexibility training into the exercise programs of healthy individuals.

DETERMINANTS OF FLEXIBILITY

Hamill and Knutzen (3) suggest that several factors determine flexibility. These factors include joint structure, soft tissue around the joint, and length of the muscles being stretched. Not surprisingly then, flexibility is largely determined by how well joints facilitate movement. To better understand the importance of these factors, study Figure 19.1 carefully. Figure 19.1 depicts an anterior view *(left panel)* and cross-sectional view *(right panel)* of a typical joint—the human knee.

Notice that the knee is padded with fat and is secured into place by ligaments. These tissues influence knee ROM both at the joint itself and elsewhere in the lower extremity. There are several examples of this to consider. For example, tightness of the ligaments illustrated in the top panel or excessive fat surrounding the thigh could both inhibit knee ROM during flexion. In fact, one belief about body builders is that they are "muscle bound" and possess a more limited joint ROM as a result of the additional bulk. This is true to a certain extent because thick skeletal muscles can certainly limit ROM. Although flexibility is the theme of this chapter, it is important to understand that it is only one component of health-related fitness. If the training demands of an athlete or the natural (healthy) body composition of a client predispose them toward muscle bulk rather than flexibility, a more limited joint ROM may be tolerable.

Because muscles bring about bone movement, the reader can also see from Figure 19.1 that contraction of the quadriceps femoris would produce leg extension if the knee were bent at the start of the movement. However, a tight quadriceps femoris (perhaps as a result of soreness or poor conditioning) could restrict leg extension and limit flexibility. Notice too that the joint is restricted by the very architecture of the bones themselves. Leg extension is limited by what are termed "bony blocks," which consist of nothing more than the ends of the femur and tibia resisting hyperextension during full leg extension brought about by the quadriceps femoris. Of course, it is also important to understand that injury, disease, and poor soft tissue integrity could also contribute to hypermobility or a condition in which individuals have excessive ROM in a joint. The possibility of hypermobility can also be imagined when studying Figure 19.1.

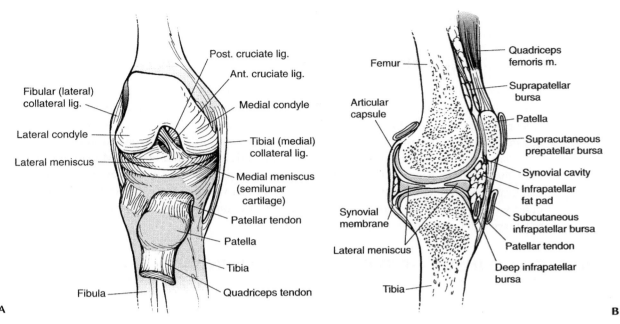

FIGURE 19.1. Typical joint anatomy. (Reprinted with permission from Hamill J, Knutzen KM. Biomechanical Basis of Human Movement. 2nd ed. Philadelphia: Lippincott Williams & Wilkins, 2003:431.)

The point of this brief anatomical review is to establish that joints have inherent structural properties that determine full ROM. Not surprisingly, these properties differ by joint and among individuals and often explain joint ROM differences expressed during testing and physical activity. Some of these factors can be controlled, while others cannot. Although the anatomical structure of the joint clearly influences ROM, there are other influences. Commonly, these influences include age, gender, and physical activity history.

Age

As we grow older, the ability to move through a full ROM becomes compromised with an overall loss of flexibility of approximately 25–30% by age 70 (4–7). The decreases in flexibility that one may experience will depend on the joint itself. Brown and Miller (8) determined a 30% loss in hamstring flexibility from the age of 20–29 to 70+ years, while Germain and Blair (6) found a 15% loss in shoulder flexion from the age of 20–30 to 70+ years.

Loss of ROM within a joint may have several causes. With age, changes occur in the framework of the connective tissue collagen fibers as demonstrated by increased rigidity of the tissue (9). This increased rigidity is attributed to tighter cross-linkage within and between collagen fibers, which makes the joint more resistant to bending (10,11). There is also a reduction of elastin as well as a deterioration of the cartilage, ligaments, tendons, synovial fluid, and muscles with age that may decrease joint ROM (12–14). Physiological changes are not the only suspect in the age-related loss of flexibility. Decreased physical activity appears to accelerate the age-related loss of physical activity (13,15).

Gender

Numerous studies suggest that females are more flexible than males owing to a different pattern of skeletal architecture and connective-tissue morphology and certain hormonal differences (2,17–20). The differences in ROM between genders may result from differences in joint and bone structures. Alter (16) has suggested that females typically have broader and shallower hips than males, which creates the possibility of a greater ROM in the pelvic region. Gelabert (19) also suggested that females generally have a greater range of extension in the elbow because of a shorter upper curve of the olecranon process of the elbow than in males. Females may also have greater potential for flexibility in trunk flexion after puberty because of a comparatively lower center of gravity and shorter leg length (21).

Physical Activity History

An individual's history of physical activity has an impact on his or her joint ROM. Studies have shown that an individual who is physically active is also more likely to have a greater ROM than a sedentary individual (22–24). Cornu et al. (22) demonstrated that volleyball players exhibited greater flexibility in wrist extension than sedentary individuals. In another sport-related study, Jaeger et al. (23) found that that elite field hockey players had significantly greater hip ROM than did sedentary individuals. Studies have not been limited to sport activity, though. In a study by Voorrips et al. (25) that examined different habitual physical activity of older women, it was found that the more active older women had significantly greater flexibility in the hip and spine than moderately active and sedentary older women.

BENEFITS AND RISKS OF FLEXIBILITY TRAINING

As with other forms of physical training, flexibility training is believed to present clients with certain benefits and risks. These benefits and risks are frequently categorized from the personal experiences of coaches, clinicians, and exercise leaders. It is important for Personal Trainers to understand, though, that while such perspectives have their place in the apprenticeship of the fitness professional, the only sound forms of training come from those rooted in an understanding of human anatomy and physiology, biomechanics, and the unique physical and psychological qualities of the client. Unfortunately, the existing science of flexibility training often presents fitness professionals with more questions than answers regarding the benefits and risks of stretching. The following two sections will provide you with a short review of what are commonly held to be the benefits and risks associated with flexibility training.

Benefits

IMPROVED ROM IN SELECTED JOINTS

Flexibility training has been shown to improve an individual's joint ROM (25–27). In a long-term study on the effects of exercise on shoulder and hip ROM by Misner et al. (27), it was found that the flexibility program used produced significant increases in shoulder extension (5.7%), shoulder transverse extension (10.4%), hip flexion (13.3%), and hip rotation (6.3%). A minor improvement (5.5%) was also observed in shoulder flexion. Improvements in flexibility could be seen in a relatively short time period. Kerrigan et al. (24) recorded improved ROM values in both static and dynamic hip extension when participants followed the program twice daily for 10 weeks. Kuukkanen et al. (26) also found improvements in spinal ROM and greater hamstring flexibility after subjects followed a 3-month program.

IMPROVED PERFORMANCE FOR ACTIVITIES OF DAILY LIVING

The extent to which individuals can live independently in the community depends on their ability to perform basic daily tasks such as self-care and essential household chores. Individuals aged 65 years and older, living independently or in nursing home facilities, are especially good candidates for training programs that help to improve overall physical functionality. These individuals allocate most of their activity time to the performance of tasks that are formally termed "activities of daily living" (ADLs). As they become older, executions of ADLs are often reported to be extremely difficult, if not impossible (27). The ability to perform ADLs has been highly correlated with joint mobility (28). In other words, ADLs are easier to perform when an individual possesses an acceptable ROM within the joint. It has also been found that flexibility training can improve ADL functioning. Klein et al. (31) found that flexibility training improved the execution of certain ADLs within an older adult population.

Risks

JOINT HYPERMOBILITY

Hypermobility syndrome is known as "congenital laxity" of ligaments and joints. This condition is characterized by extreme ROM accompanied by mild- to moderate-intensity pain (32). Although it is suggested that certain athletes (e.g., gymnasts) and individuals may possess extraordinary joint ROM, there is insufficient scientific evidence to link hypermobility to flexibility training.

DECREASED STRENGTH

There is some evidence to suggest that stretching may contribute to decreased muscular strength. In a recent study, Nelson et al. (32) found reduced muscle strength and endurance performance after short-term static stretching in physical education college students. Fowles et al. (34) found similar results after prolonged stretching of the ankle plantar flexors. This voluntary strength deficit lasted for up to an hour after stretching. In addition, Kokkonen et al. (35) demonstrated that stretching prior to the execution of a 1RM decreased the performance of the lift. Although these studies suggest that strength may be compromised following a short-term stretching session, studies need to be conducted to determine the long-term effects of stretching on strength.

INEFFECTIVENESS

In their 2004 review of the literature, Thacker et al. (36) were unable to conclude whether or not stretching before or after exercise contributed to injury prevention among competitive or recreational athletes. This was an important finding in the literature because flexibility training is often promoted as a means of reducing injury risk. Witvrouw et al. (37) also reviewed the literature regarding injury prevention and flexibility. They concluded that the type of sport activity in which an individual participates is critical when determining the value of flexibility training to reduce injury. The more explosive the skills involved in an activity, the more likely stretching may be needed to decrease injury. Interestingly, the duration of increased flexibility after stretching may not be as long as Personal Trainers may think.

In two of the more recently conducted studies, DePino et al. (38) recruited 30 male subjects and found that hamstring static stretch-induced knee ROM gains likely last no longer than approximately 3 minutes. These authors further suggest that athletes who statically stretch and then wait longer than 3 minutes before activity can expect to lose ROM gained as a result of the preceding bout of stretching. Spernoga et al. (39) also recruited 30 male subjects, used proprioceptive neuromuscular facilitation (PNF) techniques, and found increased hamstring flexibility that lasted only 6 minutes after the stretching protocol ended.

EVALUATING FLEXIBILITY

Assessment of clients' ROM is an essential component of developing their exercise programs. Goniometry assessment provides the fitness professional with several important pieces of information. These include:

➤ Immediate ROM feedback
➤ Identification of muscular imbalances
➤ Current ROM prior to the start of the exercise program
➤ Insight into the client's learning preferences and a baseline measurement from which plans can be made for future exercise goals

Following goniometry assessments for ROM, the fitness professional can make much more educated decisions about which flexibility exercises to focus on within a training session. For example, if a client could only raise his arm to a 75° angle of shoulder abduction, when the average ROM is 90° (palm facing the body), then stretches for shoulder abduction would be introduced to allow the client to achieve the norm. Keep in mind that ROM assessment is not a one-time occurrence; it should be conducted every 4 to 6 weeks to determine if the client has improved through training. If the client has improved, the Personal Trainer can be assured that the program is on the right track. However, if the client has not gained improved ROM or body alignment, a change in the program design is warranted.

THREE TYPES OF STRETCHING

Several methods exist to improve flexibility and increase joint ROM, but nearly all of them involve some form of stretching. Stretches can be performed by the client (active stretching) or by the Personal Trainer (passive stretching). Although passive stretching can be very helpful for improving flexibility, it is most safely performed by a Personal Trainer with adequate knowledge and experience to prevent injury to the client. There are generally three types of stretching that can be performed to improve flexibility: static, dynamic, and PNF, all of which are described in Chapter 6 and summarized here.

Static

Static stretching is undoubtedly the method used most commonly to improve flexibility. Static stretching can be performed actively and passively and consists of slow movements into position and holding the position for a few seconds at peak tension. For example, to actively stretch the sternocleidomastoid (neck) muscles, the client would perform a lateral flexion of the neck as depicted in Figure 19.2. This position would be held at peak tension for 10–30 seconds before returning the head upright. Static stretches can be modified too, as depicted in Figure 19.2, so that the client can better hold at peak tension or truly achieve peak tension via self-assistance and support. Further,

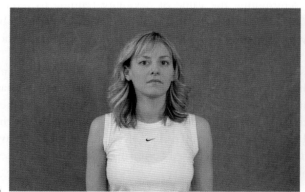

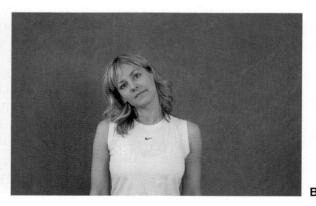

FIGURE 19.2. Stretches by body region. **A.** 1. Facing forward, tilt head to the left, moving only in the sagittal plane. 2. Hold and then return to starting position. **B.** 3. Repeat with other side. 4. A good cue for this exercise is "right ear to right shoulder." **C.** 1. Reach with one arm in opposite direction from head tilt. 2. With or without a partner, pull from top of head toward the direction of stretch, applying gentle pressure only.

lateral flexion of the neck also serves as a good example of how static stretches can be passive stretches. Through careful movements, the Personal Trainer could also guide the client's head into position and hold at peak tension for a designated period.

Despite the popularity of static stretching, little agreement has been reached among experts with respect to how long the static stretch should be held at peak tension. In its 1998 Position Stand on exercises to develop and maintain cardiorespiratory and muscular fitness and flexibility in adults, the American College of Sports Medicine suggested a hold range of 10–30 seconds (1). Recent research from Nelson and Bandy (40) supports the ACSM Position Stand—static stretches of 30 seconds, 3 days a week, for 6 weeks, significantly improved hamstring flexibility in high school–aged males compared with unstretched controls. Most of the newer published studies that have found flexibility improvements with static stretching have also used 30-second hold times.

Dynamic

Dynamic stretching is a form of stretching that incorporates movement along with muscle tension development. Dynamic stretches should only be performed as active stretches. In the broadest sense, dynamic stretches are built into every mode of exercise and physical activity. Holcomb (55) has characterized dynamic stretching as being very similar to a sport- or function-specific warm-up. As a result, it is difficult to depict examples of dynamic stretching on paper. Consider the movements of a boxer in the ring prior to a fight. Jabs he makes with the upper extremities and quick turns of the torso all serve as good examples of dynamic stretch. TaeBo® movements and medicine ball exercises provide further examples of dynamic stretching. Ideally, dynamic stretches incorporate movements that are specific to sport movements of interest, but excellent dynamic stretches can also be developed based on the flexibility needs of the medically cleared population at large (Box 19.1).

Box 19.1	**Ballistic Stretching—Understanding the Controversy**

Some flexibility experts fail to distinguish dynamic stretching from another form of movement termed "ballistic" stretching. Unfortunately, these oversights have resulted in a great deal of confusion by fitness professionals, so much so that trainees and students are often discouraged from performing dynamic stretches. As stated earlier in this section, whether the movement is a soccer ball kick or a tennis serve, physical movements usually impose dynamic stretches on the soft tissues that initiate and support them.

What ballistic stretching most often refers to is the short ROM bouncing action that produces jerky movements in an attempt to move into position and hold at peak muscle tension. For example, a client seated upright on the floor could extend his or her arms in an effort to reach toward the toes. By moving slowly into that position and holding for a few seconds at peak tension, the client would be performing an active static stretch. If the client reached toward the toes, however, and tried tapping them repeatedly with short, successive, bouncing flexions at the hip, he or she would be performing a ballistic stretch. Not unlike dynamic stretching, these movements can also be quite common during sport participation.

Considering the confusion, novice trainers might question the utility or safety of ballistic stretching. The claim is most often made that ballistic stretching is unsafe or at least ineffective for improving flexibility. Smith et al. (41) found that similar bouts of static and ballistic stretching brought on significant increases in delayed-onset muscle soreness (DOMS) in 20 male subjects unaccustomed to such exercise. However, these researchers also concluded that the static stretching actually induced significantly more DOMS than did ballistic stretching. More recently, Nelson and Kokkonen (42) concluded that acute ballistic muscle stretching inhibited maximal strength performance, but Unick et al. (43) found no statistically significant difference in vertical jump performance as a result of static or ballistic stretching among actively trained women.

No attempt is being made here to settle the questions surrounding ballistic stretching. Novice trainers should recognize that both dynamic and ballistic movements are normal components of sport activity and stay abreast of the literature as work continues to be published in this area of exercise science.

Proprioceptive Neuromuscular Facilitation

PNF involves both active and passive stretches designed to improve joint ROM. This form of stretching requires an experienced Personal Trainer and a cooperative client, but several muscle groups can be trained when PNF techniques are properly used. PNF stretching is commonly believed to elicit a relaxation response from the neuromuscular system. This response can occur in the prime mover (agonist), synergist, and antagonist muscles across a particular joint. With a stretch-induced reduction in muscle tone, joint ROM increases during subsequent stretches and eventually during physical activity. In a recent review, however, Chalmers (44) refutes this rationale and points to studies that suggest that PNF improves ROM mainly because of changes in the ability to tolerate stretching and/or changes in the viscoelastic properties of the stretched muscle.

RATIONALE FOR FLEXIBILITY TRAINING

Despite the importance of full, pain-free joint ROM for sport and physical activity, the justification for certain flexibility training techniques is controversial. Moreover, little scientific evidence exists to support or discontinue even the most common stretching habits designed for injury prevention among competitive or recreational athletes (36). Not surprisingly, the novice trainer is bound to be confused with respect to the inclusion or omission of flexibility exercises in the overall conditioning of clients.

One approach to this problem involves conducting a thorough fitness assessment of the client to determine the extent to which inflexibility limits sport and/or general physical performance. Readers are urged to read Chapter 15, which discusses postural analysis and body alignment assessment. Should ROM deficiencies be evident in the client, the basic stretching techniques described below in this chapter are those most often used to improve flexibility. While at least one early study (45) found significant improvements in flexibility with all three methods, Personal Trainers are encouraged to select an approach that best suits the needs, limitations, and abilities of the client.

GENERAL GUIDELINES TO CONSIDER WHEN DESIGNING A FLEXIBILITY TRAINING PROGRAM

There are some preliminary training guidelines unique to the design of flexibility programs. These involve warm-up, breathing, and posture.

Warm-Up

Although stretches can be performed at the start, in the middle, and/or at the finish of the workout, it is common to precede stretching with a brief, aerobic exercise warm-up. Wenos and Konin (46) have even found that active warm-up reduces the resistance to stretch. It has been established that increasing the temperature of a muscle increases the elastic properties, or the ability to stretch (10,47–49). Warm muscle tissue responds less stiffly than does cold muscle tissue. Little evidence suggests that the exercise warm-up should be altered to accommodate flexibility training exclusively. Typical warm-up exercises include stationary cycling, treadmill running, and rowing machine work.

Breathing

Proper breathing techniques are often helpful in relaxing the client and allowing movement into position more comfortably. Flexibility training is no time to perform a Valsalva maneuver (air expiration against a closed glottis). Use this time in the program design to allow the client to participate in a relaxing form of exercise, which may help to reduce stress levels and voluntary muscle tension. In general, exercisers should exhale when the body folds or contracts and inhale when the body extends.

Posture

In the design of a flexibility training program, Personal Trainers should understand the proper positioning of the stretch to target the appropriate muscle group. Focus on maintaining proper body alignment during the execution of the exercises. For example, if the client is performing a seated hamstring stretch and he or she can move further into the stretch but can only do so by rounding the upper back, this will not accomplish the goal of the stretch. Some reminders for correct postural alignment are listed below:

➤ Maintain neutral position of the spine (characterized by having a slight inward curve at the neck and low back, and a slight outward curve of the thoracic spine)
➤ Shoulders should remain back and away from the ears
➤ Hips should remain squared
➤ Avoid hyperextending or "locking out" a joint

PRECAUTIONS FOR INDIVIDUALS WITH HEALTH CONCERNS

Considering the three types of stretching presented in this chapter, there is little reason to avoid flexibility training in the apparently healthy individual. However, there are several conditions that may present challenges to the novice trainer when designing flexibility training programs. Four of these conditions are arthritis, muscular imbalance, osteoporosis, and hip fracture/replacement, and they are most commonly seen in older exercisers.

Arthritis

It is estimated that as many as 66 million individuals in the United States suffer from some form of arthritis (50). Arthritis is defined as an inflammation of a joint resulting in damage to the joint structure. There are more than 100 different types of arthritis, with the two most common types being osteoarthritis and rheumatoid arthritis. Osteoarthritis is a chronic degenerative condition that develops over time and results in abnormal wear and tear of cartilage covering the ends of the bones. Rheumatoid arthritis is classified as an autoimmune disease in which the body attacks and destroys the joint surface. In either case, flexibility training is considered the most important component of fitness for restoring physical functionality (50). Flexibility training recommendations for individuals with both types of arthritis include:

➤ Performance of flexibility exercises daily (1–2 sessions)
➤ Extended warm-ups to reduce joint stiffness
➤ Reduction of exercise intensity and duration during periods of acute inflammation or pain

Keep in mind that if the client experiences greater joint pain following a training session, the session may have been too intense for the joints and may need to be modified. To avoid overworking individuals who have taken anti-inflammatory medications (e.g., aspirin, ibuprofen, and naproxen sodium), pay close attention to their effort during exercise. Anti-inflammatory drugs may reduce the rating of self-perceived exertion.

Muscular Imbalance

Many clients possess muscular imbalances of the body, which may create postural alignment issues and injury. Repetitive movements, poor posture, and weak or tight muscles can cause these muscular imbalances. When the body experiences an imbalance in muscular forces on opposite sides of a joint, ROM may be affected (16). The obvious goal to correct the muscular imbalance would be to strengthen the weak muscle and stretch the shorter muscle.

Osteoporosis

Osteoporosis (brittle bone disease) and osteopenia (low bone density) can affect both males and females. As the bones lose density, they are more prone to fractures. The most common sites for bone loss include the spine, hips, and wrists. ROM guidelines for these populations include the following:

➤ Avoiding repetitive exercises that involve spinal flexion or twisting
➤ Suggesting exercises to help improve posture and spinal alignment

Hip Fracture/Replacement

For individuals who have recently had a hip fracture or hip replacement, it is recommended to avoid flexibility exercises that involve:

➤ Internal rotation of the hip (turning the foot inward)
➤ Hip adduction (crossing the legs beyond the midline)
➤ Hip flexion (thigh more than parallel to floor)

FLEXIBILITY PROGRAM DEVELOPMENT

Developing a flexibility training program is easy to do for a wide range of clients. Like other forms of training, flexibility programs follow the parameters of the FIDM acronym (*F*requency, *I*ntensity, *D*uration, and *M*ode). As discussed earlier, however, there is considerable controversy about nearly every constituent of flexibility training program. What follows are the FIDM recommendations condensed from the American College of Sports Medicine's current Position Stand on exercises to develop and maintain fitness and flexibility in adults (1). These parameters can be used by novice trainers to structure initial flexibility training programs. Unless otherwise indicated, the guidelines apply to all three of the stretching techniques presented in Figures 19.3 through 19.31. As the science of flexibility training progresses and personal trainer skill improves, adaptations to these parameters can be made.

Frequency

It is currently recommended that stretches be performed at least 2 to 3 days a week, including four stretch repetitions per muscle group. Bandy et al. (51) found no increase in hamstring flexibility in 93 female and male subjects when the frequency of stretching was increased from one to three times per day. Little research exists to refute the practice of stretching daily whether followed by other physical activity or not.

Intensity

Moving into position of mild discomfort before holding a stretch is the current recommendation on flexibility training intensity. Obviously, this subjective feeling of discomfort will vary from client to client. To a certain extent however, individual effort can be standardized in the laboratory using maximal voluntary isometric contractions or MVC. Feland and Marin (52) found that a submaximal form of PNF produced comparable gains in hamstring flexibility to those produced by maximal voluntary isometric contractions in 72 male subjects aged 18–27 years. These authors concluded that PNF stretching using submaximal contractions might reduce injury risk associated with PNF stretching.

Duration

Two points are at issue with respect to the parameter of duration. First, current recommendations involve stretching hold times of 10–30 seconds for active static stretches and the same for PNF techniques when preceded by a 6-second active contraction. There seems to be little additional flexibility benefit to static stretch hold times that exceed 30 seconds (53).

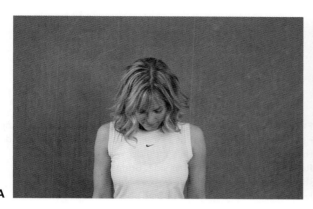

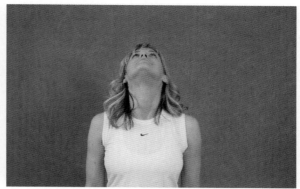

FIGURE 19.3. Forward flexion and extension. **A.** 1. Facing forward, move head forward to tuck chin into chest, hold. 2. Move slowly from this flexion position to extension. **B.** 3. Extension should involve looking up to ceiling until a 45° angle is reached, hold. 4. Avoid dropping the head back onto the upper back.

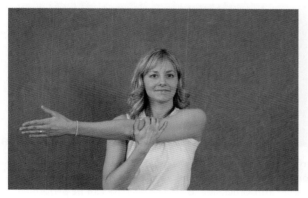

FIGURE 19.4. Arms across chest. 1. Facing forward, extend right arm and draw across chest. 2. Arm should be as straight as possible, with gentle tension developed on right shoulder. 3. Grasp right elbow with left hand. 4. Apply gentle pressure with left hand to increase tension on right shoulder. 5. Repeat with other arm/other side.

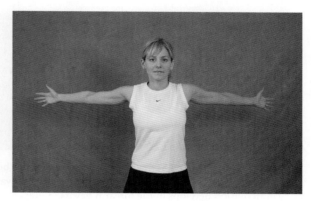

FIGURE 19.5. Chest stretch. 1. Shoulders should be relaxed, not elevated. 2. Move extended arms to the back. 3. Arms should be kept at or a little below shoulder height. 4. A good cue for this stretch is "open arms wide."

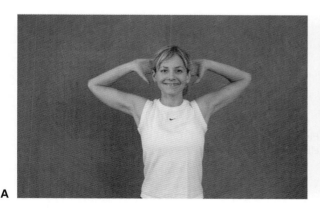

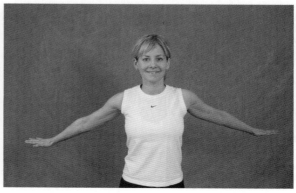

FIGURE 19.6. Chest stretch (progression). **A.** 1. Place the palms of the hand on the back of the head and bring elbow to the back. **B.** 2. Place extended arms against an open doorway, lean forward, feeling gentle tension develop across the chest.

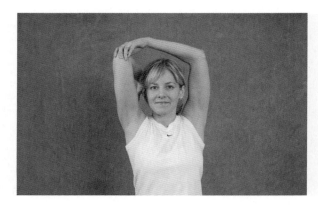

FIGURE 19.7. Elbow behind the head. 1. Facing forward, bring right arm up, bend from the elbow, and drop the hand behind the head. 2. Try to reach left shoulder with right hand. 3. Repeat with other arm/other side. Bring right hand to left shoulder and gently pull left elbow rightward to increase tension on left arm (triceps brachii).

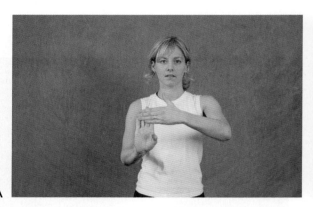

A

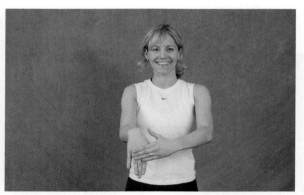

B

FIGURE 19.8. Palm up/palm down. **A.** 1. This exercise can be performed while standing or seated. 2. Extend right arm perpendicular to the body. 3. Extend wrist so the palm faces away from the body. 4. Gently pull right hand (fingertips) toward body until tension develops in the forearm flexors. 5. Repeat with other arm/other side. **B.** 1. This exercise can be performed while standing or seated. 2. Extend right arm perpendicular to the body. 3. Flex wrist so the palm faces the body. 4. Gently pull right hand with left hand until tension develops in the forearm extension.

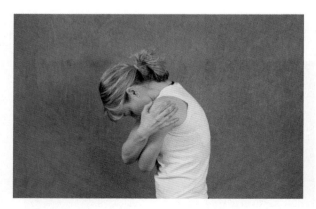

FIGURE 19.9. Arm hug. 1. Cross the arms around the body, elbows pointing forward. 2. Let the upper body round.

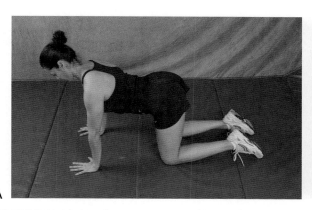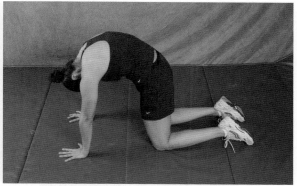

A   B

FIGURE 19.10. Kneeling cat. **A.** 1. Kneel in quadruped position. 2. Draw in abdominals and contract the gluteals. **B.** 3. Round throughout the entire spine.

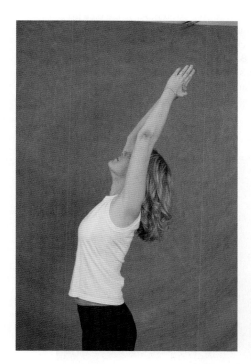

FIGURE 19.11. Pillar/overhead reach. 1. Facing forward, stand erect and extend arms above head, keeping shoulders in neutral position. 2. Interlock fingers and use the palms to press upward. 3. Stretch can also involve the trunk muscles (torso) by moving in frontal plane to one side of the body and back. 4. Hold when tension is developed in the torso on the side opposite reach.

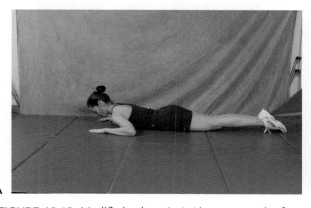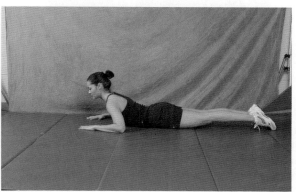

A   B

FIGURE 19.12. Modified cobra. **A.** 1. Lie prone on the floor with the head resting on the forearms and the legs extended. 2. Place the elbows directly under the shoulders with the hands facing forward. **B.** 3. Press into the forearms and raise the upper body, keeping the hips on the floor.

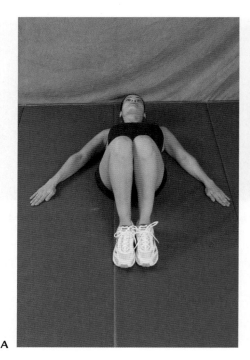

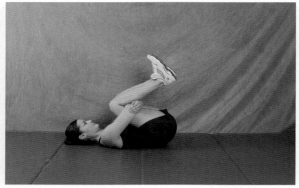

FIGURE 19.13. Supine rotational stretch. **A.** 1. Lie face up on the floor. 2. Bend knees to that the feet are flat on the floor. 3. Extend arms across the floor to stabilize upper body with movement. **B.** 4. Slowly move both legs with the knees bent to the right side of the body. 5. Maintain upper back against the floor and the abdomen oriented toward the ceiling. 6. Repeat by moving the legs to the left side.

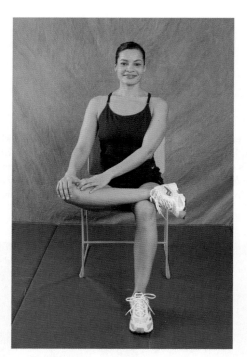

FIGURE 19.14. Seated hip rotator stretch level I. 1. Sit upright on a sturdy, non-movable chair. 2. Cross right ankle onto bent left knee. 3. Gently press down on right knee until tension develops in the outer portion of the right thigh. 4. Repeat with opposite side.

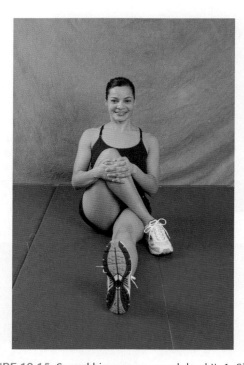

FIGURE 19.15. Seated hip rotator stretch level II. 1. Sit upright on the floor, with left leg extended and right knee bent. 2. Place the right foot over the left leg. 3. Hug the knee toward the chest. 4. Repeat on other side.

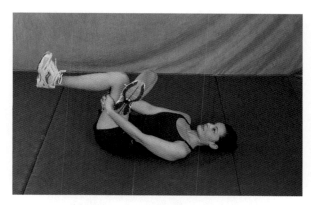

FIGURE 19.16. Supine hip rotator stretch (progression from seated). 2. Lie face up on floor with knees bent so feet are flat on the floor. 2. Cross right ankle onto bent left knee. 3. Lift left foot off the floor. 4. Wrap hands around the left leg and draw into the body. 5. Focus on opening up the right knee until tension develops in the outer portion of the right thigh. 6. Repeat on opposite side.

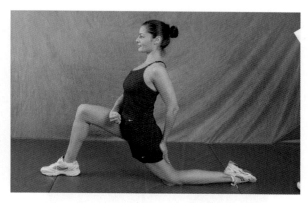

FIGURE 19.17. Kneeling hip flexors stretch. 1. Kneel on both knees with upper body lifted. 2. Plant the right foot on the floor until you reach a 90° angle with both the front and back legs. 3. Shift the weight forward while keeping the upper body lifted.

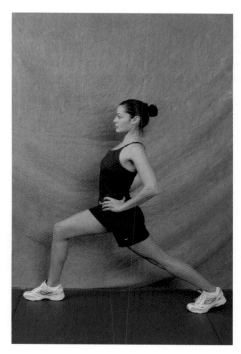

FIGURE 19.18. Standing hip flexor stretch. 1. Stand erect and keep hands on the hips. 2. Step forward with right foot into a lunge position; left heel may be elevated to facilitate this movement. 3. Shift the hips forward. 4. Maintain this position, feeling tension develop in hips, quadriceps, and buttocks. 5. Repeat with opposite side.

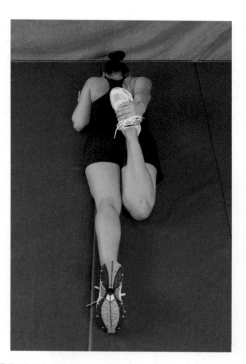

FIGURE 19.19. Prone quadriceps stretch. 1. Lie prone on the floor with legs extended. 2. Draw right heel back toward the gluteals.

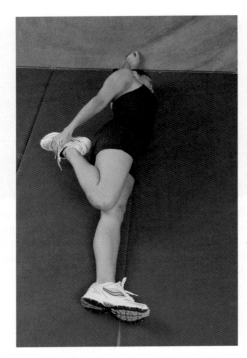

FIGURE 19.20. Side-lying quadriceps stretch (progression). 1. Lie on floor with left side of the body; the trunk should be perpendicular to the floor. 2. Bend right knee, keeping knees and hips stacked. 3. Reach with the right hand across the front of the right foot. 4. Gently pull thigh back slightly using the right arm. 5. Allow left arm to stabilize the torso by pressing against the floor. 6. Repeat with left thigh by positioning the body with the right side against the floor.

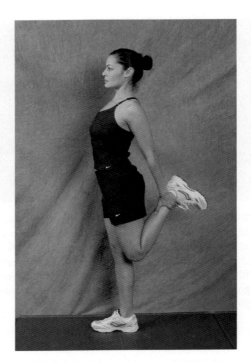

FIGURE 19.21. Standing quadriceps stretch (progression). 1. While in a standing position (a chair may be used to hold onto for support), bend the right knee toward the gluteals. 2. Grasp the right ankle with the right hand. 3. Gently pull thigh back slightly using the right arm.

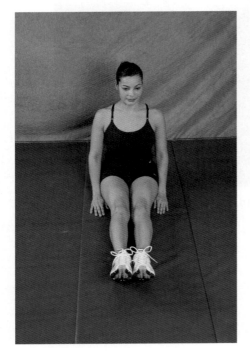

FIGURE 19.22. Seated hamstring stretch. 1. Sit upright on the floor with both legs extended and hands resting on the quadriceps. 2. Slowly walk the hands forward toward the feet, keeping the chest lifted.

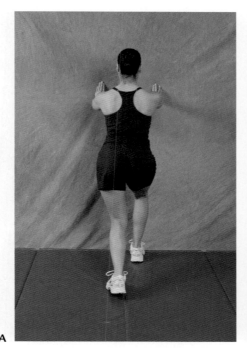 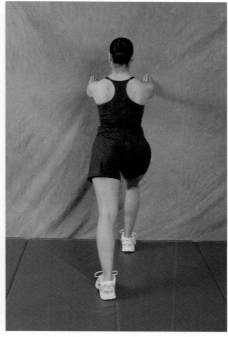

A   B

FIGURE 19.23. Standing hamstring stretch (progression). **A.** 1. Standing upright, bring the right foot slightly ahead of the left foot. 2. Slowly draw the hips back while slightly bending the left knee and extending the right knee. 3. Bring the toes of the right foot off the floor and toward the body. **B.** 4. Hold and then return to starting position. 5. Repeat with opposite leg.

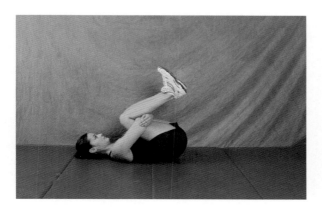

FIGURE 19.24. Supine knees to chest. 1. Lie supine on the floor. 2. Hug the knees to the chest.

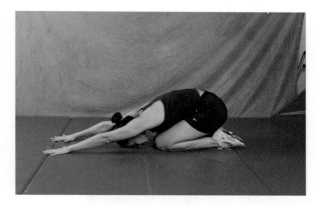

FIGURE 19.25. Child's pose. 1. Kneel in a quadruped position. 2. Sit back onto heels with arms extended.

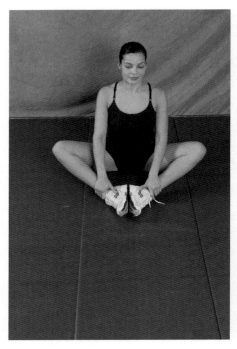

FIGURE 19.26. Butterfly stretch. 1. Sit upright on the floor with the soles of the feet together. 2. Draw the knees to the floor. 3. Lean forward from the hips.

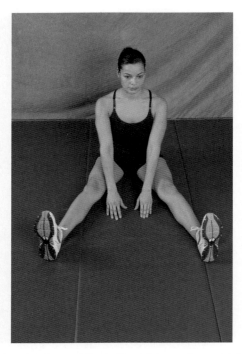

FIGURE 19.27. Straddle. 1. Sit upright on floor with both legs extended together. 2. Slowly spread legs apart so that feet are as far from each other as possible. 3. Gently reach toward center or alternate reach from right to left.

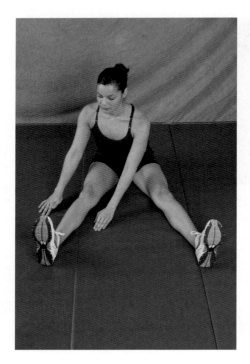

FIGURE 19.28. Seated calf stretch. 1. Sit upright with both legs extended. 2. Turn the toes toward the ceiling. 3. Draw the tops of the toes toward the upper body.

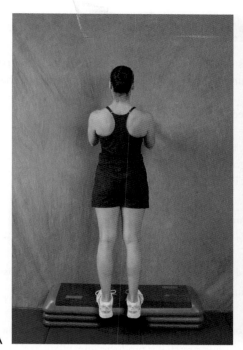
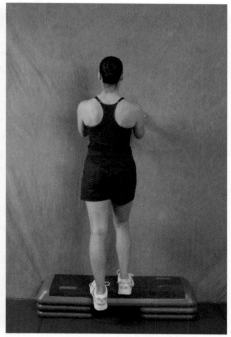

A   B

FIGURE 19.29. Standing calf step stretch. **A.** Stand erect on edge of immovable step. 2. Grasp banister or handrail for support. 3. Move heel back so that the balls of the right foot rock gently on edge of step. **B.** 4. Slowly drop heel until tension develops in right calf. 5. Slowly return to starting position and repeat with opposite side.

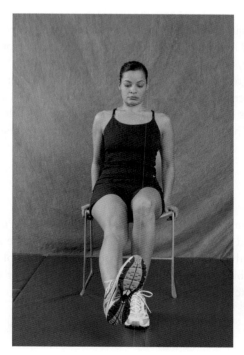

FIGURE 19.30. Dynamic foot ROM. Sit on a chair and rotate feet clockwise and counterclockwise.

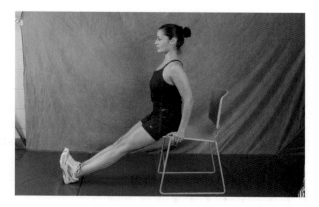

FIGURE 19.31. Dynamic foot ROM. 1. Sit upright on floor with both legs extended together. 2. Point toes away from body.

BOX 19.2	**Sample Training Program**

By incorporating the FIDM parameters discussed in this chapter, even the novice trainer can structure a basic flexibility training program for a wide range of trainees. Here is a sample training program that uses the stretches presented in this chapter.

Client: 40-year-old female, medically cleared to begin consistent exercise program
              Height = 168 cm (≈5′ 6″), weight = 68 kg (≈150 lb)
              No history of orthopedic problems, mild chronic back pain

Objectives: Improve flexibility as measured by goniometry

Session: 15-minute warm-up using a NordicTrack CX 1055 elliptical trainer
              (average heart rate ≈ 108 bpm)

Body Region	Exercise	Comments
Neck	Lateral flexion	Begin as an active stretch, move head slowly to prevent dizziness
Shoulders	Arms across chest	Avoid bending the elbow as the arm is brought across the chest
Chest	Chest stretch	Maintain relaxed shoulders
Arms	Elbow extension	
Back	Kneeling cat	Discontinue stretch if it produces immediate back pain
Torso	Modified cobra	Discontinue stretch if it produces immediate back pain
Hips	Seated hip rotator, level I	Progress to level II exercise when level I can be performed for 30 seconds without pain
Thigh (anterior)	Prone quadriceps	
Thigh (posterior)	Seated hamstring	Maintain upright posture and natural spinal curves
Calves	Standing calf step	

Trainer's notes: Be sure to follow the FIDM guidelines for flexibility training suggested in this chapter, keeping in mind that they can certainly be adapted to the progress and individual needs of the client. If one or more of the recommended parameters does not seem to be effective, adapt as needed.

This program can and should be modified as the client progresses to greater low-back ROM. Goniometer re-measures can be made every 4–6 weeks to assess the influence of the training program over time and as a result of the training session. By following the chart of stretches listed in this chapter, this client will be able to progress from these basic stretches to more complex ones. The order of exercises performed during a ses-

Mode

It is recommended that a general stretching routine be used to best improve flexibility. This means that stretches should involve the major muscle and tendon groups of the body. Some of the more commonly performed static stretches are presented in the previous pages. For an example of how these parameters can be incorporated into a flexibility training program, see Box 19.2. For more information about PNF techniques, readers are referred to Houglum (54).

SUMMARY

The purpose of this chapter is to present flexibility as an essential ingredient of health–related fitness and to provide Personal Trainers with a basic understanding of how to properly incorporate flexibility training into the exercise programs of healthy individuals. Although the science of flexibility training is often conflicting, Personal Trainers should use this aspect of flexibility training as motivation for staying abreast of the scientific literature as it develops. Moreover, Personal Trainers should make use of their good judgment and entire education in the exercise sciences to design training programs that suit the specific needs of their clients.

REFERENCES

1. American College of Sports Medicine. Position Stand: The recommended quantity and quality of exercise for developing and maintaining cardiorespiratory and muscular fitness, and flexibility in healthy adults. Med Sci Sports Exerc 1998;30:975–991.
2. Corbin CB, Welk GJ, Corbin WR, Welk KA. Fundamental Concepts of Fitness and Wellness. 2nd ed. Boston: McGraw-Hill, 2006:1–302.
3. Hamill J, Knutzen KM. Biomechanical basis of human movement. 2nd ed. Philadelphia: Lippincott Williams & Wilkins, 2003: 1–470.
4. Bassey EJ, Morgan K, Dallosso HM, Ebrahim SBJ. Flexibility of the shoulder joint measured as range of abduction in a large representative sample of men and women over 65 years of age. Eur J Appl Phys 1989;58:353–360.
5. Einkauf DK, Gondes ML, Jensen MJ. Changes in spinal mobility with increasing age in women. Phys Ther 1987;67:370–375.
6. Germain NW, Blair SN. Variability in shoulder flexion with age, activity and sex. Am Correct Ther J 1983;37:156–160.
7. Hageman PA, Blanke DJ. Comparison of gait in young women and elderly women. Phys Ther 1986;66:1382–1387.
8. Brown DA, Miller WC. Normative data for strength and flexibility of women throughout their life. Eur J Appl Phys 1998; 78:77–82.
9. Bailey AJ. Ageing of the collagen of the musculoskeletal system. Int J Sports Med 1989;10:S86–S90.
10. Wright V, Johns RJ. Observations on the measurement of joint stiffness. Arch Rheum 1960;3:328–340.
11. LaBella FS, Paul G. Structure of collagen from human tendon as influenced by age and sex. J Gerontol 1965;20:54–59.
12. Adrian MJ. Flexibility in the aging adult. In: Smith EL, Serfass RC, eds. Exercise and Aging: The Scientific Basis. Hillside, NJ: Enslow Publishers, 1981:45–57.
13. Buckwalter JA. Maintaining and restoring mobility in middle and old age: the importance of the soft tissues. Instr Course Lect 1997;46:459–469.
14. Shepard RJ. Physical Activity and Aging. Chicago: Yearbook Medical Publishers, 1978:45–48.
15. Munns K. Effects of exercise on the range of joint motion in elderly subjects. In: Smith EL, Serfass RC, eds. Exercise and Aging: The Scientific Basis. Hillside, NJ: Enslow Publishers, 1981.
16. Alter MJ. Science of Flexibility. 2nd ed. Champaign, IL: Human Kinetics, 1996.
17. Bell R, Hoshizaki T. Relationships of age and sex with joint range of motion of seventeen joint actions in humans. Can J Appl Sports Sci 1981;6:202–206.
18. Gabbard C, Tandy R. Body composition and flexibility among prepubescent males and females. J Hum Move Stud 1988; 14(4):153–159.
19. Gelabert RR. Gelabert's Anatomy for the Dancer. New York: Danad, 1966.
20. Youdas JW, Krause DA, Hollman JH, et al. The influence of gender and age on hamstring muscle length in healthy adults. J Orthop Sports Phys Ther 205;35(4):246–252.
21. Corbin CB. A Textbook of Motor Development. 2nd ed. Dubuque, IA: Brown, 1980.
22. Cornu C, Maisetti O, Ledoux I. Muscle elastic properties during wrist flexion and extension in healthy sedentary subjects and volley-ball players. Int J Sports Med 2003;24(4):277–284.
23. Jaeger M, Friewald J, Englehardt M, Lange-Berlin V. Differences in hamstring muscle stretching of elite field hockey players and normal subjects. Sortverletz Sportschaden 2003;17(2):65–70.
24. Kerrigan DC, Xenopoulos-Oddsson A, Sullivan MJ, et al. Effect of hip flexor-stretching program on gait in the elderly. Arch Phys Med Rehabil 2003;84(1):1–6.
25. Voorrips LE, Lemmink KAPM, Van Heuvelen MJG, et al. The physical condition of elderly women differing in habitual physical activity. Med Sci Sports Exerc 1993;25(10):1152–1157.
26. Kukkanen T, Malkia E. Effects of a three-month therapeutic exercise programme on flexibility in subjects with low back pain. Physiother Res Int 2000;5(1):46–61.
27. Misner JE, Massey BH, Bemben M, et al. Long-term effects of exercise on the range of motion of aging women. J Orthop Sports Phys Ther 1992;16(1):37–42.
28. Thompson CJ, Osness WH. Effects of an 8-week multimodal exercise program on strength, flexibility, and golf performance in 55 to 79-year-old men. J Aging Phys Activ 2004;12(2):144–156.
29. Guralnik JM, Simonsick EM. Physical disability in older Americans. J Gerontol 1993;48:3–10.
30. Gersten JW, Ager C, Anderson K, Cenkovich F. Relation of muscle strength and range of motion to activities of daily living. Arch Phys Med Rehabil 1970;3:137–142.
31. Klein DA, Stone WJ, Phillips WT, et al. PNF training and physical function in assisted-living older adults. J Aging Phys Activ 2002;10:476–488.
32. Finsterbush A, Pogrund H. The hypermobility syndrome: musculoskeletal complaints in 100 consecutive cases of generalized joint hypermobility. Clin Orthop 1982;168:124–127.
33. Nelson AG, Kokkonen J, Arnall DA. Acute muscle stretching inhibits muscle strength endurance performance. J Strength Cond Res 2005;19(2):338–343.
34. Fowles JR, Sale DG, MacDougall JD. Reduced strength after passive stretch of the human plantarflexors. J Appl Physiol 2000; 89(3):1179–1188.
35. Kokkonen J, Nelson AG, Cornwell A. Acute muscle stretching inhibits maximal strength performance. Res Q Exerc Sport 1998;69(4):411–415.

36. Thacker SB, Gilchrist J, Stroup DF, Kimsey CD Jr. The impact of stretching on sports injury risk: a systematic review of the literature. Med Sci Sports Exerc 2004;36(3):371–378.

37. Witvrouw E, Mahieu N, Danneels L, McNair P. Stretching and injury prevention. Sports Med 2004;34:443–449.

38. DePino GM, Webright, WG, Arnold BL. Duration of maintained hamstring flexibility after cessation of an acute static stretching protocol. J Athl Train 2000;35(1):56–59.

39. Spernoga SG, Uhl TL, Arnold BL, Gansneder BM. Duration of maintained hamstring flexibility after a one-time, modified hold-relax stretching protocol. J Athl Train 2001;36(1):44–48.

40. Nelson RT, Bandy WD. Eccentric training and static stretching improve hamstring flexibility of high school males. J Athl Train 2004;39(3):254–258.

41. Smith LL, Brunetz MH, Chenier TC, et al. The effects of static and ballistic stretching on delayed onset muscle soreness and creatine kinase. Res Q Exerc Sport 1993;64(1):103–107.

42. Nelson AG, Kokkonen J. Acute ballistic muscle stretching inhibits maximal strength performance. Res Q Exerc Sport 2001;72(4):415–419.

43. Unick J, Kieffer HS, Cheesman W, Feeney A. The acute effects of static and ballistic stretching on vertical jump performance in trained women. J Strength Cond Res 2005;19(1):206–212.

44. Chalmers G. Re-examination of the possible role of Golgi tendon organ and muscle spindle reflexes in proprioceptive neuromuscular facilitation muscle stretching. Sports Biomech 2004;3(1):159–183.

45. Lucas RC, Koslow R. Comparative study of static, dynamic, and proprioceptive neuromuscular facilitation stretching techniques on flexibility. Percept Mot Skills 1984;58(2):615–618.

46. Wenos DL, Konin JG. Controlled warm-up intensity enhances hip range of motion. J Strength Cond Res 2004;18(3):529–533.

47. Garrett WE, Best TM. Anatomy, physiology, and mechanics of skeletal muscle. In: Buckwalter JA, Einhorn TA, Simon SR, eds. Orthopaedic Basic Science Biology and Biomechanics of the Musculoskeletal System. 2nd ed. American Academy of Orthopaedic Surgeons, 2000:684–716.

48. Gillette T, Holland GJ. Relationship of body core temperature and warm-up to hamstring range of motion. J Orthop Sports Phys Ther 1991;13(3):126–131.

49. Sapega AA, Quedenfeld TC, Moyer RA, Butler RA. Biophysical factors in range-of-motion exercise. Phys Sports Med 1981;9(12):57–65.

50. Arthritis Foundation. The Facts About Arthritis. On the Internet at: http://www.arthritis.org/resources/gettingstarted/-default.asp. Accessed August 20, 2005.

51. Bandy WD, Irion JM, Briggler M. The effect of time and frequency of static stretching on flexibility of the hamstring muscles. Phys Ther 1997;77(10):1090–1096.

52. Feland JB, Marin HN. Effect of submaximal contraction intensity in contract-relax proprioceptive neuromuscular facilitation stretching. Br J Sports Med 2004;38(4):E18.

53. Bandy WD, Irion JM. The effect of time on static stretch on the flexibility of the hamstring muscles. Phys Ther 1994;74(9):845–852.

54. Houglum PA. Therapeutic Exercise for Musculoskeletal Injuries. 2nd ed. Champaign, IL: Human Kinetics, 2005.

55. Holcomb WR. Stretching and warm-up (Chapter 16). In: Baechle TR, Earle RW. Essentials of Strength Training and Conditioning. 2nd ed. Champaign, IL: Human Kinetics, 2000:321–342.

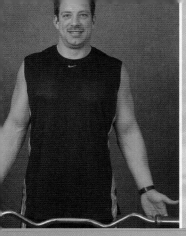

Sequencing the Personal Training Program

Neal I. Pire, MA, Director, Sports Training Academy, Ridgewood, New Jersey
Michael Rankin, M.S., Owner, Fitness Together, Waldwick, New Jersey

Chapter Outline

Optimal Client Care and Customer Service

Effective Professional Daily Habits

- Client Safety
- Planning Each Workout
- Proper Charting
- Professional Conduct in the Training Facility
- Facility Cleanliness
- Proper Exercise Protocols
- Daily Personal Trainer Improvement

Personal Training Session Criteria

- Greeting
- Warm-Up Phase
- Progression
- Continuity
- Cool-Down Phase
- Flexibility

- Monitoring Metabolic and Perceived Exertion
- Exercise Selection
- Spotting: Hands-On Interaction
- Equipment Use/Replacement
- Charting
- Adherence to Fitness Program Specifics
- Attentiveness
- Innovation and Problem-Solving Skills

Education and Motivation

The Phases of a Personal Training Session

- Preparation Phase
- Transitional Phase
- The Workout
- The Review

Training Notes

Objectives

- Provide the Personal Trainer with a "how-to" guide for the first training session as well as subsequent sessions and program variables
- Review basic customer service skills as they are applied in a fitness facility and during a personal training session
- Educate the Personal Trainer on communication skills and client–trainer relationships
- Provide the Personal Trainer with comprehensive criteria for an optimal personal training session
- Review the four phases of the personal training session: preparation, transition, workout, and review
- Provide the Personal Trainer with the purpose and template for developing useful training notes for proper documentation and effective program management

Personal training is a challenging job. Many clients have no idea where to start with their exercise program. Others take what they have read in the latest bodybuilding magazine and launch into an exercise program that is totally inappropriate for their needs. Others are simply unmotivated, which makes getting them to exercise effectively and consistently difficult, regardless of their level of knowledge and understanding.

Many clients arrive for their session with their body and minds prepared for anything but a good workout. The Personal Trainer's job is to make every minute of each session effective. This is achieved through a pre-planned series of exercises designed to meet the individual's training goals and learning objectives for that particular session. You must also maximize the trainee's physical performance within any orthopedic and/or physiological limitations or barriers.

The celebrity, the corporate executive, the model, the professional athlete, and the housewife each need and deserve the best possible training session. Results that come from productive work make each session worthwhile. The achievement of goals will encourage the client to want to continue working with the Personal Trainer or, at the very least, motivate the client to continue to exercise for a lifetime. It is the Personal Trainer's job as a professional to create this situation for each and every client. Personal Trainers must take pride in their job and train clients productively, with safety as a primary concern. Doing so ensures that both Personal Trainers and clients alike will experience their desired results.

The purpose of this chapter is to take the theoretical framework presented in the earlier chapters of this book, or the science of personal training, and demonstrate the art of personal training—how it may be applied at the "point of service"—which is the personal training session. By doing so, the Personal Trainer will be able to combine these training principles and modalities into an effective training session. This chapter also provides a framework for a Personal Trainer's job responsibilities, record-keeping procedures, and a step-by-step approach to delivering an education-based personal training session.

This chapter specifically addresses the needs and typical work activities of the Personal Trainer working in a membership fitness facility. It takes into account the barriers and situations that are common in such a work environment. The specific tenets and recommendations with regards to professionalism, customer service, and the step-by-step approach to the personal training session remain consistent regardless of the Personal Trainer's work environment.

OPTIMAL CLIENT CARE AND CUSTOMER SERVICE

It is important, first and foremost, that regardless of training venue, the highest degree of client care is essential for every Personal Trainer. It does not matter if the Personal Trainer is an employee at a fitness center or a sole proprietor running his or her own business. Safe and effective customer service is the primary responsibility of every Personal Trainer.

Table 20.1	PERSONAL TRAINER BASIC CUSTOMER SERVICE SKILLS

- **10 foot/5 foot rule:** When a customer comes within 10 feet of a Personal Trainer, the Personal Trainer will stop what he or she is doing and make eye contact. When customers come within 5 feet, the Personal Trainer will speak to them.

- **Speaking first and last—and clearly:** The Personal Trainer will initiate conversation with customers and will also have the last word with them, greeting them with "hello," etc. and ending with "have a nice day," "thank you for coming in," "my pleasure," etc. The Personal Trainer will also speak clearly and distinctly.

- **Posture:** (No slouching, hands in pocket, folded arms, etc.) The Personal Trainer will assume a professional posture, with hands at side or behind back, standing upright and alert, looking interested in the client, and with good body language.

- **Smile/pleasant expression *AND* eye contact when greeting client:** The Personal Trainer will greet the customer with eye contact and a smile or other pleasant expression.

- **Use customer's name:** The Personal Trainer will use the customer's name as often as possible.

- **Wear name tag:** The Personal Trainer will be neatly dressed in a clean and untattered uniform complete with a name tag (whenever appropriate).

- **Staff behavior is *NOT* hectic or chaotic:** The Personal Trainer will behave in a controlled and orderly fashion.

- **Staff acknowledges customers in public places:** The Personal Trainer speaks, nods, or otherwise acknowledges customers in public places.

- **The Personal Trainer speaks in a respectful tone to customers *AND* staff:** The Personal Trainer will speak to customers in a respectful tone. The Personal Trainer will also speak to staff in a respectful manner—no derogatory slurs; no religious, ethnic, or sexual jokes, comments, or epithets.

- **The Personal Trainer does not engage in distracting personal chatter or horseplay:** Personal Trainers will act in a professional manner around all customers. They will be alert to the customer's needs and proactive in their response.

- **The Personal Trainer does not eat, drink, or chew gum in public areas.**

- **The "Barney Principle":** "Please" and "thank you" are the magic words. Use common manners (staff members don't compete with customers for equipment.) Choose words that affect the customer positively ("my pleasure" vs. "no problem").

There are some customer service skills that will go a long way to provide this optimal care and will certainly enhance service delivery for every Personal Trainer. Personal Trainers should keep in mind that every person they come in contact with throughout their work day, who is not on staff, is considered a "customer." This includes all training clients, facility members, and guests (prospective clients). Table 20.1 presents basic customer service skills that every Personal Trainer should strive to perfect.

EFFECTIVE PROFESSIONAL DAILY HABITS

Client Safety

The safety of the client is of primary concern. The Personal Trainer should understand the short- and long-term physiological changes that will result from the training. The confidence that the client is placing in the Personal Trainer makes it imperative that the Personal Trainer know the client's physical limitations as ascertained from the health history and a fitness evaluation. The Personal Trainer should also be sensitive to any daily fluctuations in the client's physical status. Any medical limitation affected by exercise should be referred to the client's physician for evaluation and treatment. The Personal Trainer should apply all phases of the exercise program with safety in mind. Form, speed of contraction, weight selection, and monitoring of training intensities are all examples of safety consciousness.

Planning Each Workout

The Personal Trainer should map out specific goals and objectives in conjunction with the recommendations specified by current ACSM guidelines (1). Training programs should be planned accordingly, taking into account all structural and metabolic limitations when planning long- and short-term goals. Progressions should be planned so that each session can be as productive as possible. Clients should be pushed to their physical potential through a planned routine that is safe. Checking with clients daily on their physical/emotional readiness to exercise is crucial. This will assist the Personal Trainer in deciding on an optimal motivational approach. The Personal Trainer should be sensitive to the clients' needs and either talk to clients constantly, if they respond to that type of encouragement, or back off and keep vocal encouragement to a minimum if it is a client's preference.

Proper Charting

Proper charting is a "must-have"—not only from a customer service perspective but also from an ethical and liability standpoint. Documenting all activities and events will help the Personal Trainer provide the optimal service while limiting exposure risk. Each session should follow long- and short-term goals and objectives as agreed on at the initial fitness evaluation and interview (see Chapter 10). The Personal Trainer should record workout specifics such as appropriate weights/reps/sets, physiological data such as training HR/RPE/BP responses or changes, signs and/or symptoms that may have occurred during a session, and, in certain cases, any special routines that will assist another staff member who might train that client next. The purpose of the notes are to:

➤ Keep track of exercise programs so they can be subsequently evaluated for effectiveness based on the results of post-testing
➤ Make the client's routine somewhat consistent regardless of the instructor
➤ Reinforce long-term/short-term objectives
➤ Keep track of the trainee's progression in relation to changes in the applied program intensities

Professional Conduct in the Training Facility

The Personal Trainer must pay attention to the clients, whether he or she is working directly with them or not. It is understood that a Personal Trainer who is training a client is focused on the client alone. He or she should talk to that client only, give the client positive encouragement, and spot when necessary. A Personal Trainer who is not currently working with a client should talk to the trainees who are stretching or warming up/cooling down. Personal Trainers can take a heart rate, ask clients about their diets, and show them that they care. Proper body language is also an extremely important concept. A Personal Trainer should not sit on a piece of equipment while the client is on another piece of equipment or lean up against the wall while the client is on the treadmill. Aside from the safety factor, if the client perceives that the Personal Trainer is disinterested and not caring, the quality of the workout will be compromised. These little things will differentiate the professional Personal Trainer from others *(Fig. 20.1)*.

Facility Cleanliness

During non-training time, check the facility to make sure that all is in order, the weights are put back, and the facility looks presentable. Personal Trainers should make periodic checks of the changing rooms and locker room facilities. They should try to go out of their way, depending on the facility, to make sure that the clients know where everything is, familiarize them with the phone system, show them where the emergency alarm is, and above all make sure the room is clean.

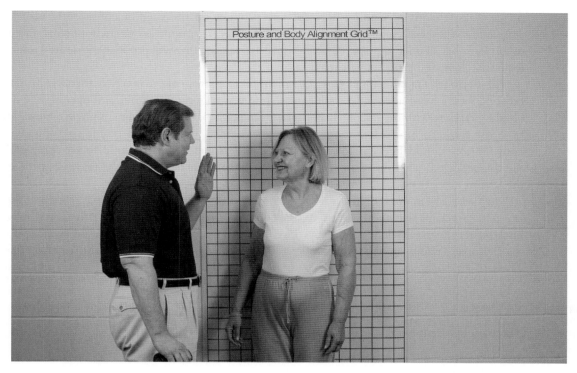

FIGURE 20.1. Proper body language is critical to the success of the Personal Trainer.

Proper Exercise Protocols

Any major changes in the client's program as outlined from the client's fitness evaluation should be indicated in the client's fitness program chart. A Personal Trainer should be sure to update the fitness program chart as soon as any change in medical or structural condition presents itself. Take the appropriate steps, speak to the client regarding those conditions that affect the program, and ask the client's permission to contact his or her physician if warranted. The more closely the Personal Trainer monitors the client's day-to-day or week-to-week variations, the more effective, safe, and valid the exercise programs will be.

Daily Personal Trainer Improvement

A Personal Trainer should set short-term and long-term career goals and make a concerted effort to reach these goals. Reading related literature, attending clinics, sharing information with other Personal Trainers, and observing other Personal Trainers with attention to detail will enhance the educational and vocational abilities of the Personal Trainer.

PERSONAL TRAINING SESSION CRITERIA

Although Personal Trainers are found in a variety of work environments, there are common work performance criteria that will set apart the professional trainer from others. The comprehensive list below outlines some of the these important work habits that should be continuously practiced and perfected.

Greeting

The Personal Trainer's appearance must be neat and professional. Personal Trainers who are not required to wear a uniform might consider developing their own to create a consistently professional image. Like effective branding does for any product on the shelf, a consistently professional appearance will speak volumes about a Personal Trainer. First impressions are important, and it is up to the Personal Trainer to portray a professional appearance that will produce the desired impression for every client and prospective client.

The Personal Trainer should greet the client in an appropriate manner. A friendly, professional greeting with a handshake and a smile goes a long way to setting the tone and opening the door to building rapport with the client. Inappropriate language (i.e., demeaning comments; racial, ethnic, or sexist epithets; or "locker-room talk") has no place in a personal training session. Personal conversation should be kept to a minimum. A Personal Trainer should focus completely on the client's needs from the moment he or she greets the client through the farewell at the end of the session.

The Personal Trainer should always greet the client and start the session on time. Starting a session late tells the client that the Personal Trainer does not value the client's time. It clearly relates an uncaring feeling to the client and displays the epitome of unprofessionalism. Like any service provider, the Personal Trainer must always exhibit good client rapport. The client must trust the Personal Trainer's guidance, skills, and knowledge to benefit from the symbiotic client–trainer relationship.

Warm-Up Phase

The Personal Trainer must select an appropriate warm-up modality that:

➤ Is relevant to any structural or metabolic limitations
➤ Is relevant to goals and structure of workout
➤ Includes:
   • A minimum of 3–5 minutes in length
   • Appropriate intensity (i.e., at low end of training zone)
   • Monitoring of heart rate and/or rating of perceived exertion (RPE)

Progression

A Personal Trainer must follow an appropriate exercise progression throughout the personal training session. Workouts should be constructed and proceed based on the following general guidelines:

➤ Cardiovascular warm-up (as detailed above)
➤ Cardiovascular aerobic or anaerobic interval work when indicated (occurs within workout content after appropriate warm-up and includes appropriate cool-down)
➤ Flexibility component after appropriate warm-up (when indicated)
➤ Strength/muscular endurance component
➤ Core strengthening
➤ Condition-specific exercises (e.g., orthopedic protocols, pregnancy protocol) should occur at a logical point within the workout (pelvic tilt or floor work exercises should be introduced within the workout without making the client move back and forth from standing/seating to a reclining position several times).

Continuity

The "flow" of the personal training session should proceed in a continuous, uninterrupted manner (i.e., the Personal Trainer should not be charting the workout while the client waits to proceed to the next exercise). The Personal Trainer must make efficient use of floor space and choice of exercise modality when the training floor is crowded. It is up to the Personal Trainer to be creative and make alternative choices of exercises in an expedient manner.

Cool-Down Phase

The Personal Trainer should build in a gradual decrease in exercise intensity at the end of any cardiovascular exercise bout for the purpose of an effective cool-down. It should be a minimum of 2 to 5 minutes in length (cool-downs are client and situation specific in almost all cases), depending on the exercise intensity, duration, time exercising, and client-specific conditions (i.e., less-fit clients should be allowed a longer cool-down period to allow heart rate and BP to decrease). Exercise heart rate and/or RPE should be monitored. Additionally, a cool-down should occur after any hard bout of exercise or at any point within the workout, prior to final flexibility and abdominal, or core, work.

Flexibility

The Personal Trainer should follow appropriate flexibility training guidelines. Flexibility training with a client should only be done after an adequate warm-up. The type of flexibility training program depends on the client's needs and orthopedic history. Clients who have specific range-of-motion concerns should have more attention given to flexibility prior to any strength training or weight work, as well. The Personal Trainer, regardless of methodology, should follow ACSM guidelines (1) and hold static stretches for a minimum of 20 to 30 seconds. Proprioceptive neuromuscular facilitation (PNF) stretches can be held for 6 to 10 seconds. However, it is vitally important to teach clients to listen to the needs of their body where stretching is concerned. Stretching exercises should include stretching of the major muscle groups as well as any specific areas of concern highlighted within the fitness assessment. Any muscle groups that may be sore from the previous workout and muscle groups worked at a high intensity during the workout should be given special consideration.

Monitoring Metabolic and Perceived Exertion

The Personal Trainer should monitor heart rate or RPE throughout various stages of the entire workout, including:

➤ Warm-up phase
➤ Cardiovascular phase
➤ During weight/resistance training
➤ Post-workout
➤ During any interval work

RPE is used for any clients taking medication that affects heart rate (e.g., beta-blockers). Heart rate and RPE should be monitored throughout the workout. All perceptual signs and responses are observed in conjunction with HR and RPE, and exercise is monitored accordingly. This is especially important for clients who have a tendency to work hard and underestimate their RPE. Clients should be monitored for ataxia (unsteadiness of gait) or other physical signs of fatigue or stress (1).

Exercise Selection

The Personal Trainer must take several factors into account when selecting appropriate exercise progressions. These factors include:

➤ Client's goals
➤ Client's advisor program
➤ Client's skill level
➤ Structural or conditional specifics

➤ Considerations on the particular training day (e.g., client is tired, sore, has been ill, hasn't trained regularly, hasn't trained in over 1 month)
➤ Availability of equipment and other activities occurring within the fitness center

Spotting: Hands-On Interaction

The Personal Trainer should provide appropriate spotting during all aspects of the exercise session. This includes:

➤ Cardiovascular work—the Personal Trainer should be in a position to monitor client's HR and RPE and give any assistance that is necessary
➤ Resistance training machines—ranges of motion, feedback on speed of movement, verbal cues, and hands-on feedback during any machine weight work
➤ Free weights—appropriate spotting occurs at all times with all clients (the Personal Trainer should be in a position to assist clients with the weights if they are not able to maintain good form or are unable to complete the activity)
➤ Core work—the Personal Trainer should assist the client and/or correct form, breathing, etc.
➤ Stretching—the Personal Trainer should direct appropriate stretching progression at the end of the session, within the context of the workout and based on client need
➤ Balancing equipment—the Personal Trainer should be properly positioned to prevent the client from falling or provide adequate support for the client during balance training drills

The hands-on interaction that occurs during the workout should be based on the client, the exercises used, the appropriate feedback needed, and the overall program. Determine whether teaching cues and safety precautions are proper and appropriate for each client.

Equipment Use/Replacement

The Personal Trainer should use a variety of equipment during the workout. Any equipment used during the workout is returned to a neat, orderly condition during the course of the workout to maintain safety and not interfere with any other workouts that are occurring within the same time frame. The variety and progression depends on several factors, including:

➤ The client's individual goals
➤ Structural or metabolic barriers and needs
➤ The previous exercise session
➤ Gym floor traffic

Charting

The Personal Trainer must document all pertinent information in the client's fitness program chart. The client's chart for the day should include specific information regarding:

➤ The day's objectives
➤ Client's subjective comments
➤ Observations made by the Personal Trainer (as relevant)
➤ A clear, and neat, write-up of the workout performed
➤ Any new exercises or new machines used and how the client felt and performed the exercises
➤ Any particular changes in the client's fitness level as noted on a specific machine (e.g., "Client ran 0.3 miles farther than usual today" or "Client wasn't able to complete usual distance on bike due to hard workout previously")
➤ Recommendations for changes/updates in fitness program
➤ Recommendation for a re-assessment
➤ Recommendations for next exercise session

Adherence to Fitness Program Specifics

The Personal Trainer should adhere to the specific fitness program recommendations as based on the initial fitness evaluation and interview. He or she should adhere to, and expand on, these recommendations within each workout. Such fitness program specifics include:

➤ Specific work or exercises for a structural and metabolic condition as recommended by a physician (e.g., perform exercises as specifically recommended for client's shoulder impingement syndrome)
➤ Exercises used within a workout based on clients' overall structural or metabolic specifics (e.g., low-back stabilization exercises included for the client who is on a low-back protocol)
➤ Exercises or workout design based on short-term and long-term goals (e.g., weight loss, workout includes CV and circuit work)

Attentiveness

Attentiveness begins the moment the client walks onto the exercise floor and finishes with the Personal Trainer saying goodbye to the client (including plans for the next session/workout and when it will occur (i.e., scheduling the client's next workout). Attention to every detail within the workout is important. Pertinent details include:

➤ Monitoring signs and symptoms
➤ Providing water and a towel, if appropriate
➤ Modification of exercises based on client's ability to perform them correctly
➤ Exercise occurring within the desired target training zone and appropriate modifications as needed during the course of the session
➤ Ensuring proper breathing and form during all exercises
➤ Adherence to fitness program-specific recommendations

Innovation and Problem-Solving Skills

The Personal Trainer must have the ability to improvise and modify any aspect of the client's workout based on:

➤ Other activities occurring within the fitness center
➤ Availability of equipment within the fitness center
➤ Specific injuries and/or limitations
➤ Exercise prescription and training recommendations for a particular sporting event
➤ Previous exercise sessions
➤ Client attitude, level of motivation, or stage of readiness

Table 20.2 serves as a checklist for Personal Trainer managers to use when evaluating other trainers' skills and execution of a personal training session (2).

EDUCATION AND MOTIVATION

Exercise the body in a logical progression. Pre-planning of the workout with consideration to muscular and systematic functions (i.e., aerobic, anaerobic power, sprint, postural problems, etc.) will make the entire session more efficient for the client. If time and machine availability make this preparation impractical, the general workout objective should be formulated and adhered to carefully. Remember to consider both the muscular and the cardiorespiratory systems in every workout.

Table 20.2 PERSONAL TRAINING SESSION EVALUATION CRITERIA / CHECKLIST

I. <u>Greeting</u>

☐ Personal Trainer's appearance is neat and professional
☐ Appropriate greeting and reception
☐ Picks up client on time
☐ Displays good client rapport

II. <u>Warm-Up Phase</u>

Appropriate CV equipment used:

☐ Relevant to any structural or metabolic limitations
☐ Relevant to workout and program goals

Includes:

☐ A minimum of 3–5 minutes in length
☐ Appropriate intensity (i.e., at low end of training zone)
☐ Monitoring and documenting intensity responses (HR, RPE)

III. <u>Exercise Selection</u>

Exercise Selection takes into account

☐ Client's goals (long-term and short-term)
☐ Overall training program
☐ Client's skill and fitness levels
☐ Any structural or metabolic conditions
☐ Any day-to-day considerations (e.g., client is tired, sore, had recent illness, inconsistent attendance, hasn't trained in over 1 month)
☐ Availability of equipment and other activities occurring within fitness center (*See Innovation)
☐ A logical rationale for exercises (order, progression, continuity, etc.) or equipment and within accepted standards of care
☐ Previous exercise sessions

IV. <u>Spotting, Hands on Interaction* and Attentiveness</u>

Spotting occurs during all aspects of the exercise session:

☐ CV work: Personal Trainer is positioned to monitor client's training HR/RPE, provide assistance
☐ Properly monitoring the range of motion in resistance training exercises, feedback on speed of movement, verbal cues, and hands-on feedback during exercises
☐ Free weights: Appropriate spotting occurs **at all times** with all clients. Personal Trainer is in a position to assist the client with the weights if they are not able to maintain good form or are unable to complete the activity.
☐ Abdominals: Personal Trainer models correct form, assists the client with form, breathing etc.
☐ Stretching: Hands-on stretching occurs at the end of the session, and within the context of the workout as needed.
☐ Balancing exercises: proper positioning to prevent client from falling
☐ Teaching cues are safe, accurate, and appropriate for the client.

* The hands-on interaction should be based upon the client, the exercises used, the appropriate feedback, and the overall program.

V. <u>Innovation and Problem-Solving Skills</u>

Ability to improvise and modify any aspect of client's workout based upon

☐ Other activities occurring within the fitness center
☐ Availability of equipment within the fitness center
☐ Specific injuries, limitations, or complaints of pain/discomfort
☐ Exercise prescription and training requests for a particular sporting event
☐ Previous exercise sessions

Table 20.2	PERSONAL TRAINING SESSION EVALUATION CRITERIA / CHECKLIST *(CONTINUED)*

VI. <u>Monitors Metabolic and Structural Considerations</u>

HR, RPE*, and/or BP are monitored throughout various stage of the entire workout:

☐ Warm-up phase
☐ CV phase
☐ Resistance phase
☐ For hypertensive clients, BP is to be monitored before, during, and after a CV bout, interval or resistance training phase.
☐ Trainer should ask for constant feedback of joint pain, fatigue, etc. from client.

* RPE is used for any **hypertensive clients** on medication that affects heart rate. Heart rate and RPE are to be monitored throughout workout with **pregnant clients.** Perceptual signs/signals (e.g., ataxia, unsteadiness of gait, or other physical signs of fatigue) should be monitored in conjunction with HR, BP, and RPE, and exercise is modified accordingly. This is especially important for clients who have a tendency to work hard and underestimate their RPE.

VII. <u>Cool-Down Phase</u>

☐ A slow decrease in exercise intensity occurs at the end of any CV bout, any hard bout of exercise, or at any point within the workout prior to final flexibility and abdominal work.
☐ 2 to 5 minutes in length; depending on the exercise intensity, time exercising, and client-specific conditions (e.g., give hypertensive client and less-fit clients a longer cool-down period to allow HR and BP to return toward pre-exercise levels without blood pooling or orthostatic hypotensive responses).
☐ Vital and perceptual signs are monitored.

VIII. <u>Flexibility Work</u>

☐ Occurs after an adequate warm-up, if necessary*
☐ Depending on the individual, at a minimum, at the end of the workout
☐ Static stretches held for 20–30 seconds; PNF stretches can be held for 6–7 seconds.
☐ Includes stretching the major muscle groups, any specific areas highlighted within the fitness assessment, or muscle groups emphasized during the workout

IX. <u>Charting / Program Update</u>

The client's session should include specific information regarding

☐ The day's objectives
☐ Client's subjective comments
☐ Relevant observations made by Personal Trainer

An update of the workout program after completion, taking into consideration

☐ New exercises/machines used and how the client felt and performed the exercises
☐ Any particular changes in the client's fitness level as noted on a specific machine (e.g., "ran .3m further than usual today," "wasn't able to complete usual distance due to hard workout")
☐ Recommendations for re-assessment, suggested exercises for next workout session, etc.
☐ Any pain or discomfort that occurred during the session
☐ Any notes for next workout.

The Personal Trainer should emphasize the muscle groups and systematic functions that are specific to the trainee's individual goals and objectives. Even though many clients are in a "general conditioning" mode, each individual has a specific area of concern to which the Personal Trainer can gear the exercise routines to make them more meaningful. Some clients, for example, want to "tone up" their hips and buttocks. Explain the effectiveness of squatting exercises in relation to this individual goal. The Personal Trainer should talk to each client about how the tailored routine he or she has designed relates to the client's training objectives. Sport-specific emphasis can be obtained by exercising the muscles specific to performing the activity (e.g., exercising the quadriceps muscles for skiing, improving flexibility for golf). When prudent, appropriate orthopedic protocols should be implemented and explained as to how they will be integrated into the client's program to improve or prevent further injury.

The Personal Trainer should take proper notes for each workout. The short-term goal for each session should be included in this procedure. Specific objectives can be listed in order of priority. Specific exercises with weights/reps/sets, and HR/RPE responses when appropriate, can also be included in the notes. Any incidental aches and pains must be recorded. Any Personal Trainer should be able to train every client with the help of the workout notes.

The Personal Trainer should emphasize correct form in all training sessions. The safety of an exercise is based in the form of execution, not the amount of weight or the number of reps. The Personal Trainer must make sure to exercise each targeted muscle group through a proper range of motion. Force the emphasis on specific targeted muscles and coach the trainee not to contract extraneous muscles. This applies especially to the lower back, the neck/shoulder area, and the forearms. Ensure that the muscles lift and support the weight. The client should not support heavy weight with the lever of the arm "locked out" (e.g., overhead press, bench press, and leg press). The Personal Trainer should teach and reinforce proper breathing techniques. The client should never hold his or her breath during any contraction. This increases intrathoracic (inside the chest) pressure and as a result increases blood pressure, which may or may not be dangerous for the specific client, but is certainly unnecessary. The client should exhale when performing a concentric contraction and inhale during the eccentric phase.

The Personal Trainer should include the proper proportion of supervised aerobic exercise in each workout. The Personal Trainer should know the appropriate training heart rate range (THR) and record RPE when applicable. These measurements of intensity should be used to guide the progression of the applied workloads. Some aerobic components can be prescribed before or after the actual supervised session. This will depend on the client's overall physical condition, daily schedule, and specific training goals and objectives. The Personal Trainer should make sure that clients understand how to operate the prescribed aerobic modality and that they can either take their own HR or gauge RPE effectively, before the client exercises without supervision. It is helpful to ask clients what additional activities they are performing outside of the facility. This will assist the Personal Trainer in the design of their training sessions. The Personal Trainer should teach each client the physiological basis of the RPE scale and explain how this will assist in monitoring exercise intensity and how it will make the sessions more efficient.

Personal Trainers must make each workout as interesting and as varied as possible. They must motivate the client in every way they can. This variation is effective both psychologically and physiologically. Attention span is increased when topics of focus are divided into small diverse blocks relative to a client's physiological, structural, and motivational status. Mixing up the routine in this manner will help the client concentrate on the workout and its quality.

It is easy to train a client who is motivated and interested in the session. The Personal Trainer's job is to ensure that interest, so that the effectiveness of each workout will be maximized. This can be achieved by incorporating static stretching in the session after a high-intensity strength set or mixing in aerobic or anaerobic intervals at specific points in the routine. The Personal Trainer should keep the client moving, minimize unnecessary conversation, and be alert to all of the overt signs of workout intensity. Personal Trainer must be creative in all of their sessions. This makes the Personal Trainer's job a lot more interesting and enjoyable.

THE PHASES OF A PERSONAL TRAINING SESSION

Many dynamics are involved in a personal training session. Although sessions may vary based on the different clients' goals and abilities, the Personal Trainer should always have a systematic approach to the personal training session. These sequential systems are not limited to the actual training session itself. Many of the systems that may be implemented will happen prior to and after the actual training session itself. These systems may be broken down into four phases: preparation phase, transitional phase, the workout, and the review.

Preparation Phase

Prior to a client's arrival, the Personal Trainer's objective should be to obtain as much information about him or her as possible. This information can be gathered while the client is on the phone scheduling the first session and should include such questions as:

➤ How did you hear about us?
➤ Are you currently exercising?
➤ What are your goals?
➤ Are there any medical conditions that a Personal Trainer should be aware of?

At the end of the conversation, the Personal Trainer should avoid commitment remorse from the client by telling the client what to expect on the first day. Here is a sample phone conversation that the Personal Trainer could use when trying to obtain information from a prospective client:

Michael: Thank you for calling the Fitness Center. How may I be of service?
Julie: Yes. I am calling to schedule my first personal training session.

Michael: Great, Julie, before I schedule that with you, I would like to ask you some questions so I can prepare a program that is specific to you. Is that okay?
Julie: Sure.

Michael: What are some of your goals?
Julie: I would like to lose some weight and tone my arms.

Michael: Are you currently exercising?
Julie: Yes. I walk and do free weights twice a week.

Michael: Wow! That's great. What are you hoping to get from this program that you are not receiving from your current program?
Julie: Well, I have been doing the same thing for over a year and I am not seeing any results.

Michael: That is quite normal, don't worry. Is there any medical condition that I should be aware of?
Julie: No.

Michael: Okay Julie, when you arrive we are going to ask you to fill out some informational paperwork prior to your session, so try to arrive about 10 minutes early. After you finish we are going to do a light warm-up before beginning the actual session. Once you complete the warm-up, I am going to take you through the workout that I will have designed for you so wear comfortable clothes. Sound good?
Julie: Yes. Thank you.

It is important to take notes during this conversation for two reasons. First, it will help the Personal Trainer develop a program that is conducive to the client's needs. Moreover, when the client arrives, the Personal Trainer can reiterate this information to the client, which shows interest and builds credibility. The first impression is the most important stage of developing a Personal Trainer–client relationship. A well-prepared Personal Trainer has a much greater chance of client retention.

On the day of the client's scheduled appointment, the Personal Trainer should be present and ready to begin well before the new client's workout time. The client's folder with the information that was obtained on the phone should be retrieved, as well as the program that the Personal Trainer prepared prior to the client's arrival. The Personal Trainer should review the exercise prescription and notes taken from the phone conversation. All pertinent forms should be on the Personal Trainer's clipboard and prepared for the session.

When the new client arrives, the Personal Trainer should be introduced with a smile, shake the client's hand, and make eye contact. The client should be invited to a waiting area or office to fill out any forms that the facility may require, such as an information sheet, medical questionnaire, or PAR-Q. Once the client finishes filling out the forms, the Personal Trainer is going to want to take a minute to review the forms with the client, looking for anything that may assist in the training process or that may have been overlooked during the initial conversation *(Fig. 20.2)*.

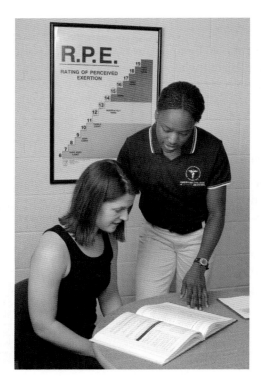

FIGURE 20.2. Personal Trainer reviewing pre-evaluation forms with a client.

It is at this point that the Personal Trainer is going to begin the transition from filling out the forms to the actual workout, also known as the transitional phase. Before we talk about the transitional phase, let's review the components of the preparation phase:

1. Ask permission to obtain as much information as possible prior to meeting the new client.
2. Inform the client about what he or she can expect during the session, to prevent commitment remorse.
3. Take notes of the conversation to aid in program development and building rapport.
4. Develop a program based on the client's goals.
5. Arrive 15 minutes prior to the session to review the client's folder.
6. Introduce yourself and ask client to fill out proper forms.
7. Review the forms with your client and begin warm-up.

Transitional Phase

Once the Personal Trainer and the client have reviewed the proper paperwork, it is time to begin the client's warm-up. Select a cardiovascular machine that is going to correspond to the client's ability. Begin slowly and after 30 seconds, ask whether the client is comfortable. Once the client is comfortable, it is time to go over exactly what he or she will be doing during the workout. Some of the key points that the Personal Trainer should convey to the client are the muscle groups that will be working, how the client will be feeling, and teaching the client to use a modified RPE scale from 1 to 10 *(Fig. 20.3)*. A sample explanation might go something like this:

Michael: Julie, typically our clients come in and train three times per week. Therefore, we will be working your entire body every time you come in. Based on your primary goal of weight loss, we are going to be moving fairly quickly from exercise to exercise with very little rest, with higher repetitions and lower weights. You are going to be out of breath and sweating. That's okay. It's very normal. After each exercise I am going to be asking you how you feel on a scale from 1 to 10, 10 being the hardest thing you have ever done in your life and 1 being the easiest. This is what I am going to use to judge if you can keep the same pace or if we need to modify the intensity in any way. So just shout out "Mike, that was a 3" or "Mike, that was a 7" so I know what is your perceived exertion is. If you have any questions at all, please feel free to ask.

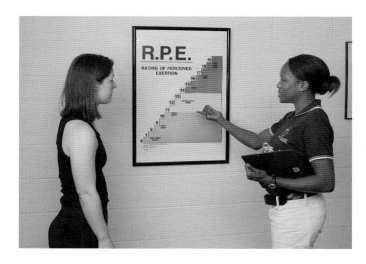

FIGURE 20.3. Personal Trainer explaining the use of the rating of perceived exertion chart to a client.

During that brief conversation *(Fig. 20.4)*, the Personal Trainer:

1. Told what muscles will be working
2. Restated the primary goal to enforce personal attention
3. Explained how the client would be feeling
4. Used a modified RPE
5. Told the client to please feel free to ask any questions

A simple conversation can bring a level of comfort between the Personal Trainer and the client. Once the Personal Trainer describes what is about to happen, he or she should make sure to set up the first exercise for the client and prepare the area where the training session will occur. Finally, check the client's heart rate to get a baseline reading for the workout. Once a baseline measurement has been established, it is time to begin the actual workout. Here is a review of the stages of the transitional phase:

1. Set up the client on a piece of cardiovascular equipment that corresponds to his or her ability.
2. After the client is set up, go over what will happen during the workout, to further develop a sense of comfort for the client. Remember to reiterate primary goals to enforce personal attention.
3. Set up the first exercise that will be performed with the client as well as the area where the Personal Trainer will be working if necessary.
4. Take the client's heart rate to determine a baseline HR.

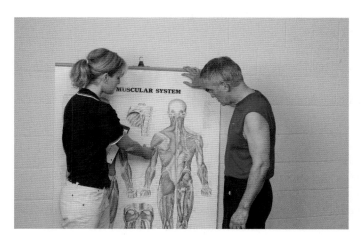

FIGURE 20.4. Personal Trainer briefing a client.

The Workout

Communication with the client is going to be extremely important throughout the workout. A Personal Trainer who is training someone for the first time cannot assume that the client knows the proper form for an exercise or where the client will be placing the hands, to spot them effectively. Before each exercise the Personal Trainer must explain the following details: proper form, proper breathing, and where the Personal Trainer will be touching the client to be able to spot them. All of these factors are imperative for the client's comfort as well as your liability. Two things that should not be incorporated in this dialogue are the amount of weight being used and the number of repetitions. If the Personal Trainer tells the client he or she is going to perform 15 repetitions and the Personal Trainer happens to overestimate the amount of weight the client can handle and he or she can only perform 10 repetitions, the client will now have a sense of failure and a "this is too hard" attitude. A sample explanation might go as follows:

> Michael: Julie, the first exercise we are going to perform is the dumbbell chest press. You are going to be lying on the bench with your hands up in the air. I am going to hand you the dumbbells and then stand behind you and spot you from your wrist. I want you to take a big deep breath in through your nose on the way down, bending your elbows and bringing your hands just above your chest. Then you are going to exhale as you push the dumbbells straight up in the air. Throughout the exercise, I want you to try and keep five points of contact: your head, shoulders, lower back, glutes, and feet. Do you have any questions?

Once again, from the simple dialogue the Personal Trainer was able to describe the proper form for the exercise, the proper breathing technique, and how the client would be spotted. Upon completion of the exercise, the client should be asked how he or she feels on a scale from 1 to 10 and then the Personal Trainer should establish a pace based on the client's first sets.

Throughout the workout, maintain constant involvement and enthusiasm. Keeping the client motivated is one of the main goals of the workout. The other key factor is time management. The Personal Trainer always wants to stay ahead of the client, having all of the weights and exercises prepared in advance. Breaks will be limited, based on the client's goals and ability. If after three exercises a client informs the Personal Trainer that he or she is at an RPE of 9 out of 10, slow down the workout by explaining the theories behind the designed workout. This will considerably slow down the pace of the workout, while the client does not get a sense of failure. Monitor the client's heart rate to determine the necessary length of the breaks.

With about 15 minutes remaining in the session, tell what exercises are remaining, so the client can mentally prepare for the finish *(Fig. 20.5)*. With approximately 10 minutes remaining, it is time to cool-down and stretch. After competing the stretching, it is time to move into the review phase, but before we do, let's review the stages of the workout:

1. Before beginning each exercise, explain to clients the proper form, proper breathing, and where you will be touching the client to spot them.
2. After each exercise, ask clients how they feel on a scale from 1 to 10.
3. Establish a pace based on the client's ability.
4. Converse during breaks if the workout needs to slow down.
5. With 15 minutes left in the workout, tell clients what exercises are remaining so they mentally prepare for the finish.
6. With 10 minutes remaining, cool-down and stretch.

The Review

Upon completion, thank the client for a good workout. Once the client is gone, the Personal Trainer must restore the training area to its proper form, racking the weights and wiping down all equipment. It is then time to record all of the information that has just been obtained throughout the workout. On the client's chart, record the client's RPE for each exercise, whether the client had any difficulty throughout any of the exercises, and any modifications that you may have for the next

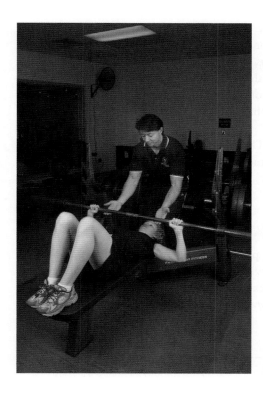

FIGURE 20.5. Personal Trainer communicating effectively with a client upon the completion of an exercise.

workout. Finally, place the folder back in the storage facility and prepare for the next client. Once again, the stages of the review phase include:

1. Thanking the client for a good workout.
2. Restoring the training room to proper form.
3. Recording information from the client's workout, including RPE and any modifications for the next workout.
4. Placing the client's folder back in the storage facility.

TRAINING NOTES

Training notes are the Personal Trainer's equivalent to medical charts. They contain valuable pieces of information that are vital to the proper treatment of each client. Although recording information and transferring data from sheet to sheet can be tedious, it is extremely important to the success of any applied training regimen. Analysis of the chart will enable the Personal Trainer to structure workouts for maximum results. The objectives for the notes are as follows:

➤ To keep track of the exercise program so that its effectiveness can be subsequently evaluated through the re-evaluation procedure
➤ To ensure that the client's program is consistent regardless of the instructor
➤ To reinforce long-term and short-term objectives
➤ To keep track of the trainee's progression in relation to changes in workout intensity

All notes should be thorough and concise. Note only relevant information and be sure to sign each session. The following types of information are a sample of what might be included in a client's training notes:

1. Subjective (SUB): Describes how the client feels on the day of a particular workout. It serves as a barometer for the Personal Trainer in structuring the physiological and psychological climate of the workout.

2. Observation (OBS): Notes any signs of tissue trauma (e.g., edema, extreme redness, ecchymosis (black and blue), or joint dysfunction (i.e., limping or impaired ROM). If any of these signs exist, it might be recommended to ask the client to see his or her physician.

3. Objectives (OBJ): Describes specific objectives for that session. It should be based on the long-term goals and short-term goals with consideration of daily SUB and OBS.

4. Workout (WO): Notes the major components of that session (i.e., modes, exercises, sets, reps, weights, workloads, HR/RPE responses, etc.).

5. Comments are noted at the end of each session. This section may include plans for the next workout (e.g., pain associated with a specific movement) or any other relevant comments.

6. Personal Trainer's signature

SUMMARY

It is obvious that, like any other "technical" job task, personal training has very specific protocols that should be followed to optimize the level of service delivered to the client. In addition to following accepted standard guidelines with regard to exercise, the Personal Trainer must also strive to deliver the highest level of customer service and accurately and completely document every aspect of the client's program and individual session.

REFERENCES

1. American College of Sports Medicine. Guidelines for Exercise Testing and Prescription. 7th ed. Baltimore: Lippincott Williams & Wilkins, 2006.
2. Plus One Training Department. Exercise Specialist Training Manual. 6th ed. New York: Plus One, 2004.

Business Principles for Personal Trainers

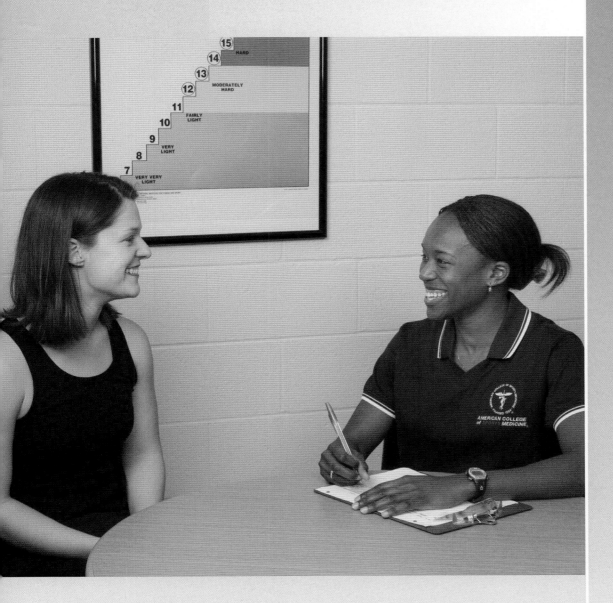

Joan Hatfield, M.S., General Manager, Personal Training Director, Plus One Health Management, Seattle, Washington
Neal I. Pire, M.A., Director, Sports Training Academy, Ridgewood, New Jersey

Chapter Outline

Objectives

- **Learn how to sell and market training services to potential clients**
- **Learn how to price training sessions**
- **Learn how to maintain professional standards that will protect a business reputation**

A Personal Trainer may be very knowledgeable and skilled in exercise science principles and their application in a personal training session, but an understanding of the business of personal training is equally important for the Personal Trainer's success. Whether associated with a personal training department or running his or her own business, a Personal Trainer needs business expertise in how to sell and market training services to potential clients, how to price training sessions, and how to maintain professional standards that will protect a business reputation. For success as a self-employed Personal Trainer, business planning, business models, and budgeting are also needed before a business can be started. Finally, business success will also depend on finding a work–life balance, as personal training can involve long days with many training sessions and interaction with many different people.

THE PERSONAL TRAINER'S POSITION

A Personal Trainer can work in several different, yet distinct settings. Some of the more common venues or "job classifications" include the solo Personal Trainer, the employee or independent contractor, and the manager or personal training business owner. The solo Personal Trainer is commonly known as a Personal Trainer who is independent of another business entity. The Personal Trainer of this type typically markets to potential clients, schedules and delivers training sessions either in the client's home, outside, or in the gym. The employee or independent contractor is typically hired or contracted by a business owner to provide training services for the business's clients. The Personal Trainer/manager/owner typically supervises the business operations and staff management of a personal training business. Whether the Personal Trainer is a sole proprietor or an employee, success will be based on how well he or she can "sell" the training services. The "Sales" section in this chapter provides a comprehensive approach to selling personal training services. Although the emphases on specific job tasks might differ from one setting to another, the goal is ultimately the same: to follow sound business practices and develop a profitable enterprise by delivering the optimal level of service to the end user, the training client.

There are various compensation models for personal training programs in the fitness center setting. Some facilities pay Personal Trainers a percentage of the revenue generated by the services they deliver. Other facilities hire Personal Trainers as hourly or salaried employees with designated work shifts and pay them an additional commission for "fee for service" sessions delivered to the members. Individual salaries or commission rates for Personal Trainers typically vary, based on education, certification, experience, seniority, job performance, and volume of revenue produced. Regardless of the compensation model, it is important that all program costs be considered during the business planning phase. General and administrative costs for marketing, administrative support, meetings, uniforms, payroll taxes, liability insurance, and continuing education can dramatically affect the profitability of the personal training program (1).

BUSINESS SUCCESS

Success in the personal training business is very much dependent on the same factors that lead to success in any such enterprise. Customer satisfaction is paramount, but an understanding of sound business practices will help ensure that a Personal Trainer keeps his or her business profitable.

Managing a Personal Training Department

If working in a health club, corporate fitness facility, or a nonprofit recreation center, a Personal Trainer may be employed to manage the personal training department, while still maintaining a schedule of training clients. This added responsibility requires good organizational skills and time management. Skills in interviewing, hiring, employee training, service pricing, marketing, sales, and policy setting are needed by the personal training manager.

Hiring Personal Trainers

The following are important steps to follow when hiring a Personal Trainer:

1. Resumes should be reviewed carefully for educational background, current certifications, recent training experience with a variety of clientele, and innovative training programs.
2. Applicants should be asked to bring copies of current fitness and CPR-AED/First Aid certifications to the interview appointment. This may prevent an undesired realization after hiring that the Personal Trainer's certifications have expired.
3. The Personal Trainer/manager should create a list of questions to ask all personal training applicants. The questions should be practical, including scenarios that require the Personal Trainer to discuss training program options for hypothetical clients.
4. The Personal Trainer's availability and scheduling preference for appointments should be clearly assessed and agreed to at the time of the interview and prior to a job offer. If the department needs an evening Personal Trainer, and the interviewee is already training elsewhere in the evening, the Personal Trainer/manager needs to know that information to effectively plan for staffing needs.
5. A practical or "hands-on" component should be a part of the interview process. The Personal Trainer should demonstrate exercises and spotting techniques on the fitness floor. Someone should be designated to be a hypothetical client. The Personal Trainer/manager should observe and assess how the Personal Trainer interacts with this person.

Setting Training Standards

The personal training manager is ultimately responsible for the safety and customer satisfaction of every personal training client. Therefore, it is necessary to set standards for delivering personal training services in a manner that is consistent with industry standards for safety and that will ensure excellent customer service that is consistently delivered. Here are some guidelines for setting the department's service standards:

1. Personal Trainers must give their undivided attention to their clients (2). This means that Personal Trainers must watch clients at all times and spot exercises with appropriate techniques. Policy parameters should be specific. Talking on cell phones, talking with other Personal Trainers or other members, and watching TV monitors are examples of unacceptable behaviors that would not meet training standards. In addition, a Personal Trainer who spends much of the training session talking about his or her personal affairs will have difficulty focusing fully on the client's workout and exercise technique (2).
2. Personal Trainers must show up for training sessions on time and end training sessions on time. Personal Trainers must respect the training client's time and schedule.
3. There should be a dress standard for the department's Personal Trainers. If possible, Personal Trainers should wear a shirt with a facility logo and the words "Personal Trainer." The shirt, along with established standards for pants and shoes, will ensure a professional look for the personal training department, while also providing advertising to other members.
4. Personal Trainers should keep written documentation of every client's workout as well as any measurements, tests, and performance tracking for that client (2). The personal training department manager should provide a standardized "training card" for the Personal Trainers to use. There

should be a designated training file where the training cards are kept that is accessible to both the training client and other Personal Trainers. If a client wants to work out without the Personal Trainer, or another Personal Trainer needs to cover a training session because of illness or vacation, the training cards are readily available.

5. A client confidentiality policy should be maintained. Personal Trainers should be reminded that they should never discuss any client's personal information with others. Personal Trainers must respect their clients' privacy and be trustworthy (2).

6. Honesty and scope of practice standards should be emphasized. If a Personal Trainer does not know the answer to a client's health- or fitness-related questions, the Personal Trainer needs to admit that he or she does not have that information. The Personal Trainer can volunteer to research the topic and provide an answer at the next training session. If the client is asking for medical advice or a diagnosis, the Personal Trainer must not overstep his or her scope of practice but should explain that the client needs to consult a physician for that information (2).

7. Personal Trainers must maintain personal training certifications, CPR certification, and liability insurance, if it is not provided by the fitness facility. Records of certification and professional liability insurance should be kept in employee files (1).

TRAINING AND EMPOWERING PERSONAL TRAINERS

Personal Trainers should be encouraged to continuously read and learn, staying current on the latest industry standards and changing trends. The Personal Trainer/manager can subscribe to trade journals and publications and make them available to his Personal Trainers. Budget permitting, some Personal Trainer/managers can provide an annual educational stipend for each Personal Trainer that will subsidize his or her participation in continuing education to maintain personal training certification. Others provide CEC-approved in-house educational sessions to make it convenient and cost effective for Personal Trainers to attend and earn credit for continuing or re-certification. Others hold weekly staff meetings with Personal Trainers and even have them take turns providing continuing education with handouts and discussion.

Managers should empower Personal Trainers by encouraging them to share training program ideas in meetings, to help plan and implement new training program approaches such as small-group training or sport-specific training, and to share ideas for how to increase clientele and sales. Personal Trainers should be included in discussions about pricing of training sessions and their compensation rates. They should be treated as professionals and their creative ideas and opinions should be valued. They should feel like an integral part of the training team.

FITNESS MANAGEMENT

A Personal Trainer may also be placed in charge of a fitness department in a health club, corporate fitness facility, or nonprofit recreation center. Other Personal Trainers may also be part of this department. In addition to overseeing the personal training sales and delivery, the fitness department manager may also be responsible for fitness equipment purchases, emergency drills, maintenance and repairs, special fitness programming events, and, in some cases, the group fitness program. Even with all of these responsibilities, the fitness manager may still be expected to retain personal training clients for additional department revenue and to supplement his or her salary in addition to that received managing the fitness department. A checklist along with some practical guidelines may include:

1. Setting a schedule for available times for training and for management responsibilities
2. Using a time-management system to stay organized
3. Training exercise specialists and Personal Trainers to follow routine procedures (such as turning in time cards) that will simplify the workload

4. Explaining tasks to other fitness staff and then delegating these tasks to those who will get them done correctly and on time (e.g., assign the planning of monthly emergency drills/procedure reviews to a fitness staff member and have this person plan and execute the drills and reviews with all fitness staff, including Personal Trainers)

5. Taking time to lead by example for both members and fitness staff by leading a healthy lifestyle of regular exercise and practicing good nutritional habits

STARTING A BUSINESS

Before starting a personal training business, there are different business models from which to choose for establishing a business entity. There are five basic business models from which to choose for a personal training business: sole proprietorship, independent contractor, partnership, corporation, and S corporation.

Sole Proprietorship

In a sole proprietorship, one person owns the business. As the simplest, least-expensive business model, often the only requirement before starting operations is a license from the state and/or local city where the business will be located. Personal income tax is paid on any business earnings. Two drawbacks to this model can be capital expenses for business start-up/expansion and personal liability for any incurred debt (3). In the eyes of the law and the Internal Revenue Service, the business and the individual are one and the same.

Independent Contractor

An independent contractor provides certain services for other individuals or businesses. Many Personal Trainers are independent contractors who provide personal training services to health clubs; the client pays the club for the services and the club pays the Personal Trainer. Personal Trainers who are independent contractors often work at multiple locations, set their own schedules, are paid by the session, and often have some control over training session format and fees. However, the percentage of the training fees that the individual contractor receives is often determined by the health club management (3). An independent contractor is similar to a sole proprietorship except the Personal Trainer actually works for another business.

Partnership

A business partnership is formed by two or more people, either with an informal agreement or with a formal written contract filed with local or state government. Partnerships are loosely governed by state and federal regulations and are subject to personal income tax based on each partner's ownership share. Forming a partnership allows pooled financial resources and talents, but ownership transfer among partners may be difficult, and each partner can be held liable if another partner fails to meet business-related obligations (3).

Corporation

A corporation is a formal business entity subject to laws, regulations, and the demands of stockholders. Governed by a charter and bylaws, a corporation is a legal entity completely separate from its owners and managers. Investors, whose personal risk for financial liability is limited, are often part of a corporation's start-up and growth. Corporation ownership can be more easily transferred than ownership in a sole proprietorship or partnership (3).

S Corporation

The S corporation (or subchapter S corporation) a popular alternative for small businesses, combines the advantages of the sole proprietorship, partnership, and corporation. The benefits include:

➤ Limited risk and exposure of personal assets
➤ No double taxation on both salary and business income
➤ Freedom for each partner to distribute dividends (3)

ADMINISTRATION

To establish and administer a business, the Personal Trainer should first develop a business plan. The business plan includes establishing a budget, developing management policies, marketing, sales, and pricing.

Establishing a Budget

A market analysis will provide valuable information useful in developing an annual operating budget. It provides the baseline data to build the budget from the ground up. Personal training businesses typically begin with determining sales goals. The sales goals are set by determining the projected number of training sessions over the course of a week, month, and year multiplied by the average rate per session. These totals will help determine expenses over each period of time, since direct expenses correlate with sessions delivered multiplied by the cost per session. To establish a budget, the Personal Trainer should consider the following:

1. Estimate business expenses (exclusive of salary) needed to operate annually, including:
    a. Gas/vehicle maintenance
    b. Income tax
    c. Liability insurance
    d. Telephone
    e. Uniforms
    f. Professional memberships/certifications
    g. Conferences and training
    h. Business supplies (computer, office supplies, postage, printing, etc.)
    i. Fitness equipment
    j. Client gifts/awards
    k. Accountant fees
2. Determine a realistic number of training hours annually that fit into a realistic schedule (factor in vacation days, personal days for medical check-ups and family emergencies, sick days, etc.)
3. Determine a charge per training session to achieve a gross annual income that will cover business expenses and personal expenses and will allow some funds to be put aside for savings and/or investments (4)

Management and Policies

To manage a business effectively, the Personal Trainer must work from a business plan, which should include the creation of a business vision, mission statement, business values, a brief description of the business services (Box 21.1), the choice of a business model, and the listing of operational policies (5) such as:

➤ Billing (Will clients prepay for each session or will you bill them monthly?)
➤ Cancellation policy (How many hours will you need without charging client?)

| BOX 21.1 | **Sample Mission Statement** |

THE PERSONAL TRAINING ACADEMY

Our Vision
✔ To grow profitably by delighting customers and achieving undisputed leadership in the field of personal training.

Our Mission
✔ To create value for shareowners through our marketplace leadership in personal training and fitness programming that helps all of our clients achieve their goals.

Our Values
✔ **INTEGRITY,** honesty, and the highest ethical standards
✔ **MUTUAL RESPECT** and trust in our working relationships
✔ **INNOVATION** and encouragement to challenge the status quo
✔ **COMMUNICATION** that is open, consistent, and two-way
✔ **TEAMWORK** and meeting our commitments to one another
✔ **CONTINUOUS IMPROVEMENT**, development, and learning in all we do
✔ **DIVERSITY** of people, cultures, and ideas
✔ **PERFORMANCE** with recognition for results

Service Description
✔ **The Personal Training Academy** provides personal training clients with the best possible physical and psychological advantage by improving their focus, discipline, and self-confidence. This is achieved through the most advanced state-of-the-art personal training techniques available; thus enhancing the client's ability to compete and achieve success both in fitness and in life.

➤ Late arrival policy (Will you charge for the entire session anyway?)
➤ Vacation policy (What will this be for both Personal Trainer and client?)
➤ Payment methods (Will client pay by cash, check, or credit card?)
➤ "Insufficient funds" check policy (Will there be a penalty and if so, what?)

Marketing

The personal training market includes different groups of people with varying needs. A market niche represents a client group with similar needs and goals. Personal Trainers often choose to focus their marketing efforts on one or several of these groups. For example, a Personal Trainer could select the niche market based on the following:

➤ Client type (e.g., gender, age, fitness level)
➤ Training needs (e.g., sport-specific training, pre-natal fitness, group training)
➤ Training location (e.g., in-home training, health club training, sport location training)

Personal Trainers should ask the following questions when selecting their market niches:

1. What is the potential for income with this market?
2. Is this market readily accessible in my geographical area?
3. Does this market fit well with my training skills and interest?
4. Can I highlight my knowledge, services, certifications, and skills in such a way to reach this market as my clientele?

One of the best ways to market personal training services is to ask for referrals from satisfied clients. Personal Trainers sometimes are hesitant to do this, but if the Personal Trainer truly believes that a client has benefited greatly from the training, then other potential clients may want to also receive these same benefits. Other ways of marketing personal training include volunteering to speak at community events and organizations and networking with other business professionals in the community. Advertising in the phone book, the newspaper, and by direct mail can be costly and may not provide a good return on the investment at first. Establishing a website and profiling the training style and qualifications is another good approach for marketing a business and staying competitive in the personal training business (6).

Personal training businesses use a variety of strategies to attract clients. Among the more popular strategies are:

1. Client referral (the most focused strategy)
   a. The focus is on generating prospects and clients
   b. The process involves existing clients providing the names of potential new clients
   c. Clients are provided with referral cards to hand in the names of prospects
   d. Incentives are typically given to clients for providing referrals
   e. It is usually an on-going strategy
2. Lead boxes (provides a very low rate of return)
   a. This strategy primarily serves as a source for leads (names)
   b. The boxes are placed in business locations that tend to serve customer bases that are demographically similar to the targeted audiences
   c. Businesses are given awards for allowing the lead boxes to be placed in their locales
3. Advertising (most expensive and lowest rate of return on investment)
   a. In general, this strategy is designed to build brand recognition in the marketplace, enhance the image of the organization, create leads, or occasionally generate prospects
   b. This technique is a shotgun approach to reaching clients (versus more targeted methods)
   c. Cable television, radio, newspapers, billboards, and external or internal signage are examples of this method
   d. The most effective type of advertising for generating leads or prospects provides a "Call to Action" and typically creates urgency by establishing a deadline
   e. It is important to know the marketing target niche before the advertising medium is selected
4. Alliances with homeowner associations (HOAs) and realtors
   a. This strategy is a good source for qualified leads and even prospects (HOAs and realtors whose customers match the organization's target market should be engaged in the process)
   b. HOAs and realtors can provide the names of new people in the area
   c. A strategy involves providing the HOAs or realtors with a certificate or letter to give to customers that offers some complimentary service (i.e., training session or pre-activity screening and goals analysis)
5. Direct mail (the return rate for this technique is usually 1 to 3% for mailed pieces and 7 to 15% for e-mails)
   a. This strategy is primarily a technique for creating leads or turning leads into prospects
   b. This method is a more focused technique than advertising
   c. Direct mail lists from agencies should be used (very targeted lists—such as zip codes or even specific delivery routes—can be obtained to best match the desired market area and demographics of the target audience)
   d. The piece that is mailed is typically simple, with an attention-grabbing call to action and normally incorporates an incentive to create urgency and generate an action response
6. Community involvement (ideal for service and relationship-driven businesses like personal training)
   a. This strategy focuses on creating relationships to uncover prospects

    b. The technique involves creating a specific image within the community and becoming a recognized professional in the community

    c. An example of this approach is to become active in community organizations, such as the local chambers of commerce, the Rotary Club, church groups, and other civic organizations

    d. Another option is hosting community events in the training facility or sponsoring community events at other locations

7. Reputation management

    a. This strategy is used to enhance the public image of the organization

    b. Over time, this approach can be a great source for prospects

    c. The technique involves developing a press kit on the Personal Trainer or the business as a whole (e.g., a background, fact sheet)

    d. This strategy requires establishing positive relationships with the local media

    e. The approach requires regularly issuing press releases of human interest involving the club and following up with the media

8. Promotional materials

    a. This strategy is normally used to help convert leads to prospects or prospects to members

    b. The materials are designed to create a positive image of the business and to help educate consumers on personal training in general, the business, and its Personal Trainers

    c. Websites, print brochures, and video brochures are examples of this technique

    d. These materials are normally given to leads and more often to prospects

9. Strategic alliances

    a. This strategy is designed to create partnerships between businesses and organizations with similar target audiences

    b. This technique is good at bringing in leads and prospects

    c. The approach involves cross-marketing between the businesses (e.g., a Personal Trainer might partner with a home fitness equipment retailer offering equipment purchasers a complimentary "orientation to the purchased equipment," with the objective of converting them into personal training clients; the retailer has a "value-added service"—the Personal Trainer—which might be an inducement for the customer to purchase the equipment)

    d. The customers of each business become potential customers for the other partner (an alliance group) (1)

Sales

Too often, Personal Trainers focus their "sales" efforts on creating signs, flyers, and brochures, hoping that clients will flock to them for training. The mistake often made is that such efforts are "low-percentage" marketing activities that offer a low return on the investment of time, money, and effort. In addition, these activities do not close the sale for the Personal Trainer; they only weed-out potential prospects for the Personal Trainer's services. The Personal Trainer is depending on the client to respond to the marketing piece. The key to sales success is for the Personal Trainer to use available resources, proactively cultivate warm-market "suspects" to convert them into prospects, and finally ask the prospect for the sale.

Before going into the sales process, "sale" must first be defined. A sale is simply an agreement—a quid pro quo—between the Personal Trainer, the client, and at times the facility where the training sessions will take place. A sale is not an imposition on the client. All too often, a Personal Trainer is "apologetic" when asking for the sale. In actuality, every sale is a "win–win" situation, because all participants position themselves to get what they want. Clients are securing the direction, expertise, or motivation they desire, and the Personal Trainer is contracting his or her professional services. The ingredient needed to fulfill the sale is commitment. The client must commit to what was agreed to at the point of sale (i.e., showing up prepared for the training session at the scheduled time), and

Table 21.1	BENEFITS OF PERSONAL TRAINING

Client achieves results more quickly
Reduces the risk of injury to the client
Increases the client's motivational levels
Provides more focused workouts for the client
Uses client's time more efficiently

the Personal Trainer must commit to deliver on the service "promise" to the client (i.e., delivering a safe, individualized, goal-oriented workout).

In the gym or fitness center environment, the Personal Trainer's primary source of business is the membership base. This captive audience is the Personal Trainer's main resource for "prospects." It is important for the Personal Trainer to be established as an expert and to build rapport with the members, creating a warm market for the Personal Trainer to target, market to, and ultimately, to ask for the sale.

Before approaching members on the exercise floor, Personal Trainers should have a clear understanding of what their objective is and what value they bring to the potential client. It is important to be empathetic and see things through the eyes of the member. Why should the member consider personal training? What is in it for the member? The Personal Trainer should know what the benefits of personal training are to the client (Table 21.1).

The Personal Trainer needs to be aware of the prospect's questions and concerns. What are the prospect's perceptions? Will personal training help get the participant more fit? Will it help the participant look better? Will it help the participant be healthier? These are all valuable benefits and perceived outcomes for the participant, but ultimately, even a prospect who perceives these outcomes as real still might not make the commitment to purchase training sessions. Why? It is because it is all about the prospect's emotions. The Personal Trainer must consider how the prospect feels about his or her goals and how he or she will feel when they are fulfilled.

Effective sales generation is simply a step-by-step process outlined on the following pages (and in Table 21.2), which could be used for a facility-based Personal Trainer.

Table 21.2	THE FITNESS FACILITY-BASED PERSONAL TRAINER'S SALES CHECKLIST

Be proactive. Approach prospects and always Remember To Smile—*be positive and upbeat, no matter how bad a day you are having*
Top priority is to build rapport—to develop a relationship of mutual trust and confidence
Sell *benefits* of Personal Training but key into *how they'll feel* when achieving those benefits
Be empathetic—see their world as if it were your own
Be genuine—exude sincerity
Be warm—treat prospects with respect
It's a win–win! • Clients—take control of their goals by hiring an expert's assistance • Personal Trainers—practice their profession, increase their earning potential, and add valuable experience, which enhances their value to the employer or facility and the fitness industry in general • The facility enhances the service delivered to clients by providing 1-on-1 management of the member • You must *ask* for the sale!—*It is a numbers game. The more prospects you ask, the more sales you'll make*

Step 1. Making contact—*"Getting a foot in the door."* A Personal Trainer needs to proactively approach a facility member or client exercising on the gym floor. The Personal Trainer should greet the member with a smile and offer his or her expertise based on their observations of the member.

Sample "openings" may include:

- "Hi! May I help you with your exercise program?"
- "Hey Mark, let me show you a more effective way to do this exercise"
- "Hello Linda, I noticed you're really focusing on your lower body. Can I show you a great new combination of exercises for your hips and thighs?"

Step 2. Building rapport—*"Trust me?" Yes!!!* Personal Trainers must build rapport and trust so that prospects believe in them and their ability help the client achieve established goals. A Personal Trainer builds trust by taking a personal interest in the prospect, making mental notes of the prospect's likes, dislikes, or personal information that the prospect may share with the Personal Trainer.

Sample rapport-building "blurbs" include:

- "Hi John, you haven't been here since before Thanksgiving..."
- "Hello Marie, how was your business trip?"
- "Hi Jessica, did your daughter decide between colleges?"

Step 3. Assessing Need—*"The Personal Trainer needs to "shut up and listen!!!"* The best salespersons are seldom the best talkers—they're usually the best listeners. The Personal Trainer should key into: *"What's in it for the prospect?"* and focus on not just "what" the prospect wants, but also learn **why** the prospect wants it.

Step 4. The Tease—This is how Personal Trainers continues to build trust and demonstrate and build their value. The simplest way is to assist a prospect with an exercise or make program suggestions. A Personal Trainer can spot the prospect as he or she is progressing through a workout and suggest a "better way." The Personal Trainer can also demonstrate a new exercise or literally "train" the client for 5 or 10 minutes, just giving the prospect a "taste" of what it is like to work with him or her. This sampling of the Personal Trainer's prowess is the "tease" that should keep the prospect wanting more.

Step 5. Presenting a Winning Proposition—*"Asking for the Sale."* The Personal Trainer must present a winning solution to the prospect's need before asking for the sale. This "frames" the pitch so that the prospect responds affirmatively when asked for the sale.

- "You really want to lose the 10 pounds by your High School Reunion in June, don't you?"
- "If I can show you how I can help you reach your goal, would that interest you?"

Step 6. "The Close"—The Personal Trainer should give the prospect "either–or" choices, never "yes" or "no." A sample "yes-or-no" proposal may include something like "Marie, would you like to set-up a training appointment?" A sample "either–or" proposal might be "Marie, you're usually here in the morning, I'm available to help you any two mornings per week at 6 AM or 7 AM. Which works best for you?" Giving the prospect a choice between two "yeses" increases the likelihood that the Personal Trainer will close the sale.

Step 7. The Fall-back—*Opening the Backdoor*—*"The Tickler File."* Every prospect that says "no" becomes a "future prospect." The Personal Trainer should maintain a database of contact and personal information (e.g., likes, dislikes, occupation) of these prospects for further rapport building, always looking for the opportunity to once again ask for the sale. The Personal Trainer should continue to deliver a service (e.g., assistance on the training floor) and communicate through every available vehicle (in person, phone, email, etc.) increasing his value as a Personal Trainer. Photocopying clips of fitness articles that prospects might be interested in and providing them to clients, emailing a web-based link to a pertinent website, or even a press release with the Personal Trainer's own "success story" are all examples of how to effectively "drip" on prospects to build a Personal Trainer's value. Personal Trainers in a fitness center setting should also do whatever they can to keep the prospect coming in to work out, even if the prospect continues to train on his or her own. Doing so helps to maintain the Personal Trainer's "warm market," so that the prospect remains a prospect and is also a source of referrals to the Personal Trainer.

Step 8. Keep in mind—*It's a "numbers game."* An insurance company study conducted several years back showed that even the worst approach to selling can be successful, if the salesperson simply goes through the numbers, and "keeps asking."

Pricing

Once the framework for the personal training business is complete, specific pricing and budgets can be established. Typical direct expenses include salaries, payroll taxes, and benefits. Operational expenses include marketing expenses, program materials, and facility use charges. Pricing is typically established through consideration of a number of factors. It is essential to consider the general business objectives (e.g., profit, overall client retention, the projected number of clients, and average number of sessions per client per unit of time) before establishing pricing. To conduct programs within established budgetary guidelines, revenues and expenses should be reviewed regularly (1).

Ultimately, what a Personal Trainer charges for training services depends on market forces. Completing a market analysis will help determine perceived value in the marketplace and thus price point. Some key elements of a market analysis include:

➤ Demographic study—How many potential clients are there in the geographical area?
➤ Competitive analysis—What are other Personal Trainers charging for their services?
➤ Consumer survey—What is the prospective client's perceived value?
➤ Demand projections—How large is the market?
➤ Financial considerations—Based on budgetary projections, what is the required revenue per unit sale? What volume is required to meet budget?
➤ Focus group information—What are the perceived needs of the prospect base?

Business Planning

Budgets are necessary to forecast financial expectations and goals, provide accountability, track progress of actual versus projected results, and allow justification and scrutiny. Completing an accurate, reliable, and analyzable budget without a computer is not easy. Simple software programs like QuickBooks, or MYOB (Manage Your Own Business) are available and recommended, even for the solo Personal Trainer; they will help organize business finances and make tax reporting easier (1).

Although there are many resources available for the Personal Trainer/manager/owner, it remains prudent to enlist the guidance of a legal and accounting professional. The Internal Revenue Service website is a great resource for obtaining specific tax forms and information. It is accessible at: http://www.irs.gov/.

PROFESSIONAL STANDARDS

A Code of Ethics for ACSM Certified and Registered Professionals has been established that helps to guide the ethical practice of Personal Trainers. This code (Box 21.2) helps to bring the profession of personal training in line with other professions and healthcare disciplines.

BOX 21.2	**Responsibility to the Public**

CODE OF ETHICS FOR ACSM CERTIFIED AND REGISTERED PROFESSIONALS

The purpose of this Code of Ethics is intended to aid all certified and registered American College of Sports Medicine Credentialed Professionals (ACSMCP) to establish and maintain a high level of ethical conduct, as defined by standards by which an ACSMCP may determine the appropriateness of his or her conduct. Any existing professional, licensure, or certification affiliations that ACSMCPs have with governmental, local, state or national agencies or organizations will take precedence relative to any disciplinary matters that pertain to practice or professional conduct.

This Code applies to all ACSMCPs, regardless of ACSM membership status. Any cases in violation of this Code will be referred to the ACSM Committee on Certification and Registry Boards (CCRB)

- ACSMCPs shall be dedicated to providing competent and legally permissible services within the scope of the Knowledge, Skills, and Abilities (KSAs) of their respective credential. These services shall be provided with integrity, competence, diligence, and compassion.
- ACSMCPs provide exercise information in a manner that is consistent with evidence-based science and medicine.
- ACSMCPs respect the rights of clients, colleagues, and health professionals, and shall safeguard client confidences within the boundaries of the law.
- Information relating to the ACSMCP–client relationship is confidential and may not be communicated to a third party not involved in that client's care without the prior written consent of the client or as required by law.
- ACSMCPs are truthful about their qualifications and the limitations of their expertise and provide services consistent with their competencies.

Responsibility to the Profession

- ACSMCPs maintain high professional standards. As such, an ACSMCPs should never represent himself/herself, either directly or indirectly, as anything other than an ACSMCP unless he/she holds other license/certification that allows him/her to do so.
- ACSMCPs practice within the scope of their knowledge, skills, and abilities. ACSMCPs will not provide services that are limited by state law to provision by another health care professional only.
- An ACSMCP must remain in good standing relative to governmental requirements as a condition of continued credentialing.
- ACSMCPs take credit, including authorship, only for work they have actually performed and give credit to the contributions of others as warranted.
- Consistent with the requirements of their certification or registration, ACSMCPs must complete approved, additional educational course work aimed at maintaining and advancing their knowledge, skills and abilities.

Principles and Standards for Candidates of the Certification Exam

Candidates applying for an ACSM Credentialing examination must comply with candidacy requirements and to the best of their abilities, accurately complete the application process.

Public Disclosure of Affiliation

Any ACSMCP may disclose his or her affiliation with ACSM Credentialing in any context, oral or documented, provided it is currently accurate. In doing so, no ACSMCP may imply College endorsement of whatever is associated in context with the disclosure, unless expressively authorized by the College. Disclosure of affiliation in connection with a commercial venture may be made provided the disclosure is made in a professionally dignified manner, is not false, misleading or deceptive, and does not imply licensure or the attainment of specialty or diploma status. ACSMCPs may disclose their credential status. ACSMCPs may list their affiliation with ACSM Credentialing on their business cards without prior authorization (ACSM

continued >

Box 21.2. Sample Session Plan, cont.

Health/Fitness Director®, ACSM Health/Fitness Instructor®, ACSM Group Fitness Exercise Leader®, ACSM Program Director®, ACSM Exercise Specialist®, ACSM Exercise Test Technologist®, ACSM Registered Clinical Exercise Physiologist®, ACSM certified Personal Trainer[SM]). ACSMCPs and the institutions employing an ACSMCP may inform the public of an affiliation as a matter of public discourse or presentation.

Discipline

Any ACSMCP may be disciplined or lose his or her certification or registry for conduct which, in the opinion of the Executive Committee of the ACSM Committee on Certification and Registry Boards, goes against the principles set forth in this Code. The ACSM Code will review such cases. Such cases will be reviewed by the ACSM Committee on Ethics and Professional Conduct, which will include a liaison from the ACSM Committee on Certification and Registry Boards as appointed by the Chair of the Committee on Certification and Registry Boards. The ACSM Committee on Certification and Registry Boards will make an action recommendation to the Executive Committee of the ACSM Committee on Certification and Registry Boards for final review and approval.

SUMMARY

It is no longer true that the best "technical Personal Trainer" is the most successful. Whether the Personal Trainer is "going solo" or is a manager of a large personal training department within a fitness center, today's Personal Trainers need to be proficient in both exercise science and business management. Only by combining these varied skills can they ensure their success and that of their clients.

REFERENCES

1. American College of Sports Medicine. ACSM's Resource Manual for Guidelines for Exercise Testing and Prescription. 5th ed. Baltimore: Lippincott Williams & Wilkins, 2006.
2. American College of Sports Medicine. ACSM's Resources for the Personal Trainer. 1st ed. Baltimore: Lippincott Williams Wilkins, 2005.
3. Holland T. Ten important personal training guidelines. Am Fitness 2001;19(1):42.
4. Miller W. ONE-ON-ONE: choosing a market niche. Strength Cond 1994;16(4):68–69.
5. Schreiber K. ONE-ON-ONE: setting up a budget for a personal training business. Strength Cond 1994;16(5):64–65.
6. American College of Sports Medicine Code of Ethics for ACSM Certified and Registered Professionals. On the Internet at http://www.acsm.org/certification/generalinfo.htm. Accessed July 1, 2005.

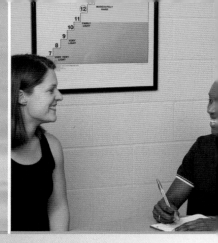

CHAPTER
22

Legal Issues and Responsibilities

Shirley Archer, M.A., J.D., Health Educator, Author, and Fitness Professional, Health Improvement Program, Stanford Prevention Research Center, Stanford University School of Medicine, Palo Alto, California

Chapter Outline

Objectives

- **Understand the primary areas of potential liability**
- **Understand the role of industry standards and guidelines**
- **Learn practical strategies to manage risk**

A Personal Trainer must understand legal issues and responsibilities before assuming the task of training any person. Regardless of the Personal Trainers' business model, whether associated with a personal training department or running their own business, Personal Trainers need to know what the areas are for potential liability that affects their practice, what industry standards and guidelines direct these areas, and what measures they can take to manage risk effectively. All physical activity involves risk of injury; accidents can and will happen. To maintain professionalism and to protect the longevity of a personal training career, a Personal Trainer needs to proactively anticipate these areas of risk and to manage them with common sense. This knowledge of, and commitment to, safety and injury prevention not only minimizes the likelihood of professional liability but also improves quality of service and may save lives.

This chapter discusses liability specifically related to working with clients and does not expand into broader issues such as type of business organization, copyright, or trademark issues that are more appropriately covered in other chapters and books devoted specifically to business practices. Local rules and regulations, definitions of standards of care, and the acceptability of informed consent forms and waivers of liability vary from state to state, county to county, and even city to city. This chapter is not intended to be legal advice and should not be considered a substitute for legal counsel on specific liability issues pertaining to individual situations.

POTENTIAL AREAS OF PROFESSIONAL LIABILITY

Legal considerations affect many aspects of the personal training experience. Areas of potential exposure for liability include the physical setting where program activities occur; the equipment used; the nature and quality of training techniques, advice, and services rendered; the degree of emergency preparedness and responsiveness; and the method of keeping and protecting records. While legal principles affect the training environment, as a practical matter most cases today are settled out of court and therefore never actually create case law. To help Personal Trainers to understand the practical ramifications, this chapter is organized according to the most common types of incidents likely to occur during day-to-day business. The application of legal concepts such as negligence to particular circumstances is then examined, and the role of professional standards, guidelines, position statements, and recommendations from professional organizations is considered. Personal training is a business/invitee relationship. In these types of relationships, the ante for invitee responsibilities is raised.

Safe Premises

Although most Personal Trainers focus on educating themselves on the latest training techniques and aspects of program design, in reality, Personal Trainers are most vulnerable to professional liability for incidents that result from conditions of the physical setting where program activities occur. In general (1), any business owner who allows people to enter upon land or into a building is required to provide a reasonably safe environment under theories of tort law (Box 22.1). The area of tort law that regulates these issues is termed "premises liability." The ACSM (2) has identified six fundamental standards to which facilities must adhere (Table 22.1). Because a Personal Trainer may offer services in a variety of locations, including a health and fitness facility, the outdoors, or in a client's home, the Personal Trainer should take basic precautions to ensure that every training setting is safe.

BOX 22.1	Key Terms

Contract law: Body of law that regulates the rights and obligations of parties who enter into a contract. A contract is an agreement between two or more parties that creates an obligation to do, or not to do, something that creates a legal relationship. If the agreement is broken, the parties have the right to pursue legal remedies. A contract can be written or verbal. The important elements of a contract include an offer and an acceptance, also referred to as a "meeting of the minds" and the exchange of something of value.

Duty of care: Refers to the level of responsibility that one has to protect another from harm. In general, the legal standard is reasonable care under the circumstances, which is based on an examination of factual details.

Informed consent: A process that entails conveying complete understanding to a client or patient about his or her option to choose to participate in a procedure, test, service, or program

Negligence: A failure to conform one's conduct to a generally accepted standard or duty

Release or waiver: An agreement by a client before beginning participation, to give up, relinquish, or waive the participant's rights to legal remedy (damages) in the event of injury, even when such injury arises as a result of provider negligence

Risk management: A process whereby a service or program is delivered in a manner to fully conform to the most relevant standards of practice and that uses operational strategies to ensure day-to-day fulfillment, ensure optimum achievement of desired client outcomes, and minimize risk of harm to clients

Tort law: Body of law that regulates civil wrongdoing

* From Herbert DL, Herbert WG, Herbert TG. Legal Aspects of Preventive, Rehabilitative and Recreational Exercise Programs. 4th ed. Canton, OH: PRC Publishing, 2002; Koeberle BE. Legal Aspects of Personal Fitness Training. 2nd ed. Canton, OH: PRC Publishing, 1994; American College of Sports Medicine. ACSM's Resource Manual for Guidelines for Exercise Testing and Prescription. 5th ed. Baltimore: Lippincott Williams & Wilkins, 2006; and Cotten DJ, Cotton MB. Legal Aspects of Waivers in Sport, Recreation and Fitness Activities. Canton, OH: PRC Publishing, 1997.

SLIP AND FALL

The number one claim against fitness facilities and professionals is for injuries related to falls on the training premises, according to many insurance providers (3). Courts have consistently held that clients are entitled to "safe" conditions. Personal Trainers can foster safe conditions by a regular practice of inspection for, and correction and warning of, any hazards in the workout and access areas to

Table 22.1	ACSM STANDARDS OF CARE FOR HEALTH AND FITNESS FACILITIES

1. A facility must be able to respond in a timely manner to any reasonably foreseeable emergency event that threatens the health and safety of facility users. Toward this end, a facility must have an appropriate emergency plan that can be executed by qualified personnel in a timely manner.

2. A facility must offer each adult member a pre-activity screening that is appropriate to the physical activities to be performed by the member.

3. Each person who has supervisory responsibility for a physical activity program or area at a facility must have demonstrable professional competence in that physical activity program or area.

4. A facility must post appropriate signage alerting users to the risks involved in their use of those areas of a facility that present potential increased risk(s).

5. A facility that offers youth services or programs must provide appropriate supervision.

6. A facility must conform to all relevant laws, regulations, and published standards.

From American College of Sports Medicine. ACSM's Health/Fitness Facility Standards and Guidelines. 2nd ed. Baltimore: Lippincott Williams & Wilkins, 1997.

the workout location (4). For example, if items are on the floor that may cause a fall, the trainer should clear these away before beginning the session. If floor surfaces are wet and incapable of correction before the session occurs, the session should either be moved or rescheduled. If safety conditions require, it is always better to be conservative and reschedule rather than to continue training in the presence of known dangers. Personal Trainers who work in aquatics facilities need to be particularly vigilant about deck conditions and pool access areas, as wet surfaces increase the likelihood of a slip-and-fall incident.

In addition to routinely inspecting locations before and during training sessions, Personal Trainers should follow a procedure of proper equipment storage when equipment is not in use (3). Regardless of the training setting, encourage designating specific storage places for equipment so items are not left where people can trip over them. Different types of equipment require different types of storage. Make sure to use storage practices that not only store equipment effectively out of people's way, but also protect it from being used for inappropriate purposes. For example, many types of personal training equipment are attractive to young children and may be best stored in locked cabinets if children potentially have access.

Personal Trainers should also educate clients about appropriate clothing and footwear to prevent injury and to enhance training. Clothing should be comfortable, breathable, and allow movement. In particular, Personal Trainers need to check footwear and not allow clients to train with inadequate shoes. Factors such as poor fit, excess wear, and unsuitability to the activity all increase the risk of injury. An awareness of foot care issues is also important if the Personal Trainer works with clients who have certain types of diabetes. Personal Trainers who work with people who are new to exercise may want to create a client handout that outlines appropriate exercise apparel and other exercise safety issues. If the Personal Trainer trains clients in a setting in which protection is necessary, such as a helmet for cycling or pads for inline skating, the Personal Trainer should make sure that the client wears protective equipment (4).

Equipment Use

According to insurance providers, the second leading reason for claims against Personal Trainers is injury resulting from use of equipment (4). These cases are based on legal theories from tort law that a Personal Trainer's duty or standard of care (see Box 22.1) is to exercise reasonable care that the client does not suffer injury. A Personal Trainer who fails to take reasonable precautions, which is determined based on an evaluation of facts surrounding an incident, could be deemed to be negligent and therefore liable or responsible. Professional organizations such as the ACSM and NSCA also offer industry guidelines relating to matters of facility and equipment setup, inspection, maintenance, repair, and signage. Although these standards and guidelines do not have the force of law, they can be introduced as evidence of the Personal Trainer's duty or standard of care. Keep in mind that the law does not envision that accidents never happen; laws exist to encourage proactive safe behavior to avoid preventable accidents.

As a practical matter, when it comes to using equipment safely, the question then becomes what steps can Personal Trainers take to prevent foreseeable accidents? Personal Trainers should always use safe, reliable, and appropriate equipment and use equipment for its intended purposes according to manufacturer guidelines (5). Whenever a Personal Trainer directs a client to use equipment, the Personal Trainer should provide proper instructions and supervision. In addition, policies and procedures for routine safety inspections, maintenance, and repair should be in place and observed systematically. Personal Trainers or facility managers should keep written records to demonstrate compliance with these policies and procedures. All of these steps are likely to minimize the risk of an accident. And, if an accident occurs and everything has been done to prevent it, then it is likely to be considered the type of accident that could not have been prevented by taking reasonable precautions.

Many clients will ask Personal Trainers to recommend equipment. It is important for the Personal Trainer to work only with reliable fitness equipment dealers when recommending equipment to clients. Personal Trainers who do not have a reliable vendor with whom to work should not recommend one piece of equipment over another. The topic of product liability is complex and outside the scope of this chapter. However, the Personal Trainer should be warned that equipment product managers are now pursuing clubs and Personal Trainers for improper installation and maintenance in cases that they lose under product liability.

FREE WEIGHTS

For a concrete example of potential liability for client injury from equipment use, consider this common scenario that involves an experienced Personal Trainer supervising an apparently healthy client who is performing a squat or similar exercise with free weights. The Personal Trainer encourages the client to use a heavier weight and to perform more repetitions even though the client complains of fatigue. The client suffers a debilitating back injury and sues the Personal Trainer and fitness facility.

Under theories of negligence, the Personal Trainer owes this client a duty to exercise reasonable care to prevent injury. Reasonable steps that a Personal Trainer can take to avoid this type of incident include fostering open communications with the client to encourage feedback and listening when the client communicates that he or she is reaching fatigue. Personal Trainers should know how to spot signs of fatigue and be conservative when implementing program progressions.

Another step that a Personal Trainer could take is to keep detailed records of numbers of repetitions, sets, and weight loads on specific training days. In this manner, a client can follow a reasonable plan of progression that minimizes injury risk. Before implementing progression in a program, Personal Trainers can discuss the client's feeling of readiness to increase intensity and further evaluate whether the timing is appropriate for such a change. If specific records are maintained, the Personal Trainer is also in a position to evaluate whether or not a client's response to a particular exercise session is abnormal and requires referral to a physician (6).

WEIGHT MACHINES

Even though machines carry a reduced risk of injury because the client's body is more stable and movement is more restricted than with free weights, injuries still occur. Most injuries happen when a client is encouraged to handle a weight that is too heavy; a weight plate slips and falls because a pin was not properly inserted; or a cable breaks. Weight plates have fallen and crushed ankles and feet, or hit people in the head. Clients suffer physical injuries and sue the Personal Trainer, fitness facility, and equipment manufacturer.

Here again, a Personal Trainer can exercise reasonable care to ensure that the client does not suffer this type of injury through a consistent practice of regular inspections and correction of any known hazards such as worn or faultily maintained equipment; through keeping records of what weight the client has been able to lift, the number of repetitions, and sets; and through following a conservative plan to increase intensity in close communication with the client. When working with weight training equipment, the Personal Trainer can develop a procedure of instruction and supervision for each exercise that includes an equipment and body scan to check for proper equipment set-up and body alignment. Creating this type of instructional technique so that an inspection becomes a routine part of each and every exercise can go a long way toward preventing accidents.

Factors that courts have looked at in equipment-related cases include whether or not the equipment has been maintained appropriately and used for its intended purpose per specific manufacturer guidelines. In particular, courts examined whether or not parts had been replaced in a timely manner and whether or not facility owners had ensured that routine inspections and maintenance were conducted and documented (3). Regardless of the setting, a Personal Trainer should be proactive in learning about equipment safety inspections, maintenance, and record-keeping policies as well as the procedures for reporting the need for repairs. Before putting a client on any piece of equipment, the Personal Trainer should have first-hand knowledge of its readiness for use.

Keep in mind that courts also examine appropriateness of use. In one case, hotel management had placed equipment in a hotel gym that was intended for private home use. The court found the hotel liable for injuries suffered by the client. A training facility should provide commercial equipment; manufacturers do not design home equipment to withstand the wear and tear of frequent use by multiple users. A Personal Trainer who owns or manages a training studio should use professional equipment.

CARDIOVASCULAR MACHINES

Treadmills are currently among the most popular form of exercise equipment in fitness facilities. Numerous cases feature instances in which a client loses control and falls from a treadmill. These cases often involve middle-aged or older adult clients who are unfamiliar with the machine's workings and unable to keep up with the movement speed. Consequences from falls include back, neck, shoulder, and other joint injuries, broken bones, and even death. Clients (or their survivors) sue the Personal Trainer, fitness facility, and equipment manufacturer (3).

Of course these examples should not discourage a Personal Trainer from using equipment to condition clients. Equipment is an essential part of creating effective training programs. These incidents simply underscore that whenever equipment is being used, Personal Trainers must remain alert to the special risks presented and take proactive steps to manage and minimize these risks. And Personal Trainers should maintain detailed records to document the steps that have been taken (4).

Scope of Practice

Another important area of potential liability for the Personal Trainer pertains to scope of practice. As fitness professionals work more closely together with healthcare providers to deliver a continuum of care to individuals, it is important to define respective roles. According to the American College of Sports Medicine's Code of Ethics for Certified and Registered Professionals, "[Personal Trainers] practice within the scope of their knowledge, skills, and abilities. [Personal Trainers] will not provide services that are limited by state law to provision by another healthcare professional only"(7). This is particularly true of Personal Trainers with advanced academic degrees or training and when working with clients who may have special exercise considerations. Both criminal and civil actions are possible for practicing without a license. An injunction against a Personal Trainer's practice is possible. An elevated standard of care is required because malpractice is certainly a viable concern.

The contemporary delivery of healthcare services itself is in a state of flux because of high costs and attempts to reduce costs by expanding the roles of paraprofessionals in the medical context. As a result, states vary widely on what constitutes the practice of medicine and what is appropriate behavior for a nurse, physician assistant, or other paraprofessional. According to fitness law experts David L. and William G. Herbert, many states have defined the practice of medicine broadly so that persons engaged in exercise testing and prescription activities could, under some circumstances, fall within the range of such statutes (8).

Personal Trainers, therefore, need to become familiar with the relevant guidelines for scope of practice that are established at their affiliated organizations and institutions. Personal Trainers who operate their own businesses would be wise to seek the advice of local counsel and to take all other steps to manage risk effectively, such as maintaining certifications, obtaining releases and waivers or consents as applicable, carrying liability insurance, and keeping detailed written records.

SUPPLEMENTS

Claims related to violations of scope of practice occur most frequently in the area of supplements. A high-profile case brought against a Personal Trainer and a large fitness chain involved a scenario in which a Personal Trainer sold supplements, including one that contained ephedra, to a client. The client, who had hypertension, died. Survivors filed a suit. In another example, a Personal Trainer sold steroids to a client, who later suffered adverse consequences and filed a claim against the Personal Trainer (3).

In another incident, a personal training company combined supplement sales with its fitness packages to increase revenue. The company eventually had a client who was allergic to an ingredient in the supplement. The problem was compounded when the client assumed that if she took more than the recommended dosage, she would see more results. She ended up in the hospital, and even though she had been a loyal client for some time, she sued the Personal Trainer and the business. The case was settled out of court, and the Personal Trainer lost his business. The problem was not that the Personal Trainer had sold the client the products, but that he had given her a written plan specifying what to eat and when to take the supplements. The fact that the client overdid it did not matter (3).

According to insurers, the problem with supplements is worsened by the fact that most supplement manufacturers do not carry any insurance coverage. Therefore, the people selling the supplements do not have any products liability coverage. Furthermore, most of the insurance policies for fitness professionals do not include protection for products liability.

In today's market, no one, even professional registered dietitians, can be certain about the ingredients in many supplements because they are not subject to government regulation. In addition, one can never be certain regarding who may have severe allergic reactions, including the risk of death, to any particular ingredient. To proactively protect client safety and to minimize the risk of professional liability, Personal Trainers should avoid selling supplements.

MEDICAL OR DIETARY ADVICE

No cases have yet been litigated to conclusion that involved a client suing a Personal Trainer for faulty medical or dietary advice, except in the case of supplements. However, remember that healthcare is a highly regulated area. The consequences of stepping over the line into the protected area of a licensed healthcare practitioner—such as a medical doctor, physical therapist, registered dietitian, or chiropractor—vary by state. You are exposed to potential liability for acting outside the scope of practice if your "advice" could be interpreted as the unauthorized practice of medicine and if this advice results in a client injury. The Personal Trainer should develop a comprehensive network of allied professionals and actively refer clients who request or require specialized services to the appropriate healthcare provider (8).

Sexual Harassment

Sexual harassment claims represent the third area of potential exposure to liability that is seeing growth in the number of claims against Personal Trainers according to insurance providers (3). Because the personal training relationship can seem "intimate," it lends itself to creating more opportunity for abusive conduct on the part of the Personal Trainer or for a misinterpretation of actions on the part of the client. Numerous cases involve a male Personal Trainer and a female client. The female client believes inappropriate touching has occurred and that she has been violated. Or a personal relationship develops between the Personal Trainer and the client that then raises questions about the legitimacy of the business services rendered. The client believes undue influence was used to create an exploitive situation.

Sexual harassment is difficult to prove and often rests on credibility. Personal Trainers, therefore, should be vigilant and act professionally at all times. One strategy to protect against a claim of inappropriate touching is to always ask a client for permission to use tactile spotting, and to avoid it unless absolutely necessary. Some Personal Trainers do not touch clients directly, but spot them through the use of another prop, such as a ball. Also, avoid situations behind closed doors where no one else is present. For example, if skinfold body composition assessments are offered, conduct the procedure in a room with other Personal Trainers, perhaps behind a folding screen, or have another Personal Trainer or staff member present. If a personal relationship develops with a client, discontinue the professional relationship and refer the client to another Personal Trainer.

Proper Qualifications

Although no specific case on the books has held that Personal Trainers have a higher standard of care based on their specific training in individual assessment, program design, and supervision, clients have filed claims after injuring themselves, based on the fact that a Personal Trainer did not have the qualifications represented in a facility's advertising literature. This claim was based on a theory of breach of contract since the facility failed to provide Personal Trainers with the level of qualification that it had promised (8).

The best evidence that a Personal Trainer can show that his or her training services meets professional standards is to maintain certification and to conduct business according to the knowledge, skills, and abilities that are expected as minimum competencies by the certifying organization. The ACSM certified Personal Trainer[SM] is defined as a fitness professional involved in developing and implementing an individualized approach to exercise leadership in healthy populations and/or those individuals with medical clearance to exercise. This certified professional is deemed to be proficient in writing appropriate exercise recommendations, leading and demonstrating safe and effective methods of exercise, and motivating individuals to begin and to continue their healthy behaviors (6).

The issue of a Personal Trainer's responsibility for advising appropriate levels of training intensity is even more critical as more people with special needs seek to work with Personal Trainers. Personal Trainers who advertise their services to targeted clientele such as older adults or people with arthritis, claiming that they are trained to serve these niche markets, need to be sure that they are sufficiently prepared to serve these clients' needs. Evidence of sufficient preparation would include additional training and experience in working with people with particular needs. Personal Trainers should therefore keep written records of all certifications, continuing education, and work-related experience.

An important precaution to ensure that a Personal Trainer delivers services that are appropriate to the client is the pre-screening health and medical history. In addition, the Personal Trainer needs to be able to assess risk and determine when a medical clearance is necessary. After all these precautionary steps are taken, the Personal Trainer needs to be able to conduct a safe fitness evaluation to determine the recommended level of training that will be safe and effective to meet the particular client's needs and goals. All of these measures should be kept in written records to document the steps taken by the Personal Trainer to create a specific exercise program (6).

The risk of exposure to liability for a Personal Trainer may be even greater when training services are delivered in a medical setting. In a 2003 Indiana case, a court held that even though a Personal Trainer was employed by a hospital and the fitness facility was owned by the hospital, the Personal Trainer was not a healthcare provider. The case, therefore, did not qualify as a medical malpractice case. The significance of this case, however, is that the client did try to sue both the fitness club and the hospital on the basis of injuries sustained while engaged in the personal training program, and the court did examine the fact that the training occurred in a setting with a close connection to a hospital. Another court might have found that this type of training did need to meet the standards of healthcare practitioners (1, 3).

Emergency Response

As yet no specific case has involved a claim against a Personal Trainer for wrongful death in a situation in which a client has had a heart attack or other medical emergency and died while under the supervision of a Personal Trainer. However, as most Personal Trainer certifications require that Personal Trainers have CPR training (and some require first aid training and automated external defibrillator [AED] training), it is possible that a claim could be filed against a Personal Trainer who failed to provide an emergency response if that failure led to a death that could have otherwise been avoided.

The American College of Sports Medicine and the American Heart Association (AHA) published a joint position stand in 1998 with recommendations for health/fitness facilities regarding the screening of clients for the presence of cardiovascular disease, appropriate staffing, emergency policies, equipment, and procedures relative to the client base of a given facility (9). In 2002, the ACSM and the AHA published a joint position stand to supplement the 1998 recommendations regarding the purchase and use of AEDs in health/fitness facilities (10). These organizations agree that a comprehensive written emergency plan is essential to promote safe and effective physical activity.

The AHA, the ACSM, and the International Health, Racquet and Sportsclub Association (IHRSA) recommend that all fitness facilities have written emergency policies and procedures, including the use of automated defibrillators, which are reviewed and practiced regularly. Staff who have responsibility for working directly with program participants and provide instruction and leadership in specific modes of exercise must be trained in CPR. These staff should know and practice regularly the facility's emergency plan and be able to readily handle emergencies. In addition, these organizations encourage health and fitness facilities to use AEDs (11).

As evidence of professional competency, Personal Trainers should keep CPR, first aid, and AED certifications current. Personal Trainers should proactively familiarize themselves with any affiliated organization's emergency plan and be ready to implement the plan's procedures in case of emergency. For Personal Trainers who operate a business, creating an emergency plan should be a top priority. Personal Trainers who provide training services outdoors or in a client's home should also have written emergency policies and procedures.

In addition to having an emergency plan, Personal Trainers should also document any accident or incident immediately, using an Incident Report Form (Box 22.2). The Personal Trainer should include only the facts surrounding the incident and not any opinions regarding what may or may not have caused the incident. In addition, the names and contact information of witnesses should be included. And, the person who experienced the incident should sign the form. Insurers will provide incident reporting forms, and the Personal Trainer should always carry one to every training session (2, 5).

Client Confidentiality

The failure to protect client confidentiality is another emerging area of potential liability for a Personal Trainer. This is rooted in the concept of preventing potential harm to a client's reputation. The Personal Trainer must keep detailed written records from the first client pre-screening to notes documenting each training session. These records are critical evidence that can document that the Personal Trainer exercised reasonable care in performing his or her professional duties. At the same time, the Personal Trainer must exercise care to protect this information. The ACSM's guidelines for the fitness testing, health promotion, and wellness area state that "A facility should ensure that its fitness testing, health promotion, and wellness has a system that provides for and protects the complete confidentiality of all user records and meetings. User records should be released only with an individual's signed authorization" (2). Before a Personal Trainer discloses any personal information, even for marketing purposes, such as a client testimonial or "before and

BOX 22.2

INCIDENT REPORT
TO BE COMPLETED BY INSTRUCTOR

Date: _____

Location/Address of Accident or Incident: _____

Name of Instructor Completing the Form: _____

Date of Accident or Incident: _____

Approximate Time of Accident or Incident: _____ : _____ am   pm

Name of Injured Person: _____ Age: _____ Sex: _____

Injured Person's Address _____

City: _____ State: _____ Zip Code: _____

Home Phone #: (   ) _____   Work Phone #: (   ) _____

How long has this person been under your instruction: _____

_____

Describe the accident/incident: _____

_____

_____

Describe possible injury (sprained ankle, etc.): _____

_____

_____

Describe type of equipment involved: _____

_____

List any type of treatment performed by you or by a doctor (include doctor, hospital name):

_____

_____

Were there any witnesses to the incident: yes _____   no _____

If yes, please have each witness write a brief statement about what happened.

YOUR SIGNATURE: _____

* From Jeff Frick, Fitness and Wellness Insurance Agency, 380 Stevens Avenue, Suite 206, Solana Beach, CA 92075.

after" photos, the Personal Trainer should get and store a signed release form. A law passed by the U.S. Congress requires healthcare professionals to have strict policies regarding the safety and security of private records (the Health Insurance Portability & Accountability Act [HIPAA] of 1996, Public Law 104-191, which amends the Internal Revenue Service Code of 1986, also known as the Kennedy-Kassebaum Act) and recently came into effect in April 14, 2003. While it is still unclear if HIPAA extends to Personal Trainers, it is wise to become familiar with this law and how it may affect the release of any personal information to a third party.

RISK MANAGEMENT STRATEGIES

Personal Trainers should manage risk exposure with a multilayered approach that incorporates a number of important strategies. As the first line of defense, Personal Trainers should create written policies, procedures, and forms that meet industry standards and guidelines and maintain detailed written records that document compliance with these policies. This strategy minimizes the likelihood that the Personal Trainer would fail to demonstrate that he or she exercised reasonable care under the circumstances. In other words, the Personal Trainer should make every effort to not be negligent.

The second strategy involves using a release, waiver, or informed consent, depending on which legal document is recognized under the laws of the place where the Personal Trainer conducts business (12). The purpose of these documents is either *(a)* to demonstrate that the Personal Trainer fully informed the client of all of the potential risks of physical activity and the client decided to undertake the activity and waive the Personal Trainer's responsibility or *(b)* to demonstrate that the client knowingly waived his or her right to file a claim against the Personal Trainer even if the Personal Trainer is negligent. The Personal Trainer should keep these records indefinitely and in a safe place. Consent forms are not infinity contracts so provisions should also be made for an annual signing of these important documents.

A third strategy is to carry professional liability insurance (4, 8). This transfers the risk to the insurer. In that instance, even if the Personal Trainer is negligent, the insurance company assumes responsibility for resolving any claims. Most insurers of Personal Trainers provide coverage for certified professionals. A fourth strategy is to incorporate the business to protect personal assets from any potential claims. A fifth strategy is to cultivate strong relationships with your clients and colleagues. Clients are much less likely to sue if they perceive a Personal Trainer as caring, responsible, and responsive to their needs. And, the final strategy is to consult local legal counsel to ensure that your business practices meet the requirements of your specific location (3).

Written Policies, Procedures, and Forms

Personal Trainers should conduct their business according to written policies, procedures, and forms that ensure that their business practices conform to the standards set by professional organizations (1–6, 8). In addition to policies discussed in the business practices chapter, every Personal Trainer should have also have risk management policies that include a written emergency plan and a pre-activity screening procedure. The most important forms for a Personal Trainer include the following:

1. Pre-activity screening form such as a PAR-Q
2. Health History Questionnaire
3. Physician's Statement and Medical Clearance
4. Fitness Assessment or Evaluation Form
5. Client Progress Notes
6. Incident Reports

In the event that a Personal Trainer is encouraging a client to train independently on equipment in a particular fitness facility, an equipment orientation form for the client to sign to indicate that he or she has received instruction on the proper set up and use of weight training equipment would be useful to document equipment instruction.

Informed Consent, Release, or Waiver

In numerous states, courts are holding up waivers more and more as valid means of protection against litigation. In 2001, a California case was dismissed after a court held that the waiver form signed by a facility member when she joined protected the facility and its owners from liability when the member filed a lawsuit claiming that she slipped and injured herself. This case is consistent with other California cases (3). Depending on where a Personal Trainer lives, he or she may need to have a document entitled one of the following:

➤ Assumption of the Risk
➤ Informed Consent
➤ Release or Waiver of Liability

An Assumption of the Risk or Informed Consent document essentially explains the risks of participating in physical activity to a prospective client. The client then agrees that he or she knowingly understands these risks, appreciates these risks, and voluntarily assumes responsibility for taking those risks.

A Waiver or Release of Liability document states that the client knowingly waives or releases the Personal Trainer from liability for any acts of negligence on the part of the Personal Trainer. In other words, the prospective client waives his or her right to sue the Personal Trainer, even if the Personal Trainer is negligent (12). A Personal Trainer needs to consult with an attorney in his or her location to determine which type of document is the standard practice for his or her state.

Professional Liability Insurance

In today's litigious environment, for the most protection, a Personal Trainer should carry professional liability insurance ($2 million per occurrence is the recommended amount), even when working in a business as an employee, where the Personal Trainer may be covered under the business owner's policy. The reason for this is that it is not unusual for a single claim to result in a million dollar judgment. Purchasing the best protection enables the Personal Trainer to practice responsibly and feel confident that his or her business will not be destroyed by one mishap.

Professional liability insurance provides a broad spectrum of protection from claims such as those arising from negligence, breach of contract, or even sexual harassment, and it can provide coverage for both injuries to a person or to property. Insurance professionals are expert at handling claims and will take care of all of the details, enabling the Personal Trainer to continue to operate his or her business (3).

SUMMARY

The personal training industry is in a rapid state of growth and redefinition as more healthcare providers acknowledge the need for exercise training as part of a program of preventive healthcare. In addition, the wellness trend is fueling more and more individuals to assume responsibility for their personal health and to consult with experts such as Personal Trainers to provide training services that enhance the quality of their daily lives. Personal Trainers have great opportunities to work in a variety of settings and make a powerful difference in the lives of clients.

More professional opportunities, however, increase expectations of responsible professional conduct. More professional responsibility means more potential exposure to liability for failing to act responsibly. Today's Personal Trainer must understand these potential areas of risk exposure and the legal issues and industry standards and guidelines that surround these issues to deliver services confidently and to proactively manage risk. This professionalism in all aspects of doing business not only increases the personal and professional rewards of life as a Personal Trainer, but also ensures lasting business success amid the growing complexity of our modern legal environment. Ultimately, the purpose of liability is to protect individuals. The most successful Personal Trainers will always keep in mind that the core of personal training is ultimately personal: to protect the best interests of the client at all times and in all ways. To this end, the ACSM has developed a Code of Ethics for ACSM Certified and Registered Professionals (see Box 21.2) that will help to establish the Personal Trainer profession.

REFERENCES

1. Herbert DL, Herbert WG, Herbert TG. Legal Aspects of Preventive, Rehabilitative and Recreational Exercise Programs. 4th ed. Canton, OH: PRC Publishing, 2002.
2. American College of Sports Medicine. ACSM's Health/Fitness Facility Standards and Guidelines. 2nd ed. Baltimore: Lippincott Williams & Wilkins, 1997.
3. Archer S. Reward carries risk: a liability update. IDEA Personal Trainer 2004;15(4):30–34.
4. Koeberle BE. Legal Aspects of Personal Fitness Training. 2nd ed. Canton, OH: PRC Publishing, 1994.
5. American College of Sports Medicine. ACSM's Certification Review. 2nd ed. Baltimore: Lippincott Williams & Wilkins, 2006.
6. American College of Sports Medicine. ACSM's Guidelines for Exercise Testing and Prescription. 7th ed. Baltimore: Lippincott Williams & Wilkins, 2006.
7. American College of Sports Medicine Code of Ethics for ACSM Certified and Registered Professionals. On the Internet at http://www.acsm.org/certification/generalinfo.htm. Accessed May 2, 2005.
8. American College of Sports Medicine. ACSM's Resource Manual for Guidelines for Exercise Testing and Prescription. 5th ed. Baltimore: Lippincott Williams & Wilkins, 2006.
9. Balady GJ, et al. Recommendations for cardiovascular screening, staffing and emergency policies at health/fitness facilities. Circulation 1998;97(22):2283–2293.
10. Balady GJ, et al. Automated external defibrillators in health/fitness facilities: supplement to the AHA/ACSM recommendations for cardiovascular screening, staffing and emergency policies at health/fitness facilities. Circulation 2002;105(9):1147–1150.
11. McInnis K, Herbert W, et al. Low compliance with national standards for cardiovascular emergency preparedness at health clubs. Chest 2001;120(1):283–288.
12. Cotten DJ, Cotton MB. Legal Aspects of Waivers in Sport, Recreation and Fitness Activities. Canton, OH: PRC Publishing, 1997.

Appendix: American College of Sports Medicine Certifications

This appendix details information about American College of Sports Medicine (ACSM) Certification and Registry Programs as well as a complete listing of the current knowledge, skills, and abilities (KSAs) that compose the foundations of these certification and registry examinations. The mission of the ACSM Committee on Certification and Registry Boards is to develop and provide high-quality, accessible, and affordable credentials and continuing education programs for health and exercise professionals who are responsible for preventive and rehabilitative programs that influence the health and well-being of all individuals.

ACSM CERTIFICATIONS AND THE PUBLIC

The first of the ACSM clinical certifications was initiated nearly 30 years ago in conjunction with publication of the first edition of the *Guidelines for Exercise Testing and Prescription*. That era was marked by rapid development of exercise programs for patients with stable coronary artery disease (CAD). ACSM sought a means to disseminate accurate information on this healthcare initiative through expression of consensus from its members in basic science, clinical practice, and education. Thus, these early clinical certifications were viewed as an aid to the establishment of safe and scientifically based exercise services within the framework of cardiac rehabilitation.

Over the past 30 years, exercise has gained widespread favor as an important component in programs of rehabilitative care or health maintenance for an expanding list of chronic diseases and disabling conditions. The growth of public interest in the role of exercise in health promotion has been equally impressive. In addition, federal government policymakers have revisited questions of medical efficacy and financing for exercise services in rehabilitative care of selected patients. Over the past several years, recommendations from the U.S. Public Health Service and the U.S. Surgeon General have acknowledged the central role for regular physical activity in the prevention of disease and promotion of health.

The development of the health/fitness certifications in the 1980s reflected ACSM's intent to increase the availability of qualified professionals to provide scientifically sound advice and supervision regarding appropriate physical activities for health maintenance in the apparently healthy adult population. Since 1975, more than 30,000 certificates have been awarded. With this consistent growth, ACSM has taken steps to ensure that its competency-based certifications will continue to be regarded as the premier program in the exercise field. For example, since 2002 ACSM has provided guidelines to assist colleges and universities with establishing standardized curricula that are focused on the knowledge, skills, and abilities (KSAs) requisite in the examinations for the ACSM Health/Fitness Instructor®, ACSM Exercise Specialist® and ACSM Registered Clinical Exercise Physiologist®.

Additionally, the ACSM University Connection Endorsement Program is designed to recognize institutions with educational programs that meet all of the KSAs specified by the ACSM Committee on Certification and Registry Boards (CCRB). Other examples include publishing a periodical addressing professional practice issues targeted to those who are certified, *ACSM's Certified News*, and oversight of continuing education requirements for maintenance of certification. Continuing education credits can be accrued through ACSM-sponsored educational programs such as ACSM workshops (ACSM Health/Fitness Instructor® and ACSM Exercise Specialist®), regional chapter and annual meetings, and other educational programs approved by the ACSM Professional Education Committee. These enhancements are intended to support the continued professional growth of those who have made a commitment to service in this rapidly growing health and fitness field.

Recently, ACSM, as a founder member of the multi-organizational Committee on Accreditation for the Exercise Sciences (CoAES), assisted with the development of standards and guidelines for educational programs seeking accreditation under the auspices of the Commission on Accreditation of Allied Health Education Programs (CAAHEP). Additional information on outcomes-based, programmatic accreditation can be obtained by visiting www.caahep.org, and specific information regarding the standards and guidelines can be obtained by visiting www.coaes.org. Because the standards and guidelines refer to the KSAs that follow, reference to specific KSAs as they relate to given sets of standards and guidelines are noted when appropriate.

ACSM also acknowledges the expectation from successful candidates that the public will be informed of the high standards, values, and professionalism implicit in meeting these certification requirements. The College has formally organized its volunteer committee structure and national office staff to give added emphasis to informing the public, professionals, and government agencies about issues of critical importance to ACSM. Informing these constituencies about the meaning and value of ACSM certification is one important priority that will be given attention in this initiative.

ACSM CERTIFICATION PROGRAMS

The ACSM Certified Personal Trainer[SM] is a fitness professional involved in developing and implementing an individualized approach to exercise leadership in healthy populations and/or those individuals with medical clearance to exercise. Using a variety of teaching techniques, the Personal Trainer is proficient in leading and demonstrating safe and effective methods of exercise by applying the fundamental principles of exercise science. The ACSM Certified Personal Trainer[SM] is familiar with forms of exercise used to improve, maintain, and/or optimize health-related components of physical fitness and performance. The ACSM Certified Personal Trainer[SM] is proficient in writing appropriate exercise recommendations, leading and demonstrating safe and effective methods of exercise, and motivating individuals to begin and to continue with their healthy behaviors.

The ACSM Health/Fitness Instructor[®] (HFI) is a professional qualified to assess, design, and implement individual and group exercise and fitness programs for low-risk individuals and individuals with controlled disease. The HFI is skilled in evaluating health behaviors and risk factors, conducting fitness assessments, writing appropriate exercise prescriptions, and motivating individuals to modify negative health habits and maintain positive lifestyle behaviors for health promotion.

The ACSM Exercise Specialist[®] (ES) is a is a healthcare professional certified by ACSM to deliver a variety of exercise assessment, training, rehabilitation, risk factor identification, and lifestyle management services to individuals with or at risk for cardiovascular, pulmonary, and metabolic disease(s). These services are typically delivered in cardiovascular/pulmonary rehabilitation programs, physicians' offices, or medical fitness centers. The ACSM Exercise Specialist[®] is also competent to provide exercise-related consulting for research, public health, and other clinical and non-clinical services and programs.

The ACSM Registered Clinical Exercise Physiologist[®] (RCEP) is an allied health professional who works with persons with chronic diseases and conditions in which exercise has been shown to be beneficial. The RCEP performs health, physical activity, and fitness assessments, and prescribes exercise and physical activity primarily in hospitals or other health provider settings.

Certification at a given level requires the candidate to have a knowledge and skills base commensurate with that specific level of certification. In addition, the HFI level of certification incorporates the KSAs associated with the ACSM Certified Personal Trainer[SM] certification, and the ES level of certification incorporates the KSAs associated with the HFI certification, as illustrated in Appendix Figure 1. In addition, each level of certification has minimum requirements for experience, level of education, or other certifications.

Level	Requirements	Recommended Competencies
ACSM Certified Personal Trainer[SM]	• 18 years of age or older • High school diploma or equivalent (GED) • Possess current Adult CPR certification that has a practical skills examination component *(such as the American Heart Association or the American Red Cross.)*	• Demonstrate competence in the KSAs required of the ACSM Certified Personal Trainer[SM] as listed in the current edition of the *ACSM's Guidelines for Exercise Testing and Prescription* • Adequate knowledge of and skill in risk factor and health status identification, fitness appraisal, and exercise prescription • Demonstrate ability to incorporate suitable and innovative activities that will improve an individual's functional capacity • Demonstrate the ability to effectively educate and/or communicate with individuals regarding lifestyle modification
ACSM Health/Fitness Instructor®	• An Associate's Degree or a Bachelor's degree in a health-related field from a regionally accredited college/university (candidates are eligible to sit for the examination if they are in the last term of their degree program), AND • Possess current Adult CPR certification that has a practical skills examination component *(such as those of the American Heart Association or the American Red Cross.)*	• Demonstrate competence in the KSAs required of the ACSM Health/Fitness Instructor® as listed in the current edition of the *ACSM's Guidelines for Exercise Testing and Prescription* • Work-related experience within the health and fitness field • Adequate knowledge of, and skill in, risk factor and health status identification, fitness appraisal, and exercise prescription • Demonstrate ability to incorporate suitable and innovative activities that will improve an individual's functional capacity • Demonstrate the ability to effectively educate and/or counsel individuals regarding lifestyle modification • Knowledge of exercise science including kinesiology, functional anatomy, exercise physiology, nutrition, program administration, psychology, and injury prevention
ACSM Exercise Specialist®	• A Bachelor's degree in an allied health field from a regionally accredited college of university (candidates are eligible to sit for the examination if they are in the last term of their degree program); AND • Minimum of 600 hours of practical experience in a clinical exercise program (e.g., cardiac/pulmonary rehabilitation programs, exercise testing, exercise prescription, electrocardiography, patient education and counseling, disease management of cardiac, pulmonary, and metabolic diseases, and emergency management); AND • Current certification as a Basic Life Support Provider or CPR for the Professional Rescuer *(available through the American Heart Association or the American Red Cross)*	• Demonstrate competence in the KSAs required of the ACSM Exercise Specialist® and ACSM Health/Fitness Instructor®, as listed in the current edition of *ACSM's Guidelines for Exercise Testing and Prescription.* • Ability to demonstrate extensive knowledge of functional anatomy, exercise physiology, pathophysiology, electrocardiography, human behavior/psychology, gerontology, graded exercise testing for healthy and diseased populations, exercise supervision/leadership, patient counseling, and emergency procedures related to exercise testing and training situations

APPENDIX FIGURE 1 CONTINUED

Level	Requirements	Recommended Competencies
ACSM Registered Clinical Exercise Physiologist®	• Master's degree in exercise science, exercise physiology, or kinesiology from a regionally accredited college or university • Current certification as a Basic Life Instructor®, as listed in the current edition of Support Provider or CPR for the Professional Rescuer *(available through the American Heart Association or the American Red Cross)* • Minimum of 600 clinical hours are required with hours in each of the clinical practice areas, which may be completed as part of a formal degree program in exercise physiology: cardiovascular 200; pulmonary 100; metabolic 120; orthopedic/musculoskeletal 100; neuromuscular 40; immunological/hematological 40. These hours may be obtained with patients with co-morbid conditions. For example, time spent working with a patient who has coronary heart disease and Parkinson's disease may be counted in two practice areas IF you were providing exercise evaluation or programming specific to each of the conditions.	• Demonstrate competence in the KSAs required of the ACSM Registered Clinical Exercise Physiologist®, ACSM Exercise Specialist®, and ACSM Health/Fitness *ACSM's Guidelines for Exercise Testing and Prescription.* • The RCEP is an allied health professional who uses exercise and physical activity to assess and treat patients at risk of, or with, chronic diseases or conditions for which exercise has been shown to provide therapeutic and/or functional benefit. Patients for whom RCEP services are appropriate may include, but are not limited to, persons with cardiovascular, pulmonary, metabolic, cancerous, immunological, inflammatory, orthopedic, musculoskeletal, neuromuscular, gynecological, and obstetrical diseases and conditions. The RCEP provides scientific, evidence-based primary and secondary preventive and rehabilitative exercise and physical activity services to populations ranging from children to older adults. The RCEP performs exercise screening, exercise testing, exercise prescription, exercise and physical activity counseling, exercise supervision, exercise and health education/promotion, and evaluation of exercise and physical activity outcome measures. The RCEP works individually and as part of an interdisciplinary team in clinical, community, and public health settings. The practice and supervision of the RCEP is guided by published professional guidelines, standards, and applicable state and federal regulations. The practice of clinical exercise physiology is restricted to patients who are referred by, and are under the care of, a licensed physician.

How to Obtain Information and Application Materials

The certification programs of ACSM are subject to continuous review and revision. Content development is entrusted to a diverse committee of professional volunteers with expertise in exercise science, medicine, and program management. Expertise in design and procedures for competency assessment is also represented on this committee. Administration of certification is the responsibility of the ACSM National Center. Inquiries concerning certifications, application requirements, fees, and examination test sites and dates may be made to:

ACSM Certification Resource Center
1-800-486-5643
Website: www.lww.com/acsmcrc
E-mail: certification@acsm.org

KNOWLEDGE, SKILLS, AND ABILITIES (KSAS) UNDERLINING ACSM CERTIFICATIONS

Minimal competencies for each certification level are outlined below. Certification examinations are constructed on the basis of these KSAs. Two companion ACSM publications, *ACSM's Resource Manual for Guidelines for Exercise Testing and Prescription, fifth edition,* and *ACSM's Certification Review Book, second edition,* may also be used to gain further insight into the topics identified here. However, neither the *Guidelines for Exercise Testing and Prescription* nor either of the above-mentioned resource manuals provides all of the information upon which the ACSM Certification examinations are based. Each may prove to be beneficial as a review of specific topics and as a general outline of many of the integral concepts to be mastered by those seeking certification.

CLASSIFICATION/NUMBERING SYSTEM FOR KNOWLEDGE, SKILLS, AND ABILITIES (KSAS)

The system for classifying and numbering KSAs has been changed. It is designed to be easier for certification candidates to use, with all of the KSAs for a given certification/credential listed in their entirety across a given Practice area and/or Content Matter area for each level of certification. Within the KSA set for each certification/credential, individual KSAs are numbered with a **three-part number** as follows:

First number—denotes Practice Area (1.x.x)
Second number—denotes Content Area (x.1.x)
Third number—denotes the sequential number of each KSA (x.x.1), within each Content Area

The Practice Areas (the first number) are numbered as follows:

1.x.x	General Population/Core
2.x.x	Cardiovascular
3.x.x	Pulmonary
4.x.x	Metabolic
5.x.x	Orthopedic/Musculoskeletal
6.x.x	Neuromuscular
7.x.x	Immunological

The Content Matter Areas (the second number) are numbered as follows:

x.1.x	Exercise Physiology and Related Exercise Science
x.2.x	Pathophysiology and Risk Factors
x.3.x	Health Appraisal, Fitness and Clinical Exercise Testing
x.4.x	Electrocardiography and Diagnostic Techniques
x.5.x	Patient Management and Medications
x.6.x	Medical and Surgical Management
x.7.x	Exercise Prescription and Programming
x.8.x	Nutrition and Weight Management
x.9.x	Human Behavior and Counseling
x.10.x	Safety, Injury Prevention, and Emergency Procedures
x.11.x	Program Administration, Quality Assurance, and Outcome Assessment
x.12.x	Clinical and Medical Considerations (ACSM-certified Personal Trainer™ only)

EXAMPLES by Level of Certification/Credential:

ACSM Certified Personal Trainer^{SM} KSAs

1.1.10	Knowledge to describe the normal acute responses to cardiovascular exercise

In this example, the **practice** area is <u>General Population/Core</u>; the **content matter** area is <u>Exercise Physiology and Related Exercise Science</u>; and this KSA is the **tenth** KSA within this content matter area.

ACSM Health/Fitness Instructor® KSAs

1.3.8	Skill in accurately measuring heart rate, blood pressure, and obtaining rating of perceived exertion (RPE) at rest and during exercise according to established guidelines

In this example, the **practice** area is <u>General Population/Core</u>; the **content matter** area is <u>Health Appraisal, Fitness and Clinical Exercise Testing</u>; and this KSA is the **eighth** KSA within this content matter area.

ACSM Exercise Specialist® KSAs★

1.7.17	**Design strength and flexibility programs for individuals with cardiovascular, pulmonary, and/or metabolic diseases, elderly, and children**

In this example, the **practice** area is <u>General Population/Core</u>; the **content matter** area is <u>Exercise Prescription and Programming</u>; and this KSA is the **seventeenth** KSA within this content matter area. Furthermore, because this specific KSA appears in **bold** text, it covers multiple practice areas and content areas.

★*A special note about ACSM Exercise Specialist® KSAs:*

Like the other certifications presented thus far, the ACSM Exercise Specialist® KSAs are categorized by content area. However, some ES KSAs cover multiple practices areas within each area of content. For example, a number of them describe a specific topic with respect to both exercise testing and training, which are two distinct content areas. Rather than write out each separately (which would have greatly expanded the KSA list length) they have been listed under a single content area. When reviewing these KSAs, please note that KSAs in **bold** text cover multiple content areas. Each ES KSA begins with a 'l' as the practice area. However, where appropriate, some KSAs mention specific patient populations (i.e., practice area). If a specific practice area is not mentioned within a given KSA, then it applies equally to each of the general population, cardiovascular, pulmonary, and metabolic practice areas. Note that "metabolic patients" are defined as those with at least one of the following: overweight or obese, diabetes (type I or II), metabolic syndrome. Each KSA describes either a single or multiple knowledge (K), skill (S), or ability (A) or a combination of K, S, or A that an individual should have mastery of to be considered a competent ACSM Exercise Specialist®. Finally, as stated earlier, the ACSM Exercise Specialist® candidate is also responsible for the mastery of both the ACSM Health/Fitness Instructor® and the ACSM Certified Personal Trainer^{SM} KSAs.

ACSM Registered Clinical Exercise Physiologist KSAs

7.6.1	"List the drug classifications commonly used in the treatment of patients with a National Institutes of Health (NIH) disease, name common generic and brand names of drugs within each class, and explain the purposes, indications, major side effects, and the effects, if any, on the exercising individual."

The **practice** area is <u>Immunological</u>; the **content matter** area is <u>Medical and Surgical Management</u>; and this KSA is the **second** KSA within this content matter area.

ACSM Certified Personal Trainer℠ Knowledge, Skills, and Abilities (KSAs):

Blue. **EXERCISE PHYSIOLOGY AND RELATED EXERCISE SCIENCE** CH. 6/7.

(116) 1.1.1 Knowledge of the basic structures of bone, skeletal muscle, and connective tissues

1.1.2 Knowledge of the basic anatomy of the cardiovascular system and respiratory system

(114) 1.1.3 Knowledge of the definition of the following terms: inferior, superior, medial, lateral, supination, pronation, flexion, extension, adduction, abduction, hyperextension, rotation, circumduction, agonist, antagonist, and stabilizer

1.1.4 Knowledge of the plane in which each muscle action occurs

(110) 1.1.5 Knowledge of the interrelationships among center of gravity, base of support, balance, stability, and proper spinal alignment

1.1.6 Knowledge of the following curvatures of the spine: lordosis, scoliosis, and kyphosis

1.1.7 Knowledge to describe the myotatic stretch reflex

1.1.8 Knowledge of the biomechanical principles for the performance of the following activities: walking, jogging, running, swimming, cycling, weight lifting, and carrying or moving objects

1.1.9 Ability to define aerobic and anaerobic metabolism

1.1.10 Knowledge to describe the normal short-term responses to cardiovascular exercise

1.1.11 Knowledge to describe the normal short-term responses to resistance training

1.1.12 Knowledge of the normal long-term physiological adaptations associated with cardiovascular exercise

1.1.13 Knowledge of the normal long-term physiological adaptations associated with resistance training

1.1.14 Knowledge of the physiological principles related to warm-up and cool-down

1.1.15 Knowledge of the common theories of muscle fatigue and delayed-onset muscle soreness (DOMS)

1.1.16 Knowledge of the physiological adaptations that occur at rest and during submaximal and maximal exercise following long-term aerobic and anaerobic exercise training

1.1.17 Knowledge of the physiological principles involved in promoting gains in muscular strength and endurance

1.1.18 Knowledge of blood pressure responses associated with short-term exercise, including changes in body position

1.1.19 Knowledge of how the principle of specificity relates to the components of fitness

1.1.20 Knowledge of the concept of detraining or reversibility of conditioning and its implications in fitness programs

✓1.1.21 Knowledge of the physical and psychological signs of overtraining and to provide recommendations for these problems

1.1.22 Knowledge of the following terms: progressive resistance, isotonic/isometric, concentric, eccentric, atrophy, hypertrophy, sets, repetitions, plyometrics, Valsalva maneuver

(120) 1.1.23 Ability to identify the major bones and muscles. Major muscles include, but are not limited to, the following: trapezius, pectoralis major, latissimus dorsi, biceps, triceps, rectus abdominis, internal and external obliques, erector spinae, gluteus maximus, quadriceps, hamstrings, adductors, abductors, and gastrocnemius

(115) 1.1.24 Ability to identify the major bones. Major bones include, but are not limited, to the clavicle, scapula, sternum, humerus, carpals, ulna, radius, femur, fibula, tibia, and tarsals.

(118) 1.1.25 Ability to identify the joints of the body

1.1.26 Knowledge of the primary action and joint range-of-motion for each major muscle group

✓1.1.27 Ability to locate the anatomical landmarks for palpation of peripheral pulses

Green **HEALTH APPRAISAL, FITNESS, AND CLINICAL EXERCISE TESTING**

1.3.1 Knowledge of, and ability to discuss, the physiological basis of the major components of physical fitness: flexibility, cardiovascular fitness, muscular strength, muscular endurance, and body composition

1.3.2 Knowledge of the importance of a health/medical history

1.3.3 Knowledge of the value of a medical clearance prior to exercise participation

1.3.4 Knowledge of the categories of participants who should receive medical clearance prior to administration of an exercise test or participation in an exercise program

✗1.3.5 Knowledge of relative and absolute contraindications to exercise testing or participation

1.3.6 Knowledge of the limitations of informed consent and medical clearance prior to exercise testing

1.3.7 Knowledge of the advantages/disadvantages and limitations of the various body composition techniques including, but not limited to, air displacement, plethysmography, hydrostatic weighing, Bod Pod, bioelectrical impedence

1.3.8   Skill in accurately measuring heart rate and obtaining rating of perceived exertion (RPE) at rest and during exercise according to established guidelines

1.3.9   Ability to locate common sites for measurement of skinfold thicknesses and circumferences (for determination of body composition and waist–hip ratio)

1.3.10   Ability to obtain a basic health history and risk appraisal and to stratify risk in accordance with ACSM Guidelines

1.3.11   Ability to explain and obtain informed consent

1.3.12   Ability to instruct participants in the use of equipment and test procedures

1.3.13   Knowledge of the purpose and implementation of pre-activity fitness testing, including assessments of cardiovascular fitness, muscular strength, muscular endurance, flexibility, and body composition

1.3.14   Ability to identify appropriate criteria for terminating a fitness evaluation and to demonstrate proper procedures to be followed after discontinuing such a test

EXERCISE PRESCRIPTION AND PROGRAMMING

1.7.1   Knowledge of the benefits and risks associated with exercise training in prepubescent and postpubescent youth

1.7.2   Knowledge of the benefits and precautions associated with resistance and endurance training in older adults

1.7.3   Knowledge of specific leadership techniques appropriate for working with participants of all ages

1.7.4   Knowledge of how to modify cardiovascular and resistance exercises on the basis of age and physical condition

1.7.5   Knowledge of, and ability to describe, the unique adaptations to exercise training with regard to strength, functional capacity, and motor skills

1.7.6   Knowledge of common orthopedic and cardiovascular considerations for older participants and the ability to describe modifications in exercise prescription that are indicated

1.7.7   Knowledge of selecting appropriate testing and training modalities according to the age and functional capacity of the individual

1.7.8   Knowledge of the recommended intensity, duration, frequency, and type of physical activity necessary for development of cardiorespiratory fitness in an apparently healthy population

1.7.9   Knowledge to describe, and the ability to demonstrate (such as technique and breathing), exercises designed to enhance muscular strength and/or endurance of specific major muscle groups

1.7.10   Knowledge of the principles of overload, specificity, and progression and how they relate to exercise programming

1.7.11   Knowledge of the components incorporated into an exercise session and the proper sequence (i.e., pre-exercise evaluation, warm-up, aerobic stimulus phase, cool-down, muscular strength and/or endurance, and flexibility)

1.7.12   Knowledge of special precautions and modifications of exercise programming for participation at altitude and in different ambient temperatures, humidity, and environmental pollution

1.7.13   Knowledge of the importance and ability to record exercise sessions and performing periodic evaluations to assess changes in fitness status

1.7.14   Knowledge of the advantages and disadvantages of implementation of interval, continuous, and circuit training programs

1.7.15   Knowledge of the concept of "Activities of Daily Living" (ADLs) and its importance in the overall health of the individual

1.7.16   Knowledge of Progressive Adaptation in resistance training and its implications on program design and periodization

1.7.17   Understanding of personal training client's "personal space" and how it plays into a trainer's interaction with the client

1.7.18   Skill to teach and demonstrate the components of an exercise session (i.e., warm-up, aerobic stimulus phase, cool-down, muscular strength/endurance, flexibility)

1.7.19   Skill to teach and demonstrate appropriate modifications in specific exercises for the following groups: older adults, pregnant and postnatal women, obese persons, and persons with low back pain

1.7.20   Skill to teach and demonstrate appropriate exercises for improving range of motion of all major joints

1.7.21   Skill in the use of various methods for establishing and monitoring levels of exercise intensity, including heart rate, RPE, and METs

1.7.22   Knowledge of, and ability to apply, methods used to monitor exercise intensity, including heart rate and rating of perceived exertion

1.7.23　Ability to describe modifications in exercise prescriptions for individuals with functional disabilities and musculoskeletal injuries

1.7.24　Ability to differentiate between the amount of physical activity required for health benefits and the amount of exercise required for fitness development

1.7.25　Ability to determine training heart rates using two methods: percentage of age-predicted maximum heart rate and heart rate reserve (Karvonen)

1.7.26　Ability to identify proper and improper technique in the use of resistive equipment such as stability balls, weights, bands, resistance bars, and water exercise equipment

1.7.27　Ability to identify proper and improper technique in the use of cardiovascular conditioning equipment (e.g., stairclimbers, stationary cycles, treadmills, elliptical trainers)

1.7.28　Ability to teach a progression of exercises for all major muscle groups to improve muscular strength and endurance

1.7.29　Ability to modify exercises on the basis of age and physical condition

1.7.30　Ability to explain and implement exercise prescription guidelines for apparently healthy clients or those who have medical clearance to exercise

1.7.31　Ability to adapt frequency, intensity, duration, mode, progression, level of supervision, and monitoring techniques in exercise programs for apparently healthy clients or those who have medical clearance to exercise

1.7.32　Ability to design resistive exercise programs to increase or maintain muscular strength and/or endurance

1.7.33　Ability to periodize a resistance training program for continued muscular strength development

1.7.34　Ability to evaluate, prescribe, and demonstrate appropriate flexibility exercises for all major muscle groups

1.7.35　Ability to design training programs using interval, continuous, and circuit training programs

1.7.36　Ability to describe the advantages and disadvantages of various commercial exercise equipment in developing cardiorespiratory fitness, muscular strength, and muscular endurance

NUTRITION AND WEIGHT MANAGEMENT

1.8.1　Knowledge of the role of carbohydrates, fats, and proteins as fuels for aerobic and anaerobic metabolism

1.8.2　Knowledge to define the following terms: obesity, overweight, percent fat, Body Mass Index, lean body mass, anorexia nervosa, bulimia nervosa, and body fat distribution

1.8.3　Knowledge of the relationship between body composition and health

1.8.4　Knowledge of the effects of diet plus exercise, diet alone, and exercise alone as methods for modifying body composition

1.8.5　Knowledge of the importance of an adequate daily energy intake for healthy weight management

1.8.6　Knowledge of the importance of maintaining normal hydration before, during, and after exercise

1.8.7　Knowledge of the USDA Food Pyramid

1.8.8　Knowledge of the female athlete triad

1.8.9　Knowledge of the myths and consequences associated with inappropriate weight loss methods (e.g., saunas, vibrating belts, body wraps, electric simulators, sweat suits, fad diets)

1.8.10　Knowledge of the number of kilocalories in 1 gram of carbohydrate, fat, protein, and alcohol

1.8.11　Knowledge of the number of kilocalories equivalent to losing 1 pound of body fat

1.8.12　Knowledge of the guidelines for caloric intake for an individual desiring to lose or gain weight

1.8.13　Knowledge of common nutritional ergogenic aids, the purported mechanism of action, and any risk and/or benefits (e.g., carbohydrates, protein/amino acids, vitamins, minerals, sodium bicarbonate, creatine, bee pollen, etc.)

1.8.14　Ability to describe the health implications of variation in body fat distribution patterns and the significance of the waist-to-hip ratio

HUMAN BEHAVIOR AND COUNSELING

1.9.1　Knowledge of at least five behavioral strategies to enhance exercise and health behavior change (e.g., reinforcement, goal setting, social support)

1.9.2　Knowledge of the stages of motivational readiness

1.9.3　Knowledge of the 3 stages of learning: Cognitive, Associative, Autonomous

1.9.4　Knowledge of specific techniques to enhance motivation (e.g., posters, recognition, bulletin boards, games, competitions). Define extrinsic and intrinsic reinforcement and give examples of each.

1.9.5   Knowledge of the different types of learners (Auditory, Visual, Kinesthetic) and how to apply teaching and training techniques to optimize a client's training session

1.9.6   Knowledge of the types of feedback and ability to use communication skills to optimize a client's training session

SAFETY, INJURY PREVENTION, AND EMERGENCY PROCEDURES

1.10.1   Knowledge of, and skill in obtaining, basic life support and cardiopulmonary resuscitation certification

1.10.2   Knowledge of appropriate emergency procedures (e.g., telephone procedures, written emergency procedures, personnel responsibilities) in a health and fitness setting

1.10.3   Knowledge of basic first aid procedures for exercise-related injuries, such as bleeding, strains/sprains, fractures, and exercise intolerance (dizziness, syncope, heat injury)

1.10.4   Knowledge of basic precautions taken in an exercise setting to ensure participant safety

1.10.5   Knowledge of the physical and physiological signs and symptoms of overtraining

1.10.6   Knowledge of the effects of temperature, humidity, altitude, and pollution on the physiological response to exercise

1.10.7   Knowledge of the following terms: shin splints, sprain, strain, tennis elbow, bursitis, stress fracture, tendonitis, patellofemoral pain syndrome, low back pain, plantar fasciitis, and rotator cuff tendonitis

1.10.8   Knowledge of hypothetical concerns and potential risks that may be associated with the use of exercises such as straight leg sit-ups, double leg raises, full squats, hurdlers stretch, yoga plough, forceful back hyperextension, and standing bent-over toe touch

1.10.9   Knowledge of safety plans, emergency procedures, and first aid techniques needed during fitness evaluations, exercise testing, and exercise training

1.10.10   Knowledge of the cPT's responsibilities, limitations, and the legal implications of carrying out emergency procedures

1.10.11   Knowledge of potential musculoskeletal injuries (e.g., contusions, sprains, strains, fractures), cardiovascular/pulmonary complications (e.g., tachycardia, bradycardia, hypotension/hypertension, tachypnea), and metabolic abnormalities (e.g., fainting/syncope, hypoglycemia/hyperglycemia, hypothermia/hyperthermia)

1.10.12   Knowledge of the initial management and first aid techniques associated with open wounds, musculoskeletal injuries, cardiovascular/pulmonary complications, and metabolic disorders

1.10.13   Knowledge of the components of an equipment maintenance/repair program and how it may be used to evaluate the condition of exercise equipment to reduce the potential risk of injury

1.10.14   Knowledge of the legal implications of documented safety procedures, the use of incident documents, and ongoing safety training

1.10.15   Skill in demonstrating appropriate emergency procedures during exercise testing and/or training

1.10.16   Ability to identify the components that contribute to the maintenance of a safe environment

1.10.17   Ability to assist or "spot" a client in a safe and effective manner during resistance exercise

(Yellow) PROGRAM ADMINISTRATION, QUALITY ASSURANCE, AND OUTCOME ASSESSMENT

1.11.1   Knowledge of the cPT's role in administration and program management within a health/fitness facility

1.11.2   Knowledge of, and the ability to use, the documentation required when a client shows abnormal signs or symptoms during an exercise session and should be referred to a physician

1.11.3   Knowledge of professional liability and most common types of negligence seen in training environments

1.11.4   Understand the practical and legal ramifications of the employee versus independent contractor classifications as they relate to personal trainers

1.11.5   Knowledge of appropriate professional conduct, practice standards, and ethics in relationships dealing with clients, employers, and other allied health/medical/fitness professionals

1.11.6   Knowledge of the types of exercise programs available in the community and how these programs are appropriate for various populations

1.11.7   Knowledge of, and ability to implement, effective, professional business practices and ethical promotion of personal training services

(Pink) CLINICAL AND MEDICAL CONSIDERATIONS

1.12.1   Knowledge of cardiovascular, respiratory, metabolic, and musculoskeletal risk factors that may require further evaluation by medical or allied health professionals before participation in physical activity

1.12.2   Knowledge of risk factors that may be favorably modified by physical activity habits

1.12.3   Knowledge of the risk factor concept of coronary artery disease (CAD) and the influence of heredity and lifestyle on the development of CAD

1.12.4   Knowledge of how lifestyle factors, including nutrition, physical activity, and heredity, influence blood lipid and lipoprotein (i.e., cholesterol: high-density lipoprotein and low-density lipoprotein) profiles

1.12.5   Knowledge of cardiovascular risk factors or conditions that may require consultation with medical personnel before testing or training, including inappropriate changes of resting or exercise heart rate and blood pressure; new-onset discomfort in chest, neck, shoulder, or arm; changes in the pattern of discomfort during rest or exercise; fainting or dizzy spells; and claudication

1.12.6   Knowledge of respiratory risk factors or conditions that may require consultation with medical personnel before testing or training, including asthma, exercise-induced bronchospasm, extreme breathlessness at rest or during exercise, bronchitis, and emphysema

1.12.7   Knowledge of metabolic risk factors or conditions that may require consultation with medical personnel before testing or training, including body weight more than 20% above optimal, BMI >30, thyroid disease, diabetes or glucose intolerance, and hypoglycemia

1.12.8   Knowledge of musculoskeletal risk factors or conditions that may require consultation with medical personnel before testing or training, including acute or chronic back pain, osteoarthritis, rheumatoid arthritis, osteoporosis, tendonitis, and low back pain

1.12.9   Knowledge of the basic principles of electrical conduction of the heart, its phases of contraction, and its implications

1.12.10 Knowledge of common drugs from each of the following classes of medications and describe their effects on exercise: antianginals, antihypertensives, antiarrhythmics, bronchodilators, hypoglycemics, psychotropics, and vasodilators

1.12.11 Knowledge of the effects of the following substances on exercise: antihistamines, tranquilizers, alcohol, diet pills, cold tablets, caffeine, and nicotine

ACSM Health/Fitness Instructor® Knowledge, Skills, and Abilities (KSAs):

GENERAL POPULATION/CORE: EXERCISE PHYSIOLOGY AND RELATED EXERCISE SCIENCE

1.1.1   Knowledge of the basic structures of bone, skeletal muscle, and connective tissues

1.1.2   Knowledge of the basic anatomy of the cardiovascular system and respiratory system

1.1.3   Knowledge of the definition of the following terms: inferior, superior, medial, lateral, supination, pronation, flexion, extension, adduction, abduction, hyperextension, rotation, circumduction, agonist, antagonist, and stabilizer

1.1.4   Knowledge of the plane in which each muscle action occurs

1.1.5   Knowledge of the interrelationships among center of gravity, base of support, balance, stability, and proper spinal alignment

1.1.6   Knowledge of the following curvatures of the spine: lordosis, scoliosis, and kyphosis

1.1.7   Knowledge to describe the myotatic stretch reflex

1.1.8   Knowledge of fundamental biomechanical principles that underlie performance of the following activities: walking, jogging, running, swimming, cycling, weight lifting, and carrying or moving objects

1.1.9   Ability to define aerobic and anaerobic metabolism

1.1.10 Knowledge of the role of aerobic and anaerobic energy systems in the performance of various activities

1.1.11 Knowledge of the following terms: ischemia, angina pectoris, tachycardia, bradycardia, arrhythmia, myocardial infarction, cardiac output, stroke volume, lactic acid, oxygen consumption, hyperventilation, systolic blood pressure, diastolic blood pressure, and anaerobic threshold

1.1.12 Knowledge to describe normal cardiorespiratory responses to static and dynamic exercise in terms of heart rate, blood pressure, and oxygen consumption

1.1.13 Knowledge of how heart rate, blood pressure, and oxygen consumption responses change with adaptation to long-term exercise training

1.1.14 Knowledge of the physiological adaptations associated with strength training

1.1.15 Knowledge of the physiological principles related to warm-up and cool-down

1.1.16 Knowledge of the common theories of muscle fatigue and delayed-onset muscle soreness (DOMS)

1.1.17 Knowledge of the physiological adaptations that occur at rest and during submaximal and maximal exercise following long-term aerobic and anaerobic exercise training

1.1.18 Knowledge of the differences in cardiorespiratory response to short-term graded exercise between conditioned and unconditioned individuals

1.1.19   Knowledge of the structure of the skeletal muscle fiber and the basic mechanism of contraction

1.1.20   Knowledge of the characteristics of fast- and slow-twitch fibers

1.1.21   Knowledge of the sliding filament theory of muscle contraction

1.1.22   Knowledge of twitch, summation, and tetanus with respect to muscle contraction

1.1.23   Knowledge of the physiological principles involved in promoting gains in muscular strength and endurance

1.1.24   Knowledge of muscle fatigue as it relates to mode, intensity, duration, and the accumulative effects of exercise

1.1.25   Knowledge of the basic properties of cardiac muscle and the normal pathways of conduction in the heart

1.1.26   Knowledge of the response of the following variables to short-term static and dynamic exercise: heart rate, stroke volume, cardiac output, pulmonary ventilation, tidal volume, respiratory rate, and arteriovenous oxygen difference

1.1.27   Knowledge of blood pressure responses associated with short-term exercise, including changes in body position

1.1.28   Knowledge of, and ability to describe, the implications of ventilatory threshold (anaerobic threshold) as it relates to exercise training and cardiorespiratory assessment

1.1.29   Knowledge of, and ability to describe, the physiological adaptations of the respiratory system that occur at rest and during submaximal and maximal exercise following long-term aerobic and anaerobic training

1.1.30   Knowledge of how each of the following differs from the normal condition: dyspnea, hypoxia, and hypoventilation

1.1.31   Knowledge of how the principle of specificity relates to the components of fitness

1.1.32   Knowledge of the concept of detraining or reversibility of conditioning and its implications in fitness programs

1.1.33   Knowledge of the physical and psychological signs of overtraining and to provide recommendations for these problems

1.1.34   Knowledge of, and ability to describe, the changes that occur in maturation from childhood to adulthood for the following: skeletal muscle, bone structure, reaction time, coordination, heat and cold tolerance, maximal oxygen consumption, strength, flexibility, body composition, resting and maximal heart rate, and resting and maximal blood pressure

1.1.35   Knowledge of the effect of the aging process on the musculoskeletal and cardiovascular structure and function at rest, during exercise, and during recovery

1.1.36   Knowledge of the following terms: progressive resistance, isotonic/isometric, concentric, eccentric, atrophy, hypertrophy, sets, repetitions, plyometrics, Valsalva maneuver

1.1.37   Knowledge of, and skill to demonstrate, exercises designed to enhance muscular strength and/or endurance of specific major muscle groups

1.1.38   Knowledge of, and skill to demonstrate, exercises for enhancing musculoskeletal flexibility

1.1.39   Ability to identify the major bones and muscles. Major muscles include, but are not limited to, the following: trapezius, pectoralis major, latissimus dorsi, biceps, triceps, rectus abdominis, internal and external obliques, erector spinae, gluteus maximus, quadriceps, hamstrings, adductors, abductors, and gastrocnemius

1.1.40   Ability to identify the major bones. Major bones include, but are not limited to, the clavicle, scapula, sternum, humerus, carpals, ulna, radius, femur, fibula, tibia, and tarsals

1.1.41   Ability to identify the joints of the body

1.1.42   Knowledge of the primary action and joint range-of-motion for each major muscle group

1.1.43   Ability to locate the anatomical landmarks for palpation of peripheral pulses

PATHOPHYSIOLOGY AND RISK FACTORS

1.2.1   Knowledge of the physiological and metabolic responses to exercise associated with chronic disease (heart disease, hypertension, diabetes mellitus, and pulmonary disease)

1.2.2   Knowledge of cardiovascular, respiratory, metabolic, and musculoskeletal risk factors that may require further evaluation by medical or allied health professionals before participation in physical activity

1.2.3   Knowledge of risk factors that may be favorably modified by physical activity habits

1.2.4   Knowledge to define the following terms: total cholesterol (TC), high-density lipoprotein cholesterol (HDL-C), TC/HDL-C ratio, low-density lipoprotein cholesterol (LDL-C), triglycerides, hypertension, and atherosclerosis

1.2.5   Knowledge of plasma cholesterol levels for adults as recommended by the National Cholesterol Education Program

1.2.6   Knowledge of the risk factor concept of CAD and the influence of heredity and lifestyle on the development of CAD

1.2.7   Knowledge of the atherosclerotic process, the factors involved in its genesis and progression, and the potential role of exercise in treatment

1.2.8   Knowledge of how lifestyle factors, including nutrition, physical activity, and heredity, influence lipid and lipoprotein profiles

HEALTH APPRAISAL, FITNESS AND CLINICAL EXERCISE TESTING

1.3.1   Knowledge of, and ability to discuss, the physiological basis of the major components of physical fitness: flexibility, cardiovascular fitness, muscular strength, muscular endurance, and body composition

1.3.2   Knowledge of the importance of a health/medical history

1.3.3   Knowledge of the value of a medical clearance prior to exercise participation

1.3.4   Knowledge of the categories of participants who should receive medical clearance prior to administration of an exercise test or participation in an exercise program

1.3.5   Knowledge of relative and absolute contraindications to exercise testing or participation

1.3.6   Knowledge of the limitations of informed consent and medical clearance prior to exercise testing

1.3.7   Knowledge of the advantages/disadvantages and limitations of the various body composition techniques including air displacement, plethysmography, hydrostatic weighing, skinfolds, and bioelectrical impedence

1.3.8   Skill in accurately measuring heart rate and blood pressure and obtaining rating of perceived exertion (RPE) at rest and during exercise according to established guidelines

1.3.9   Skill in measuring skinfold sites, skeletal diameters, and girth measurements used for estimating body composition

1.3.10 Skill in techniques for calibration of a cycle ergometer and a motor-driven treadmill

1.3.11 Ability to locate the brachial artery and correctly place the cuff and stethoscope in position for blood pressure measurement

1.3.12 Ability to locate common sites for measurement of skinfold thicknesses and circumferences (for determination of body composition and waist–hip ratio)

1.3.13 Ability to obtain a health history and risk appraisal that includes past and current medical history, family history of cardiac disease, orthopedic limitations, prescribed medications, activity patterns, nutritional habits, stress and anxiety levels, and smoking and alcohol use

1.3.14 Ability to obtain informed consent

1.3.15 Ability to explain the purpose and procedures for monitoring clients prior to, during, and after cardiorespiratory fitness testing

1.3.16 Ability to instruct participants in the use of equipment and test procedures

1.3.17 Ability to describe the purpose of testing, determine an appropriate submaximal or maximal protocol, and perform an assessment of cardiovascular fitness on the cycle ergometer or the treadmill

1.3.18 Ability to describe the purpose of testing, determine appropriate protocols, and perform assessments of muscular strength, muscular endurance, and flexibility

1.3.19 Ability to perform various techniques of assessing body composition, including the use of skinfold calipers

1.3.20 Ability to analyze and interpret information obtained from the cardiorespiratory fitness test and the muscular strength and endurance, flexibility, and body composition assessments for apparently healthy individuals and those with stable disease

1.3.21 Ability to identify appropriate criteria for terminating a fitness evaluation and to demonstrate proper procedures to be followed after discontinuing such a test

1.3.22 Ability to modify protocols and procedures for cardiorespiratory fitness tests in children, adolescents, and older adults

1.3.23 Ability to identify individuals for whom physician supervision is recommended during maximal and submaximal exercise testing

ELECTROCARDIOGRAPHY AND DIAGNOSTIC TECHNIQUES

1.4.1   Knowledge of how each of the following differs from the normal condition: premature atrial contractions and premature ventricular contractions

1.4.2   Ability to locate the appropriate sites for the limb and chest leads for resting, standard, and exercise (Mason Likar) electrocardiograms (ECGs), as well as commonly used bipolar systems (e.g., CM-5)

PATIENT MANAGEMENT AND MEDICATIONS

1.5.1 Knowledge of common drugs from each of the following classes of medications and describe the principal action and the effects on exercise testing and prescription: antianginals, antihypertensives, antiarrhythmics, bronchodilators, hypoglycemics, psychotropics, and vasodilators

1.5.2 Knowledge of the effects of the following substances on exercise response: antihistamines, tranquilizers, alcohol, diet pills, cold tablets, caffeine, and nicotine

EXERCISE PRESCRIPTION AND PROGRAMMING

1.7.1 Knowledge of the relationship between the number of repetitions, intensity, number of sets, and rest with regard to strength training

1.7.2 Knowledge of the benefits and risks associated with exercise training in prepubescent and postpubescent youths

1.7.3 Knowledge of the benefits and precautions associated with resistance and endurance training in older adults

1.7.4 Knowledge of specific leadership techniques appropriate for working with participants of all ages

1.7.5 Knowledge of how to modify cardiovascular and resistance exercises on the basis of age and physical condition

1.7.6 Knowledge of the differences in the development of an exercise prescription for children, adolescents, and older participants

1.7.7 Knowledge of, and ability to describe, the unique adaptations to exercise training in children, adolescents, and older participants with regard to strength, functional capacity, and motor skills

1.7.8 Knowledge of common orthopedic and cardiovascular considerations for older participants and the ability to describe modifications in exercise prescription that are indicated

1.7.9 Knowledge of selecting appropriate testing and training modalities according to the age and functional capacity of the individual

1.7.10 Knowledge of the recommended intensity, duration, frequency, and type of physical activity necessary for development of cardiorespiratory fitness in an apparently healthy population

1.7.11 Knowledge of, and the ability to describe, exercises designed to enhance muscular strength and/or endurance of specific major muscle groups

1.7.12 Knowledge of the principles of overload, specificity, and progression and how they relate to exercise programming

1.7.13 Knowledge of the various types of interval, continuous, and circuit training programs

1.7.14 Knowledge of approximate METs for various sport, recreational, and work tasks

1.7.15 Knowledge of the components incorporated into an exercise session and the proper sequence (i.e., pre-exercise evaluation, warm-up, aerobic stimulus phase, cool-down, muscular strength and/or endurance, and flexibility)

1.7.16 Knowledge of special precautions and modifications of exercise programming for participation at altitude and in different ambient temperatures, humidity, and environmental pollution

1.7.17 Knowledge of the importance of recording exercise sessions and performing periodic evaluations to assess changes in fitness status

1.7.18 Knowledge of the advantages and disadvantages of implementation of interval, continuous, and circuit training programs

1.7.19 Knowledge of the types of exercise programs available in the community and how these programs are appropriate for various populations

1.7.20 Knowledge of the concept of "Activities of Daily Living" (ADLs) and its importance in the overall health of the individual

1.7.21 Skill to teach and demonstrate the components of an exercise session (i.e., warm-up, aerobic stimulus phase, cool-down, muscular strength/endurance, flexibility)

1.7.22 Skill to teach and demonstrate appropriate modifications in specific exercises for the following groups: older adults, pregnant and postnatal women, obese persons, and persons with low back pain

1.7.23 Skill to teach and demonstrate appropriate exercises for improving range of motion of all major joints

1.7.24 Skill in the use of various methods for establishing and monitoring levels of exercise intensity, including heart rate, RPE, and METs

1.7.25 Ability to identify and apply methods used to monitor exercise intensity, including heart rate and rating of perceived exertion

1.7.26 Ability to describe modifications in exercise prescriptions for individuals with functional disabilities and musculoskeletal injuries

1.7.27   Ability to differentiate between the amount of physical activity required for health benefits and the amount of exercise required for fitness development

1.7.28   Ability to determine training heart rates using two methods: percentage of age-predicted maximum heart rate and heart rate reserve (Karvonen)

1.7.29   Ability to identify proper and improper technique in the use of resistive equipment such as stability balls, weights, bands, resistance bars, and water exercise equipment

1.7.30   Ability to identify proper and improper technique in the use of cardiovascular conditioning equipment (e.g., stairclimbers, stationary cycles, treadmills, elliptical trainers)

1.7.31   Ability to teach a progression of exercises for all major muscle groups to improve muscular strength and endurance

1.7.32   Ability to communicate effectively with exercise participants

1.7.33   Ability to design, implement, and evaluate individualized and group exercise programs on the basis of health history and physical fitness assessments

1.7.34   Ability to modify exercises on the basis of age and physical condition

1.7.35   Knowledge and ability to determine energy cost, $\dot{V}O_2$, METs, and target heart rates and apply the information to an exercise prescription

1.7.36   Ability to convert weights from pounds (lb) to kilograms (kg) and speed from miles per hour (mph) to meters per minute ($m \cdot min^{-1}$)

1.7.37   Ability to convert METs to $\dot{V}O_2$ expressed as $mL \cdot kg^{-1} \cdot min^{-1}$, $L \cdot min^{-1}$, and/or $mL \cdot kg \ FFW^{-1} \cdot min^{-1}$

1.7.38   Ability to determine the energy cost in METs and kilocalories for given exercise intensities in stepping exercise, cycle ergometry, and during horizontal and graded walking and running

1.7.39   Ability to prescribe exercise intensity on the basis of $\dot{V}O_2$ data for different modes of exercise, including graded and horizontal running and walking, cycling, and stepping exercise.

1.7.40   Ability to explain and implement exercise prescription guidelines for apparently healthy clients, increased-risk clients, and clients with controlled disease

1.7.41   Ability to adapt frequency, intensity, duration, mode, progression, level of supervision, and monitoring techniques in exercise programs for patients with controlled chronic disease (e.g., heart disease, diabetes mellitus, obesity, hypertension), musculoskeletal problems, pregnancy and/or postpartum, and exercise-induced asthma

1.7.42   Ability to design resistive exercise programs to increase or maintain muscular strength and/or endurance

1.7.43   Ability to evaluate flexibility and prescribe appropriate flexibility exercises for all major muscle groups

1.7.44   Ability to design training programs using interval, continuous, and circuit training programs

1.7.45   Ability to describe the advantages and disadvantages of various commercial exercise equipment in developing cardiorespiratory fitness, muscular strength, and muscular endurance

1.7.46   Ability to modify exercise programs on the basis of age, physical condition, and current health status

NUTRITION AND WEIGHT MANAGEMENT

1.8.1   Knowledge of the role of carbohydrates, fats, and proteins as fuels for aerobic and anaerobic metabolism

1.8.2   Knowledge to define the following terms: obesity, overweight, percentage fat, lean body mass, anorexia nervosa, bulimia, and body fat distribution

1.8.3   Knowledge of the relationship between body composition and health

1.8.4   Knowledge of the effects of diet plus exercise, diet alone, and exercise alone as methods for modifying body composition

1.8.5   Knowledge of the importance of an adequate daily energy intake for healthy weight management

1.8.6   Knowledge of the difference between fat-soluble and water-soluble vitamins

1.8.7   Knowledge of the importance of maintaining normal hydration before, during, and after exercise

1.8.8   Knowledge of the USDA Food Pyramid

1.8.9   Knowledge of the importance of calcium and iron in women's health

1.8.10   Knowledge of the myths and consequences associated with inappropriate weight loss methods (e.g., saunas, vibrating belts, body wraps, electric simulators, sweat suits, fad diets)

1.8.11   Knowledge of the number of kilocalories in 1 gram of carbohydrate, fat, protein, and alcohol

1.8.12   Knowledge of the number of kilocalories equivalent to losing 1 pound of body fat

1.8.13   Knowledge of the guidelines for caloric intake for an individual desiring to lose or gain weight

1.8.14   Knowledge of common nutritional ergogenic aids, the purported mechanism of action, and any risk and/or benefits (e.g., carbohydrates, protein/amino acids, vitamins, minerals, sodium bicarbonate, creatine, bee pollen)

1.8.15   Knowledge of nutritional factors related to the female athlete triad syndrome (i.e., eating disorders, menstrual cycle abnormalities, and osteoporosis)

1.8.16   Knowledge of the NIH Consensus Statement regarding health risks of obesity, Nutrition for Physical Fitness Position Paper of the American Dietetic Association, and the ACSM Position Stand on proper and improper weight loss programs

1.8.17   Ability to describe the health implications of variation in body fat distribution patterns and the significance of the waist-to-hip ratio

HUMAN BEHAVIOR AND COUNSELING

1.9.1   Knowledge of at least five behavioral strategies to enhance exercise and health behavior change (e.g., reinforcement, goal setting, social support)

1.9.2   Knowledge of the five important elements that should be included in each counseling session

1.9.3   Knowledge of specific techniques to enhance motivation (e.g., posters, recognition, bulletin boards, games, competitions). Define extrinsic and intrinsic reinforcement and give examples of each.

1.9.4   Knowledge of extrinsic and intrinsic reinforcement, with examples of each

1.9.5   Knowledge of the stages of motivational readiness

1.9.6   Knowledge of three counseling approaches that may assist less motivated clients to increase their physical activity

1.9.7   Knowledge of symptoms of anxiety and depression that may necessitate referral to a medical or mental health professional

1.9.8   Knowledge of the potential symptoms and causal factors of test anxiety (i.e., performance, appraisal threat during exercise testing) and how it may affect physiological responses to testing

SAFETY, INJURY PREVENTION, AND EMERGENCY PROCEDURES

1.10.1   Knowledge of and skill in obtaining basic life support and cardiopulmonary resuscitation certification

1.10.2   Knowledge of appropriate emergency procedures (e.g., telephone procedures, written emergency procedures, personnel responsibilities) in a health and fitness setting

1.10.3   Knowledge of basic first aid procedures for exercise-related injuries, such as bleeding, strains/sprains, fractures, and exercise intolerance (dizziness, syncope, heat injury)

1.10.4   Knowledge of basic precautions taken in an exercise setting to ensure participant safety

1.10.5   Knowledge of the physical and physiological signs and symptoms of overtraining

1.10.6   Knowledge of the effects of temperature, humidity, altitude, and pollution on the physiological response to exercise

1.10.7   Knowledge of the following terms: shin splints, sprain, strain, tennis elbow, bursitis, stress fracture, tendonitis, patellar femoral pain syndrome, low back pain, plantar fasciitis, and rotator cuff tendonitis

1.10.8   Knowledge of hypothetical concerns and potential risks that may be associated with the use of exercises such as straight leg sit-ups, double leg raises, full squats, hurdlers stretch, yoga plough, forceful back hyperextension, and standing bent-over toe touch

1.10.9   Knowledge of safety plans, emergency procedures, and first aid techniques needed during fitness evaluations, exercise testing, and exercise training

1.10.10   Knowledge of the health/fitness instructor's responsibilities, limitations, and the legal implications of carrying out emergency procedures

1.10.11   Knowledge of potential musculoskeletal injuries (e.g., contusions, sprains, strains, fractures), cardiovascular/pulmonary complications (e.g., tachycardia, bradycardia, hypotension/hypertension, tachypnea), and metabolic abnormalities (e.g., fainting/syncope, hypoglycemia/hyperglycemia, hypothermia/hyperthermia)

1.10.12   Knowledge of the initial management and first aid techniques associated with open wounds, musculoskeletal injuries, cardiovascular/pulmonary complications, and metabolic disorders

1.10.13   Knowledge of the components of an equipment maintenance/repair program and how it may be used to evaluate the condition of exercise equipment to reduce the potential risk of injury

1.10.14   Knowledge of the legal implications of documented safety procedures, the use of incident documents, and ongoing safety training

1.10.15   Skill to demonstrate exercises used for people with low back pain

1.10.16   Skill in demonstrating appropriate emergency procedures during exercise testing and/or training

1.10.17   Ability to identify the components that contribute to the maintenance of a safe environment

PROGRAM ADMINISTRATION, QUALITY ASSURANCE, AND OUTCOME ASSESSMENT

1.11.1 Knowledge of the health/fitness instructor's role in administration and program management within a health/fitness facility

1.11.2 Knowledge of, and the ability to use, the documentation required when a client shows signs or symptoms during an exercise session and should be referred to a physician

1.11.3 Knowledge of how to manage of a fitness department (e.g., working within a budget, training exercise leaders, scheduling, running staff meetings)

1.11.4 Knowledge of the importance of tracking and evaluating member retention

1.11.5 Ability to administer fitness-related programs within established budgetary guidelines

1.11.6 Ability to develop marketing materials for the purpose of promoting fitness-related programs

1.11.7 Ability to create and maintain records pertaining to participant exercise adherence, retention, and goal setting

1.11.8 Ability to develop and administer educational programs (e.g., lectures, workshops) and educational materials

CARDIOVASCULAR: PATHOPHYSIOLOGY AND RISK FACTORS

2.2.1 Knowledge of cardiovascular risk factors or conditions that may require consultation with medical personnel before testing or training, including inappropriate changes of resting or exercise heart rate and blood pressure; new-onset discomfort in chest, neck, shoulder, or arm; changes in the pattern of discomfort during rest or exercise; fainting or dizzy spells; and claudication

2.2.2 Knowledge of the causes of myocardial ischemia and infarction

2.2.3 Knowledge of the pathophysiology of hypertension, obesity, hyperlipidemia, diabetes, chronic obstructive pulmonary diseases, arthritis, osteoporosis, chronic diseases, and immunosuppressive disease

2.2.4 Knowledge of the effects of the above diseases and conditions on cardiorespiratory and metabolic function at rest and during exercise

PULMONARY: PATHOPHYSIOLOGY AND RISK FACTORS

3.2.1 Knowledge of respiratory risk factors or conditions that may require consultation with medical personnel before testing or training, including asthma, exercise-induced bronchospasm, extreme breathlessness at rest or during exercise, bronchitis, and emphysema

METABOLIC: PATHOPHYSIOLOGY AND RISK FACTORS

4.2.1 Knowledge of metabolic risk factors or conditions that may require consultation with medical personnel before testing or training, including body weight more than 20% above optimal, BMI >30, thyroid disease, diabetes or glucose intolerance, and hypoglycemia

ORTHOPEDIC/MUSCULOSKELETAL: PATHOPHYSIOLOGY AND RISK FACTORS

5.2.1 Knowledge of musculoskeletal risk factors or conditions that may require consultation with medical personnel before testing or training, including acute or chronic back pain, osteoarthritis, rheumatoid arthritis, osteoporosis, tendonitis, and low back pain

NOTE: The KSAs listed above for the ACSM Health/Fitness Instructor® are the same KSAs for educational programs seeking undergraduate (bachelor's degree) academic accreditation through the CoAES. Specifically, these programs are typically Exercise Science, Kinesiology, and/or Physical Education departments with professional development tracks for those students interested in careers in the fitness industry. For more information, please visit www.coaes.org.

ACSM Exercise Specialist® Knowledge, Skills, and Abilities (KSAs):

EXERCISE PHYSIOLOGY AND RELATED EXERCISE SCIENCE

1.1.1 **Describe coronary anatomy**

1.1.2 **Describe the physiological effects of bed rest and discuss the appropriate physical activities that might be used to counteract these changes**

1.1.3   Identify the cardiorespiratory responses associated with postural changes

1.1.4   Describe activities that are primarily aerobic and anaerobic

1.1.5   Identify the metabolic equivalent (MET) requirements of various occupational, household, sport/exercise, and leisure time activities

1.1.6   Knowledge of the unique hemodynamic responses of arm versus leg exercise and of static versus dynamic exercise

1.1.7   Define the determinants of myocardial oxygen consumption and the effects of exercise training on those determinants

1.1.8   Determine maximal oxygen (O_2) consumption and describe the methodology for measuring it

1.1.9   Plot the normal resting and exercise values associated with increasing exercise intensity (and how they may differ for diseased populations) for the following: heart rate, stroke volume, cardiac output, double product, arteriovenous O_2 difference, O_2 consumption, systolic and diastolic blood pressure, minute ventilation, tidal volume, breathing frequency, V_d/V_t, V_E/VO_2, and V_E/VCO_2

1.1.10   Discuss the effects of isometric exercise in individuals with cardiovascular, pulmonary, and/or metabolic diseases or with low functional capacity

1.1.11   Knowledge of acute and chronic adaptations to exercise for apparently healthy individuals (low risk) and for those with cardiovascular, pulmonary, and metabolic diseases

1.1.12   Describe the effects of variation in environmental factors (e.g., temperature, humidity, altitude) for normal individuals and those with cardiovascular, pulmonary, and metabolic diseases

PATHOPHYSIOLOGY AND RISK FACTORS

1.2.1   Summarize the atherosclerotic process, including current hypotheses regarding onset and rate of progression and/or regression

1.2.2   Compare and contrast the differences between typical, atypical, and vasospastic angina

1.2.3   Describe the pathophysiology of the healing myocardium and the potential complications after acute myocardial infarction (MI) (extension, expansion, rupture)

1.2.4   Describe silent ischemia and its implications for exercise testing and training

1.2.5   Examine the role of diet on cardiovascular risk factors such as hypertension, blood lipids, and body weight

1.2.6   Describe the lipoprotein classifications and define their relationship to atherosclerosis or other diseases

1.2.7   Describe the cardiorespiratory and metabolic responses that accompany or result from pulmonary diseases at rest and during exercise

1.2.8   Describe the influence of exercise on cardiovascular risk factors

1.2.9   Describe the normal and abnormal cardiorespiratory responses at rest and exercise

1.2.10   Identify the mechanisms by which functional capacity and cardiovascular, pulmonary, metabolic, and neuromuscular adaptations occur in response to exercise testing and training in healthy and disease states

1.2.11   Describe the cardiorespiratory and metabolic responses in myocardial dysfunction and ischemia at rest and during exercise

HEALTH APPRAISAL, FITNESS AND CLINICAL EXERCISE TESTING

1.3.1   Describe common procedures and apply knowledge of results from radionuclide imaging (e.g., thallium, technetium, sestamibi, single photon emission computed tomography (SPECT)

1.3.2   Knowledge of exercise testing procedures for various clinical populations including those individuals with cardiovascular, pulmonary, and metabolic diseases, in terms of exercise modality, protocol, physiological measurements, and expected outcomes

1.3.3   Describe anatomical landmarks as they relate to exercise testing and programming

1.3.4   Locate and palpate anatomical landmarks of radial, brachial, carotid, femoral, popliteal, and tibialis arteries

1.3.5   Select an appropriate test protocol according to the age and functional capacity of the individual

1.3.6   Identify individuals for whom physician supervision is recommended during maximal and submaximal exercise testing

1.3.7   Conduct pre-exercise test procedures

1.3.8   Describe basic equipment and facility requirements for exercise testing

1.3.9   Instruct the test participant in the use of the RPE scale and other appropriate subjective rating scales, such as the dyspnea and angina scales

1.3.10   Obtain informed consent and describe its purpose

1.3.11   Describe the importance of accurate and calibrated testing equipment (e.g., treadmill, ergometers, electrocardiograph, and sphygmomanometers)

1.3.12   Measure physiological and subjective responses (e.g., symptoms, ECG, blood pressure, heart rate, RPE and other scales, oxygen saturation, and oxygen consumption) at appropriate intervals during the test

1.3.13   Describe the effects of age, weight, level of fitness, and health status on the selection of an exercise test protocol

1.3.14   Ability to measure oxygen consumption during an exercise test

1.3.15   Ability to provide testing procedures and protocol for children and the elderly with or without various clinical conditions

1.3.16   Obtain and interpret medical history and physical examination findings as they relate to health appraisal and exercise testing

1.3.17   Accurately record and interpret right and left arm pre-exercise blood pressures in the supine and upright positions

1.3.18   Describe and analyze the importance of the absolute and relative contraindications of an exercise test

1.3.19   Select and perform appropriate procedures and protocols for the exercise test, including modes of exercise, starting levels, increments of work, ramping versus incremental protocols, length of stages, and frequency of data collection

1.3.20   Describe and conduct immediate post-exercise procedures and various approaches to cool-down

1.3.21   Record, organize, perform, and interpret necessary calculations of test data

1.3.22   Describe the differences in the physiological responses to various modes of ergometry (e.g., treadmill, cycle and arm ergometers) as they relate to exercise testing and training

1.3.23   Describe normal and abnormal chronotropic and inotropic responses to exercise testing and training

1.3.24   Describe and apply Baye's theorem as it relates to pretest likelihood of CAD and the predictive value of positive or negative diagnostic exercise ECG results

1.3.25   Compare and contrast obstructive and restrictive lung diseases and their effect on exercise testing and training

1.3.26   Identify orthopedic limitations (e.g., gout, foot drop, specific joint problems) as they relate to modifications of exercise testing and programming

1.3.27   Identify neuromuscular disorders (e.g., Parkinson's disease, multiple sclerosis) as they relate to modifications of exercise testing and programming

1.3.28   Describe the aerobic and anaerobic metabolic demands of exercise testing and training in individuals with cardiovascular, pulmonary, and/or metabolic diseases undergoing exercise testing or training

1.3.29   Identify the variables measured during cardiopulmonary exercise testing (e.g., heart rate, blood pressure, rate of perceived exertion, ventilation, oxygen consumption, ventilatory threshold, pulmonary circulation) and their potential relationship to cardiovascular, pulmonary, and metabolic disease

1.3.30   Discuss the appropriate use of static and dynamic exercise for individuals with cardiovascular, pulmonary, and metabolic disease

ELECTROCARDIOGRAPHY AND DIAGNOSTIC TECHNIQUES

1.4.1   Summarize the purpose of coronary angiography

1.4.2   Describe myocardial ischemia and identify ischemic indicators of various cardiovascular diagnostic tests

1.4.3   Describe the differences between Q-wave and non-Q-wave infarction

1.4.4   Identify the ECG patterns at rest and responses to exercise in patients with pacemakers and ICDs

1.4.5   Identify resting and exercise ECG changes associated with the following abnormalities: bundle branch blocks and bifascicular blocks; atrioventricular blocks; sinus bradycardia and tachycardia; sinus arrest; supraventricular premature contractions and tachycardia; ventricular premature contractions (including frequency, form, couplets, salvos, tachycardia); atrial flutter and fibrillation; ventricular fibrillation; myocardial ischemia, injury, and infarction

1.4.6   Define the ECG criteria for initiating and/or terminating exercise testing or training

1.4.7   Identify ECG changes that correspond to ischemia in various myocardial regions

1.4.8   Describe potential causes of various cardiac arrhythmias

1.4.9   **Identify potentially hazardous arrhythmias or conduction defects observed on the ECG at rest, during exercise, and recovery**

1.4.10   Describe the diagnostic and prognostic significance of ischemic ECG responses and arrhythmias at rest, during exercise, or at recovery

1.4.11   Identify resting and exercise ECG changes associated with cardiovascular disease, hypertensive heart disease, cardiac chamber enlargement, pericarditis, pulmonary disease, and metabolic disorders

1.4.12   Administer and interpret basic resting spirometric tests and measures including $FEV_{1.0}$, FVC, and MVV

1.4.13   Locate the appropriate sites for the limb and chest leads for resting, standard, and exercise (Mason Likar) electrocardiograms (ECGs), as well as commonly used bipolar systems (e.g., CM-5)

1.4.14   **Obtain and interpret a pre-exercise standard and modified (Mason-Likar) 12-lead ECG on a participant in the supine and upright positions**

1.4.15   Ability to minimize ECG artifact

1.4.16   Describe the diagnostic and prognostic implications of the exercise test ECG and hemodynamic responses

1.4.17   Identify ECG changes that typically occur due to hyperventilation, electrolyte abnormalities, and drug therapy

1.4.18   Identify the causes of false-positive and false-negative exercise ECG responses and methods for optimizing sensitivity and specificity

1.4.19   **Identify and describe the significance of ECG abnormalities in designing the exercise prescription and in making activity recommendations**

1.4.20   **Explain indications and procedures for combining exercise testing with radionuclide or echocardiographic imaging**

PATIENT MANAGEMENT AND MEDICATIONS

1.5.1   List indications for use of streptokinase, tissue plasminogen activase, and other thrombolytic agents

1.5.2   **Describe mechanisms and actions of medications that may affect exercise testing and prescription**

1.5.3   Recognize medications associated in the clinical setting, their indications for care, and their effects at rest and during exercise (e.g., antianginals, antihypertensives, antiarrhythmics, bronchodilators, hypoglycemics, psychotropics, vasodilators, anticoagulant and antiplatelet drugs, and lipid-lowering agents)

MEDICAL AND SURGICAL MANAGEMENT

1.6.1   Describe percutaneous coronary and peripheral interventions (e.g., PTCA, stent) as an alternative to medical management or bypass surgery

1.6.2   **Describe indications and limitations for medical management and interventional techniques in different subsets of individuals with CAD and PAD**

EXERCISE PRESCRIPTION AND PROGRAMMING

1.7.1   Describe basic joint movements, muscle actions, and points of insertion as they relate to exercise programming

1.7.2   **Compare and contrast benefits and risks of exercise for individuals with CAD risk factors and for individuals with cardiovascular, pulmonary, and/or metabolic diseases**

1.7.3   **Design appropriate exercise prescription in environmental extremes for normal individuals and those with cardiovascular, pulmonary, and metabolic diseases**

1.7.4   **Design, implement, and supervise individualized exercise prescriptions for people with chronic disease and disabling conditions**

1.7.5   **Design a supervised exercise program beginning at hospital discharge and continuing for up to 6 months for the following conditions: MI, angina: LVAD, congestive heart failure, PCI, CABG, medical management of CAD, chronic pulmonary disease, weight management, diabetes and cardiac transplants**

1.7.6   **Knowledge of the concept of "Activities of Daily Living" (ADLs) and its importance in the overall rehabilitation of the individual**

1.7.7   **Prescribe exercise using nontraditional modalities (e.g., bench stepping, elastic bands, isodynamic exercise, water aerobics) for individuals with cardiovascular, pulmonary, or metabolic diseases**

1.7.8   Discuss equipment adaptations necessary for different age groups

1.7.9   Identify individuals who require exercise testing prior to exercise training

1.7.10   Organize GXT and clinical data and counsel patients regarding issues such as ADLs, return to work, and physical activity

1.7.11   Describe relative and absolute contraindications to exercise training

1.7.12   Identify characteristics that correlate or predict poor compliance with exercise programs and strategies to increase exercise adherence

1.7.13   Describe the importance of warm-up and cool-down sessions with specific reference to angina and ischemic ECG changes and for overall patient safety

1.7.14   Identify and explain the mechanisms by which exercise may contribute to preventing or rehabilitating individuals with cardiovascular, pulmonary, and metabolic diseases

1.7.15   Describe common gait abnormalities as they relate to exercise testing and programming

1.7.16   Describe the principle of specificity of training as it relates to the mode of exercise testing and training

1.7.17   Design strength and flexibility programs for individuals with cardiovascular, pulmonary, and/or metabolic diseases, the elderly, and children

1.7.18   Determine appropriate testing and training modalities according to the age and functional capacity of the individual

1.7.19   Describe the indications and methods for ECG monitoring during exercise testing and training

1.7.20   Describe the importance of, and appropriate methods for, resistance training in older individuals

1.7.21   Ability to modify exercise testing and training to the limitations of peripheral arterial disease (PAD)

NUTRITION AND WEIGHT MANAGEMENT

1.8.1   Describe and discuss dietary considerations for cardiovascular and pulmonary diseases, chronic heart failure, and diabetes that are recommended to minimize disease progression and optimize disease management

1.8.2   Compare and contrast dietary practices used for weight reduction and address the benefits, risks, and scientific support for each practice. Examples of dietary practices are high-protein/low-carbohydrate diets, Mediterranean diet, and low-fat diets such as the American Heart Association recommended diet

1.8.3   Calculate the effect of caloric intake and energy expenditure on weight management

HUMAN BEHAVIOR AND COUNSELING

1.9.1   List and apply five behavioral strategies as they apply to lifestyle modifications such as exercise, diet, stress, and medication management

1.9.2   Describe signs and symptoms of maladjustment and/or failure to cope during an illness crisis and/or personal adjustment crisis (e.g., job loss) that might prompt a psychological consult or referral to other professional services

1.9.3   Describe the general principles of crisis management and factors influencing coping and learning in illness states

1.9.4   Identify the psychological stages involved with the acceptance of death and dying and ability to recognize when it is necessary for a psychological consult or referral to a professional resource

1.9.5   Recognize observable signs and symptoms of anxiety or depressive symptoms and the need for a psychiatric referral

1.9.6   Describe the psychological issues to be confronted by the patient and by family members of patients who have cardiovascular disease and/or who have had an acute MI or cardiac surgery

1.9.7   Identify the psychological issues associated with an acute cardiac event versus those associated with chronic cardiac conditions

SAFETY, INJURY PREVENTION, AND EMERGENCY PROCEDURES

1.10.1   Respond appropriately to emergency situations (e.g., cardiac arrest, hypoglycemia and hyperglycemia, bronchospasm, sudden-onset hypotension, serious cardiac arrhythmias, implantable cardiac defibrillator (ICD) discharge, transient ischemic attack (TIA) or stroke, MI) that might arise before, during, and after an exercise test and/or exercise session

1.10.2   List medications that should be available for emergency situations in exercise testing and training sessions

1.10.3   Describe the emergency equipment and personnel that should be present in an exercise testing laboratory and rehabilitative exercise training setting

1.10.4   **Describe the appropriate procedures for maintaining emergency equipment and supplies**

1.10.5   **Describe the effects of cardiovascular, pulmonary, and metabolic diseases on performance and safety during exercise testing and training**

1.10.6   **Risk stratify individuals with cardiovascular, pulmonary, and metabolic diseases, using appropriate materials and understanding the prognostic indicators for high-risk individuals**

PROGRAM ADMINISTRATION, QUALITY ASSURANCE, AND OUTCOME ASSESSMENT

1.11.1   **Discuss the role of outcome measures in chronic disease management programs such as cardiovascular and pulmonary rehabilitation programs**

1.11.2   Identify and discuss various outcome measurements that could be used in a cardiac or pulmonary rehabilitation program

1.11.3   Identify and discuss specific outcome collection instruments that could be used to collect outcome data in a cardiac or pulmonary rehabilitation program

ACSM Registered Clinical Exercise Physiologist® Knowledge, Skills, and Abilities (KSAs):

GENERAL POPULATION/CORE: EXERCISE PHYSIOLOGY AND RELATED EXERCISE SCIENCE

1.1.1   Describe the short-term responses to aerobic and resistance exercise training on the function of the cardiovascular, respiratory, musculoskeletal, neuromuscular, metabolic, endocrine, and immune systems

1.1.2   Describe the long-term effects of aerobic, resistance, and flexibility exercise training on the structure and function of the cardiovascular, respiratory, musculoskeletal, neuromuscular, metabolic, endocrine, and immune systems

1.1.3   List typical values in sedentary and trained persons for oxygen uptake, heart rate, mean arterial pressure, systolic and diastolic blood pressure, cardiac output, stroke volume, minute ventilation, respiratory rate, and tidal volume at rest and during submaximal and maximal exercise

1.1.4   Describe the physiological determinants of $\dot{V}O_2$, MVO_2, and mean arterial pressure and explain how these determinants may be altered with aerobic and resistance exercise training

1.1.5   Explain how environmental factors may affect the physiological responses to exercise, including ambient temperature, humidity, air quality (e.g., CO, ozone, air pollution) and altitude, and describe appropriate alterations in exercise recommendations due to environmental conditions and patient health status

1.1.6   Explain the health benefits of a physically active lifestyle and the hazards of sedentary behavior and summarize key recommendations of U.S. national reports of physical activity (e.g., U.S. Surgeon General, Institute of Medicine, ACSM, AHA)

1.1.7   Explain the physiological adaptations to exercise training that may result in improvement or maintenance of health, including metabolic (e.g., metabolic syndrome, glucose and lipid metabolism), cardiovascular (e.g., atherosclerosis), musculoskeletal (e.g., bone density), neuromuscular, pulmonary (e.g., lung function), and immune system (e.g., colds, acute illness) health

1.1.8   Explain the mechanisms underlying the physiological adaptations to aerobic and resistance exercise training including those resulting in changes in, or maintenance of, maximal and submaximal oxygen consumption, lactate and ventilatory (anaerobic) threshold, myocardial oxygen consumption, heart rate, blood pressure, ventilation (including ventilatory [anaerobic] threshold), muscle structure, bioenergetics (e.g., substrate use), and immune function

1.1.9   Explain the physiological effects of physical inactivity, including bed rest, and methods that may counteract these effects

1.1.10   Recognize and respond to abnormal signs and symptoms during exercise

GENERAL POPULATION/CORE: HEALTH APPRAISAL, FITNESS AND CLINICAL EXERCISE TESTING

1.3.1   Conduct pre-test procedures including explaining test procedures to the patient and obtaining informed consent, obtaining a focused medical history and results of prior tests and physical examination, disease-specific risk factor assessment (e.g., CVD, metabolic and pulmonary diseases), presenting concise information to other healthcare providers and third party payers

1.3.2   Conduct a brief physical examination including evaluation of peripheral edema, measuring blood pressure, peripheral pulses, respiratory rate, and auscultating heart and lung sounds

1.3.3   Calibrate laboratory equipment used frequently in the practice of clinical exercise physiology (e.g., motorized/computerized treadmill, mechanical cycle ergometer and arm ergometer, electrocardiograph, spirometer, respiratory gas analyzer [metabolic cart])

1.3.4   Administer exercise tests consistent with U.S. nationally accepted standards for testing (i.e., ACSM, AHA)

1.3.5   Identify contraindications to an exercise session

1.3.6   Appropriately select and administer functional tests to measure patient outcomes and functional status including the 6-minute walk, Get Up and Go, Berg Balance Scale, Physical Performance Test

1.3.7   Evaluate patient outcomes from serial outcome data collected before, during, and after exercise interventions

1.3.8   Interpret the variables that may be assessed during clinical exercise testing, including maximal oxygen consumption, resting metabolic rate, ventilatory volumes and capacities, respiratory exchange ratio, ratings of perceived exertion and discomfort (chest pain, dyspnea, claudication), ECG, heart rate, blood pressure, rate pressure product, ventilatory (anaerobic) threshold, oxygen saturation, breathing reserve, muscular strength, muscular endurance, and other common measures used for diagnosis and prognosis of disease

1.3.9   Determine atrial and ventricular rate from rhythm strip and 12-lead ECG and explain the clinical significance of abnormal atrial or ventricular rate (e.g., tachycardia, bradycardia)

1.3.10   Identify ECG changes associated with drug therapy, electrolyte abnormalities, subendocardial and transmural ischemia, myocardial injury, and infarction and explain the clinical significance of each

1.3.11   Identify SA, AV, and bundle branch blocks from a rhythm strip and 12-lead ECG, and explain the clinical significance of each

1.3.12   Identify sinus, atrial, functional, and ventricular dysrhythmias from a rhythm strip and 12-lead ECG and explain the clinical significance of each

1.3.13   Identify contraindications to exercise testing

1.3.14   Determine an individual's pre-test and post-test probability of CHD, identify factors associated with test complications, and apply appropriate precautions to reduce risks to the patient

1.3.15   Extract and interpret clinical information needed for safe exercise management of individuals with chronic disease

1.3.16   Identify probable disease-specific endpoints for testing in a patient with chronic disease or disability

1.3.17   Select and use appropriate techniques for preparation and measurement of ECG, heart rate, blood pressure, oxygen saturation, RPE, symptoms (e.g., angina, dyspnea, claudication), expired gases, and other measures as needed before, during, and following exercise, pharmacological, echocardiographic, and radionuclide tests

1.3.18   Select and administer appropriate exercise tests to evaluate functional capacity, strength, and flexibility in patients with chronic disease

1.3.19   Discuss strengths and limitations of various methods of measures and indices of body composition

1.3.20   Appropriately select, apply, and interpret body composition tests and indices

GENERAL POPULATION/CORE: EXERCISE PRESCRIPTION AND PROGRAMMING

1.7.1   Adapt exercise prescriptions for patients with comorbid conditions and disease complications

1.7.2   Design and supervise comprehensive exercise programs for outpatients with chronic disease

1.7.3   Determine the appropriate level of supervision and monitoring recommended for individuals with known disease on the basis of chronic disease risk stratification (e.g., cardiovascular, metabolic, musculoskeletal, etc.) and current health status

1.7.4   Develop and supervise an appropriate exercise prescription (e.g., aerobic, strength, and flexibility training) for individuals with co-morbid disease

1.7.5   Implement appropriate precautions prior to, during, and following exercise in patients with chronic disease according to health status, medical treatment, environmental conditions, and other relevant factors

1.7.6   Instruct individuals with chronic disease in techniques for performing physical activities safely and effectively in an unsupervised exercise setting

1.7.7   Modify the exercise prescription or discontinue exercise on the basis of patient symptoms, current health status, musculoskeletal limitations, and environmental considerations

GENERAL POPULATION/CORE: HUMAN BEHAVIOR AND COUNSELING

1.9.1   Summarize contemporary theories of health behavior change including social cognitive theory, theory of reasoned action, theory of planned behavior, Transtheoretical model, and health belief model and apply techniques to promote healthy behaviors including physical activity
1.9.2   Describe characteristics associated with poor adherence to exercise programs
1.9.3   Describe the psychological issues associated with acute and chronic illness such as depression, social isolation, hostility, aggression, and suicidal ideation
1.9.4   Counsel patients with chronic diseases and conditions on topics such as disease processes, treatments, diagnostic techniques, and lifestyle management
1.9.5   Select and apply behavioral techniques such as goal setting, relapse prevention, and social support, which enhance adoption of, and adherence to, healthy behaviors including exercise
1.9.6   Explain factors that may increase anxiety prior to or during exercise testing and describe methods to reduce anxiety
1.9.7   Recognize signs and symptoms of failure to cope during personal crises such as job loss, bereavement, and illness

GENERAL POPULATION/CORE: SAFETY, INJURY PREVENTION, AND EMERGENCY PROCEDURES

1.10.1   List routine emergency equipment, drugs, and supplies present in an exercise testing laboratory and therapeutic exercise session area
1.10.2   Provide immediate responses to emergencies (i.e., first responder), including basic cardiac life support, AED, joint immobilization, activation of EMS
1.10.3   Verify operating status of emergency equipment including defibrillator, laryngoscope, oxygen, etc.
1.10.4   Explain Universal Precautions procedures and apply as appropriate
1.10.5   Develop and implement a plan for responding to emergencies

GENERAL POPULATION/CORE: PROGRAM ADMINISTRATION, QUALITY ASSURANCE, AND OUTCOME ASSESSMENT

1.11.1   Describe appropriate staffing for exercise programs and exercise testing laboratories on the basis of factors such as patient health status, facilities, and program goals
1.11.2   List necessary equipment and supplies for exercise programs and exercise testing laboratories
1.11.3   Select, document, and report treatment outcomes using patient-relevant results of tests (e.g., exercise tests, physical work simulations, biomarkers, and other laboratory tests) and surveys (e.g., physical functioning and health-related quality of life)
1.11.4   Explain legal issues pertinent to healthcare delivery by licensed and non-licensed healthcare professionals providing rehabilitative services and exercise testing (e.g., torts, contracts, informed consent, negligence, malpractice, liability, standards of care) and legal risk management techniques
1.11.5   Identify patients requiring referral to a physician or allied health services such as physical therapy, dietary counseling, stress management, weight management, psychosocial and social services
1.11.6   Develop a plan for patient discharge from a therapeutic exercise program, including community referrals

CARDIOVASCULAR: EXERCISE PHYSIOLOGY AND RELATED EXERCISE SCIENCE

2.1.1   Describe the indications for, physiologic responses to, and potential complications of pharmacological and pacing stress testing in individuals with cardiovascular diseases
2.1.2   Describe the potential benefits and hazards of aerobic, resistance, and flexibility exercise in individuals with cardiovascular diseases
2.1.3   Explain how cardiovascular diseases may affect the physiological responses to exercise training on the ischemic cascade and the components of the Fick equation

CARDIOVASCULAR: PATHOPHYSIOLOGY AND RISK FACTORS

2.2.1   Explain current hypotheses regarding the pathophysiology of atherosclerosis, including the etiology and rate of progression of disease
2.2.2   Describe the epidemiology, pathophysiology, risk factors, and key clinical findings of cardiovascular diseases
2.2.3   Explain the ischemic cascade and its effect on myocardial function

CARDIOVASCULAR: HEALTH APPRAISAL, FITNESS AND CLINICAL EXERCISE TESTING

2.3.1	Describe common techniques used to diagnose cardiovascular disease, including echocardiography, radionuclide imaging, angiography, pharmacological testing, and biomarkers (e.g., troponin, CK, etc.) and explain the indications, limitations, risks, and normal and abnormal results for each
2.3.2	Explain how cardiovascular disease may affect physical examination findings
2.3.3	List the key clinical findings during a physical examination of a patient with cardiovascular disease
2.3.4	Recognize and respond to abnormal signs and symptoms in individuals with cardiovascular diseases such as pain, peripheral edema, dyspnea, fatigue

CARDIOVASCULAR: MEDICAL AND SURGICAL MANAGEMENT

2.6.2	Explain the common medical and surgical treatments of cardiovascular diseases including pharmacological therapy, revascularization procedures, ICD, pacemakers, and transplant
2.6.3	Summarize key recommendations current U.S. clinical practice guidelines for the prevention, treatment, and management of cardiovascular diseases (e.g., AHA, ACC, NHLBI)
2.6.4	List the drug classifications commonly used in the treatment of individuals with cardiovascular diseases, name common generic and brand names drugs within each class, and explain the purposes, indications, major side effects, and the effects, if any, on the exercising individual
2.6.5	Explain how treatments for cardiovascular disease, including preventive care, may affect the rate of progression of disease
2.6.6	Apply current U.S. national guidelines for primary and secondary prevention of heart disease (e.g., lipoproteins, obesity, pharmacological, behavioral) to identify and manage cardiovascular risk

CARDIOVASCULAR: EXERCISE PRESCRIPTION AND PROGRAMMING

2.7.1	Develop an appropriate exercise prescription (e.g., aerobic, strength, and flexibility training) for individuals with cardiovascular disease
2.7.2	Design and adapt exercise prescriptions for individuals with cardiovascular disease to accommodate physical disabilities and complications due to cardiovascular diseases
2.7.3	Design and supervise comprehensive outpatient exercise programs for individuals with cardiovascular disorders
2.7.4	Instruct an individual with cardiovascular disease and disabilities in techniques for performing physical activities safely and effectively in an unsupervised exercise setting

PULMONARY: EXERCISE PHYSIOLOGY AND RELATED EXERCISE SCIENCE

3.1.1	Describe the potential benefits and hazards of aerobic, resistance, and flexibility exercise in individuals with pulmonary diseases
3.1.2	Explain how pulmonary diseases may affect the physiological responses to aerobic, resistance, and flexibility exercise
3.1.3	Explain how scheduling of exercise relative to meals can affect dyspnea
3.1.4	Explain how pulmonary diseases may affect range of motion, muscular strength, and endurance

PULMONARY: PATHOPHYSIOLOGY AND RISK FACTORS

3.2.1	Describe the epidemiology, pathophysiology, risk factors, and key clinical findings of pulmonary diseases
3.2.2	Explain the common medical and surgical treatments of pulmonary diseases including pharmacological therapy, surgery, and transplant

PULMONARY: HEALTH APPRAISAL, FITNESS AND CLINICAL EXERCISE TESTING

3.3.1	Explain how pulmonary disease may affect physical examination findings
3.3.2	List the key clinical findings during a physical exam of a patient with pulmonary disease
3.3.3	Have knowledge of lung volumes and capacities (e.g., tidal volume, residual volume, inspiratory volume, expiratory volume, total lung capacity, vital capacity, functional residual capacity, peak flow rate) and how they may differ between normal persons and patients with pulmonary disease
3.3.4	Recognize and respond to abnormal signs and symptoms in individuals with pulmonary diseases such as wheezing, cough, sputum, edema, dyspnea, and fatigue

PULMONARY: MEDICAL AND SURGICAL MANAGEMENT

3.6.1   Describe the epidemiology, pathophysiology, risk factors, and key clinical findings of pulmonary diseases

3.6.2   List the drug classifications commonly used in the treatment of individuals with pulmonary diseases and disabilities, name common generic and brand name drugs within each class, and explain the purposes, indications, major side effects, and the effects, if any, on the exercising individual

3.6.3   Explain how treatments for pulmonary disease, including preventive care, may affect the rate of progression of disease

3.6.4   List the risk factors for pulmonary disease and explain methods of reducing risk

PULMONARY: EXERCISE PRESCRIPTION AND PROGRAMMING

3.7.1   Develop an appropriate exercise prescription (e.g., aerobic, strength, flexibility training) for individuals with chronic pulmonary diseases

3.7.2   Design and adapt exercise prescriptions for individuals with chronic pulmonary diseases to accommodate physical disabilities and complications due to pulmonary diseases

3.7.3   Design and supervise comprehensive outpatient exercise programs for individuals with chronic pulmonary disease

3.7.4   Instruct an individual with pulmonary disease in proper breathing techniques and exercises and methods for performing physical activities safely and effectively in an unsupervised exercise setting

METABOLIC: PATHOPHYSIOLOGY AND RISK FACTORS

4.2.1   Describe the epidemiology, pathophysiology, risk factors, and key clinical findings of metabolic diseases (e.g., renal failure, diabetes, hyperlipidemia, obesity, frailty)

4.2.2   Explain current hypotheses regarding the pathophysiology of metabolic diseases, including the etiology and rate of progression of disease

4.2.3   Describe the potential benefits and hazards of aerobic, resistance, and flexibility exercise in individuals with metabolic diseases.

4.2.4   Explain how metabolic diseases may affect the physiologic responses to aerobic, resistance, and flexibility exercise.

4.2.5   Describe the probable effects of dialysis treatment on exercise performance, functional capacity, and safety, and explain methods for preventing adverse effects

4.2.6   Describe the probable effects of hypo/hyperglycemia on exercise performance, functional capacity, and safety, and explain methods for preventing adverse effect

METABOLIC: HEALTH APPRAISAL, FITNESS AND CLINICAL EXERCISE TESTING

4.3.1   Describe common techniques used to diagnose metabolic diseases including biomarkers, glucose tolerance testing, GFR, and explain the indications, limitations, risks, and normal and abnormal results for each

4.3.2   List the key clinical findings during a physical exam of a patient with metabolic disease(s)

4.3.3   Explain appropriate techniques for monitoring blood glucose before, during, and after an exercise session

4.3.4   Recognize and respond to abnormal signs and symptoms in individuals with metabolic diseases such as hypo/hyperglycemia, peripheral neuropathies, fluid overload, loss of appetite, low hematocrit, and hypotension, and orthopedic problems

METABOLIC: MEDICAL AND SURGICAL MANAGEMENT

4.6.2   Summarize key recommendations of current U.S. clinical practice guidelines (e.g., ADA, NIH, NHLBI) for the prevention, treatment, and management of metabolic diseases (e.g., renal failure, diabetes, hyperlipidemia, obesity, frailty)

4.6.3   Explain the common medical and surgical treatments of metabolic diseases including pharmacologic therapy, surgery, and transplant

4.6.4   List the drug classifications commonly used in the treatment of patients with metabolic disease, name common generic and brand names drugs within each class, and explain the purposes, indications, major side effects, and the effects, if any, on the exercising individual

4.6.5   Explain how treatments for metabolic diseases, including preventive care, may affect the rate of progression of disease

4.6.6   Apply current U.S. national guidelines for prevention of metabolic diseases to identify and manage disease complications and reduce cardiovascular risk (i.e., ADA)

4.6.7   Apply current U.S. national guidelines for primary prevention of heart disease (e.g., lipoproteins, obesity, pharmacologic, behavioral) to identify and manage cardiovascular risk

METABOLIC: EXERCISE PRESCRIPTION AND PROGRAMMING

4.7.1   Develop an appropriate exercise prescription (e.g., aerobic, strength, flexibility training) for individuals with metabolic disease

4.7.2   Design, adapt, and supervise an exercise prescription for patients with complications due to metabolic diseases (e.g., amputations, retinopathy, autonomic neuropathies, vision impairment, hypotension, and hypertension and during hemodialysis treatments)

4.7.3   Design and supervise comprehensive outpatient exercise programs for individuals with metabolic diseases

4.7.4   Instruct individuals with metabolic diseases in techniques for performing physical activities safely and effectively in an unsupervised exercise setting

ORTHOPEDIC/MUSCULOSKELETAL: EXERCISE PHYSIOLOGY AND RELATED EXERCISE SCIENCE

5.1.1   Describe the potential benefits and hazards of aerobic, resistance, and flexibility exercise in individuals with musculoskeletal diseases and disabilities (e.g., low back pain, arthritis, osteoporosis/fibromyalgia, and tendonitis/impingement syndrome, amputation)

5.1.2   Explain how musculoskeletal diseases may affect the physiologic responses to aerobic, resistance, and flexibility exercise

5.1.3   Describe the appropriate use of rest, spinal extension–flexion exercises versus lumbar stabilization, and the appropriate dose of avoidance of physical activity in patients with back pain

5.1.4   Explain how musculoskeletal diseases and disabilities may affect functional capacity, range of motion, balance, agility, muscular strength, and endurance

ORTHOPEDIC/MUSCULOSKELETAL: PATHOPHYSIOLOGY AND RISK FACTORS

5.2.1   Describe the epidemiology, pathophysiology, risk factors, and key clinical findings of orthopedic/musculoskeletal diseases and disabilities (e.g., low back pain, arthritis, osteoporosis, tendonitis/impingement syndrome, and amputation)

ORTHOPEDIC/MUSCULOSKELETAL: HEALTH APPRAISAL, FITNESS AND CLINICAL EXERCISE TESTING

5.3.1   Recognize and respond to abnormal signs and symptoms in individuals with musculoskeletal diseases and disabilities such as pain and muscle weakness

ORTHOPEDIC/MUSCULOSKELETAL: MEDICAL AND SURGICAL MANAGEMENT

5.6.1   List the drug classifications commonly used in the treatment of patients with musculoskeletal diseases and disabilities, name common generic and brand name drugs within each class, and explain the purposes, indications, major side effects, and the effects, if any, on the exercising individual

5.6.2   Explain how treatments for musculoskeletal disease, including preventive care, may affect the rate of progression of disease

ORTHOPEDIC/MUSCULOSKELETAL: EXERCISE PRESCRIPTION AND PROGRAMMING

5.7.1   Explain exercise training concepts specific to industrial or occupational rehabilitation, which includes work hardening, work conditioning, work fitness, and job coaching

5.7.2   Design, adapt, and supervise an exercise prescription (aerobic, strength, and flexibility training) to accommodate patients with complications due to musculoskeletal diseases and disabilities (e.g., low back pain, arthritis, osteoporosis, tendonitis/impingement syndrome, and amputation)

5.7.3   Instruct an individual with musculoskeletal diseases and disabilities in techniques for performing physical activities safely and effectively in an unsupervised exercise setting

NEUROMUSCULAR: EXERCISE PHYSIOLOGY AND RELATED EXERCISE SCIENCE

6.1.1   Describe the potential benefits and hazards of aerobic, resistance, and flexibility exercise in individuals with neuromuscular diseases and disabilities (e.g., multiple sclerosis, muscular dystrophy, Parkinson's disease, polio and post-polio syndrome, stroke and head injury, cerebral palsy, amyotrophic lateral sclerosis, peripheral neuropathy, spinal cord injury, epilepsy)

6.1.2   Explain how neuromuscular diseases may affect the physiological responses to aerobic, resistance, and flexibility exercise

6.1.3   Describe the effects of non-motor complications, such as fatigue, on exercise performance in patients with neuromuscular diseases and disabilities

6.1.4   Explain how neuromuscular diseases and disabilities may affect range of motion, balance, agility, muscular strength and endurance

NEUROMUSCULAR: HEALTH APPRAISAL, FITNESS AND CLINICAL EXERCISE TESTING

6.3.1   Recognize and respond to abnormal signs and symptoms in individuals with neuromuscular diseases and disabilities such as muscle weakness, cognitive deficit, and fatigue

NEUROMUSCULAR: EXERCISE PRESCRIPTION AND PROGRAMMING

6.7.1   Adapt the exercise prescription on the basis of the functional limits and benefits of assistive devices (e.g., wheelchairs, crutches, and canes)

6.7.2   Develop an appropriate exercise prescription (e.g., aerobic, strength, flexibility training) for individuals with neuromuscular diseases and disabilities including those treated with surgery

6.7.3   Design, adapt, and supervise aerobic, strength training, and flexibility exercise routines to accommodate patients with complications due to neuromuscular diseases and disabilities (e.g., multiple sclerosis, muscular dystrophy, Parkinson's disease, polio and post-polio syndrome, stroke and head injury, cerebral palsy, amyotrophic lateral sclerosis, peripheral neuropathy, spinal cord injury, and epilepsy)

6.7.4   Instruct an individual with neuromuscular disease and disabilities in techniques for performing physical activities safely and effectively in an unsupervised exercise setting

IMMUNOLOGICAL: EXERCISE PHYSIOLOGY AND RELATED EXERCISE SCIENCE

7.1.1   Describe the immediate and long-term influence of medical therapies for NIH on cardiopulmonary and musculoskeletal responses to exercise training

7.1.2   Describe the potential benefits and hazards of aerobic, resistance, and flexibility exercise in individuals with NIH disease (e.g., cancer, anemia, bleeding disorders, AIDS, organ transplant, chronic fatigue syndrome)

7.1.3   Explain how NIH diseases may affect the physiological responses to aerobic, resistance, and flexibility exercise

7.1.4   Explain how cancer therapy (e.g., surgery, radiation, and chemotherapy) may affect functional capacity, range of motion, and the physiological responses to exercise

7.1.5   Apply current U.S. national guidelines for primary and secondary prevention of NIH disease (e.g., ACS, NIH)

IMMUNOLOGICAL: PATHOPHYSIOLOGY AND RISK FACTORS

7.2.1   Describe the epidemiology, pathophysiology, risk factors, and key clinical findings of NIH diseases (e.g., cancer, anemia, bleeding disorders, AIDS, organ transplant, chronic fatigue syndrome)

IMMUNOLOGICAL: HEALTH APPRAISAL, FITNESS AND CLINICAL EXERCISE TESTING

7.3.1   Recognize and respond to abnormal signs and symptoms in individuals with NIH diseases such as fatigue, dyspnea, and tachycardia

IMMUNOLOGICAL: MEDICAL AND SURGICAL MANAGEMENT

7.6.1   List the drug classifications commonly used in the treatment of patients with NIH disease, name common generic and brand name drugs within each class, and explain the purposes, indications, major side effects, and the effects, if any, on the exercising individual

7.6.2   Summarize key recommendations of current U.S. clinical practice guidelines (e.g., ACS, NIH) for the prevention, treatment and management of NIH diseases (e.g., cancer, anemia, bleeding disorders, AIDS, organ transplant, chronic fatigue syndrome)

7.6.3   Explain the common medical and surgical treatments of NIH diseases including pharmacologic therapy and surgery

IMMUNOLOGICAL: EXERCISE PRESCRIPTION AND PROGRAMMING

7.7.1   Develop an appropriate exercise prescription (e.g., aerobic, strength, flexibility training) for individuals with NIH disorders (e.g., cancer, anemia, bleeding disorders, AIDS, organ transplant, chronic fatigue syndrome)

7.7.2   Design, adapt, and supervise the exercise prescription to accommodate patients with physical disabilities and complications due to NIH diseases

7.7.3   Design and supervise comprehensive outpatient exercise programs for individuals with immunological/hematological disorders (e.g., cancer, anemia, bleeding disorders, AIDS, organ transplant, chronic fatigue syndrome)

7.7.4   Instruct an individual with immunological/hematological diseases and disabilities in techniques for performing physical activities safely and effectively in an unsupervised exercise setting

NOTE: **The KSAs listed above for the ACSM Registered Clinical Exercise Specialist® are the same KSAs for educational programs in Clinical Exercise Physiology seeking graduate (master's degree) academic accreditation through the CoAES. For more information, please visit www.coaes.org.**

Additional KSAs are required (in addition to the ACSM Health/Fitness Instructor® KSAs) for programs seeking academic accreditation in Applied Exercise Physiology. The KSAs that follow, IN ADDITION TO the ACSM Health/Fitness Instructor® KSAs listed earlier, represent the KSAs for educational programs in Applied Exercise Physiology seeking graduate (master's degree) academic accreditation through the CoAES. For more information, please visit www.coaes.org.

GENERAL POPULATION/CORE: EXERCISE PHYSIOLOGY AND RELATED EXERCISE SCIENCE

1.1.1   Ability to describe modifications in exercise prescription for individuals with functional disabilities and musculoskeletal injuries

1.1.2   Ability to describe the relationship between biomechanical efficiency, oxygen cost of activity (economy), and performance of physical activity

1.1.3   Knowledge of the muscular, cardiorespiratory, and metabolic responses to decreased exercise intensity

GENERAL POPULATION/CORE: PATHOPHYSIOLOGY AND RISK FACTORS

1.2.1   Ability to define atherosclerosis, the factors causing it, and the interventions that may potentially delay or reverse the atherosclerotic process

1.2.2   Ability to describe the causes of myocardial ischemia and infarction

1.2.3   Ability to describe the pathophysiology of hypertension, obesity, hyperlipidemia, diabetes, chronic obstructive pulmonary diseases, arthritis, osteoporosis, chronic diseases, and immunosuppressive disease

1.2.4   Ability to describe the effects of the above diseases and conditions on cardiorespiratory and metabolic function at rest and during exercise

GENERAL POPULATION/CORE: HEALTH APPRAISAL, FITNESS AND CLINICAL EXERCISE TESTING

1.3.1   Knowledge of the selection of an appropriate behavioral goal and the suggested method to evaluate goal achievement for each stage of change

1.3.2   Knowledge of the use and value of the results of the fitness evaluation and exercise test for various populations

1.3.3   Ability to design and implement a fitness testing/health appraisal program that includes, but is not limited to, staffing needs, physician interaction, documentation, equipment, marketing, and program evaluation

1.3.4   Ability to recruit, train, and evaluate appropriate staff personnel for performing exercise tests, fitness evaluations, and health appraisals

GENERAL POPULATION/CORE: MEDICAL AND SURGICAL MANAGEMENT

1.5.1   Ability to identify and describe the principal action, mechanisms of action, and major side effects from each of the following classes of medications: antianginals, antihypertensives, antiarrhythmics, bronchodilators, hypoglycemics, psychotropics, and vasodilators

GENERAL POPULATION/CORE: HUMAN BEHAVIOR AND COUNSELING

1.9.1   Knowledge of, and ability to apply, basic cognitive-behavioral intervention such as shaping, goal setting, motivation, cueing, problem solving, reinforcement strategies, and self-monitoring

1.9.2   Knowledge of the selection of an appropriate behavioral goal and the suggested method to evaluate goal achievement for each stage of change

GENERAL POPULATION/CORE: SAFETY, INJURY PREVENTION, AND EMERGENCY PROCEDURES

1.10.1   Ability to identify the process to train the exercise staff in cardiopulmonary resuscitation

1.10.2   Ability to design and evaluate emergency procedures for a preventive exercise program and an exercise testing facility

1.10.3   Ability to train staff in safety procedures, risk reduction strategies, and injury care techniques

1.10.4   Knowledge of the legal implications of documented safety procedures, the use of incident documents, and ongoing safety training

GENERAL POPULATION/CORE: PROGRAM ADMINISTRATION, QUALITY ASSURANCE, AND OUTCOME ASSESSMENT

1.11.1   Ability to manage personnel effectively

1.11.2   Ability to describe a management plan for the development of staff, continuing education, marketing and promotion, documentation, billing, facility management, and financial planning

1.11.3   Ability to describe the decision-making process related to budgets, market analysis, program evaluation, facility management, staff allocation, and community development

1.11.4   Ability to describe the development, evaluation, and revision of policies and procedures for programming and facility management

1.11.5   Ability to describe how the computer can assist in data analysis, spreadsheet report development, and daily tracking of customer use

1.11.6   Ability to define and describe the total quality management (TQM) and continuous quality improvement (CQI) approaches to management

1.11.7   Ability to interpret applied research in the areas of exercise testing, exercise programming, and educational programs to maintain a comprehensive and current state-of-the-art program

1.11.8   Ability to develop a risk factor screening program, including procedures, staff training, feedback, and follow-up

1.11.9   Knowledge of administration, management, and supervision of personnel

1.11.10   Ability to describe effective interviewing, hiring, and employee termination procedures

1.11.11   Ability to describe and diagram an organizational chart and show the relationships between a health/fitness director, owner, medical advisor, and staff

1.11.12   Knowledge of, and ability to describe, various staff training techniques

1.11.13   Knowledge of, and ability to describe, performance reviews and their role in evaluating staff

1.11.14   Knowledge of the legal obligations and problems involved in personnel management

1.11.15   Knowledge of compensation, including wages, bonuses, incentive programs, and benefits

1.11.16   Knowledge of methods for implementing a sales commission system

1.11.17   Ability to describe the significance of a benefits program for staff and demonstrate an understanding in researching and selecting benefits

1.11.18   Ability to write and implement thorough and legal job descriptions

1.11.19   Knowledge of personnel time management techniques
1.11.20   Knowledge of administration, management, and development of a budget and of the financial aspects of a fitness center
1.11.21   Knowledge of the principles of financial management
1.11.22   Knowledge of basic accounting principles such as accounts payable, accounts receivable, accrual, cash flow, assets, liabilities, and return on investment
1.11.23   Ability to identify the various forms of a business enterprise such as sole proprietorship, partnership, corporation, and S corporation
1.11.24   Knowledge of the procedures involved with developing, evaluating, revising, and updating capital and operating budgets
1.11.25   Ability to manage expenses with the objective of maintaining a positive cash flow
1.11.26   Ability to understand and analyze financial statements, including income statements, balance sheets, cash flows, budgets, and pro forma projections
1.11.27   Knowledge of program-related break-even and cost/benefit analysis
1.11.28   Knowledge of the importance of short-term and long-term planning
1.11.29   Knowledge of the principles of marketing and sales
1.11.30   Ability to identify the steps in the development, implementation, and evaluation of a marketing plan
1.11.31   Knowledge of the components of a needs assessment/market analysis
1.11.32   Knowledge of various sales techniques for prospective members
1.11.33   Knowledge of techniques for advertising, marketing, promotion, and public relations
1.11.34   Ability to describe the principles of developing and evaluating product and services and establishing pricing
1.11.35   Knowledge of the principles of day-to-day operation of a fitness center
1.11.36   Knowledge of the principles of pricing and purchasing equipment and supplies
1.11.37   Knowledge of facility layout and design
1.11.38   Ability to establish and evaluate an equipment preventive maintenance and repair program
1.11.39   Ability to describe a plan for implementing a housekeeping program
1.11.40   Ability to identify and explain the operating policies for preventive exercise programs, including data analysis and reporting, confidentiality of records, relationships with healthcare providers, accident and injury reporting, and continuing education of participants
1.11.41   Knowledge of the legal concepts of tort, negligence, liability, indemnification, standards of care, health regulations, consent, contract, confidentiality, malpractice, and the legal concerns regarding emergency procedures and informed consent
1.11.42   Ability to implement capital improvements with minimal disruption of client or business needs
1.11.43   Ability to coordinate the operations of various departments, including, but not limited to, the front desk, fitness, rehabilitation, maintenance and repair, day care, housekeeping, pool, and management
1.11.44   Knowledge of management and principles of member service and communication
1.11.45   Skills in effective techniques for communicating with staff, management, members, healthcare providers, potential customers, and vendors
1.11.46   Knowledge of, and ability to provide, strong customer service
1.11.47   Ability to develop and implement customer surveys
1.11.48   Knowledge of the strategies for management conflict
1.11.49   Knowledge of the principles of health promotion and ability to administer health promotion programs
1.11.50   Knowledge of health promotion programs (e.g., nutrition and weight management, smoking cessation, stress management, back care, body mechanics, and substance abuse)
1.11.51   Knowledge of the specific and appropriate content and methods for creating a health promotion program
1.11.52   Knowledge of, and ability to access, resources for various programs and delivery systems
1.11.53   Knowledge of the concepts of cost-effectiveness and cost-benefit as they relate to the evaluation of health promotion programming
1.11.54   Ability to describe the means and amounts by which health promotion programs might increase productivity, reduce employee loss time, reduce healthcare costs, and improve profitability in the workplace

Index

Page numbers in *italics* designate figures; page numbers followed by the letter "t" designate tables; page numbers followed by the letter "b" designate text boxes; (*see also*) designates related topics or more detailed subtopics.

A

ABCDE approach, 191–192
Abdominis muscles, *136,* 172
Abduction, 358, *359,* 360t, 361t, 362t, 363t
    defined, 114
    hip, 351, *352*
    shoulder (glenohumeral joint), 348–349
Academic accreditation, 528–529
Academic Motivation Model (ARCS),
    61–62
Accelerated Learning for the 21st Century (Rose
    & Nicholl), 32
Acceptance, 219
Accessibility, 192
Accidents, as liability issue, 494, 495t
Accountability, behavior change and,
    209–210, 225
Accreditation, academic, 528–529
Achilles tendonitis, 166
Achilles tendon rupture, 164
Acid(s)
    ascorbic (vitamin C), 250, 251t
    fatty, 249
    folic (folate), 252t
    pantothenic, 252t
    pyruvic (pyruvate), 259t
Acid–base balance, 246
Acromioclavicular joint, *129,* 131
    separation, 140
Acromioclavicular ligament, *129, 130*
Acromion, *129, 130*
ACSM/AHA recommendations,
    cardiovascular disease, 494
ACSM career pathway, 19–22, *20, 21*
ACSM Certification and Registry Boards, 14
ACSM Certification and Registry Programs,
    499–531, 500, *501–502* (*see also*
    KSAs; *individual certifications*)
    continuing education credits, 499–500
    history, 499–500
    information and application source, 502
    KSAs, 503–531
ACSM's Certification Review Book, 503
ACSM Certified Health Fitness Instructor®,
    6
ACSM Certified Personal Trainer^SM, 5–6
    certification program, 500, *501*
    KSAs, 506–510
ACSM Code of Ethics, 484–485b
ACSM Committee on Certification and
    Registry Boards, 15
ACSM Credentialed Professionals, 13–14
    discipline, 15

examination candidate standards, 14
    principles and standards, 13–15
    public disclosure of affiliation, 14–15
ACSM examination blueprint, 10–11, 11t
ACSM Exercise Specialist®
    certification program, 500, *501*
    KSAs, 516–521
ACSM facilities standards of care, 488t
*ACSM's Guidelines for Exercise Testing and
    Prescription,* 10
ACSM Health/Fitness Instructor®
    certification program, 500, *501*
    KSAs, 510–516
ACSM liability Insurance, 279
*ACSM's Medicine & Science in Sports &
    Exercise,* 373
ACSM participation screening algorithm, 303t
ACSM Position Stand
    on cardiorespiratory training, 405
    on static stretching, 437
ACSM Registered Clinical Exercise
    Physiologist®, 6
    KSAs, 521–525, 521–530
ACSM Exercise Specialist®, certification
    program, 500, *502*
ACSM's Resource Manual for Guidelines for
    Exercise Testing and Prescription,
    9, 503
ACSM risk categories, 301–302t, 303t, 309
ACSM risk stratification categories, 302t
ACSM risk stratification system, 13
ACSM role and educational continuum,
    10, 11t
ACSM University Connection Endorsement
    Program, 499–500
Actin, 96–97
Action-based goals, 292 (*see also* SMART
    goals)
Action stage, of behavior change, 211
Activation, neuromuscular, 123, 126
Active assistive stretching, 369
Active learning, 32
Active listening, 220
Active range of motion, 100, 341 (*see also*
    Goniometry)
Active stretching, 369
Activities of daily living (ADLs), flexibility
    and, 434–435
Activity (*see* Physical activity)
Adaptability, trainer, 193
Adaptation, central, 407
Adaptation principle, 407
Adaptations, to exercise (*see* Exercise
    adaptations)

Adduction, 358, *359,* 360t, 361t, 362t, 363t
    defined, 114
    hip, 352
Adductor muscles, *120, 121*
Adenosine triphosphate (ATP), *93,* 93–95
ADLs (activities of daily living), flexibility
    and, 434–435
Adults, physical activity level, 4, 4t
Advertising, 479
Advice, liability issues, 492
AED (automated external defibrillator)
    training, 494
Aerobic and anaerobic metabolism, 92–93
Aerobic capacity (*see* $\dot{V}O_2$)
    maximum (*see* $\dot{V}O_{2max}$)
Aerobic (oxidative) enzymes, 103–104
Aerobic oxidation, *94,* 94–95
Aerobic training (*see* Cardiorespiratory
    training)
Affective strategies, for behavior change,
    213–215, *214*
Afferent (sensory) fibers, 102
Affiliation, public disclosure of, 14–15
Age, flexibility and, 433
Agonist muscles, 123, 358, *359,* 360t, 361t,
    362t, 363t
AHA/ACSM Health/Fitness Facility
    Pre-Participation Screening
    Questionnaire, 299, *305*
Alignment
    body, 334–339 (*see also* Postural analysis)
    postural, 111, *113*
All-or-none principle, 97
Alpha-tocopherol (vitamin E), 253t
Alveoli, 89, *89*
Ambivalence, 229
American Association of Cardiovascular and
    Pulmonary Rehabilitation, 298
American College of Sports Medicine
    (*see* ACSM *entries*)
American Heart Association (AHA), 298
    (*see also* AHA *entries*)
Amphiarthrodial joints, 117
Anabolic hormones, 245
Anaerobic glycolysis, *94, 94*
Anatomical locations, 358
Anatomical position, 110, *111,* 112t
Anatomy
    body position, 110–111, *111,* 112t, *113*
    fingers, 143–145, *144, 145*
    hand, 143–145, *144, 145*
    joint movement, *113,* 114, 126, 127t,
        128t (*see also* Joint movements)
    lower extremity, 145–166

Take before July 1